Thyroid Cancer

Diagnosis and Treatment

Thyroid Cancer
Diagnosis and Treatment

Edited by

Orlo H. Clark, M.D.

Professor and Vice Chair, Chief of Surgery, Department of Surgery,
University of California, San Francisco, California;
Chief of Surgery, Department of Surgery,
Mount Zion Medical Center,
San Francisco, California

Shiro Noguchi, M.D., Ph.D.

Chief Executive Officer,
Noguchi Thyroid Clinic and Hospital Foundation,
Beppu, Oita, Japan

COVER ILLUSTRATION BY EMILIE CLARK

Quality Medical Publishing, Inc.

ST. LOUIS, MISSOURI
2000

Printed in the United States of America.

PUBLISHER Karen Berger

PROJECT MANAGEMENT Shepherd, Inc.

MANUSCRIPT EDITOR Suzanne Wakefield

COVER DESIGN David Berger

Quality Medical Publishing, Inc.
11970 Borman Drive, Suite 222
St. Louis, Missouri 63146
Telephone: 1-800-348-7808
Web site: http://www.qmp.com

LIBRARY OF CONGRESS CATALOGING-IN-PUBLICATION DATA

Thyroid cancer : diagnosis and treatment / edited by Orlo H. Clark, Shiro Noguchi.
p. ; cm.
Includes bibliographical references and index.
ISBN 1-57626-116-6 (alk. paper)
1. Thyroid gland—Cancer. I. Clark, Orlo H. II. Noguchi, Shiro.
[DNLM: 1. Thyroid Neoplasms—diagnosis. 2. Thyroid Neoplasms—therapy. WK 270 T54943 2000]
RC280.T6 T55 2000
616.99'444—dc21 99-057674

S/W/W
5 4 3 2 1

Contributors

Sylvia L. Asa, M.D., Ph.D.
Professor, Department of Laboratory Medicine and Pathobiology, University of Toronto, Toronto, Ontario, Canada; Consultant, Endocrine Pathology, Department of Pathology and Laboratory Medicine, Mount Sinai Hospital, Toronto, Ontario, Canada

Yvan C. Bédard, M.D., Ph.D.
Associate Professor, Department of Laboratory Medicine and Pathobiology, University of Toronto, Toronto, Ontario, Canada; Head, Electron Microscopy and Cytopathology, Department of Pathology and Laboratory Medicine, Mount Sinai Hospital, Toronto, Ontario, Canada

Ralph R. Cavalieri, M.D.
Professor Emeritus, Departments of Medicine and Radiology, University of California, San Francisco, California; Consultant, Departments of Nuclear Medicine and Endocrinology, Veterans Administration Medical Center, San Francisco, California

Orlo H. Clark, M.D.
Professor and Vice Chair, Chief of Surgery, Department of Surgery, University of California, San Francisco, California; Chief of Surgery, Department of Surgery, Mount Zion Medical Center, San Francisco, California

Cornelia Dotzenrath, M.D.
Assistant Professor, Department of Surgery, Heinrich-Heine-Universität, Düsseldorf, Germany

Quan-Yang Duh, M.D.
Professor in Residence, Department of Surgery, University of California, San Francisco, California; Staff Surgeon, Surgical Service, Department of Veterans Affairs Medical Center, San Francisco, California

Peter E. Goretzki, M.D.
Professor of Surgery, Department of Surgery, Heinrich-Heine-Universität, Düsseldorf, Germany

Charles B. Higgins, M.D.
Professor, Department of Radiology, University of California, San Francisco, California

Jeffrey F. Moley, M.D.
Chief of Endocrine and Oncologic Surgery, Department of Surgery, Washington University, St. Louis, Missouri

Tsukasa Murakami, M.D.
Department of Endocrinology, Noguchi Thyroid Clinic and Hospital Foundation, Beppu, Oita, Japan

Shiro Noguchi, M.D., Ph.D.
Chief Executive Officer, Noguchi Thyroid Clinic and Hospital Foundation, Beppu, Oita, Japan

Hans D. Röher, M.D.
Professor and Surgery-Chairman, Department of Surgery, Heinrich-Heine-Universität, Düsseldorf, Germany

Irving B. Rosen, M.D.
Professor, Department of Surgery, University of Toronto; Attending Surgeon, Co-Chair—Head and Neck Oncology, Department of Surgery, Mount Sinai Hospital; Emeritus Consultant, Department of Surgery, Princess Margaret Hospital, Toronto, Ontario, Canada

Gregory P. Sadler, M.D.
Department of Surgery, John Radcliff Hospital, Oxford, England

Klaus M. Schulte, M.D.
Department of Surgery, Heinrich-Heine-Universität, Düsseldorf, Germany

Dietmar Simon, M.D.
Associate Professor, Department of Surgery, Heinrich-Heine-Universität, Düsseldorf, Germany

Eu Young Soh, M.D.
Associate Professor, Department of Surgery, Ajou University Medical Center, Suwon, Korea

Patrick A. Treseler, M.D.
Clinical Professor, Department of Pathology, University of California, San Francisco, California

Shinya Uchino, M.D., Ph.D.
Department of Surgery, Noguchi Thyroid Clinic and Hospital Foundation, Beppu, Oita, Japan

Shin Watanabe, M.D.
Department of Surgery, Noguchi Thyroid Clinic and Hospital Foundation, Beppu, Oita, Japan

Hiroto Yamashita, M.D., Ph.D.
Research and Laboratory Department, Noguchi Thyroid Clinic and Hospital Foundation, Beppu, Oita, Japan

Hiroyuki Yamashita, M.D., Ph.D.
Department of Surgery, Noguchi Thyroid Clinic and Hospital Foundation, Beppu, Oita, Japan

Foreword

Two of the world's leading thyroid cancer experts, Shiro Noguchi of Beppu, Japan, and Orlo Clark of San Francisco have combined forces with their colleagues to produce the definitive text on this subject. Although thyroid cancer is a rare disease, it is a topic worthy of study; research and clinical work in this area has had widespread implications. Many of the new techniques and breakthroughs in understanding disease processes as a whole have grown out of advances in thyroidology, which continues to pioneer medical advances.

A compendium such as this allows the reader to gain a wider perspective of this topic. This book recalls John Keats' line, "I stood tip-toe upon a little hill." In similar fashion, this book permits us to climb a metaphoric hill and view the spectrum of progress to date in the understanding of thyroid cancer and its treatment. I heartily commend this work to you.

Selwyn Taylor, M.D., F.R.C.S.

Emeritus Dean,
Royal Postgraduate Medical Center,
Hammersmith Hospital,
London, England

Preface

Thyroid cancer is the most common endocrine neoplasm, excluding ovarian neoplasms. Despite the overall excellent outcome for patients diagnosed with this disease, death is a more common outcome than with other endocrine cancers. This text is written to help clarify the best methods for the immediate management of patients with thyroid neoplasms for all of the team members involved in the care of patients with this diagnosis. General, head and neck, and endocrine surgeons as well as surgical residents who treat patients with thyroid neoplasms are our intended audience as are thyroidologists, endocrinologists, nuclear medicine specialists, and other physicians.

This book reflects contributions from an international group of authorities. Together they provide a rationale for the various approaches to the management of thyroid nodules and thyroid cancer. Although there is general agreement regarding the evaluation of the patient with a thyroid nodule, the extent of thyroid gland resection, the need for central or lateral neck dissection, the use of postoperative radioiodine therapy, external radiation therapy, and TSH suppressive therapy remain controversial. In Japan, the emphasis is on subtotal thyroidectomy with regional node dissection without the use of post-thyroidectomy treatment with ^{131}I for patients with differentiated thyroid cancer of follicular cell origin. In the United States, the preferred treatment is total or near total thyroidectomy with postoperative radioiodine with TSH therapy. Prophylactic nodal dissection is not usually recommended for patients with papillary thyroid cancer in the United States.

Our text provides the data to document why various diagnostic and therapeutic methods are used. Chapters regarding cytologic and histologic evaluation, application and value of imaging studies, recent advances in the diagnosis and treatment of medullary thyroid cancer, angiogenesis, TSH suppression therapy, and thyroid oncogenes are included. Our goal is to present our readers with an international perspective on the current management of patients with thyroid neoplasms.

Orlo H. Clark, M.D.
Shiro Noguchi, M.D., Ph.D.

Acknowledgments

The writing or editing of any book requires the help of many individuals. Endocrine surgery has afforded both Professor Noguchi and I with the opportunity to interact with talented surgeons, endocrinologists, nuclear medicine physicians, radiologists, and pathologists who have provided tremendous intellectual stimulation and friendship over the years. We have benefited from the educational opportunities in our respective medical centers and countries. We also have been extremely fortunate to have been exposed to the inspired teachings of Mr. Selwyn Taylor and Professor Richard Welbourne at the Royal Postgraduate Medical Center, Hammersmith Hospital, London.

I (O.C.) would also like to pay tribute to my father, Orlo Holly Clark, M.D., and uncle, William Fischer Clark, M.D., both general surgeons, whose love of medicine and surgery and desire to help people influenced me in my career selection. My wife, Carol, deserves my greatest appreciation; she is a consummate source of inspiration and encouragement.

I (S.N.) would like to dedicate this book to my foster father, the late Dr. Akito Noguchi, and Dr. Hideo Kurihara, who introduced me to the basic skills of thyroid surgery, and to my wife, Ryoko, who has continuously encouraged me over the past 30 years.

Contents

I OVERVIEW AND EPIDEMIOLOGY, CYTOLOGIC, AND HISTOLOGIC EVALUATION

1 Overview 3
Shiro Noguchi, M.D., Ph.D.

2 Evaluation of Thyroid Nodules 21
Hiroyuki Yamashita, M.D., Ph.D.

3 Fine-Needle Aspiration Cytology and Histopathology 39
Sylvia L. Asa, M.D., Ph.D. • Yvan C. Bédard, M.D., Ph.D.

4 Occult Microcancer and Clinical Cancer 105
Hiroto Yamashita, M.D., Ph.D.

5 Illustrated Guide to Thyroid Tumors 127
Gregory P. Sadler, M.D. • Patrick A. Treseler, M.D. • Orlo H. Clark, M.D.

II IMAGING TOOLS AND TECHNOLOGY

6 Nuclear Medicine 161
Ralph R. Cavalieri, M.D.

7 Magnetic Resonance Imaging 195
Charles B. Higgins, M.D.

8 Ultrasonography 209
Tsukasa Murakami, M.D.

III DECISION MAKING: SELECTING A SURGICAL APPROACH

9 Total Thyroidectomy 229
Gregory P. Sadler, M.D. • Orlo H. Clark, M.D.

10 Partial Thyroidectomy 241
Irving B. Rosen, M.D.

11 Surgical Options 257
Shiro Noguchi, M.D., Ph.D.

IV MANAGEMENT

12 Medullary Thyroid Carcinoma 279
Jeffrey F. Moley, M.D.

13 Locally Recurrent Thyroid Carcinoma 309
Hiroyuki Yamashita, M.D., Ph.D.

14 Multidisciplinary Treatment of Nonresectable Differentiated Thyroid Carcinoma 327
Shin Watanabe, M.D. • Shiro Noguchi, M.D., Ph.D.

V ADVANCES IN MOLECULAR BIOLOGY

15 The Role of Basic Science Research 349
Orlo H. Clark, M.D.

16 Oncogenes and Tumor Suppressor Genes in Differentiated Thyroid Cancer 365
Peter E. Goretzki, M.D. • Cornelia Dotzenrath, M.D. • Klaus M. Schulte, M.D. • Dietmar Simon, M.D. • Hans D. Röher, M.D.

17 Angiogenesis and Thyroid Neoplasms 379
Quan-Yang Duh, M.D. • Eu Young Soh, M.D.

18 Genetic Basis of Medullary Thyroid Carcinoma 393
Shinya Uchino, M.D., Ph.D.

19 Thyroid-Stimulating Hormone Suppression Therapy 415
Orlo H. Clark, M.D.

Index 437

Thyroid Cancer

Diagnosis and Treatment

PART

I

Overview and Epidemiology, Cytologic, and Histologic Evaluation

CHAPTER 1

Overview

SHIRO NOGUCHI, M.D., Ph.D.

EPIDEMIOLOGY

Clinically evident thyroid cancer represents an uncommon disease in the general population, with an annual incidence of about 2 to 4 new cases per 100,000 population in countries in which adequate amounts of iodine are ingested. Microscopic thyroid carcinoma, however, is extremely prevalent. The highest prevalence rate of 35.6% was reported by Harach et al.[1] in 101 consecutive autopsies. The difference in the prevalence rate among the reported autopsy series may be partly the result of the method of examination, the diagnostic criteria, and real geographic differences (Table 1-1).

Kugimoto et al.[15] performed an epidemiologic survey of 30,359 subjects (which is 86.4% of the total inhabitants of the studied area, in Nagano, Japan), 1965 through 1967. The method of detection was palpation by experienced surgeons; they found thyroid cancer in 0.08% of males and 0.18% of females. Ishida et al.[16] examined 152,651 subjects and found 0.14% of them to have small but detectable thyroid carcinomas by mass screening. Omata et al.[17] reported an incidence of 0.58% in 19,821 subjects. The different incidence of thyroid cancer in these Japanese mass screenings is primarily related to the method of the survey. In the study of Omata et al.,[17] ultrasonographic examination, which can

TABLE 1-1 Prevalence of Cancer by Autopsy Studies

Author	Year	Geographic Area	No. of Autopsies	Prevalence (%)
Silverberg and Vidone[2]	1966	Connecticut, USA	300	2.70
Farooki[3]	1969	Philadelphia, USA	220	0.50
Sampson et al.[4]	1969	Hiroshima and Nagasaki, Japan	1096	17.90
Sampson et al.[5]	1974	Minnesota, USA	157	5.70
Fukunaga and Yatani[6]	1975	Columbia	607	5.60
	1975	Hawaii (Japanese)	298	24.20
	1975	Ontario, Canada	100	6.00
	1975	Poland	110	9.10
	1975	Sendai, Japan	102	28.40
Sobrinho-Simoes et al.[7]	1979	Portugal	600	6.50
Bondeson and Ljungberg[8]	1981	Sweden	500	8.60
Pingitore[9]	1982	Toscana, Italy	111	3.60
Arellano and Ibarra[10]	1984	Chile	274	3.60
Harach et al.[1]	1985	Finland	101	35.60
Franssila and Harach[11]	1986	Finland	93	27.00
Lang et al.[12]	1987	Hannover, Germany	1020	6.20
Ottino et al.[13]	1989	La Plata, Argentina	100	11.00
Yamamoto et al.[14]	1990	Tokushima, Japan	408	11.30

detect lesions larger than 4 mm, was used. The incidence of thyroid cancer detected by mass screenings is about 1 of 100 microscopic thyroid cancers observed in an autopsy series.[2-14] Clinically evident thyroid cancer incidences appearing in the cancer registry are also about 1 of 100 ultrasonographically detectable thyroid cancers. Therefore about 1 of 10,000 microscopic cancers may eventually become clinical carcinoma.

ETIOLOGIC FACTORS

In the vast majority of thyroid cancers, it is hard to assign a specific etiologic factor in a routine clinical setting. Genetic factors may play some role in the etiology of thyroid cancer, not to mention the medullary, but also in papillary cancer, since there is a significant difference in standardized incidence ratios by ethnicity in the United States.[18] The occurrence of thyroid cancer in recognized familial syndromes was reported as Pendred's syndrome,[19] Gardner's syndrome,[20] chemodectoma,[21] and familial adenomatous polyposis.[22] Women under 35 years of age with familial adenomatous polyposis have been estimated to have a 160-fold higher risk of thyroid carcinoma than the general population[23] and familial clusters of nonmedullary cancer are also reported.[24-39] However, a responsible gene is not yet identified.

One of the most well-studied causes is therapeutic-dose radiation for enlarged thymus, tonsils, adenoids, acne vulgaris, lymphoid hyperplasia, and hyperthyroidism in childhood. In 1949, the relationship between irradiation and thyroid cancer was first noted by Quimby and Werner.[40] Carefully designed epidemiologic studies have confirmed the relationship between radiation treatment and thyroid neoplasms. Ron et al.[41] showed that children who received 6 mGy to the thyroid had a fourfold increase in the rate of thyroid cancer. Shore et al.[42] followed up 2650 subjects who underwent irradiation for an enlarged thymus, 90% of whom were treated at 1 year of age, compared with 4800 nonirradiated siblings. Mean follow-up for the exposed subjects was 24 years. In the irradiated group, 30 had thyroid cancer, contrasting with only one in the nonirradiated group. Schneider et al.[43] followed up 3042 irradiated patients and found 37.6% had developed thyroid nodules; among those, 318 (10.5%) had thyroid cancer 3 to 42 years later. In our study of thyroid cancer patients under 20 years old, 3 of 27 had a history of diagnostic-dose irradiation (2 to 9 mGy) to the head, neck, or chest during their infancy or childhood, and one had a therapeutic dose (0.4 mGy). Sixty-nine age- and sex-matched control subjects were randomly selected from patients who visited the same hospital in the same calendar year. The only significant factor between the two groups was the history of radiation exposure. This observation is highly implicative that even a diagnostic dose of external radiation must be avoided in infancy as much as possible.[44] Patients developing thyroid cancer after exposure to neck irradiation are reported to constitute 4% to 57% in the United States.[45] Radiation-induced thyroid cancer is often accompanied by multiple benign and/or malignant lesions.[46]

Iodine deficiency or excess iodine may also increase the incidence of thyroid cancer. In rodents, thyroid cancer was produced experimentally under both conditions. A population-based, case-controlled study from Hawaii[47] indicated that seafood, including seaweed, increased the risk of thyroid cancer among women but not among men. A hospital-based, case-controlled study from northern Italy found a significant risk reduction when fish consumption was increased.[48] A decreased risk of thyroid cancer associated with the use of iodized salt was reported in northern Norway. High consumption of cruciferous vegetables was associated with increased risk for residents in an endemic goiter area.[49] A report from Norway showed that fishermen's wives have an elevated risk of thyroid cancer, which suggests the role of seafood as an etiologic factor of thyroid cancer.[50] An increase in iodine intake appeared to be associated with an increased incidence of papillary cancer of the thyroid and thyroiditis.[51,52]

Environmental pollution by hexachlorobenzene and tetrachlorodibenzo-p-dioxin is reported to have caused an increased incidence of thyroid cancer in humans. Living near volcanic lava is suspected to increase the incidence of thyroid cancer, because in Hawaii and in Iceland the prevalence rate of thyroid cancer is higher than in other parts of the world.[53,54] The incidence of thyroid cancer is different among different ethnic groups in the United States; however, in Hawaii the increase is noted regardless of ethnicity.[18]

In Switzerland and Paraguay, where severe iodine deficiency was previously common, wide prophylactic iodination led to a significant reduction of follicular and anaplastic cancers, whereas the proportion of papillary cancer appears to have increased.[55] At present there is no explanation for the mechanism of the histopathologic shift from follicular to papillary cancer and its relationship to different amounts of ingested iodine.

CLASSIFICATION

The main framework of the present classification of thyroid malignancies was devised by Woolner and Hazard and later approved by the World Health Organization.[56] Most authorities agree that any thyroid carcinoma of follicular origin that contains papillary elements (such as mixed papillary and follicular thyroid carcinomas) should be considered a papillary carcinoma, because its biologic behavior will be that of papillary carcinoma. From this standpoint the papillary structure of cancer tissue is important but is not necessarily the whole evidence of papillary cancer. The presence of characteristic nuclear changes, including a "ground glass" appearance, large size, pale staining, irregular outlines with deep grooves, inconspicuous nucleoli, and pseudoinclusions, are also considered important findings.

Papillary carcinoma is the most common thyroid malignancy in most areas of the world, except for iodine-deficient regions. From a clinical standpoint, a carcinoma that is 1 cm or less in maximum diameter is considered one of the variants of papillary carcinoma; these are known as *occult* or *microcarcinomas*. Although they occur with very high incidence in association with microscopic metastases, the prognosis is excellent. Vickery et al.[57] reported that no patients with a small cancer experienced recurrence in the resected thyroid bed or contralateral lobe. Hazard[58] reported one death among 56 patients. Hay et al.[59] reported a 6% recurrence rate after 20 years of follow-up. In our study of 867 patients, 12 recurrences (1.4%) were observed after a mean follow-up of 15.6 years; two patients died of thyroid cancer.

The follicular variant of papillary carcinoma may be composed entirely or almost entirely of follicles. Apart from the absence of papillae, these tumors resemble papillary carcinoma in clinical behavior as well as in morphologic features of the nucleus. Rare variants of papillary carcinomas are an encapsulated variant, a diffuse sclerosing variant, and an oxyphilic cell type. In the Noguchi Thyroid Clinic, 85% of thyroid malignancies were of papillary carcinomas. Papillary carcinoma tends to metastasize to the regional lymph nodes. The metastasis ratio, which is defined as the number of lymph nodes involved divided by the number of examined nodes, is well correlated with recurrence rates. Also, the size of the primary tumor is correlated with the prognosis.

The prognosis for a patient with papillary carcinoma is excellent in about 80% of cases. In the remaining 20%, the prognosis can vary.

Follicular carcinoma is defined as an epithelial cell tumor showing evidence of follicular cell differentiation but lacking the diagnostic features of papillary carcinoma. One of the most difficult distinctions in thyroid pathology is differentiating between benign follicular adenomas and encapsulated low-grade follicular carcinomas, also called *minimally invasive*.[56] Both neoplasms are encapsulated by definition, but neither extends into the surrounding thyroid gland. Paradoxically, the capsule surrounding a carcinoma is thicker than the often very thin capsule circumscribing an adenoma. The principal differentiating feature is capsular invasion, which in carcinoma involves penetration of nests or nodules of tumor into and through the capsule. Extensive invasion of vascular space is not a feature of encapsulated follicular carcinoma, but minimal vascular invasion may be seen. However, follicular carcinoma, with a greater degree of capsular and vascular invasion, is easier to diagnose and has been termed *widely invasive follicular carcinoma*. Such tumors are often less well differentiated and display features typical of malignancy. The prognosis for patients with minimally invasive follicular carcinoma is extremely good.[60] In our experience the 10-year survival rate was 99%.

Anaplastic carcinoma is one of the deadliest malignancies. Fortunately, the proportional incidence of anaplastic carcinoma has been decreasing continuously over the past 50 years. The reason for the decreasing incidence of anaplastic thyroid cancer may be related to the fact that the size of excised differentiated carcinomas has been decreasing gradually over the past 50 years and iodine intake has increased. Anaplastic carcinoma is believed to originate in preexisting well-differentiated cancers.[61-69] Nishiyama et al.[67] demonstrated that almost all anaplastic carcinomas arise from papillary or follicular carcinoma. In the past a lump on the neck was disregarded or inadequately treated, leading to repeated recurrences that finally transformed to anaplastic carcinoma.

Medullary carcinoma of the thyroid is unique; this type of carcinoma originates from a C cell or parafollicular cell, which produces calcitonin. Elevated basal or pentagastrin-stimulated serum calcitonin is used as a marker of this tumor's presence, as is the presence of carcinoembryonic antigen. There are two different types of medullary carcinoma; one is sporadic and the other is hereditary. Hereditary medullary carcinoma can be a part of MEN2 or familial medullary carcinoma, and it requires total thyroidectomy, whereas in the sporadic type a lobectomy of the affected side will be sufficient. Therefore preoperative differential diagnosis of the two types based on RET proto-oncogene is mandatory; careful history-taking and endocrinologic studies are not enough to establish differentiation.[70]

Malignant lymphoma is a malignancy arising in the thyroid in longstanding cases of Hashimoto's thyroiditis, regardless of whether they were treated with thyroid medication or not. The vast majority of them, with a few exceptions, are of the T-cell type.[71,72] We have seen a few patients who came from areas in which adult T-cell leukemia is endemic. In contrast to anaplastic carcinoma, the incidence of malignant lymphoma is increasing, possibly related in part to the increasing longevity of the general population. The proportion of anaplastic cancer and malignant lymphoma we have seen in our institution in the past 50 years is shown in Fig. 1-1.

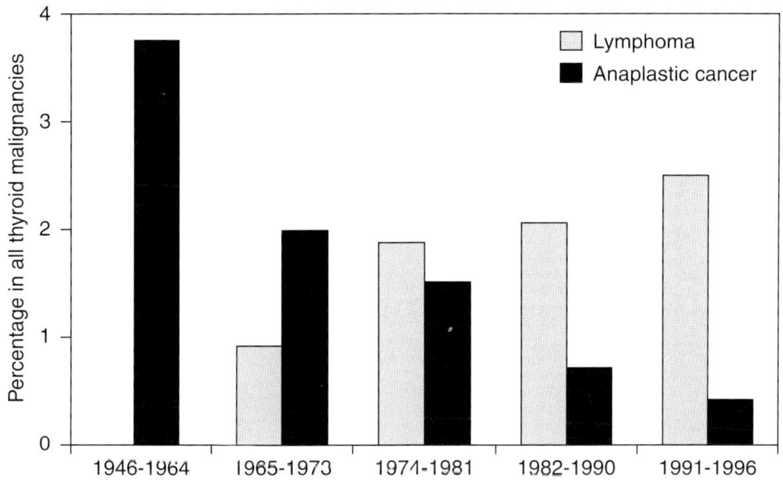

• **FIGURE 1-1** Proportion of anaplastic cancer and lymphoma.

PEDIATRIC THYROID CARCINOMAS

In general, age is an important prognostic factor in patients with differentiated thyroid carcinoma. However, this rule is not strictly applied to children and adolescents. Thyroid carcinoma can occur in patients of any age from 5 to 90 years old. In our series of 5844 patients with cancer of follicular cell origin (namely, papillary and follicular cancer), the youngest patient was 6 years old and 79 patients were under 19 years old. Distribution of pediatric thyroid cancers in this group was papillary (68), follicular (10), and one patient with anaplastic cancer. The patient with anaplastic cancer was an 18-year-old boy with a huge tumor on his neck at presentation. After 9 months, tumor recurred at the lung and neck, and he died of the disease 13 months after the initial surgery. The other young patient who died from thyroid cancer was an 18-year-old girl who had a primary tumor of 30 mm in maximum dimension that invaded the trachea, recurrent nerve, and muscular layer of the esophagus. We performed total thyroidectomy and modified radical neck dissection and found 74% of the resected nodes were involved with metastases. She died of the disease 3 years and 4 months after surgery with mediastinum and lung metastases. In our series, only one patient with papillary cancer had pulmonary metastasis at presentation. She underwent subtotal thyroidectomy with modified radical neck dissection when she was 15 years old, took thyroxine medication thereafter, and was still alive and well after 15 years and 6 months. She is persistently refusing completion thyroidectomy and radioiodine treatment, even though she has since had two children.

This observation is contrary to that of the Institute Gustave-Roussy in France.[73] They and other groups[74] also found lung metastasis in 19% of patients at initial treatment and a far higher mortality in childhood. In our series, the disease-specific 20-year survival rate of papillary cancer patients under 20 years of age was the same as for patients from 20 to 59 years of age; however, the recurrence-free survival rate was slightly lower than for patients in the 20 to 59 age group. The primary tumor is significantly larger than those found in adults; in our series, the median maximum diameter in children and adolescents was 28 mm, whereas in adults it was 24 mm; the difference was statistically significant ($p < 0.015$). Similar observations were made by others,[74-76] but contrasting findings were cited in one report.[77] The metastasis ratio, defined by the number of involved nodes divided by the number of examined nodes, is not correlated with recurrence rate in children and adolescents. Furthermore, the size of the primary tumor is not related to the prognosis. In other words, no definite risk factor is noted in this age group. The same impression was also expressed by McClellan and Francis[78]

THYROID CANCER WITH GRAVES' DISEASE

In the past, it was believed that the presence of thyrotoxicosis was insurance against cancer of the thyroid. Serendipitous case reports of combinations of the two conditions occasionally appeared until 1977, when Hancock et al.[79] first related thyroid cancer with long-acting thyroid stimulator and long-acting thyroid stimulator protector, both of which are immunoglobulins and which were considered to be the cause of Graves' disease. Thereafter, whether or not the incidence of thyroid cancer was elevated in Graves' thyroid tissue became a controversial issue. Moreover, Filetti et al.,[80] based on their experience with six patients, hypothesized that thyroid-stimulating antibodies in patients with Graves' disease supported the growth of metastatic cancers. Belfiore et al.[81] reported that thyroid cancer in patients with Graves' disease is more aggressive than that in euthyroid patients in terms of local invasiveness, metastasis to local lymph nodes and remote organs, multifocality in the thyroid gland, and the larger size of the primary tumor. Hales et al.[82] failed to find aggressive characteristics (invasion or metastasis) or larger sized tumors. On the contrary, they observed that 10 of 16 were smaller than 10 mm. The reported incidence of cancer associated with Graves' disease is between 0.06% and 8.7%.[83]

In our series of 4374 patients with differentiated thyroid cancer operated on between 1980 and 1991, 758 patients (17.3%) also had Graves' disease. Among them, 679 (89.6%) had tumors of 10 mm or less in maximum diameter; this is significantly larger than those of euthyroid patients ($p < 0.0001$). Of the remaining 79 patients with the primary tumor larger than 11 mm, eight (10.3%) had slight adhesion to the recurrent laryngeal nerve, but resection of the nerve was not necessary. In two patients (2.6%) the tumor had invaded the muscular layer of the esophagus, but these were easily resected and no reconstruction was necessary. No patient underwent noncurative surgery. Intraglandular dissemination was found in 15 patients (19.2%; not significant) and nodal metastasis was present in 30 (38.5%). This figure is less than euthyroid cancer patients; the difference was highly significant ($p < 0.0001$). In the same period, we operated on 3617 patients with euthyroid differentiated thyroid cancers; among them, 1198 (33.1%) tumors were equal to or less than 10 mm in maximum diameter. Noncurative surgery was inevitable in 119 patients (4.9%; not significant). In 587 patients, adhesion/invasion of the tumor to the recurrent laryngeal nerve was observed (not significant), and among them, 96 patients (4.0%) required resection of the recurrent laryngeal nerve due to an invasive tumor (not significant). Adhesion or invasion of the muscular layer of the esophagus was found in 400 patients (16.5%; $p < 0.017$), but none required reconstruction. Intraglandular dissemination was found in 306 patients (12.7%), and nodal metastasis was found in 1559 patients (64.5%). The mean age of patients with Graves' disease was 46.3 years and that of euthyroid patients was 48.8 years. The higher incidence of microcancer in Graves' patients can be explained by a bias related to selection. There is no evidence to support the hypothesis that cancer that is present concomitantly with Graves' disease behaves more aggressively than that arising in euthyroid patients. Of 2966 patients operated on between 1946 and 1991 with papillary thyroid cancer greater than or equal to 10 mm in maximum diameter who underwent a curative operation and median follow-up of 14 years, 83 had Graves' disease. The 10-year disease-specific survival rate for patients who did not have Graves' disease was 96.8%; among those with Graves' disease, the survival rate was 100%. The difference was not statistically significant. Recurrence-free survival rates of these patients were 90.0% and 98.3%, respectively ($p < 0.005$). These figures appear to indicate that the concomitant presence of Graves' disease might protect the growth of papillary cancer rather than induce aggressiveness. An immunochemical study supporting this hypothesis has been published recently.[84]

THYROID CANCER WITH HASHIMOTO'S THYROIDITIS

Lymphocytic infiltration of the stroma of papillary cancer is not uncommon; sometimes it is a marked feature, especially evident in the cores of fronds. This type of focal thyroiditis has often been confused with classical Hashimoto's thyroiditis, because definite morphologic criteria to differentiate these two types of thyroiditis is not known, and the degree of lymphocytic infiltration was expressed as "minimal," "moderate," "focal," "diffuse," and so on only when the author of the paper wanted to specify. Dailey et al.[85] reported that thyroid cancer arose in glands involved by Hashimoto's thyroiditis more frequently than would be expected. A long controversy emerged from this paper about whether chronic thyroiditis was a premalignant lesion. Pollock and Sprong[86,87] regarded Hashimoto's thyroiditis as a premalignant lesion and advocated total thyroidectomy; Schlicke et al.[88] also recommended a radical approach. Chesky et al.[89] recommended subtotal or total lobectomy followed by lifelong administration of thyroid hormone.

Meier et al.[90] reported no increased incidence of chronic thyroiditis in parenchyma of thyroid cancer. Crile and Hazard[91] reported no increased incidence and that thyroid hormone medication is an appropriate treatment for chronic thyroiditis, since more than 1000 patient-years had been treated that way and microcancers, theoretically present in a certain proportion of glands affected by struma lymphomatosa, had not developed into clinical cancer.

Hirabayashi and Lindsay[92] reported that chronic thyroiditis was not a premalignant lesion, and patients with chronic thyroiditis had a better prognosis than those without it. Harach and Williams[93] studied an endemic goiter region before and after iodine prophylaxis and concluded that increase of thyroiditis and increase of papillary cancer are both related to an iodine-rich diet. However, the two consequences of excess iodine administration are a separate effect and are not linked other than by a common cause. In 1995, Harach and Williams[93] stated that they considered it more likely that the papillary carcinoma causes the thyroiditis rather than the opposite. However, this issue is not yet settled.[94,95]

Regarding the clinical management of chronic thyroiditis, Clark et al.[96] recommended selective surgery. Their indications for surgery include a patient with a solitary or dominant thyroid nodule that is nonfunctioning or cold on radioiodine scan, with pressure symptoms, with hyperthyroidism, and with a growing diffusely enlarged goiter that is unresponsive to thyroid-stimulating hormone (TSH) suppression. Ott et al.[97] also approved selective surgery; in addition to the criteria of Clark et al., they included a history of head and neck irradiation, suspicious cytologic findings resulting from needle aspiration, suspicious lymphadenopathy, or other signs arousing suspicion of malignancy. Their suggestion for operative management is total thyroidectomy for those with a history of head and neck irradiation and thyroid lobectomy for patients with no history of irradiation, followed by contralateral lobectomy if a carcinoma is found. However, needle aspiration cytology and core needle biopsy have proved difficult to interpret and often unsatisfactory.[89,97-101] Recently, advanced 7.5 MHz and 10 MHz ultrasonography has been shown to be useful to some extent.[100]

Regarding clinical course and outcome of thyroid cancer associated with chronic thyroiditis, Meier et al.[90] observed less frequent metastasis in patients with lymphocyte infiltration. Hirabayashi and Lindsay[92] reported a better survival rate in patients with thyroiditis. Matsubayashi et al.[102] reported a better recurrence free survival rate. Similar observations were reported by others.[103,104] Lucas et al.[84] performed histochemical analysis of deposition of immunoglobulin and complements on thyroid tumor cells and found cellular deposits of IgG1, IgG4, and complement factors C3d, C4d, and C5 only for patients with papillary cancer. The results are suggestive of a tumor-specific immune response in papillary thyroid cancer with activation of classic complement cascade.

In our series of 2966 patients who underwent a curative operation between 1946 and 1991, for a papillary thyroid cancer greater than 10 mm in maximum diameter, 212 were associated with chronic thyroiditis. The 10-year disease-specific survival rate without chronic thyroiditis was 96.7%, whereas that with chronic thyroiditis was 98.8% ($p < 0.035$), and recurrence-free survival rates were 90.0% and 94.2% ($p < 0.045$), respectively. Patients with differentiated thyroid cancer appear to have a slightly more favorable prognosis when concomitant chronic thyroiditis is present.

CONCLUSION

Differentiated thyroid cancer has an indolent nature, and usually a term-long follow-up is required before a meaningful result of treatment can be obtained. However, in the past 50 years socioeconomic conditions have changed remarkably in most parts of the world, and medical technologies have particularly advanced in the last two decades. These changes in society and the progress of technology, along with increased awareness and concerns of health care in the general population, caused us to hesitate when comparing patients treated at present with those treated several decades ago. It is very important to be aware of what kinds of changes have taken place in the last 5 decades.

We divided patients into five groups based on the year of operation; the first period is from 1946 to 1964, the second from 1965 to 1973, the third from 1974 to 1981, the fourth from 1982 to 1990, and the fifth from 1991 to 1996.

Malignant lymphoma originating from the thyroid has increased from 0% in the first period to 2.47% in the fifth period ($p < 0.004$, Pearson) (see Fig. 1-1). No malignant lymphoma was observed in the years between 1946 and 1964, which might be a conservative estimate. Lymphoma originating from the thyroid was so rare in those days that a precise diagnosis was barely established before the disease had already spread widely in the neck and axillar lymph nodes. When lymphoma is widely spread at presentation, it is difficult to distinguish whether it originated from the thyroid or not. The rapid increase in incidence after 1965 may be the result of greater patient awareness of goiter, the increased longevity of the general population, and some other yet unknown factors. However, anaplastic cancer decreased from 3.75% to 0.41% in the same period ($p < 0.0001$).

The size of the primary tumor is continuously decreasing (Fig. 1-2). The size of papillary and follicular cancer at presentation has been gradually decreasing in recent years. In the period between 1946 and 1965, the average maximum diameter was 39.3 mm (excluding microcarcinoma), whereas for the patients treated between 1991 and 1996 it was 22.6 mm (see Fig. 1-2). This statistical observation in accordance with the autopsy studies of anaplastic cancer indicates that anaplastic cancer might originate from differentiated cancer through a point mutation of the p53 tumor suppressor gene.[105,106] The average age of the patients gradually increased over the past 50 years; this change is highly significant.

In general, the prognosis has improved in recent years. This is particularly true regarding the survival rate among patients with differentiated cancer from a large primary tumor (patients operated on after 1980); a 10-year disease-specific survival rate of 91.4% before 1979 increased to 95.2% after 1980. In the past the prognosis for male patients was less favorable compared with that for females; however, in recent years the difference has

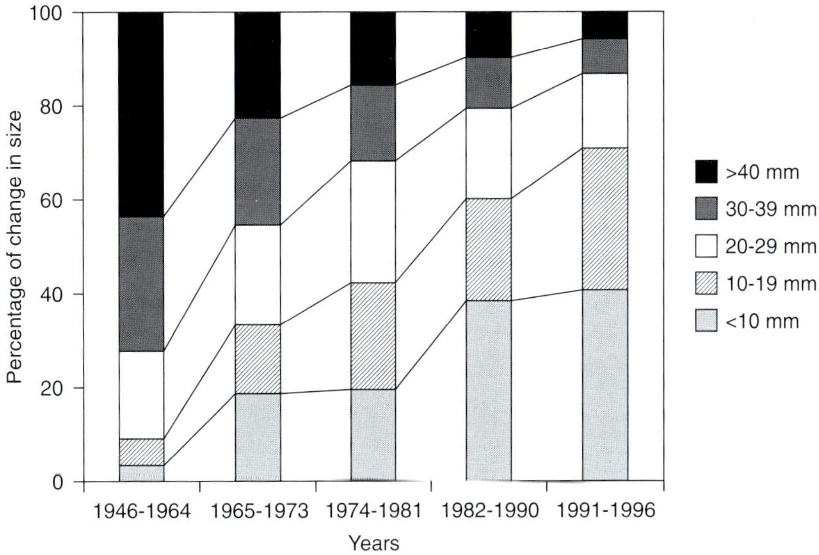

• **FIGURE 1-2** Change of tumor size (calendar years).

become smaller, because the late outcome in males has shown marked improvement. The improved survival rate cannot be attributed to one or two factors but appears related largely to the general advancement of medical technologies.

REFERENCES

1. Harach HR, Franssila KO, Wasenius VM. Occult papillary carcinoma of the thyroid. A "normal" finding in Finland. A systematic autopsy study. Cancer 56:531-538, 1985.
2. Silverberg SG, Vidone RA. Carcinoma of the thyroid in surgical and postmortem material. Analysis of 300 cases at autopsy and literature review. Ann Surg 164:291-292, 1966.
3. Farooki MA. Epidemiology and pathology of cancer of the thyroid. Int Surg 51:232-243, 1969.
4. Sampson RJ et al. Thyroid carcinoma in Hiroshima and Nagasaki. JAMA 209:65-70, 1969.
5. Sampson RJ et al. Occult thyroid carcinoma in Olmsted County, Minnesota: Prevalence at autopsy compared with that in Hiroshima and Nagasaki, Japan. Cancer 34:2074-2076, 1974.
6. Fukunaga FH, Yatani R. Geographic pathology of occult thyroid carcinoma. Cancer 36:1095-1099, 1975.
7. Sobrinho-Simoes MA, Sambade MC, Goncalves V. Latent thyroid carcinoma at autopsy. Cancer 43:1702-1706, 1979.
8. Bondeson L, Ljungberg O. Occult thyroid carcinoma at autopsy in Malmo, Sweden. Cancer 47:319-323, 1981.

9. Pingitore R. Rilievi morfologici autopsicisu 111 tiroidi clinicamente normali in un`area italiana senza edemia gozzigena. Pathologia 74:545-552, 1982.
10. Arellano L, Ibarra A. Occult carcinoma of the thyroid gland. Path Res Pract 179:88-91, 1984.
11. Franssila KO, Harach HR. Occult papillary carcinoma of the thyroid in children and young adults. A systemic autopsy study in Finland. Cancer 58:715-719, 1986.
12. Lang W, Borrusch H, Bauer L. Occult carcinomas of the thyroid. Evaluation of 1020 sequential autopsies. Am J Clin Pathol 90:72-76, 1988.
13. Ottino A, Pianzola HM, Castelletto RH. Occult papillary thyroid carcinoma at autopsy in La Plata, Argentina. Cancer 64:547-551, 1989.
14. Yamamoto Y et al. Occult papillary carcinoma of the thyroid. A study of 408 autopsy cases. Cancer 65:1173-1179, 1990.
15. Kugimoto M et al. Epidemiologic studies on thyroid cancer in Nagano prefecture, Japan. Endocrinol Jpn 14:313-319, 1976.
16. Ishida T et al. Evaluation of mass screening for thyroid cancer. Jpn J Clin Oncol 18:289-295, 1988.
17. Omata K et al. Clinico-pathological study of thyroid carcinomas detected by mass screening. Jpn J Cancer Clin 32:740-748, 1986.
18. Spitz MR et al. Ethnic patterns of thyroid cancer incidence in the United States, 1973-1981. Int J Cancer 42:549-553, 1988.
19. Elman DS. Familiar association of nerve deafness with nodular goiter and thyroid carcinoma. N Engl J Med 259:219-223, 1958.
20. Camiel MR et al. Association of thyroid carcinoma with Gardner's syndrome in siblings. N Engl J Med 259:1056-1058, 1968.
21. Albores Saavedra J, Duran ME. Association of thyroid carcinoma and chemodectoma. Am J Surg 116:887-890, 1968.
22. Harach HR, Williams GT, Williams ED. Familial adenomatous polyposis associated thyroid carcinoma: A distinct type of follicular cell neoplasm. Histopathology 25:549-561, 1994.
23. Plail RO et al. Adenomatous polyposis: an association with carcinoma of the thyroid. Br J Surg 74:377-380, 1987.
24. Robinson DW, Orr TG. Carcinoma of the thyroid and other diseases of the thyroid in identical twins. Arch Surg 70:923-928, 1965.
25. Lacour J et al. Epithelioma papillaire du corps thyroide: A propos de deux cas familiaux. Nouv Press Méd 2:2249-2252, 1973.
26. Nemec J et al. Familial occurrence of differentiated (non-medullary) thyroid cancer. Oncology 32:151-157, 1975.
27. Lote K et al. Familial occurrence of papillary thyroid carcinoma. Cancer 46:1291-1297, 1980.
28. Phade VR, Lawrence WR, Max MH. Familial papillary carcinoma of the thyroid. Arch Surg 116:836-837, 1981.
29. Flannigan GM et al. Simultaneous presentation of papillary carcinoma of thyroid in a father and son. Br J Surg 70:181-182, 1983.
30. Christensen SB, Ljungberg O. Familial occurrence of papillary thyroid carcinoma. Br J Surg 70:508-509, 1983.
31. Suzuki S, Watanabe I. Familial occurrence of papillary thyroid carcinoma. Jpn J Cancer Clin 31:414-419, 1985.

32. Stoffer SS et al. Familial papillary carcinoma of the thyroid. Am J Med Gene 25:775-782, 1986.
33. Ozaki O et al. Familial occurrence of differentiated, nonmedullary thyroid carcinoma. World J Surg 12:565-571, 1988.
34. Hrafnkelsson J et al. Papillary thyroid carcinoma in Iceland. A study of the occurrence in families and the coexistence of other primary tumours. Acta Oncol 28:785-788, 1989.
35. Fischer DK et al. Papillary carcinoma of the thyroid: Additional evidence in support of a familial component. Cancer Invest 7:323-325, 1989.
36. Szanto J et al. Coincidental papillary carcinoma of the thyroid in two sisters. Oncology 47:92-94, 1990.
37. Ron E et al. Familiar non-medullary thyroid cancer. Oncology 48:309-311, 1991.
38. Gorson D. Familial papillary carcinoma of the thyroid. Thyroid 2:131-132, 1992.
39. Grossman RF et al. Familial nonmedullary thyroid cancer. An emerging entity that warrants aggressive treatment. Arch Surg 130:892-897, 1995.
40. Quimby EH, Werner SCE. Late radiation effects in roentogen therapy for hyperthyroidism: Their possible bearing on use of radioactive iodine. JAMA 140:1046-1049, 1949.
41. Ron E et al. Thyroid cancer after exposure to external radiation: a pooled analysis of seven studies. Radiat Res 141:259-277, 1995.
42. Shore RE et al. Thyroid tumors following thymus irradiation. J Nat Cancer Inst 74:1177-1184, 1985.
43. Schneider AB, Shore FE, Weinstein RA. Radiation-induced thyroid and other head and neck tumors: Occurrence of multiple tumors and analysis of risk factors. J Clin Endocrinol Metab 63:107-112, 1986.
44. Yoshida A et al. Low-dose irradiation to head, neck, or chest during infancy as a possible cause of thyroid carcinoma in teen-agers: A matched case-control study. Jpn J Cancer Res 78:991-994, 1987.
45. Schroder DM, Chambors A, France CJ. Operative strategy for thyroid cancer. Is total thyroidectomy worth the price? Cancer 58:2320-2328, 1986.
46. Schneider AB et al. Radiation-induced thyroid carcinoma. Clinical course and results of therapy in 296 patients. Ann Intern Med 105:405-412, 1986.
47. Kanno J et al. Tumor-promoting effects of both iodine deficiency and iodine excess in the rat thyroid. Toxicol Pathol 20:226-235, 1992.
48. Franceschi S et al. Risk factors for thyroid cancer in northern Italy. Int J Epidemiol 18:578-584, 1989.
49. Galanti MR et al. Diet and the risk of papillary and follicular thyroid carcinoma: A population-based case control study in Sweden and Norway. Cancer Causes Control 8:205-214, 1997.
50. Frich L, Akslen LA, Glattre E. Increased risk of thyroid cancer among Norwegian women married to fishery workers—a retrospective cohort study. Br J Cancer 76:385-389, 1997.
51. Harach HR et al. Thyroid carcinoma and thyroiditis in an endemic goitre region before and after iodine prophylaxis. Acta Endocrinol 108:55-60, 1985.
52. Williams ED et al. Thyroid cancer in an iodide rich area: A histopathological study. Cancer 39:215-222, 1977.
53. Kolonel LN et al. An epidemiologic study of thyroid cancer in Hawaii. Cancer Causes Control 1:223-234, 1990.

54. Kung TM, Ng WL, Gibson JB. Volcanoes and carcinoma of the thyroid: A possible association. Arch Environ Health 36:265-267, 1981.
55. Franceschi S et al. The epidemiology of thyroid carcinoma. Crit Rev Oncog 4:25-52, 1993.
56. Headinger CE, Williams ED, Sobin LH. Histological typing of thyroid tumours. In Hedinger CE, eds. WHO International Histological Classification of Tumours, 2nd ed. Berlin:Springer-Verlag, 1988, pp 20-22.
57. Vickery AL, Wang CA, Walker AM. Treatment of intrathyroid papillary carcinoma of the thyroid. Cancer 60:2587-2595, 1990.
58. Hazard JB. Small papillary carcinoma of the thyroid: A study with special reference to so-called nonencapsulated sclerosing tumor. Lab Invest 9:86-97, 1960.
59. Hay ID et al. Papillary thyroid microcarcinoma: A study of 535 cases observed in a 50-year period. Surgery 112:1139-1146, 1992.
60. van Heerden JA, Hay ID, Goellner JR, et al. Follicular thyroid carcinoma with capsular invasion alone: A nonthreatening malignancy. Surgery 112:1130-1136, 1992.
61. Silliphant WM, Klinck GH, Levitin M. Thyroid carcinoma and death. A clinicopathological study of 193 autopsies. Cancer 17:513-525, 1964.
62. Wychulis AR, Beahrsa OH, Black MB. Papillary carcinoma with associated anaplastic carcinoma in the thyroid gland. Surg Gynecol Obstet 120:28-34, 1965.
63. Hutter RV et al. Spindle and giant cell metaplasia in papillary carcinoma of the thyroid. Am J Surg 110:660-668, 1965.
64. Ibanez ML et al. Thyroid carcinoma: Biologic behavior and mortality. Postmortem findings in 42 cases, including 27 cases in which the disease was fatal. Cancer 19:1039-1052, 1966.
65. Rafla S. Anaplastic tumors of the thyroid. Cancer 23:668-677, 1968.
66. Silverberg SG, Hutter RVP, Foote FW. Fatal carcinoma of the thyroid: Histology, metastasis and causes of death. Cancer 25:793-802, 1970.
67. Nishiyama RH, Dunn EL, Thompson NW. Anaplastic spindle-cell and giant-cell tumors of the thyroid gland. Cancer 30:113-127, 1972.
68. Harada T et al. Fatal thyroid carcinoma. Anaplastic transformation of adenocarcinoma. Cancer 39:2588-2596, 1977.
69. Krisch K et al. Das anaplastische Spindel- und Riesenzellkarzinom der Schilddrüse. Wien Klin Wochschr 92:122-127, 1980.
70. Lips CJ et al. Clinical screening as compared with DNA analysis in families with multiple endocrine neoplasia type 2A. N Engl J Med 331:828-835, 1994.
71. Abdul-Rahman ZH et al. T-cell lymphoma in Hashimoto's thyroiditis. Histopathology 29:455-459, 1996.
72. Suzuki Y et al. A case of primary thyroid T-cell lymphoma with infiltration of lymphoma cells in peripheral blood: Diagnosed by DNA analysis. Folia Endocrinol JP 70:1055-1062, 1994.
73. Travagli JP et al. Differentiated thyroid carcinoma in childhood. J Endocrinol Invest 18:161-164, 1995.
74. Harness JK, Thompson NW, Nishiyama RH. Childhood thyroid carcinoma. Arch Surg 102:278-284, 1971.
75. Zimmerman D et al. Papillary thyroid carcinoma in children and adults: long-term follow-up of 1039 patients conservatively treated at one institution during three decades. Surgery 104:1157-1166, 1988.

76. Schlumberger M et al. Differentiated thyroid carcinoma in childhood: long term follow-up of 72 patients. J Clin Endocrinol Metab 65:1088-1094, 1987.
77. Buckwalter JA, Gurll NJ, Thomas CJ. Cancer of the thyroid in youth. World J Surg 5:15-25, 1981.
78. McClellan DR, Francis GL. Thyroid cancer in children, pregnant women, and patients with Graves' disease. Endocrinol Metab Clin North Am 25:27-48, 1996.
79. Hancock BW et al. Thyroid carcinoma and concurrent hyperthyroidism: A study of ten patients. Cancer 39:298-302, 1977.
80. Filetti S et al. The role of thyroid-stimulating antibodies of Graves' disease in differentiated thyroid cancer. N Engl J Med 318:753-759, 1988.
81. Belfiore A et al. Increased aggressiveness of thyroid cancer in patients with Graves' disease. J Clin Endocrinol Metab 70:830-835, 1990.
82. Hales IB et al. Does Graves' disease or thyrotoxicosis affect the prognosis of thyroid cancer. J Clin Endocrinol Metab 75:886-889, 1992.
83. Farbota LM et al. Thyroid carcinoma in Graves' disease. Surgery 98:1148-1153, 1985.
84. Lucas SD et al. Tumor-specific deposition of immunoglobulin G and complement in papillary thyroid carcinoma. Hum Pathol 27:1329-1335, 1996.
85. Dailey ME, Lindsay S, Skahen R. Relation of thyroid neoplasms to Hashimoto's disease of thyroid gland. Arch Surg 70:291-297, 1955.
86. Pollock WF, Sprong DHJ. The rationale of thyroidectomy for Hashimoto's thyroiditis. West J Surg 66:17-20, 1958.
87. Pollock WF, Sprong DHJ. Surgical aspects of thyroiditis. Arch Surg 80:720-731, 1960.
88. Schlicke CP, Hill JE, Shulutz GF. Carcinoma in chronic thyroiditis. Surg Gynec Obstet 111:552-556, 1960.
89. Chesky VF, Hellwig CA, Welch JW. Cancer of the thyroid associated with Hashimoto's disease: An analysis of forty-eight cases. Am Surgeon 28:678-685, 1962.
90. Meier DW et al. Parenchymal finding in thyroidal carcinoma: pathologic study of 256 cases. J Clin Endocrinol Metab 19:162-171, 1959.
91. Crile GJ, Hazard JB. Incidence of cancer in struma lymphomatosa. Surg Gynec Obstet 115:101-103, 1962.
92. Hirabayashi RN, Lindsay S. The relation of thyroid carcinoma and chronic thyroiditis. Surg Gynecol Obstet 121:243-252, 1965.
93. Harach HR, Williams ED. Thyroid cancer and thyroiditis in the goitrous region of Salta, Argentina, before and after iodine prophylaxis. Clin Endocrinol 43:701-706, 1995.
94. Okayasu I et al. Association of chronic lymphocytic thyroiditis and thyroid papillary carcinoma. A study of surgical cases among Japanese, and white and African Americans. Cancer 76:2312-2318, 1995.
95. McLeod MK et al. Hashimoto's thyroiditis revisited: the association with thyroid cancer remains obscure. World J Surg 12:509-516, 1988.
96. Clark OH, Greenspan FS, Dunphy JE. Hashimoto's thyroiditis and thyroid cancer: indications for operation. Am J Surg 140:65-71, 1980.
97. Ott RA et al. The incidence of thyroid carcinoma in Hashimoto's thyroiditis. Am Surgeon 53:442-445, 1987.
98. Holmes HJ, Kreutner A, O'Brien PH. Hashimoto's thyroiditis and its relationship to other thyroid diseases. Surg Gynec Obstet 144:887-890, 1977.
99. Wartsman J et al. Hashimoto's thyroiditis simulating cancer of the thyroid. Arch Surg 16:386-388, 1981.

100. Noguchi S, Murakami N, Toda M. Thyroid cancer coexisting with chronic thyroiditis: Diagnosis and outcome. Endocr Surg 9:261-265, 1992.
101. Carson HJ, Castelli MJ, Gattuso P. Incidence of neoplasia in Hashimoto's thyroiditis: A fine needle aspiration study. Diagn Cytopathol 14:38-42, 1996.
102. Matsubayashi S et al. The correlation between papillary thyroid carcinoma and lymphocytic infiltration in the thyroid gland. J Clin Endocrinol Metab 80:3421-3424, 1995.
103. Rossi RL et al. Malignancies of the thyroid gland. The Lahey Clinic experience. Surg Clin North Am 65:211-230, 1985.
104. McConahey WM et al. Papillary thyroid cancer treated at the Mayo Clinic, 1946 through 1970: Initial manifestations, pathologic findings, therapy, and outcome. Mayo Clin Proc 61:978-996, 1986.
105. Ito T et al. Unique association of p53 mutations with undifferentiated but not with differentiated carcinomas of the thyroid gland. Cancer Res 52:1369-1371, 1992.
106. Ito T et al. Genetic alterations in thyroid tumor progression: association with p53 gene mutations. Jpn J Cancer Res 84:526-531, 1993.

CHAPTER

2

Evaluation of Thyroid Nodules

HIROYUKI YAMASHITA, M.D., Ph.D.

Thyroid nodules are common: the clinical prevalence of thyroid nodules is estimated to be 2% to 7%.[1-4] The majority of thyroid nodules are follicular adenomas, multinodular goiters, cysts, and chronic thyroiditis. The frequency of malignancies has been found to vary from 3% to 31% in thyroid nodules examined at surgery.[1,2,5-9] A variety of indirect and diagnostic techniques in addition to clinical presentation, past history of neck irradiation, and family history make it easier to select patients for surgery. All types of thyroid nodules are more common in women than in men, although the incidence of malignancy in men is higher than in women. Although the surgical indications for thyroid nodules may differ among institutions, the most important point is not to overlook malignancy in the assessment and management of thyroid nodules.

Fine-needle aspiration (FNA) has revolutionized the evaluation of thyroid nodules in the last two decades.[10-15] The limitation of FNA is the difficulty in distinguishing follicular and Hürthle cell carcinomas from follicular and Hürthle cell adenomas. At our institution, surgical indications for thyroid nodules include those that are FNA-proven or suspicious for malignancy, clinically suspicious nodules, hyperfunctioning nodules, local symptomatic nodules, substernal nodules, and a patient's cosmetic concern and anxiety about nodules. As for follicular neoplasms, as diagnosed by FNA and/or ultrasonography, we recommend surgery because of the significant incidence of malignancy (about 5%) and the diagnostic inability to differentiate between benign and malignant follicular and Hürthle cell tumors.[16] The diagnosis of follicular carcinoma requires identification of capsular and/or vascular invasion. Another complexity in the diagnosis and management of nodular thyroid diseases is the association of cancer with benign thyroid nodules.

In this chapter, I will outline current management of benign thyroid nodules and report surgical cases of follicular tumors and thyroid cancer associated with multinodular goiters treated at the Noguchi Thyroid Clinic.

DIAGNOSIS AND EVALUATION

For all patients with thyroid nodules a thorough history should be taken and a physical examination and laboratory evaluation performed. A family history of familial medullary carcinoma, though uncommon, greatly increases the risk of medullary thyroid cancer.[17,18] Papillary thyroid cancer is usually sporadic, but occasionally (in 5% to 10% of cases) may be either familial[19-21] or associated with Gardner's syndrome[22-24] or familial polyposis and Cowden's syndrome.[20,25,26] A history of exposure to head or neck irradiation in childhood is very important in countries where irradiation therapy was given for the treatment of thymic enlargement, recurrent tonsillitis, adenoiditis, and other dermatologic diseases. Numerous studies have shown the high incidence of thyroid cancer, as well as benign thyroid nodules, after exposure to low-dose irradiation therapy.[27-31] The risk of developing a cancer has been calculated to be 4.3 cancers per rem-year per 10^6 persons exposed to radiation.[32]

On physical examination, a nodule fixed to surrounding structures is highly suggestive of thyroid cancer. Firm or hard nodules may be malignant, but they can also be cysts or benign nodules with calcifications. Vocal cord paralysis due to thyroid nodules suggests the presence of an invasive thyroid cancer. However, benign nodules can also produce vocal cord paralysis.[33] Lymphadenopathy is occasionally present on the ipsilateral side of thyroid cancer. None of these findings are diagnostic of thyroid cancer so that following modalities are necessary for the assessment of thyroid nodules.

Ultrasonographic examination is commonly used for evaluation of thyroid nodules. The modality is noninvasive, sensitive, and relatively inexpensive. High-resolution ultrasonography can detect nodules more than 2 mm in size and with an experienced examiner can also diagnose fairly accurately whether a nodule is benign or malignant.[4,34,35] FNA, however, has become the most widely accepted means of determining whether a thyroid nodule is cancer, suspicious, or benign.[10-15] FNA is fast, minimally invasive, and highly reliable when an experienced cytologist is available. FNA under ultrasound guidance is also helpful for the diagnosis of a nonpalpable thyroid mass.[9,36-38] This procedure is detailed in Chapter 12. When one uses both ultrasonography and FNA, most thyroid nodules can be accurately diagnosed except for follicular and Hürthle cell neoplasms and some cystic lesions.[39-42] Aspiration of cystic lesions for cytologic examination usually reveals only a few foamy cells, hemosiderin, macrophage and usually not enough epithelial cells.

Although the risk of malignancy in a cystic nodule is generally considered to be lower than in a solid nodule, from 9% to 32% of surgical cystic lesion specimens reported were malignant.[39-41] This probably overestimates the risk of cancer, since patients with suspicious nodules are subject to surgery. At our institution, thyroglobulin (Tg) concentrations and lactic dehydrogenase (LDH) isozyme analysis, in addition to FNA, are examined for cystic lesions of the thyroid. We and others reported that the mean logarithmic value for the thyroglobulin concentration was significantly lower in malignant cyst fluid than in benign nodules, and the LDH 1 and 2 isozyme percentages were greater in the malignant group than in the benign group.[43,44]

Most patients with thyroid nodules have normal thyroid function. Measurements of serum levels of free thyroxin, triiodothyronine, thyrotropin (TSH), and antithyroid antibodies can be useful, since a suppressed TSH level would suggest a hot nodule, whereas elevated TSH levels and/or positive antithyroid antibodies would indicate underlying Hashimoto's thyroiditis. Some experts recommend using a sensitive TSH test in patients with thyroid nodules that appear to be euthyroid, because this is more cost-effective.

Radioisotope scanning using ^{131}I or ^{123}I or ^{99m}technetium has been used extensively in the assessment of thyroid nodules. With recent advances in other diagnostic tests, thyroid scintigraphy has become less important in the evaluation of thyroid nodules except for patients with follicular neoplasms by FNA. When such patients have a "hot" or functioning thyroid nodule, it is rarely malignant.

A serum Tg test may be useful for surgery selection of patients with follicular tumors (described later in this chapter). A routine serum calcitonin test is not recommended for thyroid nodules, because it does not appear to be cost-effective. Serum calcitonin levels should be measured only in patients with a positive family history of MEN2, or familial medullary thyroid cancer (MTC), or if the FNA of a nodule suggests medullary thyroid cancer. Most patients with palpable nodules and MTC also have an elevated calcitonin level.

At our institution, computed tomographic (CT) scanning and magnetic resonance imaging (MRI) are used selectively, because these procedures are relatively expensive and do not offer any benefit for the differential diagnosis of thyroid nodules. They are used for patients with known or suspected thyroid cancer to examine the extent of invasion to surrounding structures and the presence of lymphadenopathy, and for patients with substernal goiter.

SOLITARY FOLLICULAR TUMORS

Follicular adenoma has a well-developed fibrous capsule that sharply demarcates it from the surrounding normal thyroid tissue. Most follicular neoplasms present as a solitary thyroid nodule. Follicular adenomas tend to grow slowly; the capsule of surrounding normal thyroid tissue is compressed and may undergo degeneration and hemorrhage. Histologically, the follicular adenomas are classified into various subtypes according to the size of the thyroid follicles and degree of cellularity.

Atypical adenomas appear to be suspicious for malignancy but lack histologic evidence of invasion. In our 15 patients with atypical follicular adenomas treated between 1981 and 1996, none developed recurrence or died from these tumors. Hürthle cell adenomas are considered a morphologic variant of follicular adenomas. Treatment of Hürthle cell neoplasm is controversial because of the difficulties in grading tumor malignancy. Gundry et al.[45] reviewed 62 patients and found 35 malignant lesions and 26 benign tumors. Three of the 26 patients diagnosed as having benign Hürthle cell tumors died from their tumors. They concluded that Hürthle cell tumors should be treated aggressively with total thyroidectomy, regardless of their pathologic characteristics. Azadian et al.[46] reported similar results and advocated total thyroidectomy for all patients with Hürthle cell tumors, as well as jugular node sampling and adjuvant radioiodine therapy for cancer. Gosain and Clark[47] reported that 71 of 84 patients examined had Hürthle cell adenomas and had a natural history consistent with a benign tumor. However, one in four of the patients with Hürthle cell carcinoma died of the disease.[47] They advocated total thyroidectomy only for patients with histologically proven carcinomas (capsular or vascular invasion), in accordance with the recommendations of many other investigators.[48-50] Grant et al.[51] from the Mayo Clinic reviewed their own experience and that in the literature. In only one of their 272 patients who had Hürthle cell neoplasia that appeared to be benign, the tumor recurred as a result of this neoplasm.

In our institution, 187 patients with Hürthle cell tumors were treated between 1980 and 1994, 153 (82%) of the 187 were Hürthle cell adenomas diagnosed by the same criteria as follicular tumors. None of the 153 patients had eventual metastatic diseases. Furthermore, none of 34 patients with

Hürthle cell carcinoma died of cancer. We treated patients with Hürthle cell tumors, which are usually diagnosed by preoperative FNA, with the same procedure with which we treat patients who have other follicular tumors. Although techniques have been reported to improve the accuracy of discrimination between benign and malignant tumors,[52,53] in our opinion the results of such techniques are not yet accurate enough to be used clinically. Recently Umbricht et al.[54] reported that telomerase activity was found in all 11 follicular carcinomas and in 8 of 33 benign follicular tumors, and it was undetectable in normal thyroid tissues adjacent to the tumors in 22 patients.[54] They concluded that telomerase activity may thus provide a diagnostic marker distinguishing benign from malignant follicular thyroid tumors. Further studies are warranted to determine whether this test will allow clinicians to discriminate accurately between follicular adenoma and carcinoma.

We have surgically treated 1184 patients with follicular tumors (1130 follicular adenomas and 54 follicular carcinomas) at our institution (Figs. 2-1 through 2-3). There were 1063 women and 121 men, a mean age of 46 years (7 to 82 years), and a maximum tumor diameter of 29 mm (10 to 90 mm). Univariate analysis regarding age, gender, mean tumor size, and serum Tg were evaluated; patients with larger tumors and those with higher Tg levels

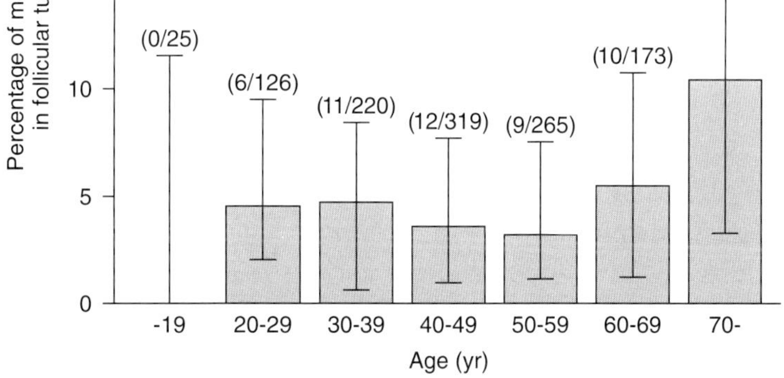

• **FIGURE 2-1** Percentage of malignancy in 1184 follicular tumors (1130 adenomas and 54 carcinomas) by age groups. Numbers in parentheses represent the number of patients with follicular cancer/total number of patients in each age decade.

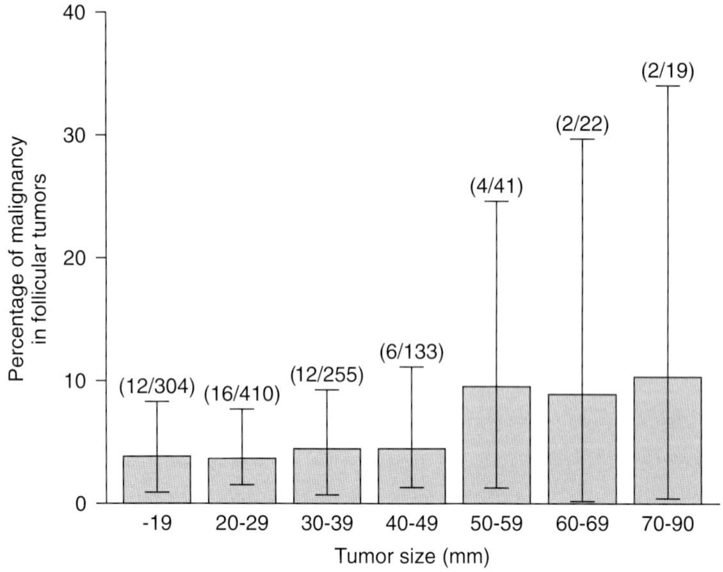

• **FIGURE 2-2** Percentage of malignancy in 1184 follicular tumors (1130 adenomas and 54 carcinomas) by tumor size. Numbers in parentheses represent the number of patients with thyroid follicular cancer/total number of patients in each group by tumor size.

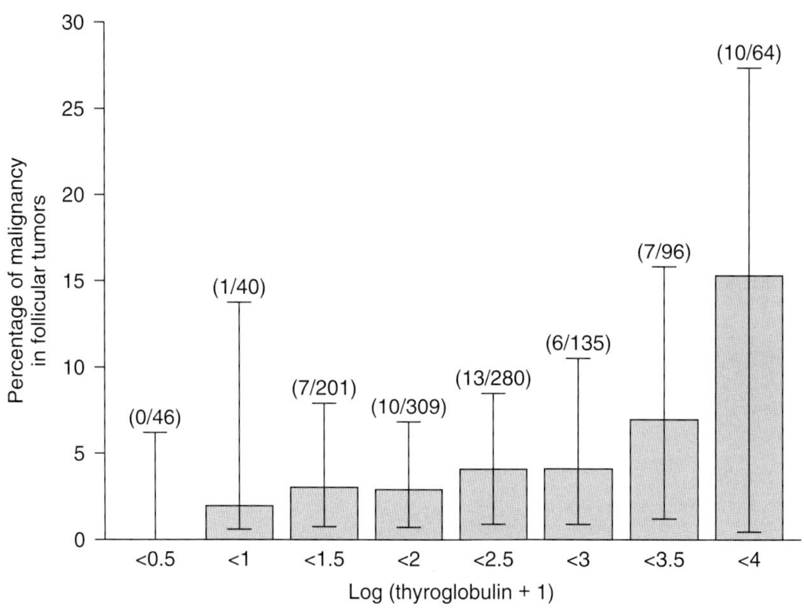

• **FIGURE 2-3** Percentage of malignancy in 1184 follicular tumors (1130 adenomas and 54 carcinomas) by serum thyroglobulin level. Numbers in parentheses represent the number of patients with thyroid follicular cancer/total number of patients in each group by preoperative serum thyroglobulin level.

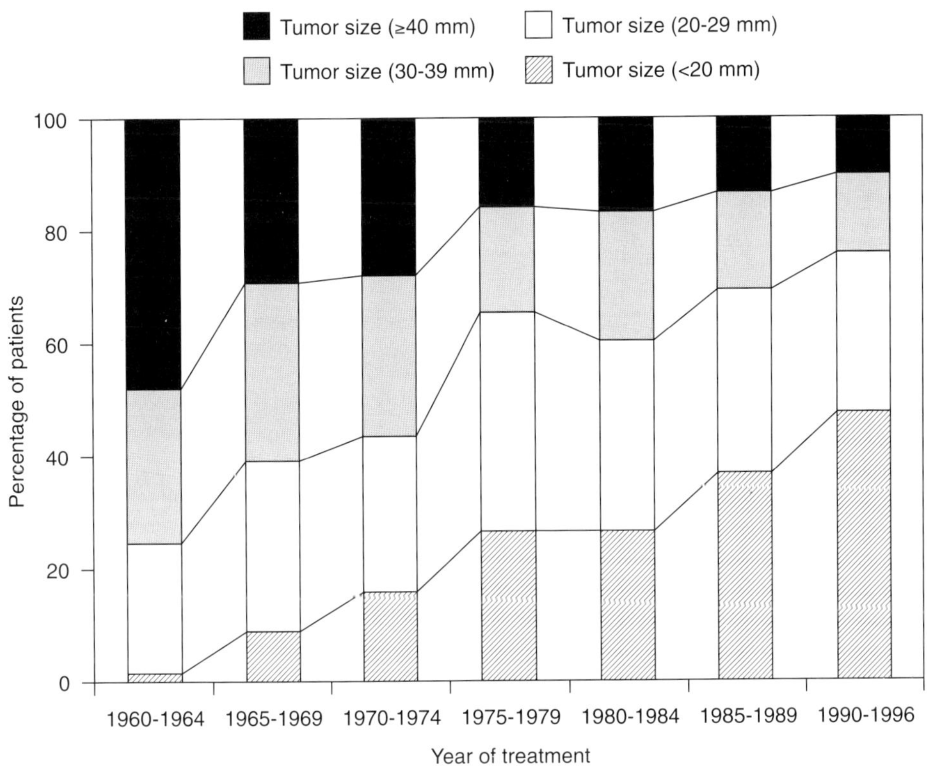

• **FIGURE 2-4** Percentage of 3410 patients with papillary thyroid cancer treated between 1960 and 1996 by tumor size.

were more likely to have cancer ($p < 0.05$). In multivariate analysis, only serum thyroglobulin level was significant ($p < 0.05$). Prognostic risk factors for 405 patients with follicular carcinomas that we have treated include age, tumor size, cell differentiation, and extracapsular invasion. Serum Tg levels were proportionally high compared with tumor size and were surprisingly high in patients with poorly differentiated tumors. Considering these results, serum Tg levels as well as tumor size and/or tumor growth during observation are important criteria to be used to select patients for thyroidectomy.

Figs. 2-4 and 2-5 show the percentages of patients with papillary cancer (Fig. 2-4) and follicular cancer (Fig. 2-5) by tumor size treated surgically at our medical center between 1960 and 1996. It clearly demonstrates that patients with papillary thyroid cancer are being diagnosed at an earlier stage, but this observation is not conclusive in patients with follicular thyroid cancer. This is most likely because many physicians follow up on their patients with follicular tumors for some time before recommending surgery. Many studies showed that tumor size is one of the significant risk factors for recurrence and death in patients with differentiated thyroid cancer.[55-58] The

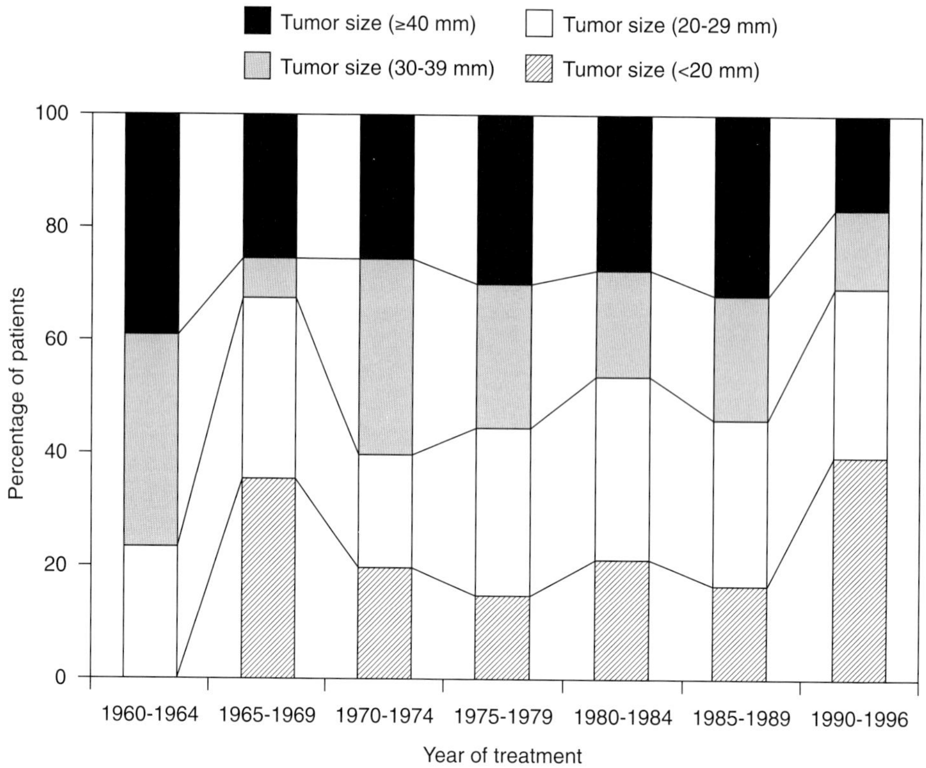

• **FIGURE 2-5** Percentage of 401 patients with follicular thyroid cancer treated between 1960 and 1996 by tumor size.

author emphasizes that physicians should be very careful when following patients with follicular thyroid tumors.

Our standard surgical procedure for a patient with follicular or Hürthle cell neoplasm is a total lobectomy of the affected thyroid lobe. Even when total thyroidectomy is indicated after a histologic diagnosis of follicular cancer has been made, or there are metastases, the remnant thyroid gland can easily be removed without or with minimal increased risk of complications. We recommend ^{131}I ablation following completion thyroidectomy in patients with invasive follicular carcinomas, because these patients have a poorer prognosis than patients with papillary thyroid cancer or those who develop distant metastases.

Of 813 patients with follicular adenomas surgically treated at our clinic, transient tetany occurred in only one patient (0.1%), transient recurrent laryngeal nerve palsy developed in 12 patients (1.5%), and reoperation for hemorrhage was required in two patients (0.2%). Six months after surgery, one patient (0.1%) had persistent recurrent laryngeal nerve palsy. This morbidity of thyroid surgery appears low when the surgeon is experienced, although there is a small risk of complications, even in patients with benign tumor.

MULTINODULAR GOITER

Multinodular goiter is a common condition in individuals in some iodine-deficient regions and is characterized histologically by the coexistence of hyperplasia and various regressive changes such as cyst formation, necrosis, hemorrhage, and calcification. The surgical indications for this disease include an association or suspicion of malignancy, compressive symptoms, hyperthyroidism, substernal goiters, and/or cosmetic appearance. Substernal goiters are usually detected by a routine chest x-ray evaluation. Vocal cord palsy is rare in association with benign multinodular goiter.[33] To manage patients with multinodular goiter, we must keep in mind an association of malignancy with benign tumors. As mentioned, FNA cytology has proved to be the most efficient and accurate diagnostic procedure and has refined the management of patients with single thyroid tumors.[10-15] However, there are problems in using this diagnostic procedure for multiple nodular glands. The incidence of thyroid cancer among individuals with multinodular goiter is higher than the general incidence of thyroid cancer; it varies from 4% to 31%.[7,8,59] According to the Third National Cancer Survey in the United States,[60] the incidence of clinical thyroid cancer was only 0.004%, whereas Maruchi et al. reported that the prevalence of thyroid cancer in Japan was 1.3 per 1000 based on their population surveys.

We have recently reported that 256 of 835 patients with histologically proven multinodular goiter had associated thyroid cancer, the incidence being 30.7%. Of the 256 patients, 137 had occult thyroid cancer (tumor size less than or equal to 10 mm) and 119 had clinical thyroid cancer (tumor size smaller than 10 mm).[8] This high incidence of coexisting thyroid cancer could be attributed to patient selection, as many of these patients underwent surgery after the diagnosis of thyroid cancer had been made by FNA cytology or after a thyroid nodule was considered suspicious by ultrasonography. The percentages and 95% confidence intervals and the mean size of the thyroid cancer of 256 patients with associated thyroid cancer in each decade are shown in Figs. 2-6 and 2-7. There were no significant differences in either the percentage of patients with associated cancer and the mean cancer size among the age groups. Furthermore, there was no correlation between the maximum size of the thyroid cancer and the age of the 256 patients.

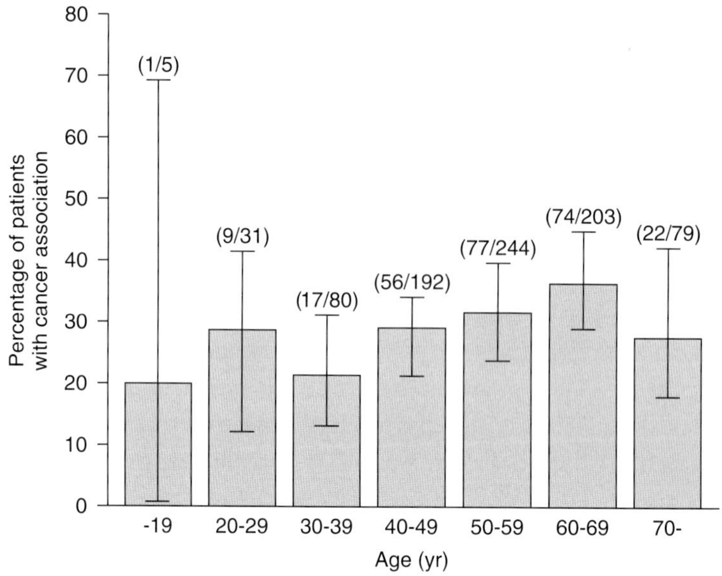

• **FIGURE 2-6** Percentages and 95% confidence intervals of 256 patients with associated cancer among a total of 835 patients with adenomatous goiter in each age decade. Numbers in parentheses represent the number of patients with thyroid cancer/ total number of patients in each age decade. (From Yamashita H et al. Thyroid cancer associated with adenomatous goiter: An analysis of the incidence and clinical factors. Surgery Today 26:495-499, 1997. Reproduced with permission.)

These results indicate that a considerable number of thyroid carcinomas would remain occult. Although we could not document any differences between benign and malignant nodules in patients with multiple nodular goiters, the frequency of calcification detected by ultrasonograph and/or neck soft exposure evaluation in the patients with clinical cancer was significantly higher than in those with occult cancer (83% vs. 57%, respectively [$p < 0.0001$]). Because the patients with clinical thyroid cancer frequently had evidence of calcification in multiple nodular glands, the detection of this cancer is a major consideration when evaluating whether surgery is appropriate in individual patients with multinodular goiter.

The extent of thyroidectomy for patients with multinodular goiter is controversial. The choice of operative procedures for multinodular goiter, including bilateral subtotal, near-total, or total thyroidectomy, must be based on the clinical situation of the patient, such as age, size and extent of the nodules, and the coexistence of cancer. We prefer bilateral subtotal lobectomy or total lobectomy of the primary affected lobe and subtotal lobectomy of the contralateral lobe to remove at least all macroscopically

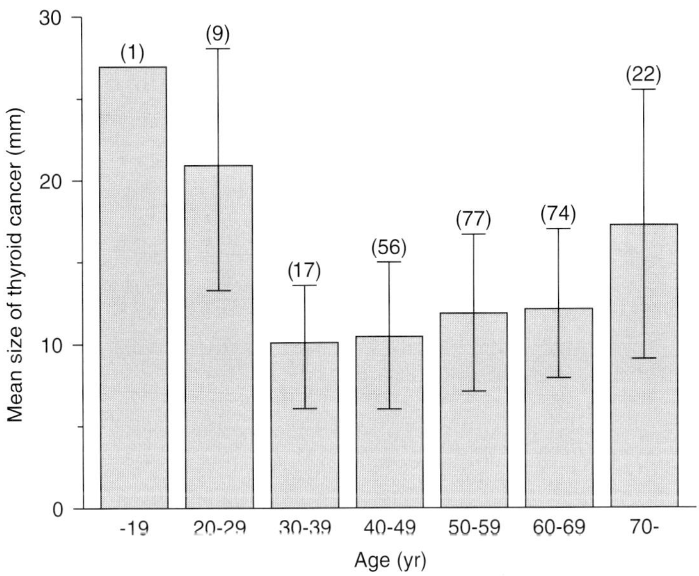

• **FIGURE 2-7** Mean size of thyroid cancer tumors among patients in each age decade. There were no significant differences in the mean size of thyroid cancer among age groups. Numbers in parentheses represent the number of patients in each age decade. (From Yamashita H et al. Thyroid cancer associated with adenomatous goiter: An analysis of the incidence and clinical factors. Surgery Today 26:495-499, 1997. Reproduced with permission.)

enlarged nodules. If coexisting cancer is noticed preoperatively or during surgery, we perform near-total or total thyroidectomy and an ipsilateral modified radical neck dissection. We choose total lobectomy with isthmectomy for patients who have unilateral nodules on gross examination. In such cases, it carries potential for the eventual development of goiter in the remnant lobe. However, the risk for necessitating reoperation in these patients is low. Even if a second surgery is indicated, resection of the untouched thyroid lobe can be performed with little morbidity. Some surgeons advocate total thyroidectomy for multinodular goiters to reduce the likelihood of goiter recurrence without increasing postoperative complications, when the surgeon is experienced in the thyroid operation.[61-63] In general, we do not favor this approach.

Of 959 patients with multiple nodular goiters surgically treated at our clinic, transient tetany occurred in 11 patients (1.1%), transient ipsilateral recurrent laryngeal nerve palsy developed in eight patients (0.8%), and reoperation for hemorrhage was required in eight patients (0.8%). Six months after surgery, four patients (0.4%) had persistent recurrent laryngeal nerve palsy. There was no mortality. In selecting the type of thyroidectomy, one must consider the benefits of extensive resection and the increased potential for complications associated with more radical procedures.

AUTONOMOUSLY FUNCTIONING THYROID NODULES

Autonomously functioning thyroid nodules (AFTN) are thyroid nodules that function independently of the normal pituitary-thyroid negative-feedback control mechanism.[64] Recently point mutations in the TSH receptor[65,66] or mutant G stimulatory proteins[67] were reported to be responsible molecular mechanisms for the development of AFTN. About 1% to 20% of all thyroid nodules are AFTN, depending on the amount of iodine intake and probably other factors.[68-70]

Baltisberger et al.[71] reported that the incidence of toxic nodular goiter decreased after the correction of mild iodine deficiency. Although AFTN are generally thought to rarely be malignant, the reported incidence varies from 1% to 11%.[72-75] At our medical center in an iodine-rich area, of 3772 patients with thyroid nodules who underwent thyroidectomy, 28 (0.7%) had AFTN with hyperthyroidism. Among these 28 patients, three had papillary thyroid carcinomas (predominantly follicular type), so that the incidence of malignancy in AFTN at our institution is 11%. This relatively low incidence can be explained by the exclusion of patients who had hot nodules as seen on scintigraphic evaluation who were euthyroid. Furthermore, not all patients with thyroid nodules underwent a thyroid scan in our series; some patients with AFTN could have been missed.

Patients with AFTN can be treated successfully by either surgery or radioactive iodine. In several centers, radioactive iodine irradiation is the first choice of therapy for patients with AFTN because it is safe, simple, and cost-effective.[76] However, it often results in persistent nodularity and also may be complicated by the late development of hypothyroidism; the reported cumulative rates have ranged from 0% to 72%.[76] Long-term results following ^{131}I therapy indicate an increased incidence of hypothyroidism with time (i.e., 25% at 5 years, 33% at 10 years, and 50% at 15 years).[77] At our clinic, surgery is the first choice of treatment for AFTN, and radioactive iodine treatment is used for patients with poor risk for good surgical result and/or those who do not want surgery. Surgical treatment is the preferable treatment for most patients, because it results in rapid restoration of a euthyroid state and allows for histopathologic diagnosis.[78] As mentioned above, the possibility of malignancy cannot be ignored.[75,79] Postoperative recurrent nerve palsy may be avoided by meticulous thyroid surgery. Surgical treatment in our series has been very successful without any morbidity or mortality. If surgery is chosen, lobectomy is an adequate therapy for solitary AFTN, and subtotal, near-total, or total thyroidectomy for patients with bilateral multinodular goiters.

Treatment of AFTN with percutaneous intranodular ethanol injection has recently been used as an alternative to surgery or radioactive iodine ablation therapy.[80-83] Lippi et al.[82] treated 242 patients with toxic adenoma and 187 patients with pretoxic adenoma. Successful treatment was achieved in 66.5% of patients with toxic adenoma and in 83.4% of patients with pretoxic adenoma, when assessed after a 12-month follow-up. Several small ethanol injections (0.5 to 2 ml) were necessary to shrink the nodules and return patients to a euthyroid state. However, leakage of ethanol can cause local pain and tissue damage, and recurrent nerve palsy has been reported.[84] Because there have been few studies concerning the long-term results of this new procedure, careful selection of patients may be advisable.

CONCLUSION

When managing patients with thyroid nodules, the most important point is not to overlook malignancy. Although FNA and high-resolution ultrasonography have greatly enhanced our ability to evaluate patients with thyroid nodules, difficulties remain in distinguishing follicular carcinomas from follicular adenomas. FNA is also not reliable in patients with multinodular goiters. Further studies will be necessary to solve these problems in selecting patients with thyroid nodules for surgery.

REFERENCES

1. Maruchi N, Furihata R, Makiuchi M. Population surveys on the prevalence of thyroid cancer in a non-endemic region, Nagano, Japan. Int J Cancer 7:573-583, 1971.
2. Ishida T et al. Evaluation of mass screening for thyroid cancer. Jpn J Clin Oncol 18:289-295, 1988.
3. Belfiore A et al. The management of thyroid nodules. J Endocrinol Invest 18:155-158, 1995.
4. Tan GH, Gharib H. Thyroid incidentalomas: management approaches to nonpalpable nodules discovered incidentally on thyroid imaging. Ann Intern Med 126:226-231, 1997.

5. Cole WH, Slaughter DP, Rossiter LJ. Potential dangers of nontoxic nodular goitre. JAMA 127:883-888, 1945.
6. Ward R. California Cancer Commission Studies: Cancer of the thyroid. Calif Med 68:170-172, 1948.
7. Sugenoya A et al. Adenomatous goitre: Therapeutic strategy, postoperative outcome, and study of epidermal growth factor receptor. Br J Surg 79:404-406, 1992.
8. Yamashita H et al. Thyroid cancer associated with adenomatous goiter—an analysis of the incidence and clinical factors. Surg Today 27:495-499, 1997.
9. Scopsi L et al. Thyroid ultrasonography with fine-needle aspiration cytology for the diagnosis of thyroid cancer. J Clin Ultrasound 25:111-118, 1997.
10. Wheeler MH. Management of the solitary thyroid nodule. J Soc Med 81:437-438, 1988.
11. Grant CS et al. Long-term follow-up of patients with benign thyroid fine-needle aspiration cytologic diagnoses. Surgery 106:980-986, 1989.
12. Borman KR, Hume AT. Credibility and clinical utility of thyroid fine-needle aspiration biopsy in a teaching hospital. Am J Surg 170:638-641, 1995.
13. Carpi A et al. Needle aspiration techniques in preoperative selection of patients with thyroid nodules: A long-term study. J Clin Oncol 14:1704-1712, 1996.
14. Burch HB et al. Fine needle aspiration of thyroid nodules. Determinants of insufficiency rate and malignancy yield at thyroidectomy. Acta Cytol 40:1176-1183, 1996.
15. Lucas A et al. Fine-needle aspiration cytology of benign nodular thyroid disease. Value of reaspiration. Eur J Endocrinol 132:677-680, 1995.
16. Tahara K et al. Diagnosis of thyroid follicular tumors using serum thyroglobulin. Thyroidol Clin Exp 10:1-6, 1998.
17. Hazard J, Hawk W, Crile G. Medullary (solid) carcinoma of the thyroid—a clinicopathologic entity. J Clin Endocrinol Metab 19:152-161, 1959.
18. Sizemore GW, Carney JA, Heath H. Epidemiology of medullary carcinoma of the thyroid gland: a 5-year experience (1971-1976). Surg Clin North Am 57:633-645, 1977.
19. Ozaki O et al. Familial occurrence of differentiated, nonmedullary thyroid carcinoma. World J Surg 12:565-571, 1988.
20. Grossman RF et al. Familial nonmedullary thyroid cancer. An emerging entity that warrants aggressive treatment. Arch Surg 130:892-899, 1995.
21. Kraimps JL et al. Familial papillary carcinoma of the thyroid. Surgery 121:715-718, 1997.
22. Camiel MR et al. Association of thyroid carcinoma with Gardner's syndrome in siblings. N Engl J Med 278:1056-1058, 1968.
23. Bell B, Mazzaferri EL. Familial adenomatous polyposis (Gardner's syndrome) and thyroid carcinoma. A case report and review of the literature. Dig Dis Sci 38:185-190, 1993.
24. Tanaka Y et al. A case of Gardner's syndrome associated with thyroid carcinoma. Nippon Geka Gakkai Zasshi 95:716-718, 1994.
25. Plail RO et al. Adenomatous polyposis: An association with carcinoma of the thyroid. Br J Surg 74:377-380, 1987.
26. Harach HR, Williams GT, Williams ET. Familial adenomatous polyposis associated thyroid carcinoma: A distinct type of follicular cell neoplasm. Histopathology 25:549-561, 1994.
27. Favus MJ et al. Thyroid cancer occurring as a late consequence of head-and-neck irradiation. Evaluation of 1056 patients. New Engl J Med 294:1019-1025, 1976.

28. Auguste LJ, Sako K. Radiation and thyroid carcinoma: Radiotherapy, head and neck regions, thyroid carcinoma. Head Neck Surg 7:217-224, 1985.
29. Calandra DB et al. Total thyroidectomy in irradiated patients. A twenty-year experience in 206 patients. Ann Surg 202:356-360, 1985.
30. DeGroot LJ. Clinical review 2: Diagnostic approach and management of patients exposed to irradiation to the thyroid. J Clin Endocrinol Metab 69:925-928, 1989.
31. Fjälling M et al. Benign and malignant thyroid nodules after neck irradiation. Cancer 58:1219-1224, 1986.
32. Maxon HR et al. Ionizing irradiation and the induction of clinically significant disease in the human thyroid gland. Am J Med 63:967-978, 1977.
33. Collazo-Clavell ML et al. Relationship between vocal cord paralysis and benign thyroid disease. Head Neck 17:24-30, 1995.
34. Massol J et al. Management of the thyroid nodule. Preliminary results of a practice survey of 685 general practitioners and specialists. Ann Endocrinol 54:220-225, 1993.
35. Hopkins CR, Reading CC. Thyroid and parathyroid imaging. Semin Ultrasound CT MR 16:279-295, 1995.
36. Boland GW et al. Efficacy of sonographically guided biopsy of thyroid masses and cervical lymph nodes. Am J Roentgenol 161:1053-1056, 1993.
37. Cochand PB et al. The diagnostic value of fine-needle aspiration biopsy under ultrasonography in nonfunctional thyroid nodules: A prospective study comparing cytologic and histologic findings. Am J Med 97:152-157, 1994.
38. Yokozawa T et al. Thyroid cancer detected by ultrasound-guided fine-needle aspiration biopsy. World J Surg 20:848-853, 1996.
39. Ashcraft MW, Van Herle AJ. Management of thyroid nodules. II: Scanning techniques, thyroid suppressive therapy, and fine needle aspiration. Head Neck Surg 3:297-322, 1981.
40. Hammer M, Wortsman J, Folse R. Cancer in cystic lesions of the thyroid. Arch Surg 117:1020-1023, 1982.
41. Rosen IB, Provias JP, Walfish PG. Pathologic nature of cystic thyroid nodules selected for surgery by needle aspiration biopsy. Surgery 100:606-613, 1986.
42. MacDonald L, Yazdi HM. Nondiagnostic fine needle aspiration biopsy of the thyroid gland: A diagnostic dilemma. Acta Cytol 40:423-428, 1996.
43. Clark OH, et al. Diagnosis and treatment of thyroid, parathyroid, and thyroglossal duct cysts. J Clin Endocrinol Metab 48:983-988, 1979.
44. Morita M et al. Thyroglobulin and lactic dehydrogenase isozymes in cystic fluid of thyroid nodules. Endocr J 41:227-233, 1994.
45. Gundry SR et al. Total thyroidectomy for Hürthle cell neoplasm of the thyroid. Arch Surg 18:529-532, 1983.
46. Azadian A et al. Management considerations in Hürthle cell carcinoma. Surgery 118:711-715, 1995.
47. Gosain AK, Clark OH. Hürthle cell neoplasms. Malignant potential. Arch Surg 119:515-519, 1984.
48. Caplan RH, Abellera RM, Kisken WA. Hürthle cell tumors of the thyroid gland. A clinicopathologic review and long-term follow-up. JAMA 251:3114-3117, 1984.
49. Heppe H et al. Hürthle cell tumors of the thyroid gland. Surgery 98:1162-1165, 1985.
50. Chen HY, Benjamin LB, Chen MF. Hürthle cell tumor. Int Surg 81: 168-170, 1996.
51. Grant CS et al. Benign Hurthle cell tumors of the thyroid: A diagnosis to be trusted? World J Surg 12:488-495, 1988.

52. De Micco C et al. Fine-needle aspiration of thyroid follicular neoplasm: diagnostic use of thyroid peroxidase immunocytochemistry with monoclonal antibody 47. Surgery 116:1031-1035, 1994.
53. Henry J-F et al. Thyroperoxidase immunodetection for the diagnosis of malignancy on fine-needle aspiration of thyroid nodules. World J Surg 18:529-534, 1994.
54. Umbricht CB et al. Telomerase activity—a marker to distinguish follicular thyroid adenoma from carcinoma. Cancer Res 57:2144-2147, 1997.
55. Noguchi S, Murakami N, Kawamoto H. Classification of papillary cancer of the thyroid based on prognosis. World J Surg 18:552-557, 1994.
56. Cady B, Rossi R. An expanded view of risk-group definition in differentiated thyroid carcinoma. Surgery 104:947-953, 1988.
57. Hay ID et al. Ipsilateral lobectomy versus bilateral lobar resection in papillary thyroid carcinoma: a retrospective analysis of surgical outcome using a novel prognostic scoring system. Surgery 102:1088-1095, 1987.
58. Mazzaferri EL, Jhiang SM. Long-term impact of initial surgical and medical therapy on papillary and follicular thyroid cancer. Am J Med 97:418-428, 1994.
59. Koh KBH, Chang KW. Carcinoma in multinodular goitre. Br J Surg 79:266-267, 1992.
60. Culter SJ, Young JL. Third national cancer survey, incidence data. Washington DC: National Cancer Institute, Department of Health, Education, and Welfare. NIH monograph. Washington DC 1975, p 775.
61. Reeve TS et al. Total thyroidectomy—the preferred option for multinodular goiter. Ann Surg 206:782-786, 1987.
62. Perzik S. The place of total thyroidectomy in the management of 909 patients with thyroid disease. Am J Surg 132:480-483, 1976.
63. Colin FJ, Russell MB. Management of benign nonendemic goiter. In Clark OH, Duh Q-Y eds. Textbook of Endocrine Surgery. 1st ed. Philadelphia: WB Saunders, 1997, pp 22-31.
64. Van SJ et al. Pathogenesis of autonomous thyroid nodules: in vitro study of iodine and adenosine 3′,5′-monophosphate metabolism. J Clin Endocrinol Metab 66:570-579, 1988.
65. Van Sande J et al. Somatic and germline mutations of the TSH receptor gene in thyroid diseases. J Clin Endocrinol Metab 80:2577-2585, 1995.
66. Takeshita A et al. Rarity of oncogenic mutations in the thyrotropin receptor of autonomously functioning thyroid nodules in Japan. J Clin Endocrinol Metab 80:2607-2611, 1995.
67. Russo D et al. Genetic alterations in thyroid hyperfunctioning adenomas. J Clin Endocrinol Metab 80:1347-1351, 1995.
68. Bransom CJ et al. Solitary toxic adenoma of the thyroid gland. Br J Surg 66:590-595, 1979.
69. Hamburger JI. Evolution of toxicity in solitary nontoxic autonomously functioning thyroid nodules. J Clin Endocrinol Metab 50:1089-1093, 1980.
70. Laurberg P et al. Hyperfunctioning thyroid nodules. Thyroidology 3:1-6, 1991.
71. Baltisberger BL, Minder CE, Bürgi H. Decrease of incidence of toxic nodular goitre in a region of Switzerland after full correction of mild iodine deficiency. Eur J Endocrinol 132:546-549, 1995.
72. Croom RD et al. Autonomously functioning thyroid nodules in childhood and adolescence. Surgery 102:1101-1107, 1987.

73. Melliere D, Etienne G, Becquemin JP. Operation for hyperthyroidism. Methods and rationale. Am J Surg 155:395-399, 1988.
74. Pacini F et al. Thyroid carcinoma in thyrotoxic patients treated by surgery. J Endocrinol Invest 11:107-112, 1988.
75. Castelli V et al. Occurrence of papillary carcinoma in a hyperfunctioning thyroid nodule: Report of a case and diagnostic considerations. Thyroidology 6:69-72, 1994.
76. Clerc J et al. Radioiodine therapy of the autonomous thyroid nodule in patients with or without visible extranodular activity. J Nucl Med 36:217-223, 1995.
77. Goldstein R, Hart IR. Follow-up of solitary autonomous thyroid nodules treated with 131I. N Engl J Med 309:1473-1476, 1983.
78. David E et al. Management of the hot thyroid nodule. Am J Surg 170:481-483, 1995.
79. De Rosa G et al. Thyroid carcinoma mimicking a toxic adenoma. Eur J Nucl Med 17:179-184, 1990.
80. Livraghi T et al. Treatment of autonomous thyroid nodules with percutaneous ethanol injection: 4-year experience. Radiology 190:529-533, 1994.
81. Di Lelio A et al. Treatment of autonomous thyroid nodules: Value of percutaneous ethanol injection. Am J Roentgenol 164:207-213, 1995.
82. Lippi F et al. Treatment of solitary autonomous thyroid nodules by percutaneous ethanol injection: Results of an Italian multicenter study. J Clin Endocrinol Metab 81:3261-3264, 1996.
83. Nakada K et al. Percutaneous ethanol injection therapy for autonomously functioning thyroid nodule. Ann Nucl Med 10:171-176, 1996.
84. Martino E et al. Percutaneous ethanol injection: What is its role in the management of nodular lesions of endocrine glands? Eur J Endocrinol 132:300-301, 1995.

CHAPTER

3

Fine-Needle Aspiration Cytology and Histopathology

SYLVIA L. ASA, M.D., Ph.D.
YVAN C. BÉDARD, M.D., Ph.D.

The thyroid gland derives from an endodermal thickening in the midline of the floor of the embryonic foregut. By the end of the first month of gestation, this diverticulum develops caudally and enlarges laterally to form a bilobed structure. It maintains contact with the foregut via the thyroglossal duct, which opens to the base of tongue. By 6 to 7 weeks of gestation, this duct disintegrates, but remnants of the caudal end form a pyramidal lobe of the gland in about 75% of adult thyroid glands. By about 12 weeks of gestation, follicles and colloid are identified, iodine is concentrated, and hormone synthesis is detectable; after 12 weeks, pituitary thyrotropin (thyroid-stimulating hormone [TSH]) and thyroxine (T_4) are measurable.

The mature gland is a butterfly-shaped organ with lateral lobes that measure about 5 cm superoinferiorly, 3 cm mediolaterally, and 2 cm anteroposteriorly. There is a thin isthmus joining the two lobes, and it often merges with a pyramidal lobe superiorly. In nongoitrous regions of the world, the average adult thyroid weighs 15 to 35 g.

The parenchyma is usually divided into lobules by fibrous septa that carry vascular channels and nerves. The functional unit is the follicle, a spherical structure measuring from 50 to 500 μm in diameter, lined by a single layer of follicular epithelial cells and storing colloid. Follicular epithelial cells vary from flat attenuated cells to cuboidal to tall columnar cells depending on the degree of stimulation by TSH. They harbor basal nuclei, form microvilli at the luminal surface, and form tight terminal junctions at the lumen. Their subcellular organelles include well-developed rough endoplasmic reticulum and Golgi complexes appropriate for glycoprotein synthesis. Endocytotic vesicles indicate uptake of thyroglobulin from the stored colloid. These cells are readily identified by thyroglobulin immunoreactivity. The follicles are surrounded by a basement membrane that also encases scattered C cells that do not make contact with the follicular lumen. The C cells, like other peptide hormone–secreting cells of the dispersed endocrine system, are polygonal cells characterized by immunoreactivity for neuron-specific enolase (NSE), synaptophysin, and chromogranin as well as their hormone product, calcitonin, and other peptides, including somatostatin. Ultrastructurally they contain numerous membrane-bound secretory granules that measure from 100 to 300 nm in diameter.

The ultimobranchial body derives from the fourth and fifth branchial pouches and during embryologic life comes to lie in the lateral aspects of the thyroid. The C cells are thought to derive from this structure. In addition, rests of the ultimobranchial body are found in up to 25% of adult thyroid glands[1] and up to 80% of fetal and neonatal glands.[2,3] These irregular collections of squamous or epidermoid cells, sometimes associated with mucinous cysts, are known as *solid cell nests*.[4,5] One must be careful not to overinterpret these as papillary thyroid carcinomas; their nuclei are elongated and may even show grooves, but they do not exhibit clearing of nucleoplasm and peripheral margination of chromatin.

THYROID NODULES

Thyroid nodules are extremely common in the general population; it has been estimated that about 20% of the population have a palpable thyroid nodule and approximately 70% have a nodule that can be detected by ultrasonography.[6] The prevalence of thyroid nodules is greater in women (72%) than in men (41%), and multiple nodules are more common than solitary nodules.

The differential diagnosis of the thyroid nodule includes numerous entities, nonneoplastic and neoplastic, benign and malignant.[7-10] Most of these nodules are benign, and the pathologist or cytologist plays an important role in selecting those which should undergo surgery as well as evaluating malignancies to determine appropriate management and prognosis.

Cytology

One of the most useful techniques to evaluate thyroid nodules is cytologic examination of a thyroid aspirate.[11-13] Before this technique is performed, the patient's thyroid hormone levels and autoantibodies should be determined, since the concurrent presence of clinical or subclinical hyperthyroidism or hypothyroidism may alter the interpretation of cytologic features of a thyroid lesion. Hyperthyroid patients should undergo radionucleotide scanning to determine whether the nodule or the non-nodular gland is responsible for the hormone hypersecretion. The presence of thyroid autoimmunity is a relevant factor in interpreting aspirate findings.

The thyroid aspirate is extremely useful as a first-line determinant of the pathology underlying a thyroid nodule.[14] It can clearly identify patients who will require surgery and those who are unlikely to require surgery. As detailed below, cytologic examination can impart a diagnosis of papillary carcinoma, medullary carcinoma, lymphoma, anaplastic carcinoma, or metastatic tumor.[15] An unequivocal cytologic diagnosis of papillary carcinoma allows definitive surgical management. Medullary carcinoma will of necessity entail evaluation to rule out pheochromocytoma and total thyroidectomy and total thyroidectomy with central neck cleanout. Anaplastic carcinoma will usually be treated with debulking surgery followed by radiation. A diagnosis of lymphoma will direct management away from definitive surgery; open biopsy may be required to obtain adequate tissue for lymphoma typing, but chemotherapy and/or radiotherapy is usually considered the treatment of choice. In contrast to these clearly malignant lesions, the majority of thyroid aspirates yield a benign diagnosis of either *thyroiditis* or *colloid nodule*, a benign hyperplastic process with abundant colloid storage. Patients with one of these cytologic diagnoses can be followed clinically with relative safety. Endocrinologists discuss the use of thyroid hormone suppression for some of these patients and in some instances, the size of a thyroid nodule can be reduced with hormonal manipulation.

An adequate aspirate, according to various authors, is a sample that contains two slides with 6 to 10 groups of follicular cells or two pools of isolated cells (e.g., lymphocytes).[15-17] A management dilemma arises when an *indeterminate cytologic aspirate* is obtained. In some instances, the aspirate yields insufficient tissue for analysis and requires a repeat study. In others, a diagnosis of "degenerating lesion" is obtained when the aspirate reveals hemorrhage and hemosiderin-laden macrophages, indicating that there has been involution (Fig. 3-1). In these instances, the true nature of the underlying lesion cannot be determined with accuracy.

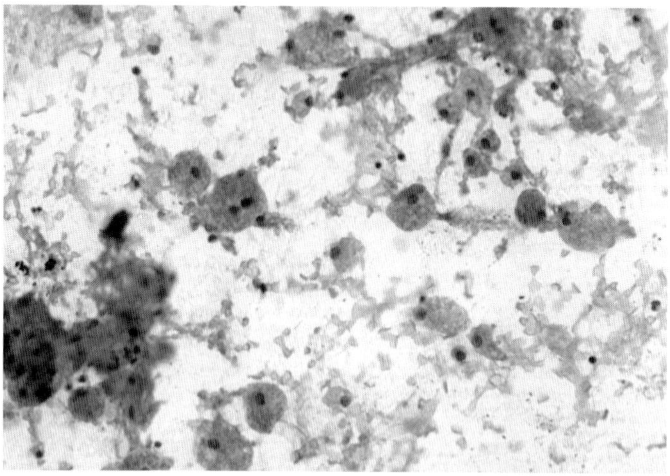

• **FIGURE 3-1** Fine-needle aspirate of a degenerating lesion yields abundant hemorrhage and hemosiderin-laden macrophages.

Another problematic area is the *follicular lesion.* Any tumor composed of well-differentiated follicular epithelial cells that do not exhibit the characteristic nuclear features of papillary carcinoma will fall into this category; these will include hyperplastic lesions as well as neoplasms that may be benign (follicular adenomas) or malignant (follicular carcinomas). These diagnoses cannot be distinguished on the basis of cytology alone; in all of these lesions, the follicular cells generally have evenly spaced round to oval nuclei with uniform speckled chromatin; nuclear or cellular atypia is not significant and does not reflect potential malignancy. Mitoses are also not significant. This underscores the limitation of cytology in these disorders, and the management of patients with these lesions requires clinicopathologic correlation. If the patient is not thought to have a high likelihood of malignancy (e.g., those with multinodular disease that is most consistent with sporadic nodular goiter), the patient can be watched before proceeding to surgery. If there is no progression of disease or if thyroid hormone replacement therapy results in regression of the nodule, surgery is usually not indicated. In contrast, a cellular follicular lesion that appears to be a solitary nodule or a lesion in a patient who has risk factors predisposing to thyroid tumor formation (e.g., previous head and neck irradiation or a rapidly enlarging nodule) should proceed to surgery at this point. Resection of the lesion by thyroid lobectomy and histologic examination will yield a more definitive diagnosis concerning the benign or malignant nature of a follicular lesion.

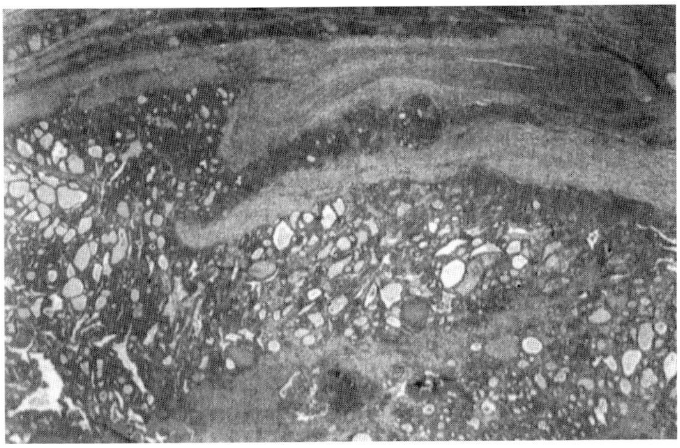

• **FIGURE 3-2** Previous fine-needle aspiration biopsy of this lesion resulted in the formation of a linear tract that simulated capsular invasion. In the center of the lesion at the bottom there is hemorrhage with granulation tissue and fibrosis. The evidence of previous needle aspiration immediately below the capsular defect and linear nature of the tract, rather than a mushrooming of tumor cells into the capsule, are features that distinguish artifact from true invasion.

Complications

Thyroid aspiration is now performed routinely by most clinicians, and the impact of this procedure on subsequent histologic morphology must be recognized. The effects of biopsy include acute and chronic changes. The acute changes in the first 3 weeks do not present a significant diagnostic problem; they include hemorrhage, granulation tissue, foreign body giant cells, hemosiderin-laden macrophages, and occasional granulomas.

The subsequent chronic changes can be more problematic. Fibrosis and trapping of lesional cells into or through a capsule can mimic capsular invasion, and displacement of tumor cells into capsular vessels can mimic vascular invasion. Total infarction can result in loss of diagnostic material. Calcifications can be mistaken for psammoma bodies. Various metaplastic changes occur. These changes have been described with the acronym WHAFFT, which stands for *worrisome histological alterations following fine-needle aspiration of the thyroid*.[18]

The distinction between WHAFFT and true invasion relies on awareness and a high index of suspicion. Usually, areas simulating invasion are associated with a linear tract that leads to a central area of fibrosis and hemosiderin deposition (Fig. 3-2), rather than a mushrooming into or through the capsule. The vascular change involves just a few cells in a vessel without associated fibrin or adherence to the vessel endothelium.[19]

Intraoperative Consultation

If a definitive diagnosis of malignancy has been established by cytologic examination, there is no compelling reason to perform an intraoperative consultation. On the other hand, patients who do not have a definitive cytologic diagnosis may benefit from intraoperative consultation with or without frozen section.

Frozen section may be useful to identify a *papillary lesion;* however, papillary hyperplasia cannot be distinguished from papillary carcinoma at frozen section. A nodule with follicular architecture may represent a follicular variant papillary carcinoma. The differential diagnosis of papillary carcinoma requires evaluation of cytologic, particularly nuclear, features that are altered by a freezing artifact. This problem can be circumvented by preparing cytologic smears of the lesion along with the usual frozen section.

Follicular lesions identified at frozen section may represent hyperplastic nodules, adenoma or carcinoma. Distinguishing these entities may be extremely difficult to achieve at frozen section. The diagnosis of malignancy, which is the only significant diagnosis that would alter intraoperative management, requires identification of capsular and/or vascular invasion; the likelihood of identifying microinvasion is exceedingly small, rather like the proverbial search for "a needle in a haystack." It requires multiple sections to analyze the entire capsule of the lesion, a procedure that is not time efficient or cost-effective intraoperative consultation.[8,20-22] A final diagnosis is usually reached on examination of numerous permanent sections.

Medullary carcinoma, lymphoma, or *anaplastic carcinoma* can generally be diagnosed at frozen section, but preoperative cytologic evaluation is equally effective. Frozen section remains useful for assessing lymph node status and tumor extension that may influence surgical management of known malignancies, and for identifying parathyroid glands intraoperatively.

An important aspect of intraoperative consultation for thyroid lesions is *tissue handling.* The pathologist can grossly examine the tissue and process samples that may require special handling, such as flow cytometry, electron microscopy, or molecular analysis.

CONGENITAL TUMORLIKE LESIONS

Thyroglossal Duct Cysts

Aberrant thyroid tissue has been described along the full course of the thyroglossal duct; excessive descent can lead to ectopic thyroid tissue in the mediastinum and pericardium. The most common sites are lingual and sublingual. These rests can be the site of cysts or fistulas that are lined by

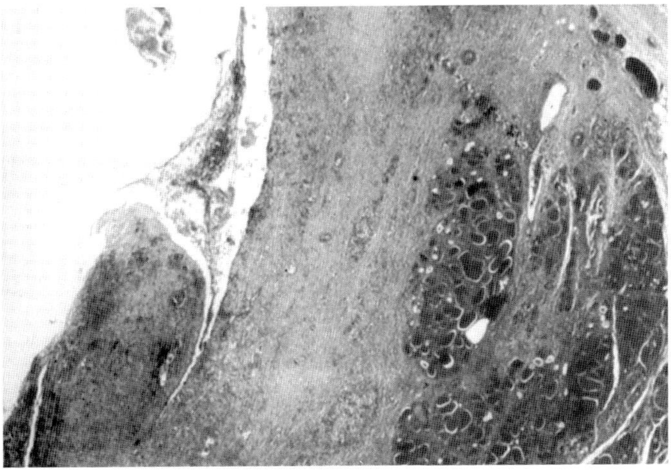

• **FIGURE 3-3** The wall of a thyroglossal duct cyst contains thyroid parenchyma with abundant colloid *(right)*. The cyst itself at left contains hemorrhagic debris, and the lining is primarily fibrous tissue with scant and degenerate epithelium lining the cyst lumen.

respiratory or squamous epithelium and harbor thyroid follicles in their wall. The epithelial lining may be obliterated by inflammatory changes.

The location and clinical presentation of these lesions are sufficiently characteristic to allow a presumptive diagnosis in most instances. Aspiration of these cysts yields proteinaceous material and foamy macrophages consistent with benign cyst contents. A definitive diagnosis of this entity cannot usually be made based on cytologic findings, since the aspirate includes the contents of the cyst and not the follicular epithelium, which is in the cyst wall (Fig. 3-3). Surgical removal allows identification of the thyroglossal remnants that may be found only after serial sectioning.

Hyperplasia and Cysts of the Ultimobranchial Body

Hyperplasia of ultimobranchial body rests occurs in chronic lymphocytic thyroiditis.[23] The reason for this association is not clear, but it is known that the more significant and severe the thyroiditis, the more common is ultimobranchial hyperplasia. The rests not only increase in number but also can undergo cystification; these branchial cleft–like cysts can present as clinically palpable thyroid nodules.[24,25] Grossly they contain thick yellow material, and their lining has a granular appearance. The features of aspiration cytology have not been described but are unlikely to be diagnostic, since the contents are largely proteinaceous material. Histologically, the cysts are lined by attenuated squamous epithelium, which ranges from one or two cells to

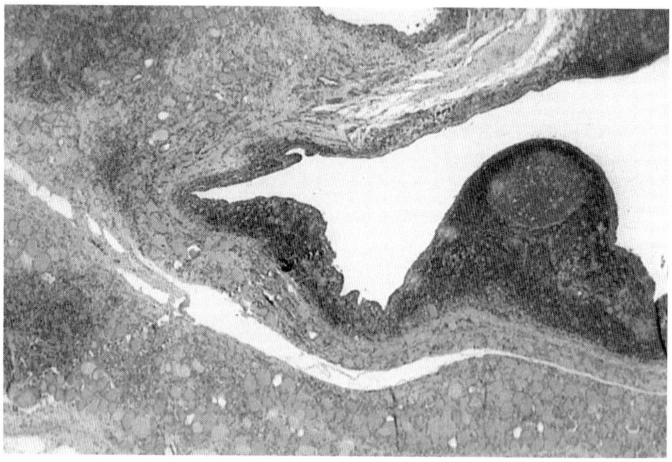

• **FIGURE 3-4** Ultimobranchial body–like cysts associated with Hashimoto's thyroiditis can give rise to clinically palpable cystic nodules. The cyst is lined by attenuated squamous epithelium that overlies dense lymphoid tissue that forms lymphoid aggregates with large germinal centers.

approximately seven cells in thickness; there is focal denudation of epithelium. There is no glandular differentiation of the cyst lining but the epithelium is immunoreactive for cytokeratins and carcinoembryonic antigen (CEA). Chromogranin, calcitonin, and thyroglobulin are not detectable within these cells. Deep to the epithelial lining there is dense lymphoid tissue, including lymphoid aggregates with large reactive germinal centers, surrounded by fibrous tissue (Fig. 3-4).

INFLAMMATORY TUMORLIKE LESIONS

Hashimoto's Thyroiditis

In 1912, Hashimoto described four patients with a well-defined clinicopathologic syndrome consisting of goiter, hypothyroidism, and lymphocytic thyroiditis. It is now generally accepted that the form of lymphocytic thyroiditis known as Hashimoto's thyroiditis is of autoimmune etiology.[26,27] Patients have antibodies to thyroglobulin and to thyroid microsomal antigen.[28] Some patients also have antibodies to a colloid component other than thyroglobulin ("second colloid antigen") and occasionally to thyroid hormones.

Patients with this disorder are most often women (the female/male ratio is 10:1) between 30 and 50 years of age. They typically develop a diffuse, lobulated, asymmetric, nontender goiter. Most patients with long-standing disease are hypothyroid. Occasionally there is a transient episode of hyperthyroidism

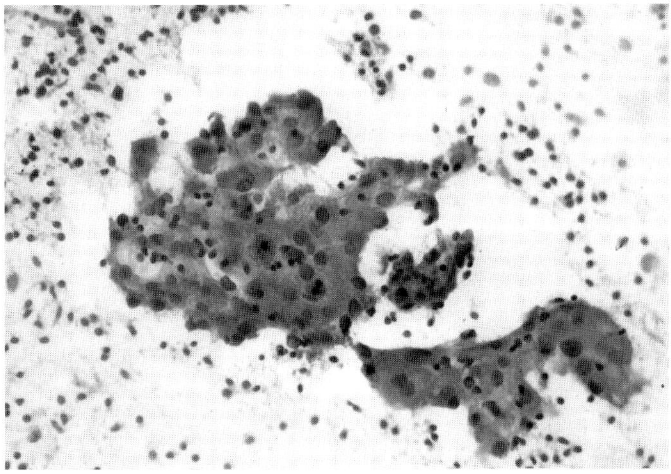

• **FIGURE 3-5** Fine-needle aspiration of nodules in Hashimoto's thyroiditis yields an admixture of epithelial cells and inflammatory cells. The epithelial cells exhibit variable degrees of Hürthle cell change with accumulation of abundant granular cytoplasm.

known as "Hashitoxicosis" early in the course of the disease; this has been attributed to release of stored hormone during tissue destruction or to stimulation by antibodies to the TSH receptor.[28]

Antibodies directed against TSH receptors have been found to be of three types.[29] Thyroid-stimulating immunoglobulin (TSI) stimulates hormone secretion by thyroid epithelial cells. Thyroid growth–stimulating immunoglobulin (TGI) selectively stimulates cell replication in the thyroid. Thyrotropin binding–inhibiting immunoglobulin (TBII) interacts with the TSH receptor and inhibits TSH binding without stimulating function or growth.

The presence of TGI in these patients and/or compensatory TSH excess resulting from tissue destruction and hypothyroidism have been implicated in the development of hyperplastic nodules that present as discrete masses in patients with this disorder. Aspiration of these lesions yields an admixture of epithelial cells and inflammatory cells (Fig. 3-5).[15] The hallmark is the Hürthle cell, a follicular epithelial cell that is characterized by abundant granular cytoplasm and a nucleus that often has a prominent "cherry pink" nucleolus. The background is composed of small and large lymphocytes, plasma cells, germinal center fragments, and macrophages with or without tingible bodies. Follicular cells and colloid are usually scant but may show nuclear atypia with irregular nuclear contours and prominent grooves.

The appearance of the thyroid involved by Hashimoto's thyroiditis is variable. The gland is usually enlarged and can weigh more than 200 g. It is composed of firm, lobulated, rubbery tissue with a homogeneous, pale gray, fleshy, cut surface that lacks colloid translucence and resembles lymphoid tissue. Microscopically, the gland is diffusely infiltrated by mononuclear inflammatory cells, including lymphocytes, plasma cells, immunoblasts, and macrophages. Lymphoid follicles contain well-formed germinal centers. The glandular epithelium exhibits variable degrees of damage. Residual follicles are either atrophic, with sparse colloid and flattened epithelium or exhibit oxyphilic metaplasia, the accumulation of abundant eosinophilic granular cytoplasm characteristic of Hürthle cells.[30] Follicular epithelial cells may also exhibit marked cytologic atypia that can be characterized by irregular nuclear membranes, grooves, and even clearing of nucleoplasm. These features, which in the face of inflammation are considered reactive, mimic papillary carcinoma.[8,10] Areas of squamous metaplasia may be found.[31] As the disease evolves, fibrosis becomes more conspicuous and in some patients there is progression to the "fibrous variant," with less prominent lymphocytic infiltration, more prominent squamous metaplasia, and intense fibrosis that almost totally replaces thyroid tissue.[32]

The nodules that usually precipitate surgical intervention are cellular areas composed of hyperplastic, colloid-depleted follicles. It is not uncommon for them to be composed predominantly of Hürthle cells, and they may be difficult to distinguish from adenomas (Fig. 3-6). The cytologic atypia that resembles that of papillary carcinoma and the fibrosis that can trap follicular epithelium create difficult diagnostic problems and in

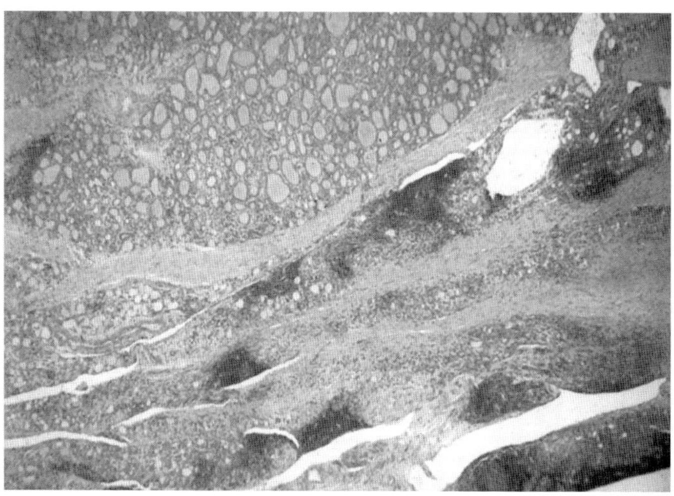

• **FIGURE 3-6** In Hashimoto's thyroiditis, the stroma exhibits chronic lymphocytic infiltration and fibrosis. Nodules are frequent *(top)* and are usually composed of small follicles with scant colloid. The epithelial cells often show Hürthle cell metaplasia.

extreme cases, papillary proliferation may be associated with "Hashitoxicosis." Distinguishing thyroid cancer from a reactive process can be extremely difficult.

Sudden and rapid enlargement of a nodule in a patient with Hashimoto's thyroiditis may indicate the development of primary thyroid lymphoma that occurs usually in this setting; this entity is discussed below.

Other Lesions

Juvenile thyroiditis is a milder form of autoimmune lymphocytic thyroiditis that has its onset during childhood or adolescence. Patients are generally euthyroid or may have transient hyperthyroidism. The morphologic abnormalities are similar to those of Hashimoto's thyroiditis but are less intense: the thyroid is smaller, it is infiltrated with fewer lymphocytes, and the epithelium is better preserved, without oncocytic change. Hyperplastic foci with papillary architecture are frequently present, but the tall, columnar epithelium does not exhibit the nuclear features of papillary carcinoma.[28] Cytologic examination reveals features of chronic lymphocytic thyroiditis with follicular epithelial cells and a sprinkling of lymphocytes in the background. Contrary to Hashimoto's thyroiditis, Hürthle cells are not seen.

Postpartum thyroiditis is a transient disorder that usually occurs in the first 6 months after delivery. It can be painful or painless and is associated with either hypothyroidism or hyperthyroidism; most cases resolve spontaneously. Cytologically and histologically, the chronic lymphocytic thyroiditis resembles Hashimoto's thyroiditis, except that Hürthle cells are infrequently seen and fibrosis is absent or minimal.[28]

de Quervain's (subacute) thyroiditis has been attributed to autoimmune phenomena; this self-limited disease is usually characterized by a painful goiter, frequently associated with hyperthyroidism, but it may also occur without pain; it has a tendency to follow upper respiratory tract viral infections.[33] A few cases seem to be due to the virus that causes mumps. The development of cell-mediated immunity to thyroid cell antigens appears to be related to release of thyroid cell fractions during tissue destruction. Morphologically there is granulomatous inflammation with lysozyme-positive macrophages and giant cells (Fig. 3-7). The inflammatory cells otherwise resemble those of Hashimoto's thyroiditis with one exception; the absence of lymphoid follicles suggests that the numerous plasma cells must originate from extrathyroid lymphocytes. Viral inclusions have not been identified.[34] On fine-needle aspiration (FNA), de Quervain's thyroiditis is characterized by inflammatory cells including lymphocytes, plasma cells and neutrophils with multinucleated giant cells, and epithelioid cells (Fig. 3-8).[15] Well-formed granulomas may be seen. There is little colloid or follicular epithelium.

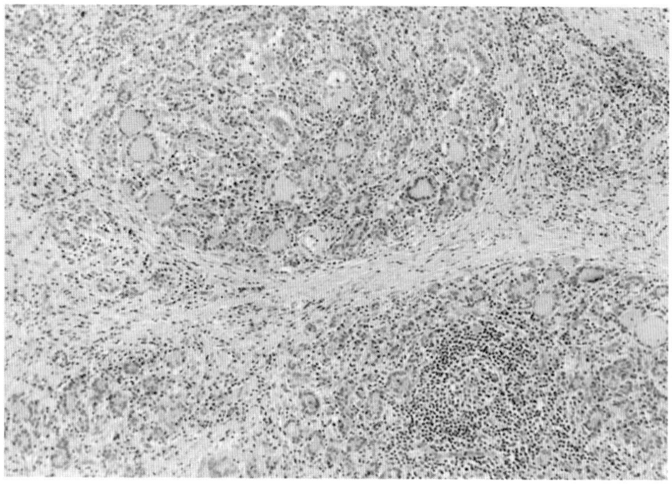

• **FIGURE 3-7** Subacute thyroiditis is characterized by granulomatous inflammation with follicular rupture and formation of multinucleate giant cells. There is stromal fibrosis.

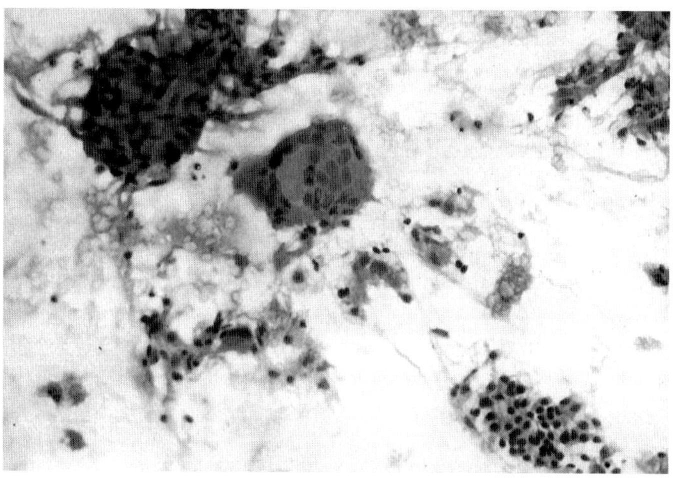

• **FIGURE 3-8** Fine-needle aspiration of subacute thyroiditis yields lymphocytes and plasma cells as well as characteristic multinucleated giant cells.

Riedel's thyroiditis, a rare, chronic sclerosing lesion also known as *ligneous thyroiditis,* is characterized by dense proliferative fibrosis that can cause pressure symptoms, including dyspnea, dysphagia, hoarseness, aphonia, and even stridor. With progressive tissue destruction, the disease gives rise to hypothyroidism and, when the parathyroid gland is involved, may also result in hypoparathyroidism.[28] The lesion may be difficult to distinguish from diffuse involvement of the thyroid by carcinoma; however, unlike the rapidly growing anaplastic carcinomas, which produce a similar clinical presentation, Riedel's thyroiditis is a slowly progressive lesion. This disorder of unknown etiology may be associated with similar fibrosclerotic processes involving lacrimal glands and orbits, parotid glands, mediastinum, lung, myocardium, retroperitoneal tissues, and bile ducts. Riedel's thyroiditis cannot be diagnosed on the basis of cytologic findings, since the gland is dense and fibrous and the fine-needle aspirate is usually acellular. Histologically, the disorder is characterized by dense fibrosis replacing thyroid parenchyma and infiltrating adjacent tissues. An inflammatory component may be present in the form of a lymphoplasmacytic infiltrate; however, it is not prominent and does not form lymphoid follicles. Vasculitis may be present. Although this may mimic the fibrous variant of Hashimoto's thyroiditis, several unique histologic features are not seen in Hashimoto's thyroiditis, including (a) extrathyroidal extension of the fibrotic process, (b) areas of uninvolved thyroid parenchyma, and (c) vasculitis.

THYROID FOLLICULAR HYPERPLASIA AND NEOPLASIA

Follicular nodules are the most commonly encountered problems in the surgical pathology of the thyroid. These lesions can be classified along the full spectrum of thyroid pathology from hyperplastic nodules to benign follicular adenomas and malignant follicular carcinomas.

Nodular Goiter

The morphology of sporadic nodular goiter is characterized by heterogeneity and variability, features that have suggested a hyperplastic rather than neoplastic pathogenesis.[35-38] The gland may achieve a weight ranging from several hundred to a thousand grams. The nodules are irregular; some are poorly circumscribed, whereas others are surrounded by scarring and condensation of thyroid stroma, creating the appearance of complete encapsulation. Focal calcification and cystic change may be evident.

On FNA, recognition of colloid is essential to the diagnosis of a colloid nodule (Fig. 3-9). Colloid has quite a varied appearance; it is a film of acellular material that may stain pink, greenish blue, or orange. The presence of blood makes the recognition of colloid even more difficult, but colloid is refractile, has a tendency to crack, and looks like crumpled plastic wrap. Follicular cells are usually in sheets with a honeycomb pattern; micro- or

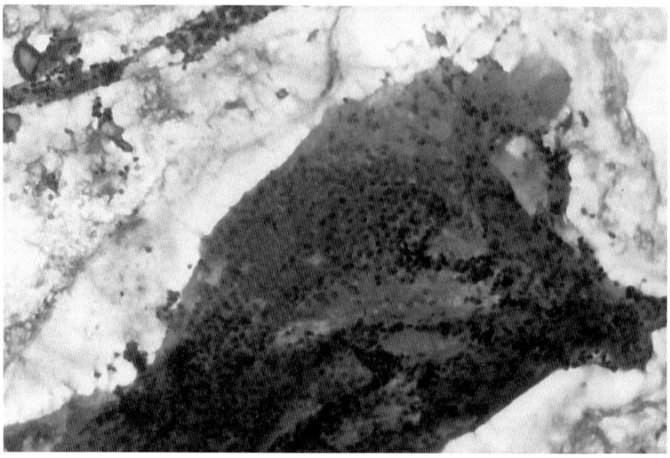

• **FIGURE 3-9** Fine-needle aspiration biopsy of a colloid nodule yields abundant background colloid and follicular cells in sheets; the follicular epithelium shows no significant atypia.

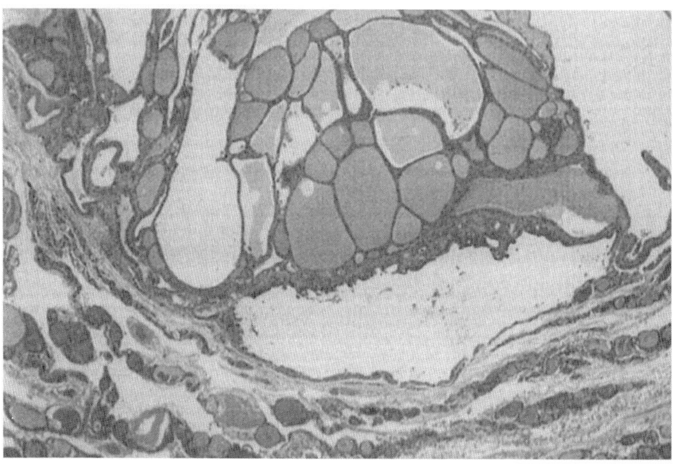

• **FIGURE 3-10** A classical colloid nodule in the setting of nodular hyperplasia is composed of large colloid-filled follicles lined by follicular epithelial cells that are markedly heterogeneous.

macrofollicles containing colloid may be seen. The nuclei of the follicular cells are often pyknotic. Associated degenerative changes are characterized by macrophages with erythrophagocytosis or hemosiderin accumulation.

Histologically, the nodules are composed of follicles of variable size and shape. Some follicles are large, with abundant colloid surrounded by flattened, cuboidal, or columnar epithelial cells (Fig. 3-10). Cellular areas are composed of small follicles lined by crowded epithelium with scant colloid

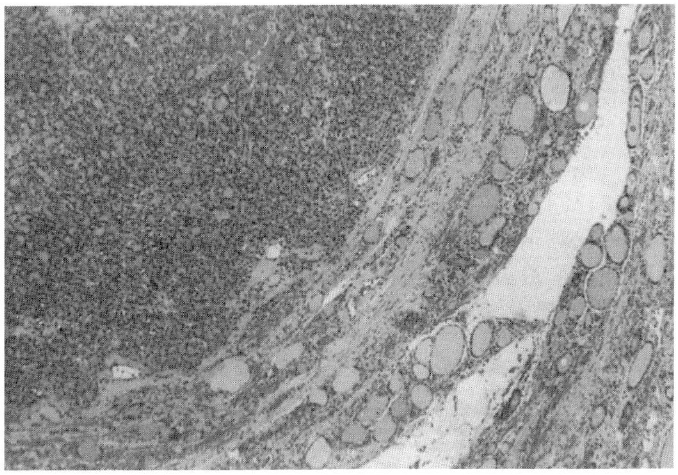

• **FIGURE 3-11** Some nodules in multinodular goiters are more cellular, with very scant colloid storage. In this case, the distinction between a cellular hyperplastic nodule and a benign follicular adenoma is strictly academic.

in a small lumen (Fig. 3-11). There may be focal necrosis, hemorrhage with hemosiderin deposition and cholesterol clefts, fibrosis, and granulation tissue. These degenerative changes are usually found in the center of large nodules, creating stellate scars.

The morphologic classification of cellular follicular nodules in nodular glands can be extremely difficult. Hyperplasia may be extremely difficult to distinguish from neoplasia. Classical guidelines that allow distinction of a hyperplastic nodule from a follicular adenoma include the following:

- Multiple lesions suggest hyperplasia, whereas a solitary lesion is likely to be neoplastic.
- A poorly encapsulated nodule is likely hyperplastic; a well-developed capsule suggests a neoplastic growth.
- Variable architecture reflects a polyclonal proliferation, whereas uniform architecture suggests a monoclonal neoplastic growth.
- Cytologic heterogeneity suggests hyperplasia; monotonous cytology is characteristic of neoplasia.
- The presence of multiple lesions in hyperplasia means that areas similar to the lesion in question will be present in the adjacent gland; in contrast, neoplasms have a distinct morphology compared with the surrounding parenchyma.
- Classically hyperplastic nodules are said not to compress the surrounding gland, whereas neoplasms result in compression of the adjacent parenchyma.

For the most part, large nodules in multinodular glands tend to be incompletely encapsulated and poorly demarcated from the internodular tissue. However, in some glands, large encapsulated lesions with relatively monotonous architecture and cytology make distinguishing hyperplasia from adenoma difficult. Many pathologists have applied nonspecific terms such as "adenomatoid nodules" to describe such lesions.

The pathophysiology of nodule formation remains poorly understood. The etiologic factors related to this disorder have long remained elusive, since the goiters do not appear to be TSH dependent.[37] The work of Stüder suggests that the initial proliferation is a polyclonal one involving cells that are intrinsically more rapidly growing than their neighbors.[35,38,39] Although the stimulus for growth is not certain, high levels of circulating thyroid growth immunoglobulins (TGI) and defects in T suppressor cell function have been documented in patients with sporadic nodular goiter[40,41] implicating autoimmunity in the pathogenesis of this disease. Drexhage et al.[40] compared immunoglobulin preparations from patients who had goitrous Graves' disease with those of patients who had sporadic nodular goiter; they found that the former are approximately 10-fold more potent in inducing growth than the latter. It has been postulated that the weaker stimuli result in proliferation of only the most sensitive of the heterogeneous follicular epithelial cell population, hence the nodularity, and that "toxic" nodular goiter results from preferential replication of cells that are highly responsive to TSH stimulation.[42,43]

Recent studies have indicated that the dominant nodules of multinodular goiters are monoclonal proliferations and therefore represent benign neoplasms.[36,44] It may be that these represent true adenomas arising in the background of a hyperplastic process that is mediated by growth-stimulating immunoglobulins. Moreover, most hyperfunctioning nodules are also now thought to represent clonal benign neoplasms with activating mutations of the TSH receptor or Gsα(see below).[45,46] The evidence of clonal proliferation in sporadic nodular goiter and the identification of ras mutations as early events in morphologically classified hyperplastic nodules in this disorder[47] indicate that the thyroid is a site for the hyperplasia-neoplasia sequence. Nevertheless, clinical experience has shown that the vast majority of these lesions remain entirely benign.

Follicular Adenoma

Solitary follicular nodules have been unequivocally shown to be monoclonal[48,49] and in the absence of invasive behavior, these lesions are considered to be benign. Follicular adenomas are described as encapsulated follicular lesions that exhibit a uniform architectural and cytologic pattern. On

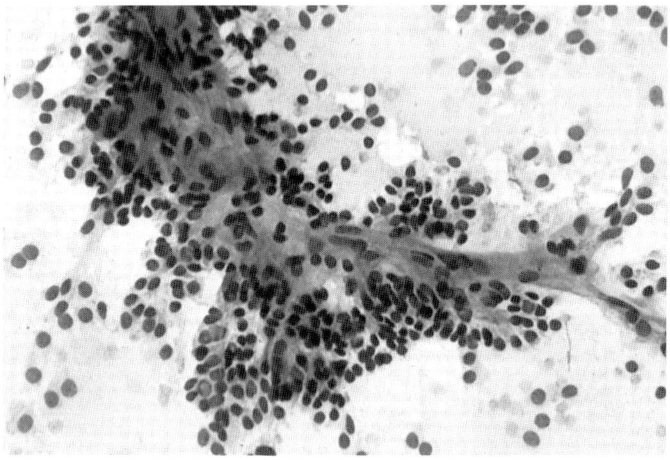

• **FIGURE 3-12** Fine-needle aspiration of a follicular lesion is usually cellular with follicular cells in sheets. The nuclei exhibit none of the morphologic features of papillary carcinoma. The distinction between follicular adenoma and follicular carcinoma cannot be made in this material.

FNA, the diagnosis of "follicular lesions" covers both follicular adenoma and follicular carcinoma; these are difficult if not impossible to distinguish, because the diagnostic criteria do not rest on cytologic characteristics. The aspirate of a follicular lesion is usually cellular, with follicular cells in sheets or microfollicular arrangements (Fig. 3-12). The colloid is scant. The follicular cells are monotonous with elongated, bland nuclei and micronucleoli. Worrisome features include nuclear crowding, altered polarity, pleomorphism, macronucleoli, and coarse chromatin. The main practical role of cytologic examination is to distinguish a colloid nodule from a follicular neoplasm based on the ratio of colloid to follicular epithelium.

Follicular adenomas can be classified histologically according to the size or presence of follicles and degree of cellularity, each adenoma tending to have a consistent microscopic pattern (Fig. 3-13). The subclassification of follicular adenomas into simple, microfollicular, trabecular, oxyphil, atypical, papillary, and signet ring cell types has no prognostic significance.

Atypical adenomas are highly cellular tumors with unusual gross and/or histologic appearances that suggest the possibility of malignancy, but these tumors lack evidence of invasion. They may have necrosis, infarction, numerous mitoses, or unusual cellularity (Fig. 3-14). Many so-called atypical adenomas are indeed papillary carcinomas. The distinction of an encapsulated follicular variant papillary carcinoma from follicular adenoma relies entirely on the indentification of appropriate cytologic characteristics. The presence of the cytologic features of papillary carcinoma described below

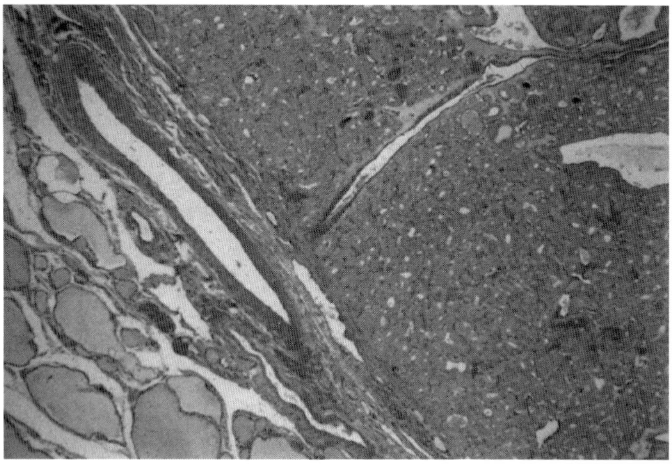

• **FIGURE 3-13** The histology of a follicular adenoma is characterized by homogeneous architecture within the lesion, lack of cytologic atypia indicating papillary differentiation, and an intact capsule without vascular invasion.

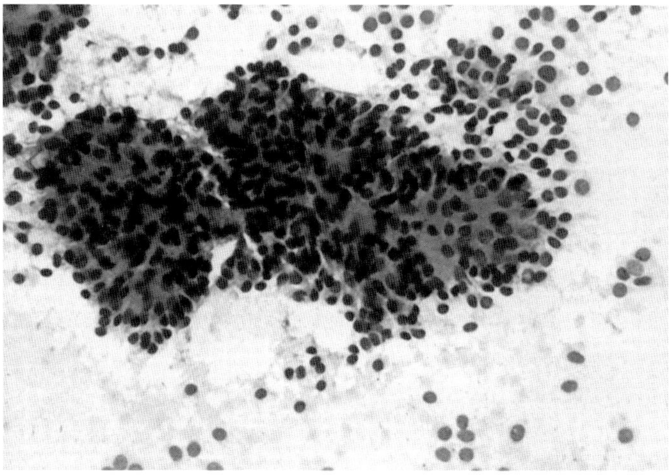

• **FIGURE 3-14** Cellular follicular lesions can exhibit variable degrees of nuclear atypia. This lesion, despite the marked cellularity and nuclear pleomorphism, was finally diagnosed as an atypical follicular adenoma.

should indicate that diagnosis, despite lack of invasion. Nevertheless, encapsulated papillary carcinomas have a very good prognosis;[50] therefore aggressive management of patients with these lesions remains controversial.

The *hyalinizing trabecular adenoma* or *paraganglioma-like adenoma of thyroid* (PLAT) is usually architecturally a follicular adenoma with trabecular architecture and elongated tumor cells, which can have abundant pale eosinophilic cytoplasm (Fig. 3-15).[51-54] There is perivascular hyaline fibrosis

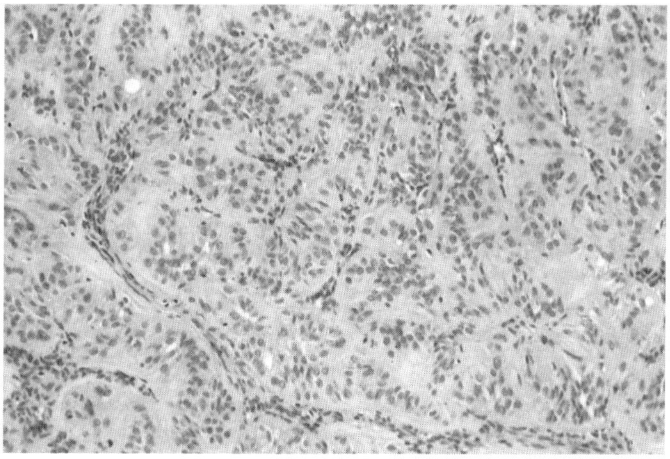

• **FIGURE 3-15** Occasional thyroid follicular adenomas are composed of elongated tumor cells with abundant pale eosinophilic cytoplasm. These lesions are known as *hyalinizing trabecular adenomas* or *paraganglioma-like adenoma of thyroid* (PLAT).

and the cytoplasmic hyaline is usually identified as cytoplasmic filaments of cytokeratin. Occasional cases are immunoreactive for S100 protein. These rare tumors were generally considered to be benign but occasional cases that exhibit capsular or vascular invasion behave in a malignant fashion and the criteria used to distinguish any type of follicular carcinoma from follicular adenoma apply to this group of tumors.[55]

Whether some solitary follicular nodules classified histologically as adenomas have the biologic potential to become carcinoma is not clear; aneuploid cell populations have been described in a significant percentage of these lesions, suggesting that some of these may represent carcinoma in situ.

Follicular Carcinoma

Follicular adenoma and follicular carcinoma of the thyroid often are identical in their clinical presentation, radiographic appearance, cytologic findings, and microscopic features. In most cases, the parenchymal component of both tumor types is essentially the same histomorphologically. The distinction between these two conditions has been considered possible only by recognition of invasion or metastasis. As indicated above, some encapsulated follicular adenomas exhibit evidence of aneuploidy and may in fact represent in situ follicular carcinomas.

Nuclear and cellular atypia and mitotic figures may be present in adenomas as well as in carcinomas and therefore cytologic characteristics are not

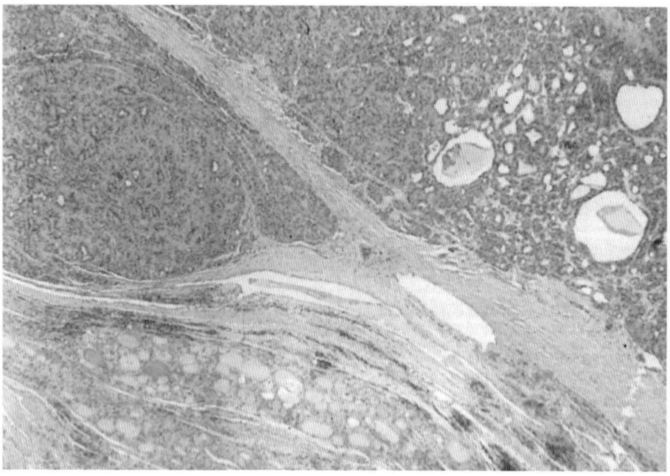

• **FIGURE 3-16** A widely invasive follicular carcinoma exhibits extensive invasion beyond the tumor capsule into the surrounding parenchyma. Usually satellite nodules such as the one illustrated at left are not difficult to recognize as grossly invasive.

helpful. Most follicular tumors are composed of cells with nuclei that are round to oval with uniformly speckled chromatin; the nuclei are evenly spaced and lack the crowded, overlapping appearance found in papillary carcinoma. As stated previously, these lesions cannot be diagnosed by FNA.

Follicular carcinoma can only be diagnosed by the pathologist on high-quality sections of well-fixed tissues that demonstrate capsular and/or vascular invasion. At the time of intraoperative consultation, frozen section will reveal only a very small number of these lesions, since the likelihood of identifying microinvasive foci on a single frozen section is low. The use of multiple frozen sections is not cost-effective in the evaluation of these lesions.[20]

Follicular carcinomas are divided into groups that reflect the biology of tumor growth and metastasis. *Widely invasive follicular carcinomas,* which are usually identifiable as invasive grossly and certainly are not difficult to recognize as invasive microscopically (Fig. 3-16), carry a poor prognosis with a 25% to 45% 10-year survival.[56,57] In contrast, the more common scenario is that of minimal capsular invasion. Patients with these tumors have an excellent prognosis with 70% to 100% survival. A diagnosis of follicular neoplasm requires very careful and thorough examination of the entire capsule of the follicular neoplasm by the pathologist.[58] *Minimally invasive follicular carcinoma* is identified by invasion through but not widely beyond the capsule (Fig. 3-17). Borderline lesions include those with invasion into the capsule beyond the bulk of the lesion but not through the full thickness of the capsule or situations in which islands of tumor are trapped within a capsule,

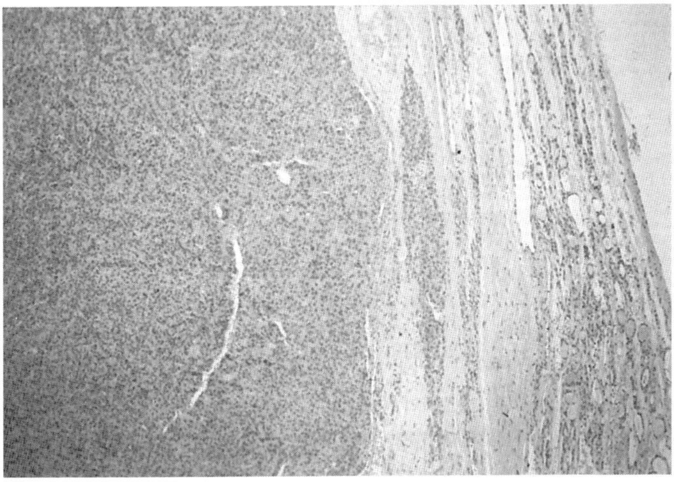

• **FIGURE 3-17** In contrast to widely invasive follicular carcinoma, a minimally invasive lesion exhibits only microscopic invasion into and through the capsule.

associated with perpendicular rupture of collagen. The finding of nests, cords, or individual tumor cells within a tumor capsule leads some pathologists to the diagnosis of minimally invasive follicular carcinoma, however, this may represent an artifact in a patient who has undergone FNA biopsy, with trapping by fibrosis or displacement of tumor cells into the capsule. Therefore pathologists should carefully search for evidence of FNA biopsy in the adjacent tissue. This would include finding focal hemorrhage, deposition of hemosiderin-laden macrophages, or the presence of granulation tissue and/or fibrosis, all of which would indicate a needle biopsy site and the possibility of artifactual invasion rather than genuine invasion.

Patients with minimally invasive follicular carcinomas are on average about 10 years younger than those with widely invasive carcinomas, and since traces of capsule are found in about 24% of widely invasive lesions, it is possible that encapsulated follicular carcinoma is a precursor of the widely invasive lesion.[59] Minimally invasive carcinomas have 10-year survival rates of up to 100%,[60] and therefore some argue that this disease does not warrant the painstaking search for microscopic invasion that distinguishes it from follicular adenoma. Nevertheless, the investigators who have reported these promising data have treated their patients for carcinoma rather than for benign disease. Rather than endorsing a cavalier approach that would entail less work for the pathologist, we must recognize the presence of potential malignancy, not only to treat the patient appropriately,[61] but also to identify the excellent prognosis that these lesions carry after appropriate management.

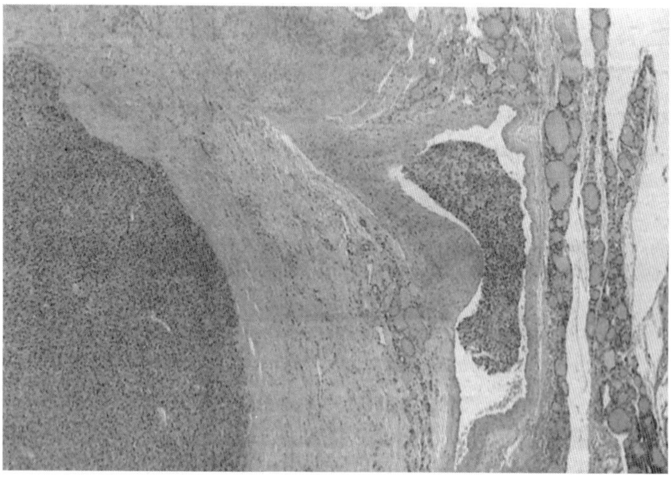

• **FIGURE 3-18** Vascular invasive follicular carcinoma is an aggressive disease. Vascular invasion is identified by careful examination of the circumference of the lesion where microscopic tumor within vascular channels, such as illustrated here, can be identified.

Vasculoinvasive follicular carcinomas are aggressive and require aggressive management. Although vascular invasion is more reliable for the diagnosis of malignancy, again the criteria are vague. Vascular invasion cannot be evaluated within the tumor; therefore, again, the circumference of the lesion is the site that warrants careful examination. Nests of tumor cells within an endothelial lumen generally are accepted as representing invasion (Fig. 3-18). However, it is recognized that artifactual implantation of tumor cells into blood vessels can occur during the surgical procedure or sectioning. Therefore endothelium covering invasive tumor cells or thrombus adherent to intravascular tumor is required by some to distinguish true invasion from artifact.

The use of elastin stains is of little value in assessing vascular invasion, since the involved vessels are usually thin-walled veins with little if any elastic tissue. Some have advocated the use of factor 8–related antigen, type IV collagen, lectin CD31 or CD34 immunohistochemistry to improve the recognition of vascular invasion in follicular carcinoma.[7-10]

It is obvious that the diagnosis of malignancy in well-differentiated encapsulated follicular tumors rests on subjective criteria. The search for objective markers of malignancy has yielded only one candidate thus far; the antibody to mesothelial cell clone called HBME-1, a marker of mesothelial cells, is immunohistochemically detected in 40% of thyroid malignancies of papillary or follicular differentiation.[62,63]

DNA aneuploidy is a well-recognized feature of human malignant tumors and it was initially hoped that ploidy analyses could help to distinguish adenomas from carcinomas of the thyroid. However, it has now been recognized that about 27% of follicular adenomas are aneuploid and about 40% of follicular carcinomas are diploid.[64] Therefore such measurements are of limited diagnostic value for the individual patient. In contrast, however, ploidy may be a useful adjunct in determining prognosis. Among histologically confirmed carcinomas, patients with thyroid tumors that have diploid DNA content tend to have a better prognosis than those with aneuploid values.[65-67]

The significance of this diagnosis must be interpreted in light of clinical data that assess the behavior of this disorder. The dominant determinant of cause-specific mortality in patients with follicular carcinoma is the presence of distant metastases.[68-70] Most studies have indicated that morbidity and mortality for patients with nonmetastatic encapsulated follicular carcinoma is very low and correlates better with patient age than with any other parameter. Some have suggested that capsular invasion alone does not alter the incidence of distant metastases or cancer-related death.

Since the incidence of follicular carcinoma is low,[71] most investigators still advocate total thyroidectomy and radioactive iodine therapy.[61,72,73] The rationale for total thyroidectomy is not bilateral carcinoma; multifocal disease in follicular carcinoma is exceedingly rare and the identification of occult papillary carcinoma in the contralateral lobe is not an indication for further surgery.[74] The only logical rationale for completion thyroidectomy is to allow selective uptake of radioactive iodine by metastatic tumor deposits rather than by residual thyroid gland. Uptake of radioactive iodine by distant metastases is a favorable prognostic factor and is improved by pretherapeutic total thyroidectomy, resulting in improved survival.[75-77] In contrast, external-beam radiotherapy is not thought to be of use in patients with differentiated thyroid carcinoma, apart from those with locally advanced tumors such as widely invasive follicular carcinomas that involve extrathyroidal soft tissues of the neck and cannot be completely resected.[77]

In the past few decades there has been a decrease in the incidence of follicular thyroid carcinoma, probably because of dietary iodine supplementation.[71] However, misdiagnosis of this tumor continues. Benign lesions, such as partly encapsulated hyperplastic nodules or nodules exhibiting pseudoinvasion after FNA,[18] are often overdiagnosed as malignant; papillary carcinomas with follicular architecture are often misinterpreted as follicular carcinoma. The clinical features, pathophysiology, and biologic behavior of follicular cancer differ significantly from those of the entities with which it is often confused. Only careful histopathologic classification will allow correct evaluation of treatment options and prognosis.

PAPILLARY LESIONS OF THE THYROID

Papillary lesions of the thyroid consist of papillary hyperplasia, benign nodules with papillary architecture, and papillary carcinoma.

Hyperplasia

Hyperplasia with the formation of true papillae occurs in diffuse and nodular forms. The former is most commonly found in untreated autoimmune hyperthyroidism or Graves' disease.

Antibodies that stimulate thyroid function give rise to Graves' disease or "autoimmune thyrotoxicosis."[29] The description of this disorder is attributed to Robert Graves in 1835; an earlier report by C.H. Parry was recorded in 1786 but was not published until its posthumous recognition in 1825.[9,28] The disease is also known as von Basedow's disease in German-speaking countries after that author's publication of 1840.[9,28] The entity is characterized by a hyperfunctioning, diffuse hyperplastic goiter, often associated with ophthalmopathy and dermopathy. It may arise at any age but has a peak incidence in the third and fourth decades. The female/male ratio is 5:1. Graves' disease has a well-defined association with other endocrine autoimmune phenomena, notably Hashimoto's thyroiditis, and there are some similarities in the clinical and morphologic features of Hashimoto's and Graves' disease.

The size of the goiter in Graves' disease does not correlate with the degree of thyrotoxicosis but is, in fact, proportional to the amount of circulating TGI; the degree of thyrotoxicosis correlates with the circulating thyroid stimulating immunoglobulins (TSI) levels.[40]

The enlarged thyroid glands of patients with Graves' disease are uniform, firm, and symmetrical; the weight varies from 35 to 90 g. Grossly the gland is red-brown, with a meaty appearance, and lacks colloid translucence. Microscopically the follicular epithelium is hypertrophied and hyperplastic. The hypertrophy results in tall columnar epithelial cells, and the severity of the altered metabolic state correlates with the height of the cells. The increased number of cells form nonbranching, fingerlike papillary projections of pseudostratified or multilayered epithelium lining a delicate fibrovascular stroma and may be so large that they virtually fill the follicles. The scant residual colloid typically has a scalloped border resulting from the accelerated proteolytic digestion of the colloid before its resorption. Inflammatory cell infiltrates, occasionally with germinal centers, constitute the only feature allowing morphologic differentiation of Graves' disease from other hyperplastic thyroid disorders.

Graves' disease rarely presents with a thyroid nodule and the development of a nodule in this setting warrants investigation for thyroid cancer.[78] Clearly, because of the cytologic atypia that resembles papillary carcinoma, the cytologist must be made aware of the clinical history before interpreting an FNA specimen.

Hyperplastic Nodules and Adenomas With Papillary Architecture

The "papillary hyperplastic nodule" of the thyroid is usually identified in girls, usually teenagers at about the age of menarche. These present as solitary nodules and it is unusual for them to be associated with clinical hyperfunction, although that might occur. These lesions are distinguished from papillary carcinoma in that they are totally encapsulated, often show central cystic change, have subfollicle formation in the centers of broad edematous papillae, and do not show nuclear features of papillary carcinoma. Although one analysis of clonality has suggested that these are polyclonal hyperplasias,[79] the detection of Gsα or TSH receptor activating mutations in such nodules suggests that they are benign neoplasms.[80-82] Some have advocated the name *papillary adenoma* for these tumors; while scientifically appropriate, this term carries historical connotations that some feel are unacceptable.[10]

In some adults, one can have a similar histologic appearance to a hot nodule that is a nodule in the thyroid associated with clinical toxicity. This is often seen in the setting of sporadic nodule goiter. Molecular analyses of clonality in nodular goiter[44] and of hyperfunctioning nodules[45,46] again support the view that these may represent benign neoplasms.

On FNA (Fig. 3-19) and on histologic evaluation (Fig. 3-20), papillary hyperplastic nodules or adenomas can be very alarming and lead to a false-positive diagnosis of papillary carcinoma. Indeed, these entities give rise to well-formed papillae, but on higher magnification, the cytologic criteria for the diagnosis of papillary carcinoma are lacking. According to Kini,[15] the minimal criteria for the cytologic diagnosis of papillary carcinoma should include syncytial-type tissue fragments, powdery nuclear chromatin, multiple micronuclei and/or macronucleoli, intranuclear cytoplasmic inclusions, and linear chromatin grooves.

Papillary Carcinoma

Papillary carcinoma comprises at least 80% of thyroid epithelial malignancies diagnosed in regions of the world where goiters are not endemic. The

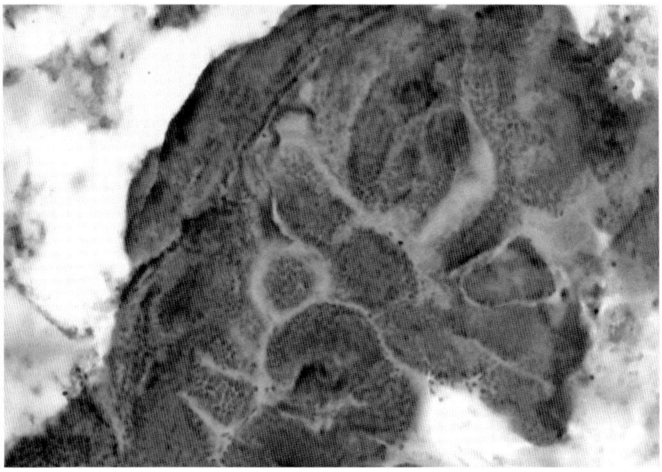

• **FIGURE 3-19** Fine-needle aspiration biopsy of a hyperfunctioning follicular adenoma reveals papillary fragments of tissue; however, the nuclear features of papillary carcinoma are not identified.

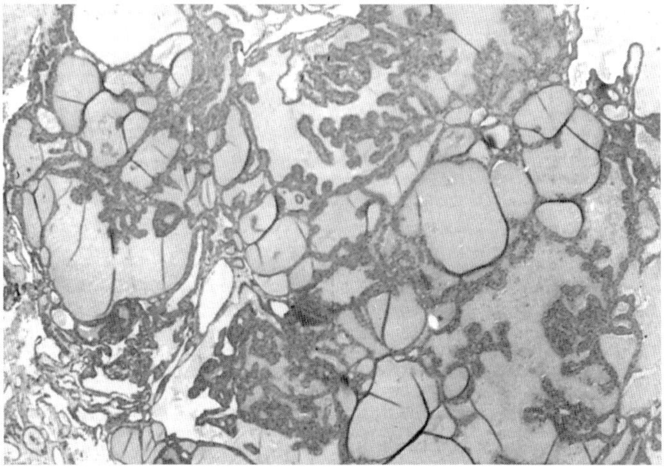

• **FIGURE 3-20** Histology of a hyperfunctioning follicular adenoma reveals papillary architecture with papillae that show orientation to the center of colloid-filled spaces. Although not seen at this magnification, the nuclei have a vesicular chromatin pattern and do not exhibit the atypia of papillary carcinoma.

terminology is misleading: papillary carcinomas can exhibit papillary architecture, but they may also have follicular or mixed papillary and follicular patterns.[8,10,83-88] It is now recognized that the diagnosis of papillary carcinoma is based on what the World Health Organization has described as "a distinctive set of nuclear characteristics."[89] In contrast to true follicular carcinomas,

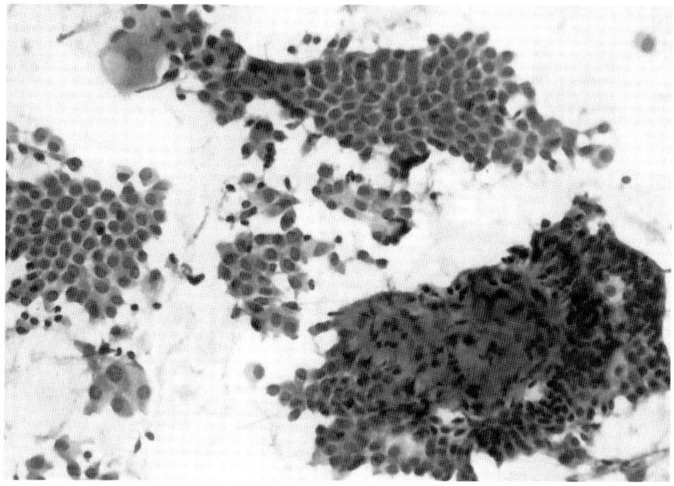

• **FIGURE 3-21** Fine-needle aspiration biopsy of papillary carcinoma can occasionally yield tissue fragments with papillary architecture. The nuclei are crowded and exhibit significant overlap and molding.

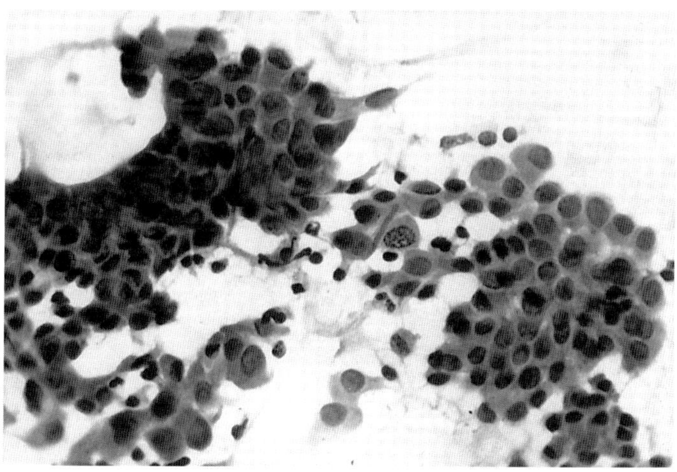

• **FIGURE 3-22** Higher magnification of the cytology of an aspirate of papillary carcinoma reveals crowded nuclei that exhibit irregularity, including prominent nuclear grooves and occasional inclusions.

these lesions are more indolent and most have an excellent prognosis with a 20-year survival rate of 90% or better.[90,91]

The defining nuclear features are readily seen on cytology of fine needle aspirates (Figs. 3-21 through 3-23). They include an alteration of the size and roundness of the normal follicular cell nucleus to one that is large and oval. Because of peripheral margination of chromatin, the center of the

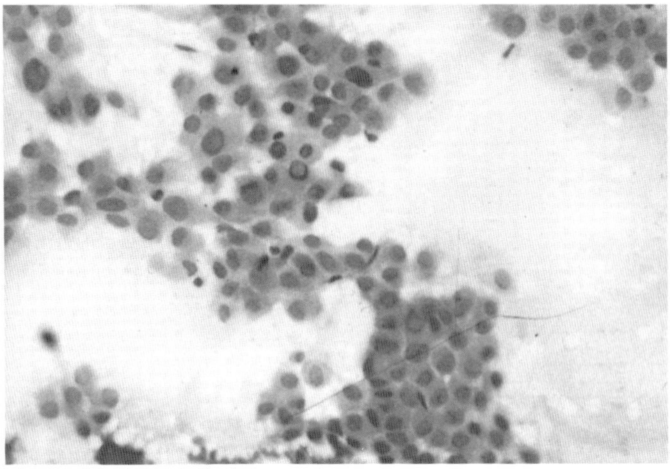

• **FIGURE 3-23** Aspiration biopsy of a papillary carcinoma reveals the characteristic cytologic features including very prominent intranuclear inclusions.

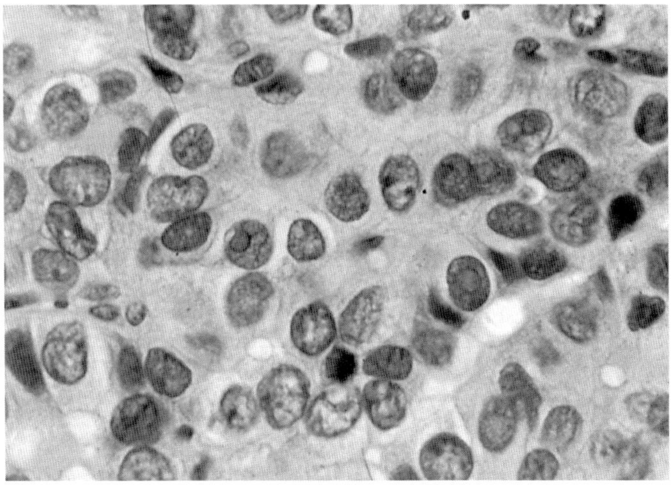

• **FIGURE 3-24** Histologic examination within a lesion that does not exhibit papillary architecture still relies on cytologic features. The prominent irregularity of nuclear contours, nuclear grooves, and intranuclear cytoplasmic pseudoinclusions provide the basis for a diagnosis of papillary carcinoma.

nucleus has a curious empty appearance that has been termed "ground glass."[92] The chromatin and nucleolus are pushed to the edge of the nucleus. The nuclear contour is strikingly irregular, resulting in intranuclear cytoplasmic pseudoinclusions and nuclear grooves (Fig. 3-24).[93,94] No one specific feature is absolutely diagnostic of papillary carcinoma; a constellation or combination of nuclear features is required for the diagnosis.

Papillary carcinomas may be multifocal. This has been interpreted as reflective of intraglandular lymphatic dissemination, but the identification of such microcarcinomas in up to 24% of the population[95] and the detection of different RET/PTC rearrangements in multifocal lesions[96] support the interpretation of multifocal primary lesions in most patients. Nevertheless, when these lesions do invade, they show a preference for lymphatic involvement with a high percentage of regional lymph node metastases. Metastases beyond the neck are unusual in common papillary carcinoma and probably only occur in about 5% to 7% of cases.

The most useful prognostic markers in papillary carcinoma are patient variables, tumor size, and extent of disease.[56,57,75,97] Patients under age 45 usually have an excellent prognosis; in contrast, those over age 45 generally have a poorer outlook. Gender has also been said in the past to be an important determinant of tumor biology, but more recent studies have suggested that there is no major difference in the behavior of papillary carcinoma in men compared to women. Tumor size is exceedingly important.[98] Tumors less than 1 cm are common and appear to be different biologically from larger tumors;[99-101] a recent study has shown that occult papillary carcinomas are identified in up to 24% of the population in thyroid glands that are removed for nonmalignant or unrelated disease.[95] In contrast, tumors greater than 1 cm are thought to be of clinical significance and those larger than 3 cm generally have a poorer prognosis than do smaller tumors. The presence of cervical lymph node metastasis, whether identified microscopically or clinically, is thought to increase the risk of recurrence of disease but has been shown to have no impact on mortality. Extrathyroidal extension, by contrast, predicts a worse prognosis, and the presence of distant metastases is the hallmark of an aggressive tumor that will bear the potential for high mortality.

Grossly, papillary carcinomas vary in size from microcarcinomas (also called small, tiny, occult, and minute) which are defined as lesions measuring less than 1 cm (usually 4 to 7 mm) to large neoplasms that extend beyond the thyroid capsule into surrounding soft tissue. Most clinical papillary carcinomas are intrathyroidal tumors confined within the capsule of the thyroid and may have an encapsulated appearance (this is usual for the follicular variant) or an irregularly infiltrative appearance. One can see gross cystic change, but usually papillary carcinoma is a firm tumor and some are calcified or even ossified.

Microscopically, papillary carcinomas classically are composed of papillae, but virtually all contain follicular elements (Fig. 3-25). Ghosts of dead papillae or infarcted papillae calcify with a concentric whorled pattern that is characteristic of psammoma bodies;[102] these are found in 40% to 50% of papillary carcinomas, either in the tumor stroma or in the surrounding nontumorous thyroid.

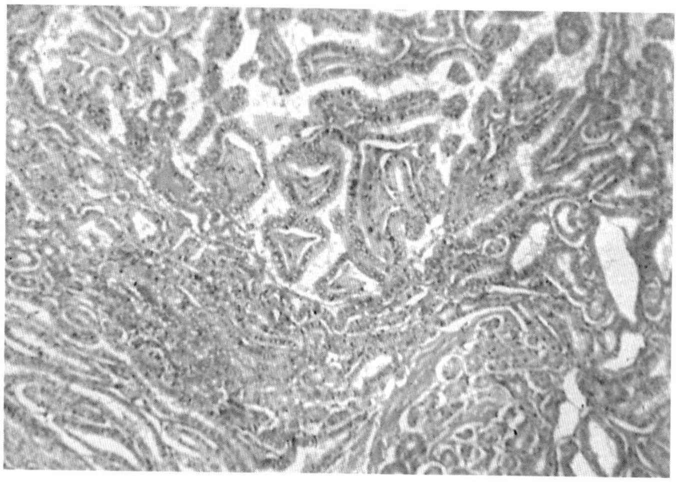

• **FIGURE 3-25** Most papillary carcinomas contain at least focal papillary architecture, but almost all exhibit areas of follicular architecture.

Inflammatory infiltrates within papillary carcinomas and in the surrounding thyroid parenchyma have been noted by several authors, although the prognostic significance of this is not clear.[103,104] Some people have postulated that this inflammatory infiltrate may indicate host-tumor immune interactions that are responsible for the general indolence of this type of thyroid carcinoma.[103]

Papillary Carcinoma Variants

Although there are reports to the contrary, in our experience the exact histologic variant of papillary carcinoma cannot be predicted from the appearance of the fine-needle aspirate.[105] Nevertheless, the histologic distinctions, which are characteristic[8,10,89,106-108] are of prognostic value.

Patients with *papillary microcarcinoma*[95] (Fig. 3-26) and *cystic and encapsulated variants of papillary carcinoma*[50] are thought to have a slightly better prognosis than those with usual papillary carcinoma.

The *follicular variant* has been recognized more frequently in the past 20 years (Fig. 3-27).[10,89,109,110] This lesion comprises about 10% to 15% of papillary cancers. It has either been misdiagnosed as follicular carcinoma or underdiagnosed as follicular adenoma or atypical adenoma. Any lesion with follicular architecture and characteristic nuclear features of papillary carcinoma should be classified as this tumor. Infiltrating areas and metastases may exhibit a more striking papillary appearance and may even have psammoma bodies. It is unclear what the ultimate biologic and clinical behavior of follicular variant is, since some of these may be underdiagnosed

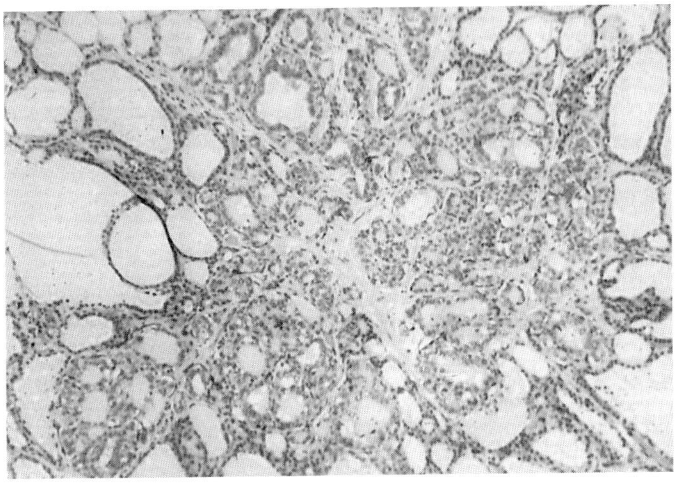

• **FIGURE 3-26** Papillary microcarcinoma is a microscopic lesion that often exhibits a stellate fibrosis and infiltrating pattern. These microscopic lesions exhibit the characteristic cytologic atypia of papillary carcinoma.

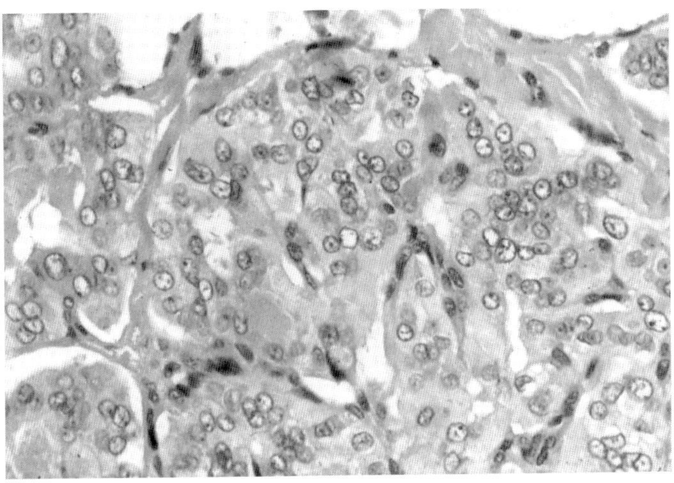

• **FIGURE 3-27** Follicular variant papillary carcinoma may exhibit only follicular architecture throughout the lesion, but the cytologic features, including clearing of nucleoplasm and peripheral margination of chromatin, identify this as a tumor that will behave similar to classical papillary carcinoma.

as atypical adenomas; it is likely that the initial reports of this tumor included the aggressive biologic spectrum of this variant.

The presence of cytologic atypia may raise the possibility of papillary carcinoma without being sufficiently convincing for unequivocal diagnosis. In such cases, immunostaining for high-molecular-weight cytokeratins may be useful. This technique, also considered controversial in the past, has recently been shown to be useful when applied to paraffin sections only if microwave antigen retrieval is used.[111] The results of these studies indicate that moderate to strong diffuse staining is confined to papillary carcinoma, whereas follicular neoplasms and hyperplastic nodules are negative or show only focal staining in areas of reaction to degeneration or previous FNA biopsy. Nevertheless, only approximately 60% of papillary carcinomas are positive; a positive stain result is therefore helpful, but negative stain results cannot be used to assist in the diagnostic process.

Diagnosis of this entity has been further advanced by the recognition of a family of gene rearrangements that are specific to papillary carcinoma.[112] The RET/PTC oncogenes (1 through 5, depending on the site of rearrangement) are the result of DNA damage with rearrangements that transpose various cellular genes adjacent to the gene encoding the intracellular tyrosine kinase domain of the RET proto-oncogene.[113-117] The rearrangements result in constitutive tyrosine kinase activation and translocation of the fusion protein to the cytoplasm.[118] Animal models have shown the tumorigenicity of these fusion proteins;[119,120] the rearrangements are common in radiation-induced tumors[121-125] but are also found in sporadic papillary carcinomas[126-129] and appear to be an early event in tumor development.[130] Immunohistochemical staining with antisera directed against the carboxy terminus of RET allow rapid and clinically useful detection of this marker of papillary carcinoma (Fig. 3-28), which is present in up to 80% of occult papillary microcarcinomas and approximately 50% of clinically detected lesions.[96] Again, a negative stain result is not useful; however, the combination of high-molecular-weight cytokeratins and RET provides a set of immunohistochemical markers that aids in the diagnosis of papillary carcinoma in equivocal cases.

The *diffuse sclerosis variant* occurs in young individuals and often presents as goiter without a specific mass lesion.[131-134] This tumor microscopically involves thyroid lymphatics, exhibits squamous metaplasia, and forms numerous psammoma bodies, giving it a very gritty appearance when examined grossly. These tumors almost always have lymph node metastases at presentation, and 25% have lung metastases as well. It is interesting that about 10% of the pediatric thyroid cancers that have occurred following the Chernobyl nuclear accident in 1986 are tumors of the diffuse sclerosis type.[135]

Aggressive variants of papillary carcinoma include the *tall cell variant* and probably related lesions, the *trabecular and columnar cell variant*.[136-141] The tall cell variant is defined as a tumor composed of cells that have a height-to-width ratio that exceeds 3:1 (Fig. 3-29). Tumors that exhibit this feature in more than 30% of the tumor mass generally tend to occur in older individuals with a median age at diagnosis of 20 years older than usual papillary

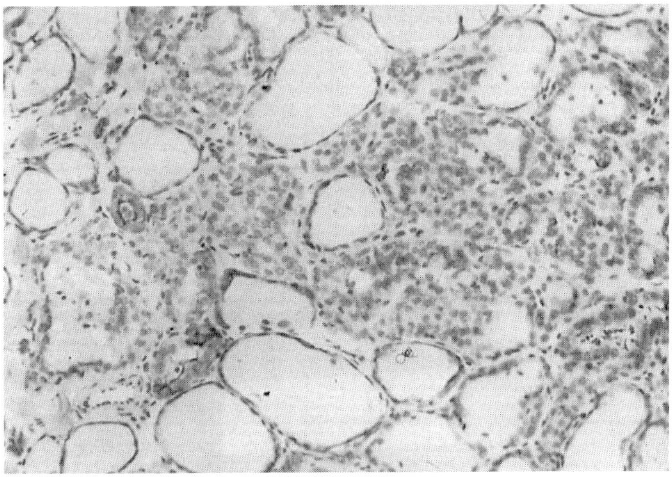

• **FIGURE 3-28** Some cases of follicular variant papillary carcinoma exhibit either focal or borderline nuclear morphology. The presence of a RET/PTC gene rearrangement, said to be specific for papillary carcinoma, can be identified by immunohistochemistry for *ret*, which exhibits a cytoplasmic pattern of reactivity in papillary carcinoma.

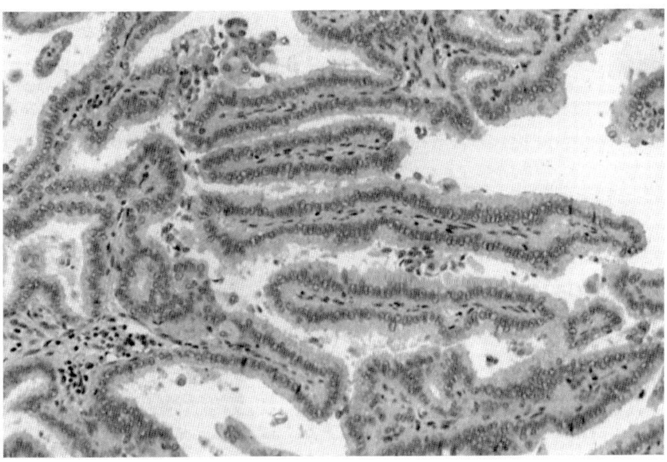

• **FIGURE 3-29** Tall cell papillary carcinoma is characterized by markedly elongated cells that exhibit a height-to-width ratio that exceeds 3:1. These tumors also have very crowded nuclear morphologic features.

carcinoma, are often large lesions greater than 5 cm, and often extend extrathyroidally.[138] In addition to lymphatic invasion, vascular invasion is not uncommonly found in these lesions. Tumor mortality rates vary up to 25% for tall cell tumors and 90% for columnar cell carcinoma.[140-142]

The management of papillary thyroid carcinoma is controversial. Most experts advocate total thyroidectomy and radioactive iodine therapy.[61-73]

The rationale for total thyroidectomy is twofold, based on the frequency of bilateral carcinoma and the need for enhancement of uptake of radioactive iodine by metastatic tumor deposits rather than residual thyroid tissue. However, as shown by the studies of Sugg et al.,[96] identification of occult papillary carcinoma in the contralateral lobe is usually not attributable to intrathyroidal dissemination, which would justify further surgery for local disease. Therefore the major indications for total thyroidectomy are to enhance uptake of radioactive iodine, and to increase the sensitive use of thyroglobulin assays to detect persistent disease.[75-77] The controversy involves the management of patients with low-risk clinical and pathologic parameters; some have advocated less-aggressive management with unilateral thyroidectomy and no radioiodine therapy in this setting.[72] Since there are no controlled clinical trials that address this issue, the answer remains an empirical one. As for follicular carcinoma, external-beam radiotherapy is not used in patients with differentiated thyroid carcinoma, apart from those with locally advanced tumors that involve extrathyroidal soft tissues of the neck and cannot be completely resected.[77,97]

HÜRTHLE CELL LESIONS

Hürthle cells in the thyroid represent a misnomer in that Dr. Hürthle originally described the parafollicular cell. The first description of oxyphilic cells in the thyroid is actually attributed to Askenazy. However, the term Hürthle cell is ingrained in the literature, and it is unlikely that the historical error will ever be corrected.

The Hürthle cell is derived from the follicular epithelium and possesses the capacity to produce thyroglobulin.[30] Morphologically it is characterized by large size, square shape, distinct cell borders, voluminous granular and eosinophilic cytoplasm, a large nucleolus, and an often prominent nucleus that may stain red with eosin. By electron microscopy, the cytoplasmic granularity is produced by large mitochondria filling the cell, consistent with oncocytic transformation.[143,144] Hürthle cells have been studied using enzyme histochemistry and have been shown to contain a high level of oxidative enzymes.[145-146]

Hürthle cells are sometimes considered to be a cause of concern in needle biopsies.[15] When they are not the major component in a thyroid aspirate, they are not diagnostic of any given lesion. Hürthle cells are found in patients with thyroiditis as well as in several forms of thyroid neoplasia including Hürthle cell papillary carcinomas. Hürthle cell adenomas and Hürthle cell follicular carcinomas are diagnosed when more than 75% of a lesion is composed of this cell type; the criteria for the diagnosis of lesions

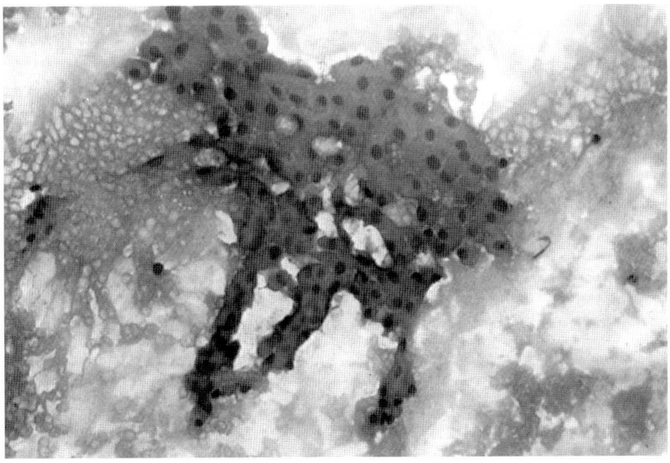

• **FIGURE 3-30** Aspiration of a Hürthle cell nodule of the thyroid reveals a monomorphous population of large polygonal cells with abundant granular cytoplasm.

that are composed predominantly of Hürthle cells are the same as those applied to follicular lesions that do not contain Hürthle cells.[147] Similar to follicular neoplasms, cytologic diagnosis of Hürthle cell tumors is reported under the generic term *Hürthle cell lesion.* The aspirate is composed of a monomorphous population of large polygonal cells with granular cytoplasm (Fig. 3-30). With the Papanicolau stain, the cytoplasm may be orange, green, or blue. The nuclei are prominent and often contain "cherry-pink" macronucleoli. The colloid is usually scant or absent. Overall, Kini[15] reports a diagnostic accuracy of 85% to 90% for Hürthle cell neoplasm and 60% for Hürthle cell carcinoma. The diagnosis of Hürthle cell papillary carcinoma (see below) is possible when the minimal cytologic criteria for papillary carcinoma are present.[148]

FNA of Hürthle cell tumors may cause them to partially or totally infarct.[149] This probably occurs because of the high metabolic activity of these cells and the delicate blood supply of these lesions, which may readily become inadequate after direct trauma. A solitary tumor of the thyroid that occurs in a patient without thyroiditis and that is purely or predominantly composed of Hürthle cells on FNA should be excised, since Hürthle cell tumors show an average malignancy rate of 30% based on histologic findings.[147]

Hyperplasia

Hürthle cells are found in the thyroid in a variety of conditions and therefore are not specific for any particular disease. Individual cells, follicles, or groups of follicles may show Hürthle cell features in radiated thyroids, in aging thyroids, in nodular goiter, and in thyroiditis as well as in long-standing autoimmune hyperthyroidism. One can see these cells in chronic lymphocytic thyroiditis, in Graves' disease, and in nodular goiter, where one can often find an entire nodule composed of oncocytes.

Adenoma

Confusion and concern arise when Hürthle cell nodules and neoplasms occur in the thyroid. Most Hürthle cell nodules are found in the setting of thyroiditis or nodular goiter and are benign and may not even be neoplastic. Lesions that arise in otherwise normal glands, that are encapsulated, and are composed of 75% or more Hürthle cells are considered to be neoplastic. They can have microfollicular, macrofollicular (rare), trabecular, or solid architecture. On occasion, especially with the solid pattern and since these lesions can be extremely vascular, they may resemble medullary thyroid carcinomas and it may be necessary to resort to immunoperoxidase stains for thyroglobulin and calcitonin to obtain the correct diagnosis.

Follicular Carcinoma

For many years it was felt that all Hürthle cell neoplasms of the thyroid should be considered malignant, since it was thought that the histologic findings could not predict clinical behavior. However, numerous studies have indicated that the criteria that apply to all follicular neoplasms of the thyroid also distinguish malignant from benign Hürthle cell lesions (Fig. 3-31).[147,150-156] The larger the Hürthle cell lesion, however, the more likely it is to show invasive characteristics; a Hürthle cell tumor that is 4 cm or greater has an 80% chance of showing histologic evidence of malignancy. Nuclear atypia (the hallmark of the Hürthle cell), multinucleation, and mitotic activity are not useful in predicting prognosis and therefore should not be used as diagnostic criteria for malignancy.

A subgroup of Hürthle cell neoplasm has been described that shows some atypical features including marked nuclear anaplasia, mitoses, spontaneous infarction, and trapping of tumor cells within the capsule in the absence of a preoperative FNA. Some authors have called these "atypical Hürthle cell adenoma" or "tumor of indeterminate malignancy." The great majority of these behave in a clinically benign fashion.

Ancillary techniques have not been helpful in distinguishing Hürthle cell lesions, which will behave as carcinomas or adenomas. Flow cytometric analyses document aneuploid cell populations in 10% to 25% of Hürthle

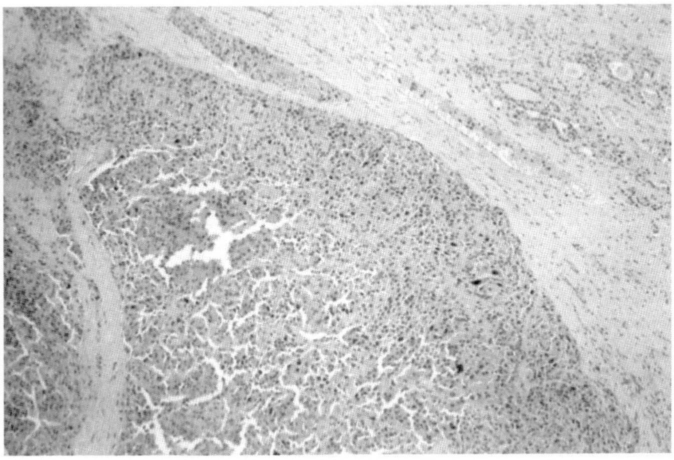

• **FIGURE 3-31** Hürthle cell carcinoma is composed of large cells with abundant granular eosinophilic cytoplasm and marked nuclear atypia. The diagnosis of malignancy rests on the demonstration of capsular invasion *(top center)* and vascular involvement *(top right)*.

cell neoplasms that are clinically and histologically classified as adenomas.[65,66,157] Virtually all of these tumors behave in a benign fashion after excision. Once a histologic diagnosis of carcinoma is made, however, aneuploidy as shown on flow cytometry may predict a more aggressive clinical behavior for that carcinoma.

The management of Hürthle cell tumors is controversial.[153,154,158-161]

Papillary Carcinoma

Many Hürthle cell tumors, whether benign or malignant, show papillary change that is really a pseudopapillary phenomenon, since Hürthle cell neoplasms have only scant stroma and may fall apart during manipulation, fixation, and processing.

True oxyphilic or Hürthle cell variant of papillary carcinoma has been reported to comprise from 1% to 11% of all papillary carcinomas.[144,162-167] These tumors have papillary architecture, but are composed predominantly or entirely of Hürthle cells.[144,168] The nuclei may exhibit the characteristics of usual papillary carcinoma[163,169] or they may instead resemble the nuclei of Hürthle cells, being large, hyperchromatic, and pleomorphic.[89,164] The clinical behavior of this rare subtype is controversial; some authors have reported that they behave like typical papillary carcinomas[89,148,166,168,169] whereas others maintain that the Hürthle cell morphology confers a more aggressive behavior[170,171] with higher rates of 10-year tumor recurrence and

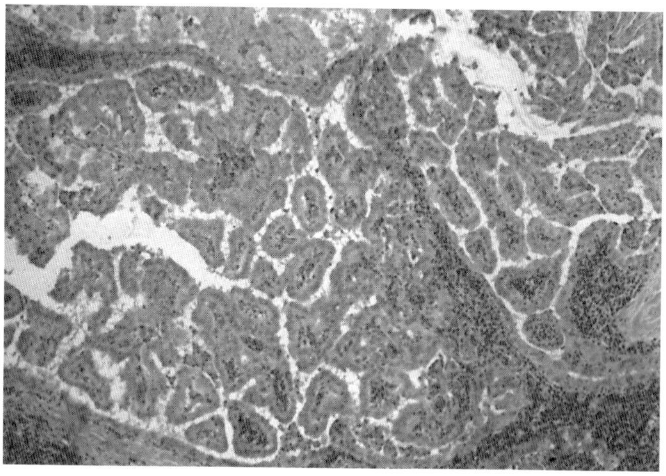

• **FIGURE 3-32** A Hürthle cell papillary carcinoma is composed of classical papillae with fibrovascular cores, lined by follicular epithelial cells that have abundant eosinophilic granular cytoplasm. This variant, which has extensive lymphocytic infiltration in the cores of the papillae, resembles Warthin's tumor of the salivary gland.

cause-specific mortality.[164] This suggestion of aggressive behavior may be attributed to inclusion of tall cell variant papillary carcinoma in the group of Hürthle cell carcinomas.

One morphologic subtype of papillary Hürthle cell carcinoma which, because of a characteristic cystic change and extensive lymphocytic infiltration into the cores of the papillae of the tumor, has a striking histologic resemblance to papillary cystadenoma lymphomatosum of the salivary gland (Fig. 3-32) has been called "Warthin-like tumor of the thyroid."[172] This lesion occurs in the setting of chronic lymphocytic thyroiditis, predominantly in women, and is associated with a similar prognosis to usual papillary carcinoma.

POORLY DIFFERENTIATED (INSULAR) CARCINOMA

Poorly differentiated or *insular carcinoma* is a tumor of follicular cell origin, which mimics the architecture of medullary thyroid carcinoma.[173-175] The tumor forms large, well-defined solid nests; it is largely devoid of follicular architecture and devoid of colloid (Fig. 3-33). The tumor cells are small and uniform in size, and there is a variable degree of mitotic activity. Sclerosis

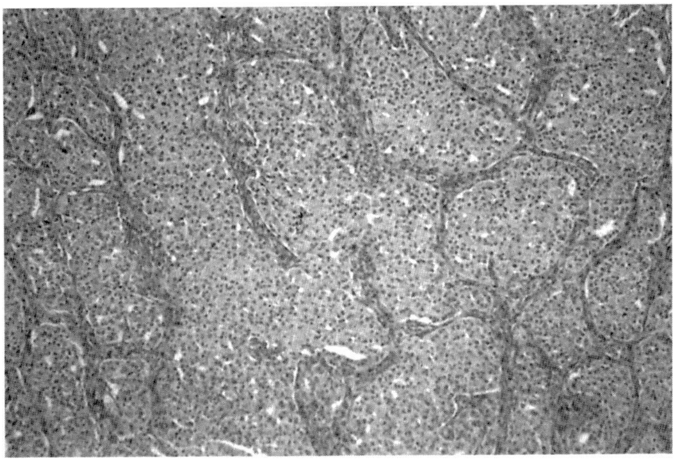

• **FIGURE 3-33** Insular carcinoma of the thyroid has a nesting architecture that resembles neuroendocrine tumors but is composed of cells of follicular differentiation. The nests may contain areas of individual tumor cell necrosis.

can mimic amyloid; however, Congo red stains yield negative results and immunohistochemical stains for calcitonin, chromogranin, and CEA are negative. By contrast, the tumor is positive for thyroglobulin, confirming the follicular cell differentiation of this tumor. Also, by contrast to anaplastic carcinomas, there is little pleomorphism and no bizarre, giant, or multinucleated cells are found; however, mitotic activity is identified and single-cell necrosis may be prominent.

The cytologic features of insular carcinoma on FNA have only sporadically been reported. The aspirate is usually very cellular, with small monomorphic cells in loose aggregates with or without follicle formation. Nuclear grooves and pseudoinclusions may be present. The tumor often resembles medullary carcinoma, but insular carcinoma is thyroglobulin positive and calcitonin negative.

Insular carcinoma behaves in an aggressive fashion and is often lethal. Metastases are frequent at the time of diagnosis. Insular carcinoma therefore occupies a position both morphologically and biologically between differentiated papillary or follicular carcinoma and anaplastic thyroid carcinoma. These tumors are not uncommonly found associated with well-differentiated carcinoma, and the insular growth is thought to represent a dedifferentiation phenomenon. Since this entity has only been recognized relatively recently and the clinical literature does not include studies of this tumor type as a separate entity, appropriate clinical management is yet to be established.

ANAPLASTIC CARCINOMA

Anaplastic or undifferentiated carcinoma accounts for 5% to 10% of all primary malignant tumors of the thyroid.[176] The incidence is decreasing and currently accounts for about 1 to 27 of all primary tumors in the USA. These tumors are rapidly growing, with massive local invasion that usually overshadows the early metastases, most frequently to lung, adrenals, and bone.[9,10] They are highly lethal with a 5-year survival rate of 7.1%[177] and a mean survival period of 6.2 to 7.2 months.[177,178]

Microscopically, anaplastic carcinomas exhibit wide variation. Three general patterns are recognized, but most tumors manifest mixed morphology:

The most common type is the *giant cell variant*. As the name suggests, these tumors are composed predominantly of large cells with abundant amphophilic or eosinophilic, often granular cytoplasm and bizarre, often multiple, hyperchromatic nuclei (Fig. 3-34). Some have round, densely acidophilic, intracytoplasmic hyaline globules. These tumors grow in solid sheets; artifactual tissue fragmentation may simulate an alveolar pattern.

The *squamoid variant* is composed of large, moderately pleomorphic epithelial cells that form nests, resembling squamous carcinoma. They may even form keratin pearls.

Spindle cell anaplastic carcinomas have a fascicular architecture and dense stromal collagen with spindle-shaped tumor cells (Fig. 3-35). They may resemble fibrosarcoma; the presence of scattered atypical cells and

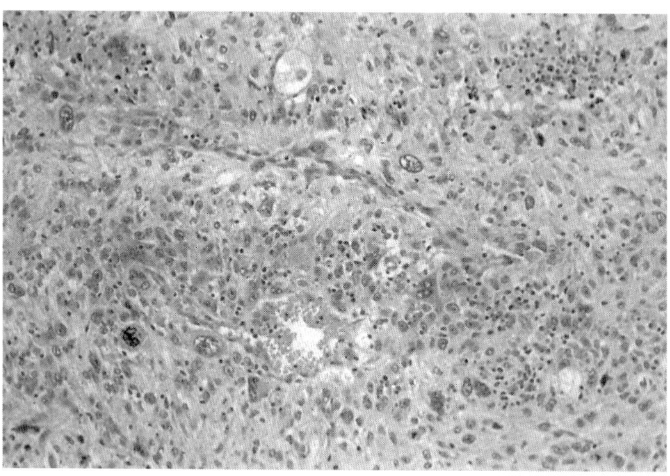

• **FIGURE 3-34** Anaplastic carcinoma of the thyroid may be composed of giant cells with abundant cytoplasm and bizarre, hyperchromatic nuclei. Focal necrosis is identified at top right and left.

inflammatory infiltrates may suggest malignant fibrous histiocytoma. Prominent vascularization may suggest hemangioendothelioma.[8,10,179]

In all three variants, mitotic figures and atypical mitoses are frequent. There is usually extensive necrosis and in some cases, necrosis may be so extensive that the only viable tumor is around blood vessels. Inflammatory infiltrates are associated with necrosis, and the osteoclast-like giant cells that are occasionally found in these tumors have been shown by immunohistochemical studies to be reactive cells of monocytic/histiocytic lineage.[180-181]

Anaplastic carcinomas are highly infiltrative. Malignant cells usually grow between residual thyroid follicles and invade skeletal muscle, adipose tissue, and other perithyroidal structures. Blood vessel invasion and thrombosis with or without tumor cell involvement is frequent.

The appearances of anaplastic carcinoma on FNA are quite varied and reflect the histologic type, with giant cells, squamoid cells, or spindle cells. There is high cellularity, with necrosis, acute inflammation, and marked cellular pleomorphism (Fig. 3-36). Mitoses are often atypical, and no colloid is seen.

Immunohistochemistry is useful in only a limited fashion in the diagnosis of these lesions. Most anaplastic carcinomas do not contain convincing reactivity for thyroglobulin and the few that are positive have only a weak or focal reaction.[178,181-185] This staining must be interpreted carefully, since it may reflect trapped nontumorous follicles or follicular cells, and since thyroglobulin is known to diffuse into nonfollicular cells.[10] The epithelial nature of the tumor cells can be verified with stains for cytokeratins and squamoid areas may exhibit reactivity for high-molecular-weight keratins

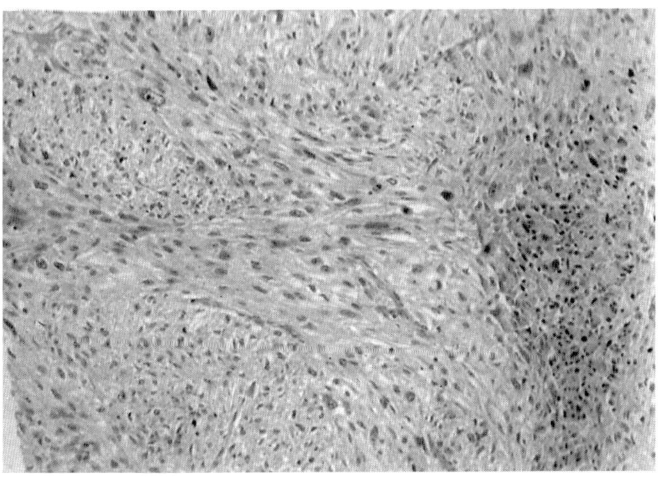

• **FIGURE 3-35** Spindle-cell anaplastic carcinomas have fascicular architecture that can mimic sarcoma. There are areas of geographic necrosis *(right)*.

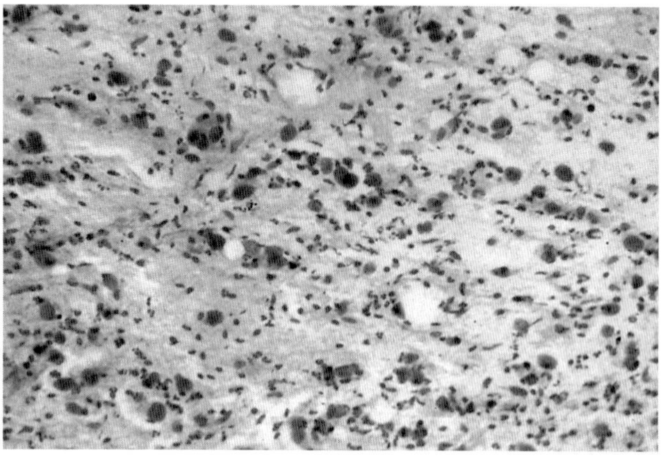

• **FIGURE 3-36** The appearance of anaplastic carcinoma on fine-needle aspiration biopsy is characterized by marked cellular pleomorphism and a background of necrotic debris with acute inflammation.

and/or epithelial membrane antigen (EMA).[178,181-183] CEA reactivity may be found in the center of squamous nests.[178,181] Anaplastic tumors have been reported to be positive for calcitonin, but this finding should alter the diagnosis to that of medullary carcinoma.[10]

p53 mutations are common in anaplastic thyroid carcinomas;[186-192] since mutated forms of this tumor suppressor gene have prolonged half-lives, the application of immunohistochemistry has yielded positive results in these tumors (Fig. 3-37).[193-194]

As demonstrated by electron microscopy,[180,182,185,195,196] there may be formation of intercellular junctions, microvilli, and basal lamina, providing evidence of epithelial differentiation. However, many tumors do not exhibit evidence of any differentiation. Their large nuclei have prominent nucleoli and clumped chromatin; usually the cytoplasm contains only poorly developed rough endoplasmic reticulum, scattered dense bodies, lipid droplets, numerous free ribosomes, mitochondria, and lysosomes. Intermediate filaments (keratin or vimentin) may form filamentous whorls that correspond to the acidophilic hyaline globules seen on light microscopy. Secretory granules are not seen in these tumors.

Most anaplastic thyroid carcinomas are aneuploid on flow cytometry; this abnormality correlates with poor outcome.[67]

Some tumors do not exhibit immunohistochemical or ultrastructural markers that allow classification as epithelial malignancies. Nevertheless, the diagnosis of anaplastic carcinoma should be favored for pleomorphic lesions in older patients if they arise in the thyroid.

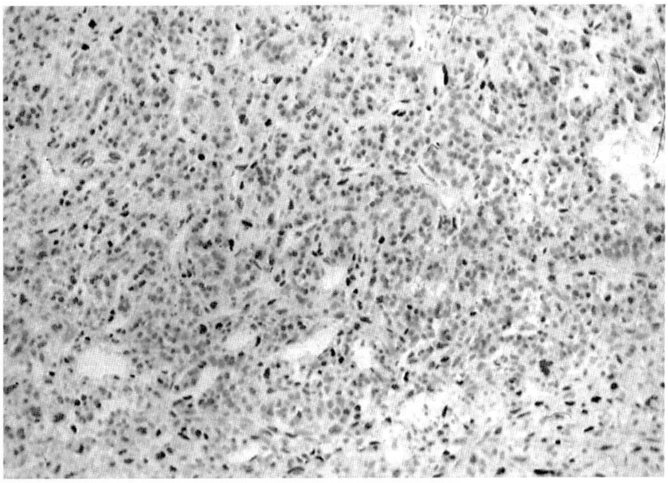

• **FIGURE 3-37** Immunohistochemical staining reveals prominent p53 nuclear reactivity in anaplastic thyroid carcinoma. This immunologic reaction usually correlates with a p53 mutation.

Small cell carcinomas and lymphomas constitute a common source of diagnostic error, often misclassified as anaplastic carcinomas.[8,10,179,182] The former are usually poorly differentiated medullary carcinomas, which can also mimic giant cell or spindle cell anaplastic carcinomas; the latter are readily identified by staining for leukocyte common antigen (LCA) and other markers of lymphoid cells. Rarely, primary intrathyroidal thymoma may be mistaken for anaplastic carcinoma.[197,198]

The reported association between well-differentiated thyroid carcinoma and anaplastic carcinoma ranges from 7% to 89% of cases, however, the lower figures are likely underestimates, attributable to inadequate sampling.[8,177,178,182,199-201] The data suggest that anaplastic carcinoma originates most often in an abnormal thyroid; the tumor has a higher incidence in regions of endemic goiter and a history of goiter is reported in over 80% of cases.[8,177] As stated above, nodular goiter is often the site of monoclonal proliferation, the first step in the hyperplasia-neoplasia sequence. However, it is difficult to document transformation of a benign lesion to a malignant tumor. Insular carcinoma appears to be intermediate in the spectrum and may represent a transition form.[174,201] The association of papillary carcinoma, particularly the more aggressive tall cell variant, with anaplastic tumors has also been described.[8,201,202] Thyroid carcinomas can exhibit an entire spectrum of differentiation through insular to anaplastic foci. The significance of microscopic anaplastic change is controversial; some people have suggested that focal microscopic anaplastic dedifferentiation does not alter prognosis, but others have shown that this finding alone is statistically significant as a marker of aggressive behavior.

The factors underlying dedifferentiation in thyroid tumors remain to be established; age and radiation have been implicated.[203,204] Clearly the vast majority of well-differentiated thyroid lesions do not undergo such transformation. A pattern of genetic mutations resulting in oncogene activation or loss of tumor suppressor gene activity has been proposed to correlate with the stepwise progression from adenoma to carcinoma and through the dedifferentiation process in the thyroid.[186,187]

C-CELL LESIONS

Medullary Carcinoma

Medullary carcinoma of the thyroid comprises 5% to 10% of all thyroid carcinomas.[10] This lesion is usually readily recognized because of its unusual cytologic and histologic features but sometimes special investigation is required to distinguish it from follicular lesions or other tumors including lymphomas and/or anaplastic carcinomas.

The aspirate from medullary carcinoma has a variable appearance. The cells may be spindle shaped, columnar, or plasmacytoid (Fig. 3-38). Nucleoli and nuclear pseudoinclusions are often seen. Amyloid is identified in up to 60% of cases as homogeneous, spherical, or rod-shaped extracellular material that polarizes with the Papanicolaou stain or the Congo red stain (Fig. 3-39). The diagnosis is confirmed by immunostaining for calcitonin or the demonstration of secretory granules on electron microscopy.

Medullary carcinoma has a wide range of histologic appearances.[7,205] Typically the tumors are composed of sheets and nests of round, polyhedral, or spindle-shaped cells that may exhibit palisading at the periphery (Fig. 3-40). The stroma is vascular and contains amyloid in more than half of these tumors. When present, amyloid provides a helpful diagnostic marker; however, amyloid may also be present in occasional nonmedullary thyroid carcinomas.[206]

Sometimes fixation artifact produces a pseudopapillary appearance. Areas of true papillary architecture may also be found, and the distinction of such lesions from papillary carcinoma can be difficult.[207] A pseudofollicular appearance frequently results from entrapped nonneoplastic thyroid follicles or rounded masses of amyloid, and true glandular variants have been described. Dedifferentiation results in a small cell tumor morphology that can mimic lymphoma. Oncocytic features may predominate and make the distinction of medullary from oncocytic follicular carcinoma difficult.

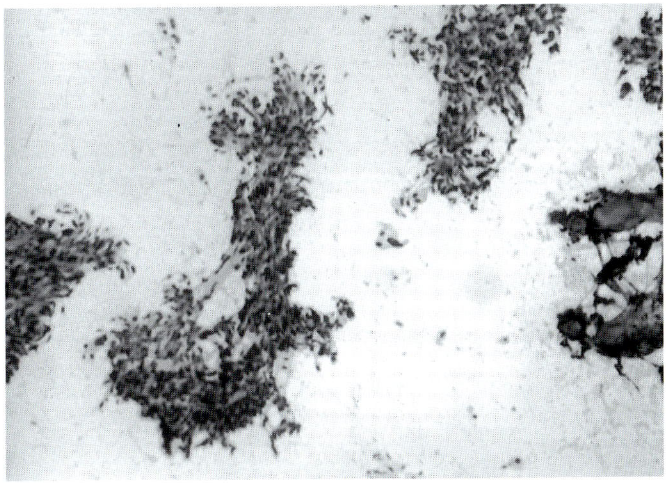

• **FIGURE 3-38** Fine-needle aspiration of a medullary thyroid carcinoma reveals clusters of spindle cells with elongated nuclear morphologic features.

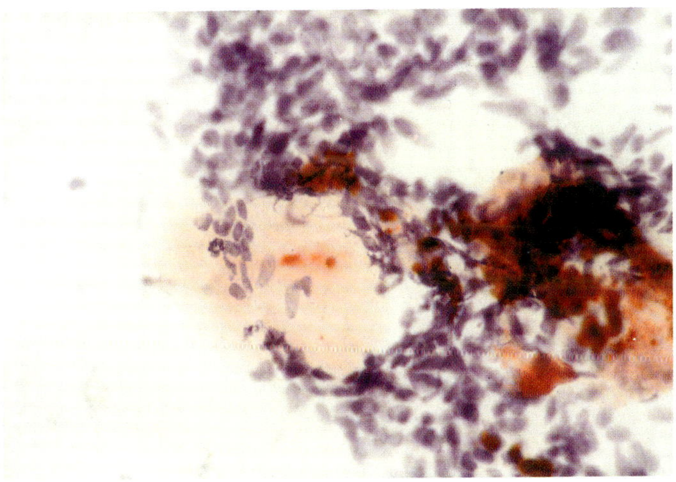

• **FIGURE 3-39** Amyloid may be detected with the Congo red stain, even on cytologic preparations of medullary thyroid carcinoma.

Foreign body giant cells may be associated with amyloid deposits and calcification may be identified. These features may result in difficult differential diagnosis. True psammoma bodies are generally not seen in these tumors but have been reported.

Staining for amyloid can be helpful. Congo red staining is typical, and the apple-green birefringence with polarized light is diagnostic. Nevertheless, as indicated, some follicular tumors may also contain amyloid stroma.

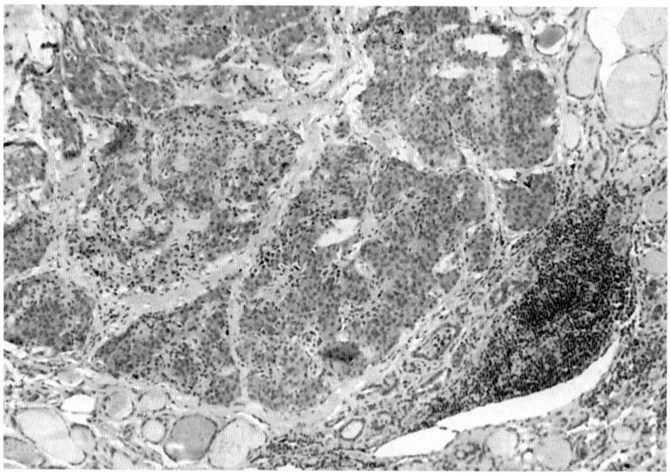

• **FIGURE 3-40** The histologic structure of medullary thyroid carcinoma is characterized by nests of tumor cells with poorly defined cell borders and areas of pale eosinophilic stroma that contain amyloid.

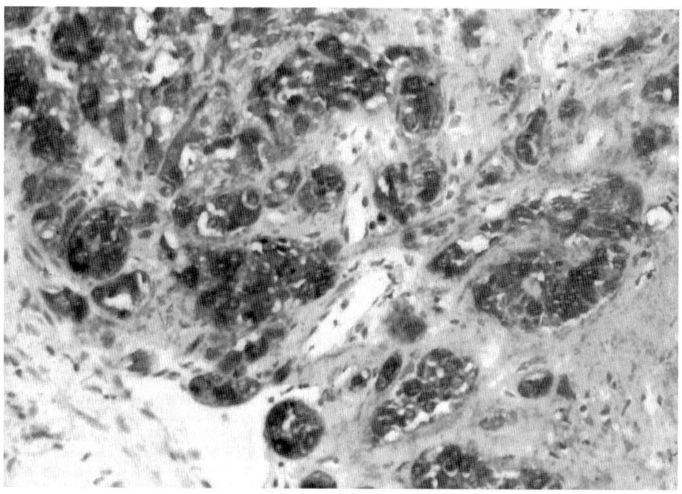

• **FIGURE 3-41** The diagnosis of medullary carcinoma is confirmed by calcitonin immune activity in tumor cells.

Immunohistochemical staining represents the "gold standard" for the diagnosis of medullary thyroid carcinoma. These tumors express cytokeratins, chromogranin A, and NSE, but the most specific diagnostic marker is calcitonin (Fig. 3-41). The number of calcitonin-positive cells varies from case to case, but the diagnosis should be questioned in the absence of calcitonin staining. The amyloid in these tumors often stains for calcitonin, probably because the amyloid protein represents deposition of a precursor of the calcitonin molecule.

These tumors also stain for CEA, and the inverse relationship between the intensity of staining for calcitonin and that for CEA may be prognostically significant: tumors containing few calcitonin-positive cells and abundant CEA immunoreactivity are said to have a worse prognosis than do the well-differentiated tumors with strong calcitonin immunoreactivity.[208,209] CEA is not identified in follicular thyroid tumors; occasional reports of positivity are attributable to use of antibodies that react with nonspecific cross-reacting antigens.[210] Therefore CEA positivity indicates the presence of medullary thyroid carcinoma or other lesions such as metastatic carcinomas or thymic carcinomas.

Medullary thyroid carcinomas also produce a number of other peptides including somatostatin, derivatives of the proopiomelanocortin molecule (ACTH, MSH, β-endorphin, and enkephalin), serotonin, glucagon, gastrin, cholecystokinin, VIP, bombesin, and α-HCG.[10,211-213] Calcitonin gene-related peptide (CGRP) is also identified in normal C cells as well as medullary thyroid carcinomas. Individual tumors may express a variety of these various hormones but none has been shown to correlate with altered prognosis.[214]

Ultrastructural examination confirms the presence of cells that do not form desmosomes but do show complex interdigitations of cell membranes. The cytoplasm contains characteristic membrane-bound secretory granules that usually are numerous and variable in size.

The importance of distinguishing this tumor from follicular lesions is twofold. The first is for diagnostic classification and management considerations in the individual patient. These tumors do not preferentially take up iodine, and therapy with radioactive iodine is not indicated. By contrast, expression of somatostatin receptors by some of these tumors[215] makes the octreoscan a feasible diagnostic tool to localize the primary lesion and to identify metastatic deposits,[216] and somatostatin analogs may have applications in the management of disseminated disease.[217] The other aspect of management involves the implications for both the patient and members of his/her family, since many of these tumors are hereditary.[218]

The inherited forms of medullary carcinoma are of three types: familial medullary thyroid carcinoma (FMTC) alone, multiple endocrine neoplasia (MEN) type 2A in which MTC is associated with pheochromocytomas, and MEN 2B in which the thyroid and adrenal proliferative disorders are associated with mucosal ganglioneuromas and a Marfanoid habitus. The inheritance of all three syndromes was mapped to the pericentromeric region of chromosome 10 by linkage analysis.[219-221] Subsequently, mutations in exons 10 and 11 of the RET proto-oncogene in patients with FMTC or MEN 2A and at codon 918 in MEN 2B[222,223] have provided a more accurate marker of germline mutation and predisposition to this disease.[224] Current recommendations suggest that family members of these kindreds have genetic screening early in life, and affected members should undergo total thyroidectomy at about 5 years of age. This age was chosen because of the early onset of medullary thyroid carcinoma in these familial forms of the disease; metastatic tumor has been found in patients as young as 6 years of age.

Sporadic medullary carcinomas also may have mutations of RET in the same codons as the familial disorders;[223,225] the mutation involved may have prognostic value.[226] The presence of RET mutations in sporadic tumors indicates the importance of analyzing DNA from white blood cells to establish that a mutation is germline and thus potentially hereditary. Other oncogenes and tumor suppressor genes have not been implicated in the pathogenesis of MCT: *ras* mutations are rare, *c-myc* and *c-erb*B are not amplified[227,228] and p53 mutations are not found in these tumors.[229]

Hyperplasia

Familial forms of medullary thyroid carcinoma usually result in multicentric disease as well as multicentric C-cell hyperplasia.[230] Many definitions of C-cell hyperplasia have been offered, all requiring immunohistochemical analysis because C cells cannot be reliably recognized with routine histologic stains. Quantitation of C cells as well as geographic mapping throughout the gland must be performed.[230,231] C cells are usually limited to the central portion of the junction between the upper and middle thirds of the lateral lobes where they are generally distributed singly rather than in clusters. Increased numbers of C cells (more than 7 cells per cluster), complete follicles surrounded by C cells, and distribution of cells beyond this geographic location are indicative of C-cell hyperplasia (Fig. 3-42).

The presence of C-cell hyperplasia usually indicates an inherited disorder rather than a sporadic lesion; however, C-cell hyperplasia can also be associated with chronic hypercalcemia, thyroid follicular nodular disease, and thyroiditis.[232-235]

The identification of oncogenic activation of RET in familial C-cell disease has raised questions about the term *C-cell hyperplasia.* In this disorder, unlike other familial cancer syndromes that result from inactivation of tumor suppressor genes, each affected member is born with an activated oncogene. Theoretically, then, every C cell has already undergone transformation, since it does not appear to require a second hit to knock out protective mechanisms. If this proves to be true, it will suggest that the term C-cell hyperplasia is a misnomer, since each C cell with its activated oncogene is a transformed cell

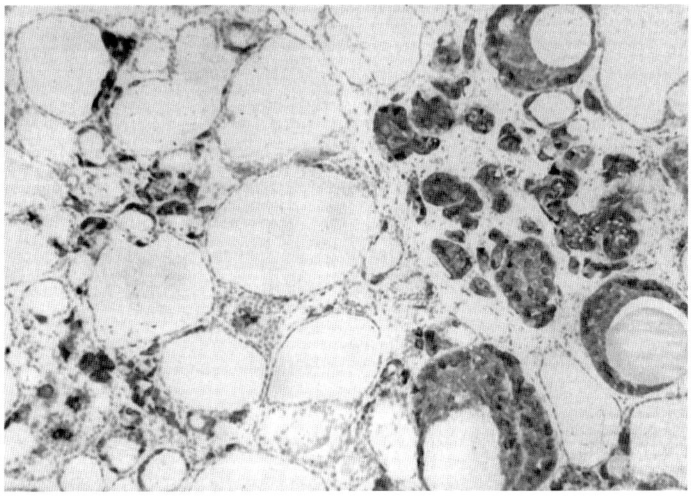

• **FIGURE 3-42** Patients with familial medullary thyroid carcinoma who carry germline mutations of the RET proto-oncogene develop C-cell hyperplasia that evolves into multifocal thyroid carcinoma.

that represents a site of neoplastic potential. This remains to be proven, however, and the mechanism of tumorigenesis in C cells of the thyroid, as it unfolds, will shed further light on the biology of neoplasia.

MIXED FOLLICULAR C-CELL LESIONS

Although controversial, mixed follicular-parafollicular cell carcinomas do occur;[236] these rare monomorphous tumors are composed of cells showing dual differentiation.[237,238] Composite tumors are composed of two intermixed well-differentiated components (Fig. 3-43), one showing thyroglobulin immunoreactivity and either papillary or follicular architecture and cytology, the other with calcitonin and CEA immunopositivity.[108,239] The diagnosis of a mixed or composite tumor can be convincing only in cases in which metastatic disease is identified, since the identification of thyroglobulin and calcitonin in a primary intrathyroidal tumor may represent the identification of a typical medullary thyroid carcinoma with trapped nontumorous elements containing thyroglobulin, or phagocytosis of thyroglobulin by medullary carcinoma cells. Moreover, the two tumors may occur separately in the same gland and metastasize together to a regional node.[240,241]

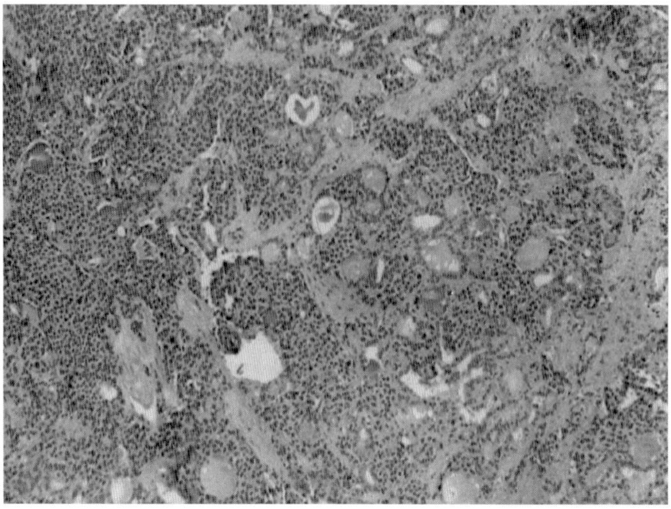

• **FIGURE 3-43** Mixed follicular–C-cell lesions are rare. This composite tumor is composed of predominantly medullary carcinoma with areas of follicular differentiation forming follicles that contain colloid. In a primary tumor this could be interpreted as infiltration of normal thyroid; however, this represents a biopsy of a lymph node metastasis.

OTHER PRIMARY EPITHELIAL MALIGNANCIES

Squamous Cell Carcinoma

Pure primary squamous carcinoma of the thyroid is rare.[10] By contrast, squamous cell malignancies may merge with papillary carcinoma that has undergone dedifferentiation.[202]

Primary Thyroid Thymoma

Branchial rests and intrathryroidal remnants of thymic tissue are considered to be the sites of origin of certain unusual tumors of the thyroid.[197,198]

The so-called SETTLE lesion (spindle epithelial tumor with thymus-like differentiation) occurs almost exclusively in young people under the age of 20 and often in children. It is a lesion of low-grade malignancy. It is composed of spindle cells with associated squamous nests.

A second lesion called CASTLE (carcinoma showing thymus-like differentiation) looks like a nasopharyngeal carcinoma in the thyroid (Fig. 3-44). These have been called variously squamous cell carcinomas of the thyroid and anaplastic carcinomas of the thyroid, but in fact they behave much less

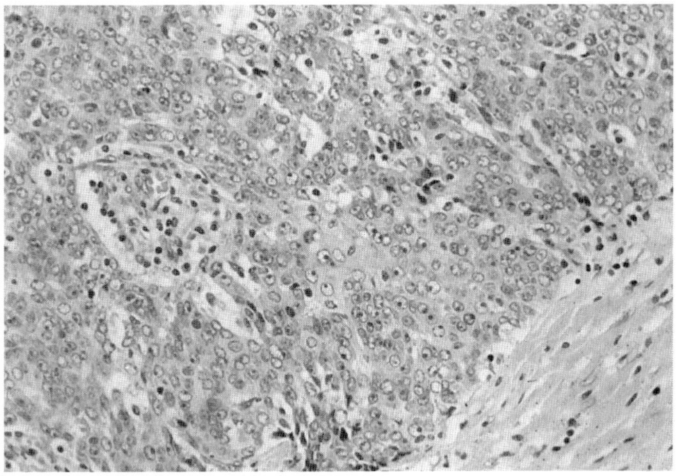

• **FIGURE 3-44** A carcinoma showing thymus-like differentiation in the thyroid was initially interpreted as anaplastic carcinoma, but after a prolonged disease-free interval, the patient presented with this local recurrence. The tumor has squamoid features with a lymphocytic infiltrate.

aggressively clinically than anaplastic carcinomas. About 50% of cases may develop metastases, often months or years following initial treatment.[197,198]

Mucoepidermoid Carcinoma

Mucoepidermoid carcinoma of the thyroid (Fig. 3-45) to some authors represents a variant of papillary carcinoma[242] and to others is a truly unusual entity arising in the thyroid.[243] Papillary carcinomas rarely if ever contain mucin, and certainly not pools of mucin. In any event, some authors have suggested that the ultimobranchial body gives rise to these tumors. Because they occur in any part of the thyroid they may not be related to ultimobranchial body rests, which are found only in the lateral thyroid;[3] occasional intrathyroidal fragments of salivary gland suggest derivation from oral elements.

Another lesion is the so-called sclerosing mucoepidermoid carcinoma of the thyroid associated with eosinophilia.[244] This has been described in association with fibrosing lymphocytic thyroiditis. Even with the presence of extrathyroidal extension and regional metastasis, they behave in an indolent fashion. These lesions are thyroglobulin and calcitonin negative and stain for cytokeratin and mucin. It is unclear why there is such extensive associated eosinophilia. The association of this lesion with the fibrosing type of chronic lymphocytic thyroiditis is also unexplained.

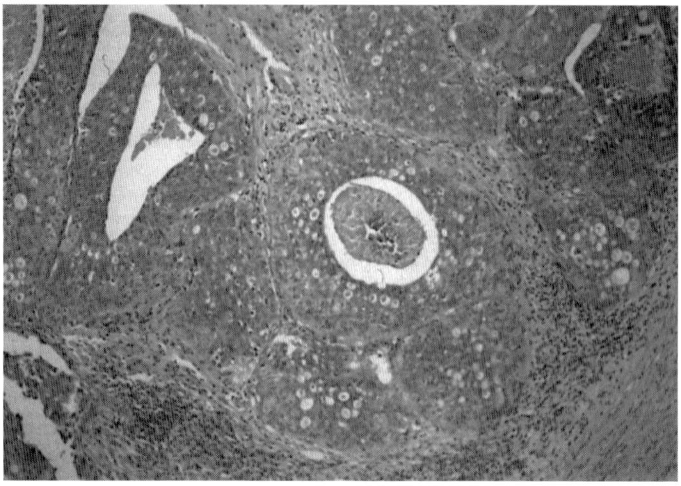

• **FIGURE 3-45** Mucoepidermoid carcinoma of the thyroid resembles mucoepidermoid carcinoma of the salivary gland. Nests of epithelial tumor cells are characterized by mucin production and central necrosis.

METASTATIC CARCINOMA

Metastatic carcinoma to the thyroid results from hematogenous spread of melanoma, breast, lung, kidney, or colon primary lesions or from direct extension of esophageal, laryngeal, or pharyngeal tumors. On FNA, the appearances will reflect the primary tumor (Fig. 3-46); often the malignant cells are admixed with benign follicular cells. These cases rarely come to surgery, but occasionally the diagnosis of metastasis is made histologically. In most cases, the histologic features are characteristic but occasionally, mainly with renal carcinoma, the differential diagnosis of a primary follicular lesion is considered. Immunohistochemical staining is useful in this setting; thyroglobulin immunoreactivity confirms a primary lesion, but the interpretation must also recognize and distinguish diffusion of this antigen from surrounding tissue.[10]

NONEPITHELIAL NEOPLASMS

Lymphomas

Primary thyroid lymphoma usually arises in the setting of autoimmune thyroiditis.[10] Most are of the non-Hodgkin's type and have a B-cell phenotype. The diagnosis is usually made on cytologic examination, which will reveal

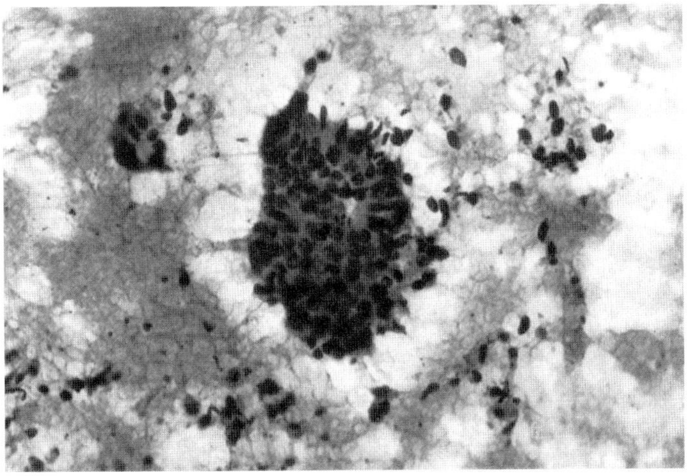

• **FIGURE 3-46** Fine-needle aspiration of metastatic carcinoma involving the thyroid gland reveals the cytologic features of the primary tumor, in this case colonic adenocarcinoma.

monotonous populations of noncohesive large cells that have nuclear atypia and prominent karyorrhexis (Fig. 3-47). The distinction from Hashimoto's thyroiditis can be difficult both on cytologic and histologic evaluation, since the two usually coexist.

While the treatment of choice is usually irradiation, many patients are offered surgical excision to make or confirm the diagnosis and to debulk the lesion. The role of postradiation chemotherapy for localized disease is controversial.

Sarcomas

The thyroid can be the site of various local sarcomas including fibrosarcoma (Fig. 3-48), liposarcoma, leiomyosarcoma, chondrosarcoma, osteosarcoma, and malignant hemangiopericytoma.[10] These lesions are similar to sarcomas elsewhere in the body; however, the diagnosis requires stringent verification. Most primary malignant thyroid tumors with a sarcoma-like appearance are undifferentiated (anaplastic) carcinomas and should be regarded as such in the absence of indisputable proof to the contrary.[89]

Angiosarcoma is a rare tumor that occurs as a primary lesion in the thyroid gland.[245] It is reported to constitute 4% (and in some reports up to 16%)[10] of thyroid malignancies in the European Alpine region, where it typically arises in a gland with multinodular goiter.

The existence of this entity has been considered controversial. Many investigators have suggested that it actually represents a vascular variant of

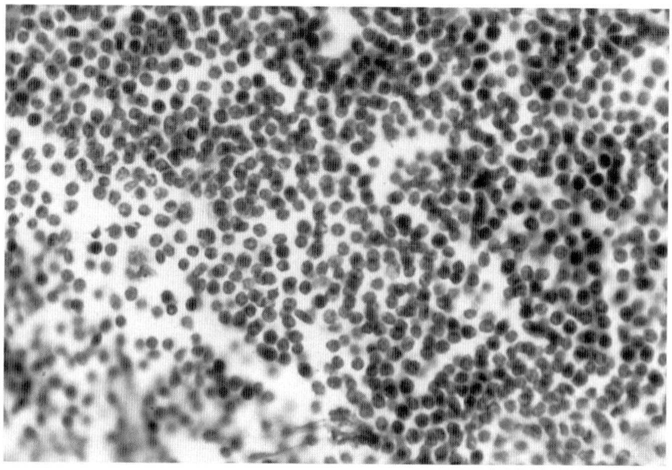

• **FIGURE 3-47** Fine-needle aspiration of a primary thyroid lymphoma reveals monotonous populations of noncohesive cells with nuclear atypia. Immunohistochemistry is useful to confirm the monoclonal nature of this tumor cell population.

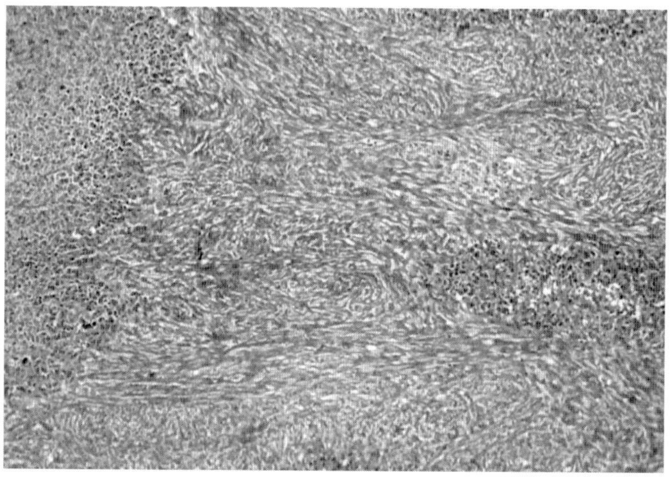

• **FIGURE 3-48** Fibrosarcoma of the thyroid can resemble a spindle cell anaplastic carcinoma; however, immunohistochemical and ultrastructural parameters confirm the mesenchymal nature of the lesion.

anaplastic carcinoma;[246] however, some tumors have been shown to contain factor VIII–related antigen and Weibel-Palade bodies within tumor cells, consistent with endothelial differentiation.[247-249] The distinction of true angiosarcoma from anaplastic carcinoma may be exceedingly difficult,[250] but the clinical implications are of dubious value, since both are highly aggressive and rapidly lethal malignancies.

CONCLUSION

Thyroid nodules are common, and their management can be difficult and controversial. Clearly the pathologist has an important role to play in their evaluation. The use of FNA biopsy has significantly improved our ability to identify specific high-risk disorders and to facilitate their management in an expeditious and cost-effective manner. Patients who require surgery for further confirmation of the disease process rely on the pathologist to correctly characterize their nodules, and pathologists are actively involved in research to clarify the pathogenesis of thyroid disease. Advances in our understanding of the molecular basis of thyroid cancer will allow more accurate characterization of specific subtypes of neoplasia and malignancy, even on single cells obtained by FNA biopsy. This should further enhance the usefulness of this technique and better guide the management of patients with a thyroid nodule.

REFERENCES

1. Harach HR. Solid cell nests of the thyroid. An anatomical survey and immunohistochemical study for the presence of thyroglobulin. Acta Anat 122:249-253, 1985.
2. Beckner ME, Shultz JJ, Richardson T. Solid and cystic ultimobranchial body remnants in the thyroid. Arch Pathol Lab Med 114:1049-1052, 1990.
3. Harach HR, Vujanic GM, Jasani B. Ultimobranchial body nests in human fetal thyroid: An autopsy, histological, and immunohistochemical study in relation to solid cell nests and mucoepidermoid carcinoma of the thyroid. J Pathol 169:465-469, 1993.
4. Harach HR. Solid cell nests of the thyroid. J Pathol 155:191-200, 1988.
5. Janzer RC, Weber E, Hedinger C. The relation between solid cell nests and C cells of the thyroid gland. An immunohistochemical and morphometric investigation. Cell Tissue Res 197:295-312, 1979.
6. Ezzat S, Sarti DA, Cain DR, et al. Thyroid incidentalomas. Prevalence by palpation and ultrasonography. Arch Intern Med 154:1838-1840, 1994.
7. Hedinger C, Williams ED, Sobin LH. The WHO histological classification of thyroid tumors: A commentary on the second edition. Cancer 63:908-911, 1989.
8. LiVolsi VA. Surgical Pathology of the Thyroid. Philadelphia: WB Saunders, 1990.
9. Murray D. The thyroid gland. In Kovacs K, Asa SL, eds. Functional Endocrine Pathology. Boston: Blackwell Scientific Publications, 1991, pp 293-374.
10. Rosai J, Carcangiu ML, DeLellis RA. Tumors of the Thyroid Gland. Atlas of Tumor Pathology, Third Series, Fascicle 5. Washington, DC: Armed Forces Institute of Pathology, 1992.
11. Hamberger JI. Diagnosis of thyroid nodules by fine needle biopsy. J Clin Endocrinol Metab 79:335-339, 1994.
12. Gharib H. Fine needle aspiration biopsy of thyroid nodules. Mayo Clin Proc 69:44-49, 1994.
13. Clark OH. Fine-needle aspiration biopsy and management of thyroid tumors. Am J Clin Pathol 108 (4 Suppl 1):S22-S25, 1997.

14. Guidelines of the Papanicolaou Society of Cytopathology for the examination of fine-needle aspiration specimens from thyroid nodules. The Papanicolaou Society of Cytopathology Task Force on Standards of Practice. Diagn Cytopathol 15:84-89, 1996.
15. Kini SR. Thyroid. New York: Igaku-Shoin, 1996.
16. Hamberger JI, Husain M. Semiquantitative criteria for fine-needle biopsy diagnosis: Reduced false-negative diagnosis. Diagn Cytopathol 4:14-17, 1988.
17. Glant MD. Procurement and processing in fine-needle aspiration biopsy. Cyto-Teleconferencing. American Society of Cytology Handbook, 1989.
18. LiVolsi VA, Merino MJ. Worrisome histologic alterations following fine needle aspiration of the thyroid. Pathol Annu 29:99-120, 1994.
19. Axiotis CA et al. Papillary endothelial hyperplasia in the thyroid following FNA. Arch Pathol Lab Med 115:240-242, 1991.
20. Bronner MP, Hamilton R, LiVolsi VA: Utility of frozen section analysis on follicular lesions of the thyroid. Endocr Pathol 5:154-161, 1994.
21. Chen H, Nicol TL, Udelsman R. Follicular lesions of the thyroid: Does frozen section evaluation alter operative management? Ann Surg 222:101-106, 1995.
22. Irish JC et al. Accuracy of pathologic diagnosis in thyroid lesions. Arch Otolaryngol Head Neck Surg 118:918-922, 1992.
23. Vollenweider I, Hedinger C. Solid cell nests (SCN) in Hashimoto's thyroiditis. Virchows Archiv 412:357-363, 1988.
24. Apel RL et al. Intrathyroidal lymphoepithelial cysts of probable branchial origin. Hum Pathol 25:1238-1242, 1994.
25. Louis DN et al. Multiple branchial cleft-like cysts in Hashimoto's thyroiditis. Am J Surg Pathol 13:45-49, 1989.
26. Volpé R. Lymphocytic (Hashimoto's) thyroiditis. In Werner SC, Ingbar SC, eds. The Thyroid. New York: Harper & Row, 1978, pp 996-1008.
27. Jansson R, Karlsson A, Forsum U. Intrathyroidal HLA-DR expression and T lymphocyte phenotypes in Graves' thyrotoxicosis, Hashimoto's thyroiditis and nodular colloid goitre. Clin Exp Immunol 58:264-272, 1984.
28. Asa SL. The pathology of autoimmune endocrine disorders. In Kovacs K, Asa SL, eds. Functional Endocrine Pathology. Boston: Blackwell Scientific Publications, 1991, pp 961-978.
29. Rees Smith B, McLachlan SM, Furmaniak J. Autoantibodies to the thyrotropin receptor. Endocr Rev 9:106-121, 1988.
30. Friedman NB. Cellular involution in thyroid gland: significance of Hürthle cells in myxedema, exhaustion atrophy, Hashimoto's disease and reaction in irradiation, thiouracil therapy and subtotal resection. J Clin Endocrinol 9:874-882, 1949.
31. Dube VE, Joyce GT. Extreme squamous metaplasia in Hashimoto's thyroiditis. Cancer 27:434-437, 1971.
32. Katzmann JA, Vickery AL: The fibrosing variant of Hashimoto's thyroiditis. Hum Pathol 5:161-170, 1974.
33. Leclerc J et al: In situ immunologic disorders in deQuervain's thyroiditis. In Medeiros-Neto G, Gaitan E, eds. Frontiers in thyroidology. New York: Plenum Publishing, 1986, pp 1365-1368.
34. Volpé R. Subacute (de Quervain's) thyroiditis. Clin Endocrinol Metab 8:81-95, 1979.
35. Studer H, Peter H-J, Gerber H. Natural heterogeneity of thyroid cells: The basis for understanding thyroid function and nodular goiter growth. Endocr Rev 10:125-135, 1989.

36. Aeschimann S et al. Morphological and functional polymorphism within clonal thyroid nodules. J Clin Endocrinol Metab 77:846-851, 1993.
37. Studer H, Ramelli F: Simple goiter and its variants: Euthyroid and hyperthyroid multinodular goiters. Endocr Rev 3:40-61, 1982.
38. Peter HJ et al. Pathogenesis of heterogeneity in human multinodular goiter. A study on growth and function of thyroid tissue transplanted onto nude mice. J Clin Invest 76:1992-2002, 1985.
39. Studer H, Hunziker HR, Ruchti C. Morphologic and functional substrate of thyrotoxicosis caused by nodular goiters. Am J Med 65:227-234, 1978.
40. Drexhage HA et al. Evidence for thyroid growth-stimulating immunoglobulin in some goitrous thyroid diseases. Lancet 2:287-292, 1980.
41. Van der Gaag RD et al. Further studies on thyroid growth-stimulating immunoglobulins in euthyroid nonendemic goiter. J Clin Endocrinol Metab 60:972-979, 1985.
42. Studer H, Peter H-J, Gerber H. Toxic nodular goitre. J Clin Endocrinol Metab 14: 351-372, 1985.
43. Wiener JD, Van der Gaag RD. Autoimmunity and the pathogenesis of localized thyroid autonomy (Plummer's disease). Clin Endocrinol 23:635-642, 1985.
44. Apel RL, Ezzat S, Bapat B, et al. Clonality of thyroid nodules in sporadic goiter. Diag Mol Pathol 4:113-121, 1995.
45. Parma J et al. Diversity and prevalence of somatic mutations in the thyrotropin receptor and Gs alpha genes as a cause of toxic thyroid adenomas. J Clin Endocrinol Metab 82:2695-2701, 1997.
46. Krohn D et al. Clonal origin of toxic thyroid nodules with constitutively activating thyrotropin receptor mutations. J Clin Endocrinol Metab 83:180-184, 1998.
47. Ezzat S et al. Prevalence of activating ras mutations in morphologically characterized thyroid nodules. Thyroid 6:409-416, 1996.
48. Hicks DG et al. Clonal analysis of solitary follicular nodules in the thyroid. Am J Pathol 137:553-562, 1990.
49. Namba H, Matsuo K, Fagin JA. Clonal composition of benign and malignant human thyroid tumors. J Clin Invest 86:120-125, 1990.
50. Evans HL. Encapsulated papillary neoplasms of the thyroid. A study of 14 cases followed for a minimum of 10 years. Am J Surg Pathol 11:592-597, 1987.
51. Carney JA, Ryan J, Goellner JR. Hyalinizing trabecular adenoma of the thyroid gland. Am J Surg Pathol 11:583-591, 1987.
52. Chan JKC, Tse CCH, Chiu HS. Hyalinizing trabecular adenoma-like lesion in multinodular goitre. Histopathology 16:611-614, 1990.
53. Katoh R, Jasani B, Williams ED. Hyalinizing trabecular adenoma of the thyroid. A report of three cases with immunohistochemical and ultrastructural studies. Histopathology 15:211-224, 1989.
54. Bronner MP, LiVolsi VA, Jennings TA. PLAT: Paraganglioma-like adenomas of the thyroid. Surg Pathol 1:383-389, 1988.
55. Sambade C et al. Hyalinizing trabecular adenoma: A misnomer for a peculiar tumor of the thyroid gland. Endocr Pathol 2:83-91, 1991.
56. Treseler PA, Clark OH. Prognostic factors in thyroid carcinoma. Surg Oncol Clin N Am 6:555-598, 1997.
57. Clark OH: Predictors of thyroid tumor aggressiveness. West J Med 165:131-138, 1996.
58. Yamashina M: Follicular neoplasms of the thyroid. Total circumferential evaluation of the fibrous capsule. Am J Surg Pathol 16:392-400, 1992.

59. Jorda M et al. Prognostic factors in follicular carcinoma of the thyroid. Arch Pathol Lab Med 117:631-635, 1993.
60. van Heerden JA et al. Follicular thyroid carcinoma with capsular invasion alone: A non-threatening malignancy. Surgery 112:1130-1138, 1992.
61. Harness JK et al. Follicular carcinoma of the thyroid gland: Trends and treatment. Surgery 96:972-980, 1984.
62. Miettinen M, Karkkainen P: Differential reactivity of HBME-1 and CD15 antibodies in benign and malignant thyroid tumours. Preferential reactivity with malignant tumours. Virchows Arch 429:213-219, 1996.
63. Sack MJ et al. HBME-1 immunostaining in thyroid fine-needle aspirations: A useful marker in the diagnosis of carcinoma. Mod Pathol 10:668-674, 1997.
64. Zedenius J et al. Follicular tumors of the thyroid gland: Diagnosis, clinical aspects and nuclear DNA analysis. World J Surg 16:589-594, 1992.
65. Galera-Davidson H et al. Correlation between automated DNA ploidy measurements of Hürthle cell tumors and their histopathologic and clinical features. Anal Quant Cytol Histol 8:158-167, 1986.
66. McLeod MK et al. Flow cytometric measurements of nuclear DNA and ploidy analysis in Hürthle cell neoplasms of the thyroid. Arch Surg 123:849-854, 1988.
67. Klemi PJ, Joensuu H, Eerola E. DNA aneuploidy in anaplastic carcinoma of the thyroid gland. Am J Clin Pathol 89:154-159, 1988.
68. Samaan NA et al. Pulmonary metastasis of differentiated thyroid carcinoma: Treatment results in 101 patients. J Clin Endocrinol Metab 65:376-380, 1985.
69. DeGroot LJ et al. Morbidity and mortality in follicular thyroid cancer. J Clin Endocrinol Metab 80:2946-2953, 1995.
70. Mizukami Y et al. Distant metastases in differentiated thyroid carcinomas: A clinical and pathologic study. Hum Pathol 21:283-290, 1990.
71. LiVolsi VA, Asa SL. The demise of follicular carcinoma of the thyroid gland. Thyroid 4:233-235, 1994.
72. Shah JP et al. Lobectomy versus total thyroidectomy for differentiated carcinoma of the thyroid: A matched-pair analysis. Am J Surg 166:331-335, 1993.
73. Singer PA et al. Treatment guidelines for patients with thyroid nodules and well-differentiated thyroid cancer. American Thyroid Association. Arch Intern Med 156:2165-2172, 1996.
74. Pasieka JL et al. The incidence of bilateral well-differentiated thyroid cancer found at completion thyroidectomy. World J Surg 16:711-717, 1992.
75. Mazzaferri EL, Jhiang SM. Long-term impact of initial surgical and medical therapy on papillary and follicular thyroid cancer. Am J Med 97:418-428, 1994.
76. Benker G et al. Survival rates in patients with differentiated thyroid carcinoma. Influence of postoperative external radiotherapy. Cancer 65:1517-1520, 1990.
77. Tsang RW et al. The effects of surgery, radioiodine, and external radiation therapy on the clinical outcome of patients with differentiated thyroid carcinoma. Cancer 82: 375-388, 1998.
78. Mazzaferri EL. Thyroid cancer and Graves' disease. J Clin Endocrinol Metab 70:826-829, 1990.
79. Namba H et al. Solitary polyclonal autonomous thyroid nodule: A rare cause of childhood hyperthyroidism. J Clin Endocrinol Metab 72:1108-1112, 1991.
80. Lyons J, Landis CA, Harsh G. Two G protein oncogenes in human endocrine tumors. Science 249:635-639, 1990.

81. Porcellini A et al. Novel mutations of thyrotropin receptor gene in thyroid hyperfunctioning adenomas. Rapid identification by fine needle aspiration biopsy. J Clin Endocrinol Metab 79:657-661, 1994.
82. van Sande J et al. Genetic basis of endocrine disease. Somatic and germline mutations of the TSH receptor gene in thyroid disease. J Clin Endocrinol Metab 80:2577-2585, 1995.
83. Vickery AL. Thyroid papillary carcinoma. Pathological and philosophical controversies. Am J Surg Pathol 7:797-807, 1983.
84. Vickery AL et al. Papillary carcinoma. Semin Diagn Pathol 2:90-100, 1985.
85. Rosai J et al. Papillary carcinoma of the thyroid. Am J Surg Pathol 7:809-817, 1983.
86. Carcangiu ML et al. Papillary carcinoma of the thyroid. A clinicopathologic study of cases treated at the University of Florence, Italy. Cancer 55:805-828, 1985.
87. LiVolsi VA. Papillary neoplasms of the thyroid. Pathologic and prognostic features. Am J Clin Pathol 97:426-434, 1992.
88. Carcangiu ML, Zampi G, Rosai J. Papillary thyroid carcinoma: A study of its many morphologic expressions and clinical correlates. Pathol Annu 20 (Part 1):1-44, 1985.
89. Hedinger C, Williams ED, Sobin LH. Histological typing of thyroid tumours. World Health Organization International Histological Classification of Tumours. Berlin: Springer-Verlag, 1988.
90. Hay ID. Papillary thyroid carcinoma. Endocrinol Metab Clin North Am 19:545-576, 1990.
91. Mazzaferri E, Jhiang S. Long-term follow-up impact of initial surgical and medical therapy on papillary and follicular thyroid cancer. Am J Med 97:418-428, 1994.
92. Hapke MR, Dehner LP. The optically clear nucleus. A reliable sign of papillary carcinoma of the thyroid? Am J Surg Pathol 3:31-38, 1979.
93. Chan JKC, Saw D. The grooved nucleus: A useful diagnostic criterion of papillary carcinoma of the thyroid. Am J Surg Pathol 10:672-679, 1986.
94. Deligeorgi-Politi H. Nuclear crease as a cytodiagnostic feature of papillary thyroid carcinoma in fine-needle aspiration biopsies. Diagn Cytopathol 3:307-310, 1987.
95. Fink A. Occult micropapillary carcinoma associated with benign follicular thyroid disease and unrelated thyroid neoplasms. Mod Pathol 9:816-820, 1996.
96. Sugg SL et al. Distinct multiple ret/PTC gene rearrangements in multifocal papillary thyroid neoplasia. J Clin Endocrin Metab 83:4116-4122, 1998.
97. Brierley JD et al. A comparison of different staging systems predictability of patient outcome. Thyroid carcinoma as an example. Cancer 79:2414-2423, 1997.
98. Noguchi M et al. Clinicopathological studies of minimal thyroid and ordinary thyroid cancers. Jpn J Surg 13:110-117, 1984.
99. Harach HR, Franssila KO, Wasenius V-M. Occult papillary carcinoma of the thyroid. A "normal" finding in Finland. A systematic autopsy study. Cancer 56:531-538, 1985.
100. Yamashita H et al. Thyroid carcinoma in benign thyroid diseases. An analysis from minute carcinoma. Acta Pathol Jpn 35:781-788, 1985.
101. Yamashita H et al. Prognosis of minute carcinoma of the thyroid. Follow-up study of 48 patients. Acta Pathol Jpn 36:1469-1475, 1986.
102. Johannessen JV, Sobrinho-Simoes M. The origin and significance of thyroid psammoma bodies. Lab Invest 43:287-296, 1980.
103. Schröder S et al. Dendritic/Langerhans cells and prognosis in patients with papillary thyroid carcinomas. Am J Clin Pathol 89:295-300, 1988.

104. Volpé R. Immunology of human thyroid disease. In Volpé R, ed. Autoimmune Diseases of the Endocrine System. Boca Raton: CRC Press, 1990, pp 73-240.
105. Leung CS, Hartwick RWJ, Bédard YC. Correlation of cytologic and histologic features in variants of papillary carcinoma of the thyroid. Acta Cytol 37:645-650, 1993.
106. Hawk WA, Hazard JB. The many appearances of papillary carcinoma of the thyroid. Cleve Clin Q 43:207-216, 1976.
107. Chan JK. Papillary carcinoma of the thyroid: Classical and variants. Histol Histopathol 5:241-257, 1990.
108. Mizukami Y et al. Mixed medullary-follicular carcinoma of the thyroid occurring in familial form. Histopathology 22:284-287, 1993.
109. Chen KTK, Rosai J. Follicular variant of thyroid papillary carcinoma: A clinicopathologic study of six cases. Am J Surg Pathol 1:123-130, 1977.
110. Tielens ET et al. Follicular variant of papillary thyroid carcinoma: A clinicopathologic study. Cancer 73:424-431, 1994.
111. Raphael SJ, Apel RL, Asa SL. Detection of high-molecular-weight cytokeratins in neoplastic and non-neoplastic thyroid tumors using microwave antigen retrieval. Mod Pathol 8:870-872, 1995.
112. Santoro M et al. Ret oncogene activation in human thyroid neoplasms is restricted to the papillary cancer subtype. J Clin Invest 89:1517-1522, 1992.
113. Fusco A et al. A new oncogene in human thyroid papillary carcinomas and their lymphnodal metastases. Nature 328:170-172, 1987.
114. Pierotti MA et al. Characterization of an inversion on the long arm of chromosome 10 juxtaposing D10S170 and RET and creating the oncogenic sequence RET/PTC. Proc Natl Acad Sci USA 89:1616-1620, 1992.
115. Minoletti F et al. The two genes generating RET/PTC3 are localized in chromosomal band 10q11.2. Genes Chromosom Cancer 11:51-57, 1994.
116. Sozzi G et al. A t(10;17) translocation creates the RET/PTC2 chimeric transforming sequence in papillary thyroid carcinoma. Genes Chromosom Cancer 9:244-250, 1994.
117. Jhiang SM, Mazzaferri EL. The ret/PTC oncogene in papillary thyroid carcinoma (Review). J Lab Clin Med 123:331-337, 1994.
118. Ishizaka Y et al. Detection of phosphorylated ret/TPC oncogene product in cytoplasm. Oncogene 7:1441-1444, 1992.
119. Jhiang SM et al. Targeted expression of the ret/PTC1 oncogene induces papillary thyroid carcinomas. Endocrinology 137:375-378, 1996.
120. Santoro M et al. Development of thyroid papillary carcinomas secondary to tissue-specific expression of the RET/PTC1 oncogene in transgenic mice. Oncogene 12:1821-1826, 1996.
121. Klugbauer S et al. High prevalence of RET rearrangement in thyroid tumors of children from Belarus after the Chernobyl reactor accident. Oncogene 11:2459-2467, 1995.
122. Nishisho I et al: Distinct pattern of ret oncogene rearrangements in morphological variants of radiation-induced and sporadic thyroid papillary carcinoma in children. Cancer Res 57:1690-1694, 1997.
123. Klugbauer S et al. A new form of RET rearrangement in thyroid carcinomas of children after the Chernobyl reactor acident. Oncogene 13:1099-1102, 1996.
124. Fugazzola L et al. Molecular and biochemical analysis of RET/PTC4, a novel oncogenic rearrangement between RET and ELE1 genes, in a post-Chernobyl papillary thyroid cancer. Oncogene 13:1093-1097, 1996.

125. Klugbauer S et al. Detection of a novel type of RET rearrangement (PTC5) in thyroid carcinomas after Chernobyl and analysis of the involved RET-fused gene RFG5. Cancer Res 58:198-203, 1998.
126. Williams GH et al. RET activation in adult and childhood papillary thyroid carcinoma using a reverse transcriptase-polymerase chain reaction approach on archival-nested material. Br J Cancer 74:585-589, 1996.
127. Jhiang SM et al. Detection of the PTC/retTPC oncogene in human thyroid cancers. Oncogene 7:1331-1337, 1992.
128. Sugg SL et al. ret/PTC-1,-2 and -3 oncogene rearrangements in human thyroid carcinomas: Implications for metastatic potential? J Clin Endocrinol Metab 81:3360-3365, 1996.
129. Mayr B et al. ret/PTC-1, -2, and -3 oncogene rearrangements in human thyroid carcinomas: Implications for metastatic potential? (Letter). J Clin Endocrinol Metab 82:1306-1307, 1997.
130. Viglietto G et al. RET/PTC oncogene activation is an early event in thyroid carcinogenesis. Oncogene 11:1207-1210, 1995.
131. Chan JKC, Tsui MS, Tse CH. Diffuse sclerosing variant of papillary carcinoma of the thyroid: a histological and immunohistochemical study of three cases. Histopathology 11:191-201, 1987.
132. Carcangiu ML, Bianchi S. Diffuse sclerosing variant of papillary thyroid carcinoma: Clinicopathologic study of 15 cases. Am J Surg Pathol 13:1041-1049, 1989.
133. Soares J, Limbert E, Sobrinho-Simoes M. Diffuse sclerosing variant of papillary thyroid carcinoma. A clinicopathologic study of 10 cases. Path Res Pract 185:200-206, 1989.
134. FujimotoY et al. Diffuse sclerosing variant of papillary carcinoma of the thyroid. Cancer 66:2306-2312, 1990.
135. Nikiforov Y, Gnepp DR. Pediatric thyroid cancer after the Chernobyl disaster: Pathomorphologic study of 84 cases (1991-1992) from the Republic of Belarus. Cancer 74:748-766, 1994.
136. Flint A, Davenport RD, Lloyd RV. The tall cell variant of papillary carcinoma of the thyroid gland. Arch Pathol Lab Med 115:169-171, 1991.
137. Hicks MJ, Batsakis JG. Tall cell carcinoma of the thyroid gland. Ann Otol Rhinol Laryngol 102:402-403, 1993.
138. Van den Brekel MWM et al. Prognostic features in tall cell papillary carcinoma and insular thyroid carcinoma. Laryngoscope 107:254-259, 1997.
139. Sobrinho-Simoes M, Nesland JM, Johannessen JV. Columnar cell carcinoma: Another variant of poorly differentiated carcinoma of the thyroid. Am J Clin Pathol 89:264-267, 1988.
140. Evans HL. Columnar-cell carcinoma of the thyroid. A report of two cases of an aggressive variant of thyroid carcinoma. Am J Clin Pathol 85:77-80, 1986.
141. Akslen L, Varhaug JE. Thyroid carcinoma with mixed tall cell and columnar cell features. Am J Clin Pathol 94:442-445, 1990.
142. Johnson TL et al. Prognostic implications of the tall cell variant of papillary thyroid carcinoma. Am J Surg Pathol 12:22-27, 1988.
143. Nesland JM et al. Hürthle cell lesions of the thyroid: A combined study using transmission electron microscopy, scanning electron microscopy and immunocytochemistry. Ultrastruct Pathol 8:131-142, 1985.
144. Sobrinho-Simoes M et al. Hürthle cell and mitochondrion-rich papillary carcinomas of the thyroid gland: An ultrastructural and immunocytochemical study. Ultrastruct Pathol 8:131-142, 1985.

145. Triggs SM, Pearse AGE. Histochemistry of oxidate enzyme systems in the human thyroid with special reference to Askanazy cells. J Pathol Bacteriol 80:353-358, 1960.
146. Clark OH, Gerend PL. Thyrotropin receptor-adenylate cyclase system in Hürthle cell neoplasms. J Clin Endocrinol Metab 39:719-723, 1985.
147. Bronner MP, LiVolsi VA. Oxyphilic (Askanazy/Hürthle cell) tumors of the thyroid. Microscopic features predict biologic behavior. Surg Pathol 1:137-150, 1988.
148. Chen KTK. Fine-needle aspiration cytology of papillary Hürthle-cell tumors of thyroid: A report of three cases. Diagn Cytopathol 7:53-56, 1991.
149. Kini SR et al. Post fine needle aspiration biopsy infarction in thyroid nodules. Mod Pathol 1:48A, 1988.
150. Johnson TL et al. Hürthle cell thyroid tumors: An immuno-histochemical study. Cancer 59:107-112, 1987.
151. Arganini M et al. Hürthle cell tumors: A twenty-five year experience. Surgery 100:1108-1114, 1986.
152. Gosain AK, Clark OH. Hürthle cell neoplasms: Malignant potential. Arch Surg 119:515-519, 1984.
153. Har-El G et al. Hürthle cell carcinoma of the thyroid gland. A tumor of moderate malignancy. Cancer 57:1613-1617, 1986.
154. Thompson NW et al. Hürthle cell lesions of the thyroid gland. Surg Gynecol Obstet 139:555-560, 1974.
155. Flint A, Lloyd RV. Hürthle cell neoplasms of the thyroid gland. Pathol Annu 25:37-52, 1990.
156. Carcangiu ML et al. Follicular Hürthle cell tumors of the thyroid gland. Cancer 68:1944-1953, 1991.
157. Ryan JJ et al. Flow cytometric DNA measurements in benign and malignant Hürthle cell tumors of the thyroid. World J Surg 12:482-487, 1988.
158. Bondeson L, Bondeson A-G, Ljungberg O. Treatment of Hürthle cell neoplasms of the thyroid. Arch Surg 118:1453, 1983.
159. Bondeson L et al. Oxyphil tumors of the thyroid. Ann Surg 194:677-680, 1981.
160. Gundry SR et al. Total thyroidectomy for Hürthle cell neoplasm of the thyroid. Arch Surg 118:529-532, 1983.
161. Watson RG et al. Invasive Hürthle cell carcinoma of the thyroid: Natural history and management. Pathol Annu 59:851-855, 1984.
162. Gardner LW. Hürthle-cell tumors of the thyroid. Arch Pathol 59:372-381, 1955.
163. González-Campora R et al. Hürthle cell and mitochondrion-rich cell tumors. A clinicopathologic study. Cancer 57:1154-1163, 1986.
164. Herrera MF et al. Hürthle cell (oxyphilic) papillary thyroid carcinoma: A variant with more aggressive biologic behavior. World J Surg 16:669-675, 1992.
165. Meissner WA, Adler A. Papillary carcinoma of the thyroid. A study of the pathology of two hundred twenty-six cases. Arch Pathol 66:518-525, 1958.
166. Tscholl-Ducommun J, Hedinger C. Papillary thyroid carcinomas. Morphology and Prognosis. Virchows Arch 396:19-39, 1982.
167. Becker ME, Heffess CS, Oertel JE. Oxyphilic papillary thyroid carcinoma. Am J Clin Pathol 103:280-287, 1995.
168. Hill JH, Werkhaven JA, DeMay RM. Hürthle cell variant of papillary carcinoma of the thyroid gland. Otolaryngol Head Neck Surg 98:338-341, 1988.
169. Berho M, Suster S. The oncocytic variant of papillary carcinoma of the thyroid. A clinicopathologic study of 15 cases. Mod Pathol 7:51, 1994.

170. Barbuto D, Carcangiu ML, Rosai J. Papillary Hürthle cell neoplasms of the thyroid gland: A study of 20 cases (abstract). Lab Invest 62:7A, 1990.
171. Wu P-C et al. Papillary thyroid carcinoma (PTC), oxyphilic cell type: A tumor misclassified by the World Health Organization (WHO)? Clin Res 39:279A, 1991.
172. Apel RL, Asa SL, LiVolsi VA. Papillary Hürthle cell carcinoma with lymphocytic stroma. "Warthin-like tumor" of the thyroid. Am J Surg Pathol 19:810-814, 1995.
173. Carcangiu ML, Zampi G, Rosai J. Poorly differentiated ("insular") thyroid carcinoma. A reinterpretation of Langhans' "wuchernde Struma." Am J Surg Pathol 8:655-668, 1984.
174. Sakamoto A, Kasai N, Sugano H. Poorly differentiated carcinoma of the thyroid. A clinicopathologic entity for a high-risk group of papillary and follicular carcinomas. Cancer 52:1849-1855, 1983.
175. Papotti M et al. Poorly differentiated thyroid carcinomas with primordial cell component. A group of aggressive lesions sharing insular, trabecular, and solid patterns. Am J Surg Pathol 17:291-301, 1993.
176. Samaan NA, Ordoñez NG. Uncommon types of thyroid cancer. Endocrinol Metab Clin North Am 19:637-648, 1990.
177. Aldinger KA et al. Anaplastic carcinoma of the thyroid. A review of 84 cases of spindle and giant cell carcinoma of the thyroid. Cancer 41:2267-2275, 1978.
178. Venkatesh YSS et al. Anaplastic carcinoma of the thyroid. A clinicopathologic study of 121 cases. Cancer 66:321-330, 1990.
179. Shvero J et al. Anaplastic thyroid carcinoma. A clinical, histologic, and immunohistochemical study. Cancer 62:319-325, 1988.
180. Gaffey MJ et al. Anaplastic thyroid carcinoma with osteoclast-like giant cells. A clinicopathologic, immunohistochemical, and ultrastructural study. Am J Surg Pathol 15:160-168. 1991.
181. Ordóñez NG et al. Anaplastic thyroid carcinoma. Immunocytochemical study of 32 cases. Am J Clin Pathol 96:15-24, 1991.
182. Carcangiu ML et al. Anaplastic thyroid carcinoma. A study of 70 cases. Am J Clin Pathol 83:135-158, 1985.
183. Hurlimann J, Gardiol D, Scazziga B. Immunohistology of anaplastic thyroid carcinoma. A study of 43 cases. Histopathology 11:567-580, 1987.
184. LiVolsi VA, Brooks JJ, Arendash-Durand B: Anaplastic thyroid tumors. Immunohistology. Am J Clin Pathol 87:434-442, 1987.
185. Pilotti S et al. A novel panel of antibodies that segregates immunocytochemically poorly differentiated carcinoma from undifferentiated carcinoma of the thyroid gland. Am J Surg Pathol 18:1054-1064, 1994.
186. Fagin JA. Genetic basis of endocrine disease 3. Molecular defects in thyroid gland neoplasia. J Clin Endocrinol Metab 75:1398-1400, 1992.
187. Farid NR, Shi Y, Zou M. Molecular basis of thyroid cancer. Endocr Rev 15:202-232, 1994.
188. Fagin JA et al. High prevalence of mutations of the p53 gene in poorly differentiated human thyroid carcinomas. J Clin Invest 91:179-184, 1993.
189. Donghi R et al. Gene p53 mutations are restricted to poorly differentiated and undifferentiated carcinomas of the thyroid gland. J Clin Invest 91:1753-1760, 1993.
190. Nakamura T et al. p53 gene mutations associated with anaplastic transformation of human thyroid carcinomas. Jpn J Cancer Res 83:1293-1298, 1992.
191. Ito T et al. Unique association of p53 mutations with undifferentiated but not with differentiated carcinomas of the thyroid gland. Cancer Res 52:1369-1371, 1992.

192. Wyllie FS et al. Structure and expression of nuclear oncogenes in multi-stage thyroid tumorigenesis. Br J Cancer 60:561-565, 1989.
193. Hosal SA et al. Immunohistochemical localization of p53 in human thyroid neoplasms: Correlation with biological behavior. Endocr Pathol 8:21-28, 1997.
194. Jossart GH et al. Immunocytochemical detection of p53 in human thyroid carcinomas is associated with mutation and immortalization of cell lines. J Clin Endocrinol Metab 81:3498-3504. 1996.
195. Gaal JM, Horvath E, Kovacs K. Ultrastructure of two cases of anaplastic giant cell tumor of the human thyroid gland. Cancer 35:1273-1279, 1975.
196. Jao W, Gould VE. Ultrastructure of anaplastic (spindle and giant cell) carcinoma of the thyroid. Cancer 35:1280-1292, 1975.
197. Asa SL et al. Primary thyroid thymoma: A distinct clinicopathologic entity. Hum Pathol 19:1463-1467, 1988.
198. Chan JKC, Rosai J. Tumors of the neck showing thymic or related branchial pouch differentiation: A unifying concept. Hum Pathol 22:349-367, 1991.
199. Spires JR, Schwartz MR, Miller RH. Anaplastic thyroid carcinoma. Association with differentiated thyroid cancer. Arch Otolaryngol Head Neck Surg 114:40-44, 1988.
200. Nishiyama RH, Dunn EL, Thompson NW. Anaplastic spindle-cell and giant-cell tumors of the thyroid gland. Cancer 30:113-127, 1972.
201. van der Laan BFAM et al. The association of well-differentiated thyroid carcinoma with insular or anaplastic thyroid carcinoma: Evidence for dedifferentiation in tumor progression. Endocr Pathol 4:215-221, 1993.
202. Bronner MP, LiVolsi VA. Spindle cell squamous carcinoma of the thyroid: An unusual anaplastic tumor associated with tall cell papillary cancer. Mod Pathol 4:637-643, 1991.
203. Yoshida A et al. Proliferative activity in thyroid tumors. Cancer 69:2548-2552, 1992.
204. Kapp DS, LiVolsi VA, Sanders MM. Anaplastic carcinoma following well-differentiated thyroid cancer: Etiological considerations. Yale J Biol Med 5:521-528, 1982.
205. Uribe M et al. Medullary carcinoma of the thyroid gland. Clinical, pathological, and immunohistochemical features with review of the literature. Am J Surg Pathol 9: 577-594, 1985.
206. Valenta LJ et al. Microfollicular thyroid carcinoma with amyloid rich stroma, resembling the medullary carcinoma of the thyroid (MCT). Cancer 39:1573-1586, 1977.
207. Harach HR, Williams ED. Glandular (tubular and follicular) variants of medullary carcinoma of the thyroid. Histopathology 7:83-97, 1983.
208. Nelkin BD et al. The molecular biology of medullary thyroid carcinoma. A model for cancer development and progression. JAMA 261:3130-3135, 1989.
209. Mendelsohn G, Wells SA, Baylin SB. Relationship of tissue carcinoembryonic antigen and calcitonin to tumor virulence in medullary thyroid carcinoma. An immunohistochemical study in early, localized and virulent disseminated stages of disease. Cancer 54:657-662, 1984.
210. Schröder S, Klöppel G. Carcinoembryonic antigen and nonspecific cross-reacting antigen in thyroid cancer. An immunocytochemical study using polyclonal and monoclonal antibodies. Am J Surg Pathol 11:100-108, 1987.
211. Williams ED, Morales AM, Horn RC. Thyroid carcinoma and Cushing's syndrome. A report of two cases with a review of the common features of the non-endocrine tumours associated with Cushing's syndrome. J Clin Pathol 21:129-135, 1968.

212. Birkenhäger JC et al. Medullary thyroid carcinoma: Ectopic production of peptides with ACTH-like, corticotrophin releasing factor-like and prolactin production-stimulating activities. Acta Endocrinol (Copen) 83:280-292, 1976.
213. Goltzman D et al. Adrenocorticotropin and calcitonin in medullary thyroid carcinoma: Frequency of occurrence and localization in the same cell type by immunohistochemistry. J Clin Endocrinol Metab 49:364-369, 1979.
214. Takami H et al. Immunohistochemical study of medullary thyroid carcinoma: Relationship of clinical features to prognostic factors in 36 patients. World J Surg 12:572-579, 1988.
215. Reubi JC et al. Somatostatin receptors and somatostatin content in medullary thyroid carcinomas. Lab Invest 64:567-573, 1991.
216. Lamberts SWJ et al. Somatostatin-receptor imaging in the localization of endocrine tumors. N Engl J Med 323:1246-1249, 1990.
217. Lamberts SWJ, Krenning EP, Reubi JC. The role of somatostatin and its analogs in the diagnosis and treatment of tumors. Endocr Rev 12:450, 1991.
218. Schimke RN, Hartmann WH. Familial amyloid-producing medullary thyroid carcinoma and pheochromocytoma: A distinct genetic entity. Ann Intern Med 63:1027-1037, 1965.
219. Goodfellow PJ. Mapping the inherited defects associated with multiple endocrine neoplasia type 2A, multiple endocrine neoplasia type 2B, and familial medullary thyroid carcinoma to chromosome 10 by linkage analysis. Endocrinol Metab Clin North Am 23:177-185, 1994.
220. Carson NL et al. The mutation for medullary thyroid carcinoma with parathyroid tumors (mTC with PTs) is closely linked to the centromeric region of chromosome 10. Am J Hum Genet 47:946-951, 1990.
221. Lairmore TC et al. Low incidence of loss of chromosome 10 in sporadic and hereditary human medullary thyroid carcinoma. Cancer Res 49:4114-4119, 1989.
222. Mulligan LM et al. Germ-line mutations of the RET proto-oncogene in multiple endocrine neoplasia type 2A. Nature 363:458-460, 1993.
223. Hofstra RMW et al. A mutation in the RET proto-oncogene associated with multiple endocrine neoplasia type 2B and sporadic medullary thyroid carcinoma. Nature 367:375-376, 1994.
224. Marsh DJ et al. A rapid screening method for the detection of mutations in the RET proto-oncogene in multiple endocrine neoplasia type 2A and familial medullary thyroid carcinoma families. Genomics 23:477-479, 1994.
225. Santoro M et al. The ret proto-oncogene is consistently expressed in human pheochromocytomas and thyroid medullary carcinomas. Oncogene 6:339-342, 1991.
226. Zedenius J et al. Mutations of codon 918 in the RET proto-oncogene correlate to poor prognosis in sporadic medullary thyroid carcinomas. J Clin Endocrinol Metab 80:3088-3090, 1995.
227. Moley JF et al. Low frequency of ras gene mutations in neuroblastomas, pheochromocytomas, and medullary thyroid cancers. Cancer Res 51:1596-1599, 1991.
228. Yang KP, Castillo SG, Nguyen CV. C-myc, N-ras, c-erb B: Lack of amplification or rearrangement in human medullary thyroid carcinoma and a derivative cell line. Anticancer Res 10:189-192, 1990.
229. Yana I, Nakamura T, Shin E. Inactivation of the p53 gene is not required for tumorigenesis of medullary thyroid carcinoma or pheochromocytoma. Jpn J Cancer Res 83:1113-1116, 1992.

230. Wolfe HJ, Melvin KEW, Cervi-Skinner SJ. C-cell hyperplasia preceding medullary thyroid carcinoma. N Engl J Med 289:437-441, 1973.
231. DeLellis RA, Wolfe HJ. The pathobiology of the human calcitonin (C)-cell: A review. Pathol Annu 16:25-52, 1981.
232. Albores-Saavedra J et al. C-cell hyperplasia in thyroid tissue adjacent to follicular cell tumors. Hum Pathol 19:795-799, 1988.
233. Biddinger PW, Brennan MF, Rosen PP. Symptomatic C-cell hyperplasia associated with chronic lymphocytic thyroiditis. Am J Surg Pathol 15:599-604, 1991.
234. Scopsi L et al. C-cell hyperplasia accompanying thyroid diseases other than medullary carcinoma: an immunocytochemical study by means of antibodies to calcitonin and somatostatin. Mod Pathol 4:297-304, 1991.
235. Libbey NP, Nowakowski KJ, Tucci JR. C-cell hyperplasia of the thyroid in a patient with goitrous hypothyroidism and Hashimoto's thyroiditis. Am J Surg Pathol 13:71-77, 1989.
236. LiVolsi VA. Mixed thyroid carcinoma: A real entity? Lab Invest 57:237-239, 1987.
237. Holm R et al. Concurrent production of calcitonin and thyroglobulin by the same neoplastic cells. Ultrastruct Pathol 10:241-248, 1986.
238. Holm R et al. Medullary thyroid carcinoma with thyroglobulin immunoreactivity. A special entity? Lab Invest 57:258-268, 1987.
239. Apel RL et al. A metastasizing composite carcinoma of the thyroid with distinct medullary and papillary components. Arch Pathol Lab Med 118:1143-1147, 1994.
240. González-Cámpora R et al. Concurrence of a symptomatic encapsulated follicular carcinoma, an occult papillary carcinoma and a medullary carcinoma in the same patient. Histopathology 21:380-382, 1992.
241. Pastolero GC, Coire CI, Asa SL. Concurrent medullary and papillary carcinomas of thyroid with lymph node metastases. Am J Surg Pathol 20:245-250, 1996.
242. Miranda R, Myint MA, Gnepp DR. Composite follicular variant of papillary carcinoma and mucoepidermoid carcinoma of the thyroid. Am J Surg Pathol 19:1209-1215, 1995.
243. Sambade C et al. Mucoepidermoid carcinoma of the thyroid revisited. Surg Pathol 3:271-280, 1990.
244. Chan JKC et al. Sclerosing mucoepidermoid thyroid carcinoma with eosinophilia. A distinctive low-grade malignancy arising from the metaplastic follicles of Hashimoto's thyroiditis. Am J Surg Pathol 15:438-448, 1991.
245. Vollenweider I et al. Malignant haemangioendothelioma of the thyroid, immunohistochemical evidence of heterogeneity. Path Res Pract 184:376-381, 1989.
246. Mills SE, Stallings RG, Austin MB. Angiomatoid carcinoma of the thyroid gland. Anaplastic carcinoma with follicular and medullary features mimicking angiosarcoma. Am J Clin Pathol 86:674-678, 1986.
247. Tötsch M et al. Malignant hemangioendothelioma of the thyroid. Its immunohistochemical discrimination from undifferentiated thyroid carcinoma. Am J Surg Pathol 14:69-74, 1990.
248. Tanda F et al. Angiosarcoma of the thyroid: A light, electron microscopic and histoimmunological study. Hum Pathol 19:742-745, 1988.
249. Beer TW. Malignant thyroid haemangioendothelioma in a non-endemic goitrous region, with immunohistochemical evidence of a vascular origin. Histopathology 20:539-541, 1992.
250. Eusebi V et al. Keratin-positive epithelioid angiosarcoma of thyroid. A report of four cases. Am J Surg Pathol 14:737-747, 1990.

CHAPTER

4

Occult Microcancer and Clinical Cancer

HIROTO YAMASHITA, M.D., Ph.D.

Since Graham's first report in 1928,[1] the presence of clinically silent cancer of the thyroid[2] has become well recognized. It is found in the thyroid tissues removed for various benign thyroid lesions (incidental cancer), in nodal metastasis (occult cancer), and in autopsy studies (latent cancer). This cancer is usually small in size and is also called microcancer, which is less than or equal to 10 mm in diameter.[3] We define thyroid cancer larger than 10 mm as *clinical cancer.* In this chapter we compare the differences between microcancers and clinical cancers to better understand the development of clinical thyroid cancers.

RATE OF INCIDENCE

One of the main differences between thyroid microcancers and thyroid clinical cancers is their rate of incidence. The incidence of thyroid cancer is different from country to country; this is related to environmental factors,[4-8] periods of the study,[9] and the methods used for the study.[10] Clinical cancer is rare, ranging from 0.5 to 10 persons per 100,000 people.[11] Thyroid microcancers, in contrast, are common, ranging from 1.5%[12] to

35.6%[13] in autopsy studies. In Japan, the incidence of thyroid microcancer is about 10% in autopsy studies,[14-15] and the incidence of clinical thyroid cancer is about 0.2% in mass screening studies.[16-18] We can thus assume that in this population only 2% of all thyroid microcancers develop into clinical cancers. The development of microcancer seems related to gender, since the incidence of clinical thyroid cancer is three to six times higher in women.[19-20] On the other hand, the incidence of thyroid microcancer in men has been reported to be almost equal to[14, 21-22] or slightly higher than that in women.[13, 23] However, the factors that cause microcancer to develop into clinical cancer and inhibit the growth of microcancer have not yet been identified.

RELATIVE INCIDENCE OF HISTOLOGICALLY CLASSIFIED THYROID CANCER

Histologically, papillary carcinoma accounts for most clinical and microcancers. However, the presence of follicular, undifferentiated, and medullary carcinoma and malignant lymphoma is also well documented in clinical cancer.[3,24] There are fewer reports regarding microscopic-sized follicular,[25-28] medullary,[28-39] and undifferentiated carcinoma[40] and malignant lymphoma.[27,41]

To compare the relative incidence of histologically classified cancer in microcancer and clinical cancer, we reclassified histologic specimens obtained from 5752 patients with thyroid cancer according to the latest World Health Organization histologic typing guidelines for thyroid tumors.[3] These patients received their primary curative treatment at the Noguchi Thyroid Clinic and Hospital Foundation between 1966 and 1996. When necessary, serial sections were stained with hematoxylin and eosin (HE) and/or immunostained with antithyroglobulin,[42] anticalcitonin,[31,43] antithyroid peroxidase,[44,45] JT-95,[45-47] and anti-LCA antibodies.[48-49] When histologically different types of cancer were present in a patient, they were counted separately. However, when more than two cancer nodules of the same histologic type were present, they were counted only once.

The incidence of histologically classified microcancer and clinical cancer is shown in Table 4-1. Sixty-six patients with clinical cancer and 38 patients with microcancers had two histologically different cancers at the same time. The incidence of papillary, follicular, medullary, and undifferentiated cancer and malignant lymphoma in the microcancers was 1844, 131, 10, 0, and 1, respectively. In clinical cancers, the numbers are 3182, 438, 57, 69, and 122, respectively.

TABLE 4-1 Relative Incidence of Histologically Documented Thyroid Cancer (Total Cases)

	Clinical Cancer		Microcancer	
	Incidence	Percent	Incidence	Percent
Papillary	3182	82	1844	93
Follicular	438	11	131	7
Lymphoma	122	3	1	
Undifferentiated	69	2	0	
Medullary	57	1	10	0.5
Squamous cell	2		0	
TOTAL	3870		1986	

Papillary Carcinoma

The relative incidence of papillary carcinoma was the highest among the clinical cancers (82%) and microcancers (93%). When the incidence of each cancer among the clinical cancers was compared with that of the microcancers in Table 4-1, the incidence of clinical papillary carcinoma was lower than that of papillary microcancer ($p < 0.01$). In other studies, the incidence of papillary carcinoma has been reported to be lower in clinical cancer than in microcancer.[14-17] Since most, if not all, clinical cancers presumably develop from microcancers, the higher incidence of papillary carcinoma in microcancer suggests a slower growth rate of the papillary microcarcinomas than other microcancers.

Medullary Carcinoma

The relative incidence of medullary carcinoma in the present series was 1.4% in clinical cancer and 0.5% in microcancer groups. Four medullary microcarcinomas coexisted with papillary microcarcinomas. Ten patients, including two with microcarcinomas, were found from examination of family members of de novo patients having a RET proto-oncogene germline point mutation. Therefore one third of the clinical medullary carcinomas and one fifth of the medullary microcarcinoma cases in the present series were hereditary forms.

It is well known that the relative incidence of clinical medullary carcinoma in thyroid malignancies in Japan is lower (about 1%)[20,50] than in Western countries (up to 10%).[30,51-54] The relative incidence of medullary microcarcinoma has been reported to be 10% and 1.6% in Sweden and Germany.[32,36] Whether the incidence of medullary microcarcinoma differs from country to country, like papillary and follicular carcinomas, warrants further study.

Malignant Lymphoma

Primary malignant lymphoma of the thyroid accounts for about 2% to 5% of all thyroid clinical cancers.[55-59] In the present series, all the malignant lymphomas coexisted with chronic thyroiditis and the relative incidence of malignant lymphoma in clinical cancer was 3.3%, consistent with former reports. However, in microcancer, the incidence of malignant lymphoma was very low (one case out of 1986 cases of thyroid microcancers). This low incidence of lymphoma in microcancers might be attributed to a failure to diagnose the lesion, because it sometimes is difficult to differentiate histologically between thyroid malignant lymphoma and chronic thyroiditis.[60-64] However, from analysis of the background lesions coexisting with the microcancers, we concluded that this low incidence was probably not completely the result of failure to detect lymphoma, but rather to the preoperative selection of patients. As mentioned, thyroid lymphoma coexists with chronic thyroiditis.[63,65-69] According to Aozasa,[70] the incidence of malignant lymphoma among patients with chronic thyroiditis is 0.1% (8/5592) (95% confidence interval 0.07 to 0.28).[71] In the present study, among 1948 patients with microcancers, only 188 were diagnosed as having chronic thyroiditis simultaneously. From these figures, the expected number of patients with malignant lymphoma among the patients with microcancers in the present series is 0.3 (95% confidence interval 0.1 to 0.53),[71] which is consistent with the present results. Therefore the low incidence of malignant lymphoma in the present series of microcancers was related to the small number of patients with chronic thyroiditis. Our studies and others document that malignant lymphomas rarely arise in the thyroid gland without the presence of chronic thyroiditis.

Undifferentiated Carcinoma

In the present series, the relative incidence of clinical undifferentiated carcinoma was 1.8%, whereas no undifferentiated carcinomas were found in the microcancer groups. This low incidence is not because lesions were overlooked: undifferentiated carcinoma is easy to recognize histologically because of its marked cellular and structural atypism. There is no information to suggest that undifferentiated carcinomas arise from benign thyroid nodules: therefore absence of undifferentiated microcarcinomas in our series is not because of nondetection nor related to the preoperative selection of the patients, but to the paucity of patients with the disease. In the literature, to our knowledge, only one case of undifferentiated microcarcinoma, 8 mm in diameter, has been reported.[40] In that case, undifferentiated microcarcinoma coexisted with a differentiated microcarcinoma. Therefore there have been no reports of undifferentiated microcarcinoma composed solely of undifferentiated cancer cells until now.

Sugitani et al.[72] reported that papillary microcarcinomas did not have overexpression of p53 protein. An overexpression of p53 protein or p53 gene mutation has been found in many undifferentiated carcinomas and is thought to be important in their development.[73-78] Since undifferentiated carcinomas usually coexist with differentiated carcinomas[79-82] and occasionally occur in patients who have had well-differentiated carcinoma,[82-84] many believe that undifferentiated carcinomas arise from preexisting differentiated carcinomas. The absence of undifferentiated carcinoma in the microcancer supports this idea.

HISTOLOGIC DIFFERENCES

The histologic criteria used for the diagnosis of microcancers are the same as those used for clinical cancers, although there are slight differences. A histologic finding, almost exclusively observed in microcarcinomas, is stromal sclerosis. Thyroid carcinomas with marked stromal fibrous sclerosis are called *sclerosing carcinomas.*[85] In clinical carcinoma, sclerosing carcinomas have been found to be very rare,[85] whereas in microcarcinomas, the incidence is high, ranging from 21% to 41%.[22,27,86-87] It has been reported to be higher in smaller microcarcinomas (less than 5 mm in diameter) than larger microcarcinomas (larger than 5 mm in diameter).[22] Therefore this type of microcarcinoma seems to grow extremely slowly and usually remains as a microcarcinoma throughout its natural history. Some may change to a fibrous nodule without cancer cells. The occasional finding of psammoma bodies in fibrous nodules without cancer cells suggests the spontaneous regression of papillary carcinomas.

Papillary Carcinoma

Papillary carcinoma is diagnosed by the presence of papillary structures and/or characteristic nuclear findings, such as intranuclear cytoplasmic inclusions or nuclear grooving. Immunohistologically, no differences were reported between papillary microcarcinomas and clinical papillary carcinomas in the location of cytoskeletal proteins, thyroglobulin,[88] thyroid peroxidase,[44-45] and JT-95.[45-47] Metastasis in the regional lymph nodes was also noted in patients with papillary microcarcinomas.[2, 89-92]

In clinical papillary carcinoma, the presence of papillary structures is one of the main diagnostic findings; therefore a papillary carcinoma solely composed of follicular structures is called a *follicular variant* of papillary carcinoma.[93] In papillary microcarcinomas, however, not the papillary structure but the nuclear findings, such as ground-glass appearance, large size, paleness, irregular outline, deep grooving, pseudoinclusion, and overlapping arrangement,[3,24] were more helpful in making a diagnosis (Fig. 4-1). This is because as Harach et al.[13] already reported the smallest papillary carcinomas are composed almost solely of follicles. Yamamoto et al.[15] also reported that papillary microcarcinomas less than 1 mm in diameter showed follicular growth patterns, whereas 70% of those larger than 3 mm in diameter showed papillary growth patterns. In clinical papillary carcinomas, papillary structures, follicular structures, and poorly differentiated structures[94-95] are observed histologically, although their mixing ratio is variable. In the present series, there were no poorly differentiated microcarcinomas. From these, we can conclude that when papillary carcinomas proliferate, they first grow as a follicle-forming tumor, then the papillae formation follows, and finally poorly developed patterns emerge. Sakamoto et al.[94] stated that the prognosis for patients with poorly differentiated carcinoma (thyroid carcinoma with poorly differentiated structure) was poorer than that of patients with well-differentiated carcinoma. The present study supports their opinion that when other prognostic factors are the same, poorly differentiated carcinomas are a late stage of papillary carcinoma.

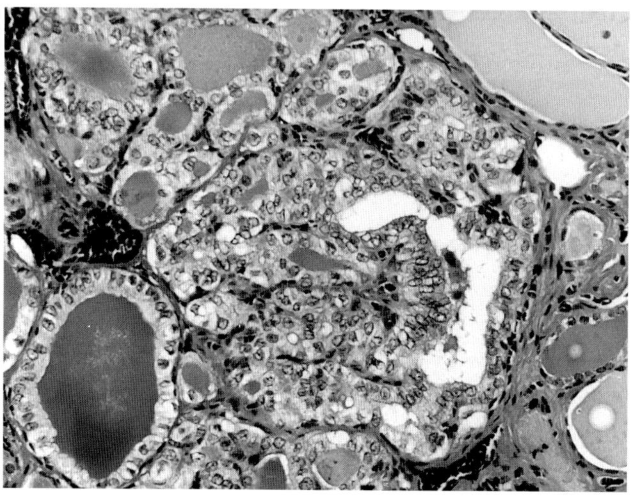

• **FIGURE 4-1** Papillary microcarcinoma. In microcarcinoma, it is not the papillary structure but the nuclear change, such as the vesicular nucleus, that is useful for diagnosis. Maximum diameter 0.75 mm. (Hematoxylin and eosin ×400.)

Follicular Carcinoma

Histologic criteria for making the diagnosis of follicular carcinoma are capsular invasion and/or vascular invasion.[3] In the present cases, no vascular invasion was found in the small encapsulated follicular tumors. Therefore diagnosis of follicular microcarcinoma was made by the presence of capsular invasion alone. Interpretation of capsular invasion is at times difficult.[24] In the present series, capsular invasion was divided into four types. In type 1, tumor cells had completely invaded the capsular wall (the same as in clinical follicular carcinoma), and most cases showed extracapsular deposits (tumor cells situated on the outside rim of the capsule—65 nodules) (Fig. 4-2).

In type 2, tumor cells showed penetration into but not through the capsule (incomplete capsular invasion) and extracapsular deposits (28 nodules). In type 3, only extracapsular deposits were observed (23 nodules) (Fig. 4-3). Follicular microcarcinomas showing marked sclerosis and/or repeated encapsulation were subclassified as type 4 (18 nodules) (Fig. 4-4). This type was reported to be a follicular carcinoma of unusual appearance by Bondeson and Ljungberg in 1981.[32] We have concluded that any encapsulated follicular nodules with one of the four types of capsular invasion described belong to the follicular carcinoma group, although others might not agree with our views. We believe that, at least, encapsulated follicular neoplasms with type 1 invasion (complete capsular invasion) can be diagnosed as a follicular microcarcinoma without further discussion.

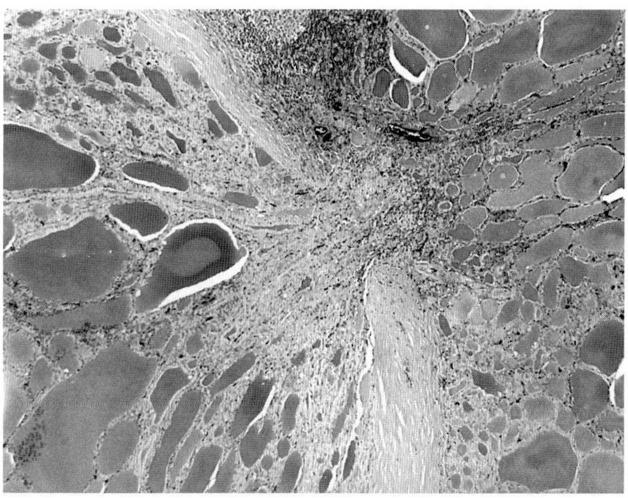

• **FIGURE 4-2** Follicular microcarcinoma, type 1. Capsular and extracapsular invasion can be seen. Maximum diameter 2.5 mm. (Hematoxylin and eosin ×100.)

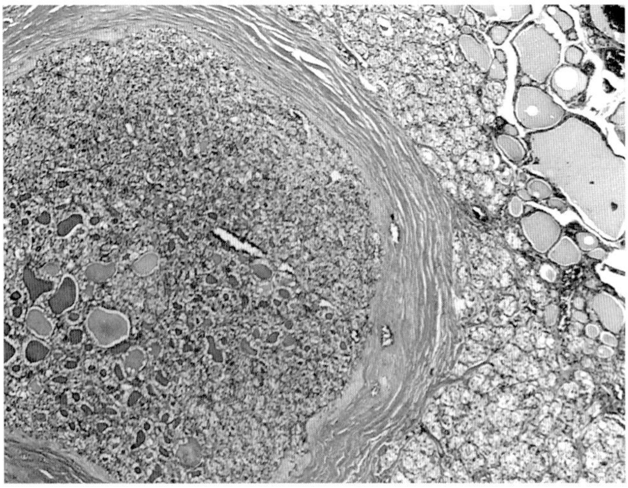

• **FIGURE 4-3** Follicular microcarcinoma, type 3. No capsular invasion, but extracapsular tumor cell deposit can be seen. Maximum diameter 1.8 mm. (Hematoxylin and eosin ×200.)

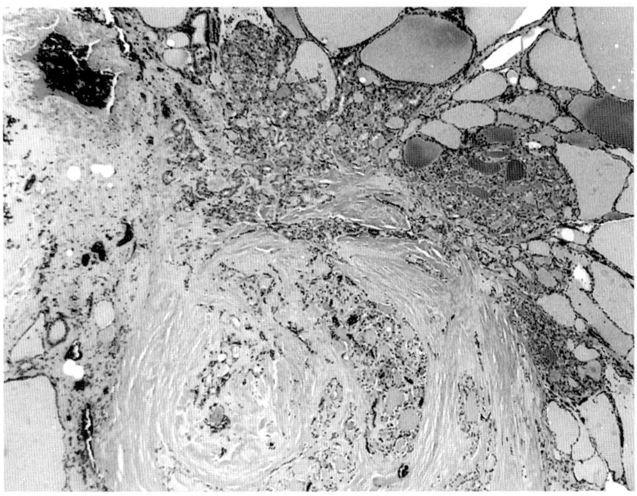

• **FIGURE 4-4** Follicular microcarcinoma, type 4 (unusual appearance). Follicular microcarcinoma with an unusual appearance shows marked sclerosis and/or repeated encapsulation. Maximum diameter 2.0 mm. (Hematoxylin and eosin ×100.)

Some experts suggest that follicular carcinomas develop from follicular adenomas. The notion of transition from follicular microcarcinoma to clinical carcinoma, to our knowledge, has not been considered.[96-97] The adenoma-carcinoma sequence theory for the thyroid follicular tumor arises partly from the paucity of follicular microcarcinomas, and also partly from analogy

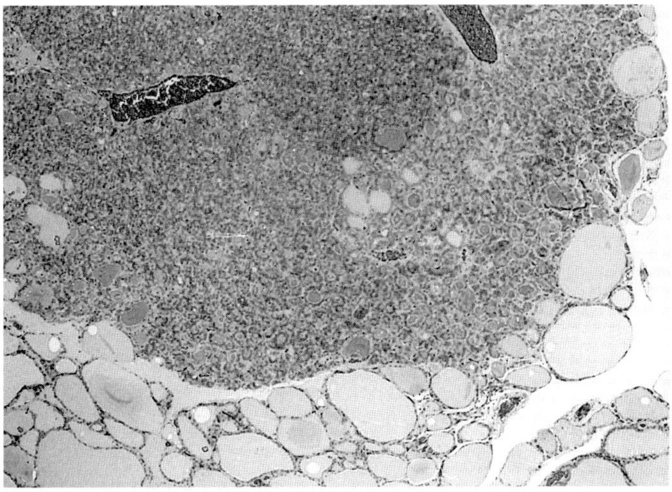

• **FIGURE 4-5** Follicular nodule with invasion. Follicle cells show monotonous proliferation without encapsulation and invasive growth to the surrounding tissue. Maximum diameter 3.1 mm. (Hematoxylin and eosin ×100.)

with the adenoma-carcinoma sequence in colorectal tumors.[98-101] The presence of follicular microcarcinomas in our series suggests that if follicular carcinomas develop from follicular adenomas, the transition must have occurred at the time of the microadenoma (10 mm or less in diameter). Some follicular carcinoma may also arise from follicular adenomas.

Follicular nodules without encapsulation were also observed. These lesions were composed of a rather homogeneous proliferation of small follicles containing follicle cells with hyperchromatic nuclei. Although rare, mitotic figures were observed. These follicular nodules resembled the hypercellular foci of follicle cells found in the adenomatous goiters and in follicular adenomas.[24] These follicular nodules, however, were different from adenomatous nodules, which are usually composed of various-sized follicles with a euchromatic nucleus. They also differ from papillary carcinomas because of their absence of papillary structures or the characteristic nuclear changes present in papillary carcinomas. Moreover, they differ from follicular carcinomas and follicular adenomas, because they are not encapsulated. Most of the follicular nodules show clear demarcation from the surrounding tissue, but some show invasive proliferation (Fig. 4-5). Such lesions might possibly be an early form of follicular carcinoma. Since the introduction of iodine supplementation to food supplies in endemic goiter areas such as Switzerland, the relative incidence of follicular carcinoma has declined while papillary carcinoma has increased.[102] Whether or not follicular microcarcinomas and other related diseases have decreased and whether or not the ras oncogene, which is relatively specific for the development of follicular carcinoma in some studies,[97] is activated in these noncancerous nodules must be studied further to clarify the early forms of the follicular carcinoma.

C-Cell Hyperplasia

C-cell hyperplasia is a noninvasive proliferation of thyroid C cells. It is defined as a multifocal proliferative condition characterized by an increased mass of C cells within the follicles of the thyroid gland.[24] The presence of additional C-cell hyperplasia has been used as a histologic marker to distinguish sporadic and heritable forms of medullary thyroid carcinoma.[24]

Apart from medullary carcinoma, C-cell hyperplasia has been reported in the thyroid gland without medullary carcinoma.[103,104] Guyetant et al.[105] reported that 20% of patients with chronic lymphocytic thyroiditis had a C-cell hyperplasia.

Perry et al.[106] stated that the C-cell hyperplasia found in hereditary medullary carcinoma was different from the C-cell hyperplasia found in the thyroid gland without medullary carcinoma. They called the former a neoplastic C-cell hyperplasia and the latter a physiologic C-cell hyperplasia, because neoplastic C cells were recognized with certainty on HE stain and indistinguishable from those of medullary thyroid carcinoma on HE stain and immunostain with anticalcitonin antibody. On the other hand, physiologic C cells were not recognized with certainty on HE stain but were recognized with the immunostain and were indistinguishable from those of normal C cells on HE stain and immunostain, except for their large number.

We examined the presence of the neoplastic C-cell hyperplasia in 55 cases of medullary thyroid carcinoma, including 30 sporadic medullary thyroid cancers and more than 200 cases of nonmedullary thyroid lesions, including 32 cases of chronic lymphocytic thyroiditis. We found additional neoplastic C-cell lesions (including C-cell hyperplasia) in 46 patients among the 55 patients with medullary thyroid carcinoma. Neoplastic C-cell hyperplasia was found even in medullary carcinoma patients without germline or somatic point mutations of the RET oncogene. We found no neoplastic C cells in patients with nonmedullary thyroid lesions. Assuming the incidence of 20% C-cell hyperplasia in chronic thyroiditis,[105] the expected number of patients having C-cell hyperplasia in 32 patients with chronic thyroiditis would be four to nine (95% confidence interval),[71] which is different from our observation. We therefore concluded that C-cell hyperplasia found in medullary thyroid carcinoma differs from the C-cell hyperplasia found in nonmedullary thyroid lesions.[107]

ASSOCIATED BENIGN LESIONS

Incidental cancer, by its definition, is found in thyroid glands with benign pathology. In our previous study using surgical material, we found that the incidence of microcancer in the thyroids of patients with adenomatous goiter was 15% (adenomatous goiter with clinical cancer was not included). This frequency was the highest among other benign lesions such as follicular adenoma and Graves' disease.[108] Yamashita et al.[109] reported that the incidence of microcancer in the thyroids with adenomatous goiter was 19%. As surgically removed thyroid tissues were used in these two reports, the preceding figures might be influenced by the preoperative selection of patients, the total amount of thyroid tissue that was removed, and the thoroughness of the histologic examination. Because the patients who have thyroid cancer, or have a nodule suspicious for cancer, are more apt to undergo surgical therapy and have more thyroid tissue removed, it is more likely that a microcancer, if present, would be identified. In an autopsy series, where these factors seem to have no influence, Yamamoto et al.[15] reported that the incidence of papillary microcancer in adenomatous goiters was 15%, a higher rate than that found in other benign diseases. On the contrary, using surgical material, Fink et al.[23] reported that there was no difference in the incidence rate of microcancer in the thyroids with benign thyroid diseases. Whether or not the incidence of microcancer in the thyroid with adenomatous goiter is higher than that in the thyroid with other benign diseases warrants further studies.

As just described, the occurrence of malignant lymphoma in chronic thyroiditis is well known. We found that an incidence of microcarcinoma was also higher in chronic thyroiditis.[108] However, we considered that this higher incidence of microcarcinoma was probably the result of the preoperative selection of the patients; we believe this because the patients with chronic thyroiditis undergo surgery when the thyroid gland becomes too large, painful, or is to be suspected to have a malignancy. In the autopsy series, Yamamoto et al.[15] did not find a high incidence of microcarcinoma in patients with chronic thyroiditis. Their findings seem to support our interpretation that a high incidence of microcarcinoma in patients with chronic thyroiditis is related to the preoperative selection of these patients for thyroidectomy.

PROGNOSIS

In clinical cancers, risk factors include undifferentiated carcinoma, the presence of distant metastasis, nodal involvement, local invasion, large tumor (greater than or equal to 4 cm), and older age (over 45 years).[110] Undifferentiated carcinoma is rare in microcancers, as described earlier. The presence of distant metastasis is also a risk factor for patients with microcancers.[25,26,111,112] However, patients with microcancers who have distant metastases at their first surgery are uncommon, and we had no such patients in the present series.

In 1990, Satge et al.[25] summarized 34 cases of small thyroid cancer (less than 15 mm in diameter) that either showed bloodborne metastases or were the cause of death. Their investigation documents that vascular or capsular invasion, lack of lymphoid infiltrate, and large cervical node metastases were risk factors for more aggressive occult cancers.[25] In one study, capsular invasion alone was not considered a risk factor for follicular carcinoma.[113] Therefore this study suggests that nodal involvement, vascular invasion, lack of lymphoid infiltrate, and old age—but not capsular invasion—are risk factors for patients with microcancer.

Most reports regarding patients with microcancers, including the present report, support a most favorable prognosis for these patients.[114] Sporadically reported fatal cases of microcancer seem to be related to elderly patients and to the presence of clinically detectable nodal metastasis (gross nodal metastasis) during the first surgery.[25] We previously reported that it was not intranodal metastasis (cancer cells contained within the lymph nodes), but extracapsular invasion through the lymph node capsule that was a risk factor for the patients with clinical papillary carcinoma.[115]

To examine the risk factors for patients with microcancers, we performed a follow-up study of 1743 patients with microcancer who had undergone primary surgery with a curative intent at the Noguchi Thyroid Clinic and Hospital Foundation between 1970 and 1994. Follow-up periods were 11.2 ± 6.32 years (mean standard deviation). Fifty-nine patients were followed for less than 3 years. Among 1743 patients, we found 31 patients with recurrence and 75 patients died. Sites of primary recurrence in the 31 patients were contralateral thyroid bed (14 patients), ipsilateral and contralateral neck nodes (eight cases each), paratracheal node (eight cases), ipsilateral thyroid bed (five cases), bones (four cases), and mediastinum (one case). More than two primary recurrence sites were noted in 13 patients. Four of the 75 patients who died were considered to have died of thyroid cancer, 63 of unrelated diseases, and in eight patients, the cause of death was unknown. One of the four patients who died of thyroid cancer developed metastasis of the spinal cord, one died from a hemorrhage of a rupture of a recurrent neck tumor, and the remaining two patients had both mediastinal and/or pulmonary metastases. Since the number of patients who died of thyroid cancer was only four among 1743 patients, and thyroid cancer-related death occurred only after the recurrence, we examined the risk factors for tumor recurrence.

TABLE 4-2 Manner of Nodal Excision and Recurrence of Microcancer

Manner of Excision	Total No. of Patients	No. of Patients With Recurrence	Recurrence Rate (%)
No nodes excised	1419	17	1.2
Prophylactic	234	5	2.1
Therapeutic	90	9	10.0
TOTAL	1743	31	1.8

The follow-up periods for the patients with and without recurrence were 13.6 ± 6.7 years and 10.9 ± 6.2 years, which were statistically significant ($p = 0.015$). However, the first recurrence in 31 patients occurred 8.1 months to 5.7 years after surgery. We used the Cox proportional hazard model for the following analysis; the difference in follow-up periods between the two groups did not affect the result of the following statistical study.

Table 4-2 shows the effects of nodal excision on preventing recurrence. Recurrence rate was the highest among the patients who underwent therapeutic nodal excision (whole model test, $p = 0.001$, full model –log likelihood 201.9615). Between the patients who underwent prophylactic nodal excision and those who did not undergo nodal excision, the rate of recurrence was higher among the patients who underwent prophylactic nodal excision, although no statistical difference was found between these two groups. The relative risk of recurrence between prophylactic excision and nonexcision was 1.7 (95% confidence interval 0.5 to 4.2) and that between therapeutic excision and nonexcision was 8.2 (95% confidence interval 3.5-20.0). This result suggests that prophylactic nodal excision is not effective for preventing recurrence. Since the patients underwent therapeutic nodal excision because of the presence of gross nodal metastasis (N[+]), we considered that not the therapeutic nodal excision but the presence of gross nodal metastasis was a risk factor for recurrence. We previously reported that it was not gross nodal metastasis but extracapsular invasion (ECI) of the metastatic deposit through the lymph node capsule that was a risk factor for patients with clinical papillary carcinoma.[114] Therefore we examined whether ECI was also related to the recurrence of microcancers.

Table 4-3 shows the results of univariate analysis between recurrence and 10 factors including nodal factors such as ECI through the lymph node capsule, N(+) (gross nodal metastasis), n(+) (microscopically confirmed nodal metastasis), and the number of examined lymph nodes per patient; coexisting benign lesions such as Graves' disease, adenomatous goiter,

TABLE 4-3 Univariate Analysis (Cox Proportional Hazard Model) for Recurrence of Microcancer

Factors	Recurrence Yes	Recurrence No	p	Full Model –Log L
No. of patients	31	1712		
With ECI	9	53	0.00	199.7648
With N(+)	9	81	0.00	202.4266
With n(+)	11	191	0.00	206.1527
With Graves' disease	3	735	0.00	202.0806
With AG	15	476	0.00	206.9375
With CT	3	156	0.64	211.3943
With FA	7	445	0.69	211.4975
No. of examined nodes Per patient	8.1 ± 14.0	2.7 ± 8.2	0.02	208.9473
Age at surgery	50.4 ± 11.6	45.7 ± 13.0	0.00	206.6643
Gender (M/F)	1/30	185/1527	0.09	210.1321

ECI, Extracapsular invasion of nodal metastasis; N(+), presence of gross nodal metastasis; n(+), presence of nodal metastasis confirmed by microscopic study; AG, adenomatous goiter; CT, chronic thyroiditis; FA, follicular adenoma (Reduced model –log likelihood 211.4975).

chronic thyroiditis, and follicular adenoma; and patients' age and gender. Among these 10 factors, seven were statistically significant for recurrence. Since recurrence was noted in only 31 patients, at most two variables were available for multivariate proportional hazard regression analysis.[115-116] We performed multivariate analysis between the recurrence and all combinations of two factors that were statistically significant (see Table 4-3). The two-variable model, having a maximum recurrence likelihood[117] contained ECI and Graves' disease (full model –log likelihood 193.9495, reduced model –log likelihood 211.4975).

Other factors that were significant in Table 4-3 were correlated significantly either with ECI or Graves' disease. Therefore we considered that the presence of ECI and the absence of Graves' disease were risk factors for tumor recurrence. When Graves' disease was present, the risk ratio for tumor recurrence was $\frac{1}{6}$ (95% confidence interval $\frac{1}{24}$ to $\frac{1}{2}$) times higher than that without Graves' disease. When an ECI was present, the risk ratio was 7 (95% confidence interval 2.9 to 14.0) times higher than without an ECI. Thus the mechanism through which Graves' disease prevents the recurrence of microcancer must be studied further. ECI was also found in three of four patients who had died of thyroid cancer. We therefore believe that ECI, even in patients with microcancers, predicts a more aggressive tumor and poorer prognosis.

In clinical thyroid cancers, age at the time of diagnosis has been considered one of the main prognostic factors.[110] However, Gilliland et al.[118] reported that in clinical thyroid cancers, the age at the time of the diagnosis was a stronger predictor of survival for patients with follicular and medullary carcinomas, but not for those with papillary carcinoma. Schelfhout et al.[119] also stated that in clinical thyroid cancers, the age at the time of diagnosis appeared to be less important than the tumor stage as a prognostic factor. In our series, the effect of age on recurrence was inversely correlated with the presence of Graves' disease (correlation coefficient −0.3544; $p = 0.0000$). Therefore age by itself was not an important factor in the present series of microcarcinomas.

From an analysis of 867 surgically treated consecutive patients with small cancer of the thyroid, Noguchi et al.[111] stated that although small thyroid cancer could be fatal, a total thyroidectomy was not necessary. Even modified radical neck dissection was unnecessary in patients with occult thyroid cancers until the presence of gross nodal metastasis was found. The present study showed that not the gross nodal metastasis, but ECI through the lymph node capsule was a risk factor. However, ECI of nodal metastases is usually not seen preoperatively and is usually only observed histologically around nodes with large metastatic deposits. (In the present study, the correlation coefficient between ECI and N [+] was 0.6131; $p = 0.0001$). It is reasonable to regard patients with gross nodal metastasis as being at higher risk.[111]

Including our one case, there have been several reports of fatal microcancers without lymphadenopathy.[25-26, 120-126] This results from ECI from the microscopic-sized nodal metastasis or unknown factors not related to the nodal metastases and must be further investigated.

CONCLUSION

From the difference between the incidence of microcancer in the autopsy studies and that of the clinical cancer obtained in mass screening studies, it is roughly calculated that only 2% of thyroid microcancers developed into the clinical cancer. A comparison of the relative incidence of histologically classified thyroid tumors in the microcancers and clinical cancers in our series suggests that papillary cancer grows more slowly (including possible spontaneous regression) than other cancers. Malignant lymphomas and undifferentiated carcinomas were rarely present as microcancers. The small number of microscopic malignant lymphomas in our series is probably the result of the fact that only a few of our patients had chronic thyroiditis. The small number of undifferentiated carcinomas is probably because these develop as a transformation from well-differentiated thyroid carcinomas, not from de novo mutations.

A histologic finding almost exclusively observed in microcarcinoma is sclerosing carcinoma. Sclerosing microcarcinoma seems to show extremely slow growth or even spontaneous regression. From the relationship between the size and histologic pattern, papillary carcinoma seems to start as a follicle-forming tumor and then papillary structures and poorly differentiated patterns develop. In follicular microcarcinoma, no vascular invasion was seen, suggesting that follicular carcinomas with vascular invasion are at a more advanced stage than in tumor development. Benign nonencapsulated follicular nodules with invasive growth are possibly an early stage of follicular microcarcinoma.

Although the term C-cell hyperplasia has been used for the lesions associated with medullary carcinoma and with nonmedullary lesions, C-cell hyperplasia found in medullary thyroid carcinoma differs from that found in nonmedullary thyroid lesions. The former was found only in the thyroid glands containing medullary carcinoma and not in nonmedullary thyroid tumors. The incidence of incidental microcancer (microcancer found in the thyroid tissue removed for various benign lesions) was reported to be the highest among the patients with adenomatous goiter. In one report, however, no difference in incidence was found. Our studies suggested that extracapsular invasion of nodal metastasis in patients with microcancer is a risk factor for a more aggressive tumor.

REFERENCES

1. Graham A. The malignant thyroid. Proc Inter-State Post-Grad M Assem North Am 3:264-269, 1928.
2. Woolner LB et al. Occult papillary carcinoma of the thyroid gland: A study of 140 cases observed in a 30 year period. J Clin Endocrinol 20:89-105,1960.
3. Hedinger C, Williams ED, Sobin LH. Histological Typing of Thyroid Tumours, 2nd ed. Berlin: Springer-Verlag, 1980, pp 9-11.
4. Chesky VE, Dreese WC, Hellwig CA. Hemangioendothelioma of the thyroid. J Clin Endocrinol Metabol 13:801-808, 1953.
5. Sampson RJ et al. Occult thyroid carcinoma in Olmsted County, Minnesota: Prevalence at autopsy compared with that in Hiroshima and Nagasaki, Japan. Cancer 34:2072-2076, 1974.
6. Fukunaga FH, Yatani R. Geographic pathology of occult thyroid carcinoma. Cancer 36:1095-1099, 1975.
7. Williams ED et al. Thyroid cancer in an iodide rich area: A histopathological study. Cancer 39:215-222, 1977.
8. Avetisian IL et al. Thyroid pathology in residents of the Kiev region, Ukraine, during pre-post periods. J Environ Pathol Toxicol Oncol 15:233-237, 1996.

9. Agrawal S et al. Histologic trends in thyroid cancer 1969-1993: A clinico-pathologic analysis of the relative proportion of anaplastic carcinoma of the thyroid. J Surg Oncol 63:251-255, 1996.
10. Martinez-Tello F et al. Occult carcinoma of the thyroid. Cancer 71:4022-4029, 1993.
11. Waterhouse J, Muir C, Shanmugaratnam K, Powell J, eds. Cancer Incidence in Five Continents, vol. IV. IARC Scientific Publication No 42. Lyon: IARC Press, 1982.
12. Delides GS et al. Occult thyroid carcinoma in a Greek population. Neoplasma 34:119-125, 1987.
13. Harach HR, Franssila KO, Wasenius VM. Occult papillary carcinoma of the thyroid. A "normal" finding in Finland. A systematic autopsy study. Cancer 56:531-538, 1985.
14. Takahashi S. Clinico-pathological study on thyroid latent carcinoma. Nihon Naibunpitu Gakkai Zasshi 45:65-79, 1968.
15. Yamamoto Y et al. Occult papillary carcinoma of the thyroid: A study of 408 autopsy cases. Cancer 65:1173-1179, 1990.
16. Makiuchi M. Thyroid carcinoma among Japanese. Nihon Rinsho 40:1172-1182, 1982.
17. Omata K et al. Detection of thyroid cancer in mass screening using ultrasonic echography and aspiration biopsy cytology. J Jpn Soc Clin Cytol 24:680-685, 1985.
18. Ishida T et al. Evaluation of mass screening for thyroid cancer. Jpn J Clin Oncol 182:289-295, 1988.
19. Livolsi VA. Surgical pathology of the thyroid. Philadelphia: WB Saunders, 1990, pp 136-172.
20. The Japanese society of thyroid surgery: Tumor registry of thyroid malignancy (1977-1995). Abstracts of the 30th meeting of the Japanese society of thyroid surgery, 1997.
21. Sugano H. Natural history of human cancer. Gan No Rinsho 29:475-482, 1983.
22. Yamashita H et al. Minute carcinoma of the thyroid and its development to advanced carcinoma. Acta Pathol Jpn 35:377-383, 1985.
23. Fink A et al. Occult micropapillary carcinoma associated with benign follicular thyroid disease and unrelated thyroid neoplasms. Mod Pathol 9:816-820, 1996.
24. Rosai J, Carcangiu M L, DeLellis R A. Atlas of Tumor Pathology, Third series. Tumor of the thyroid gland, Fascicle 5. Washington, DC: Armed Forces Institute of Pathology, 1992.
25. Satge D et al. Microcarciome thyroidien d'évolution fatale. Arch Anat Cytol Path 38:143-151, 1990.
26. Lissak B et al. Solitary skin metastasis as the presenting feature of differentiated thyroid microcarcinoma: Report of two cases. J Endocrinol Invest 18:813-816, 1995.
27. Sako H et al. Histological study of minute papillary carcinoma of the thyroid. Nihon Rinsyo Geka Zassi 57:2088-2093, 1996.
28. Russo F et al. Studio clinico-pathologico del microcarcinoma della tiroide. Minerva Chir 52:891-900, 1997.
29. Woolner LB et al. Classification and prognosis of thyroid carcinoma. A study of 885 cases observed in a thirty year period. Am J Surg 102:354-387, 1961.
30. Ljungberg O. On medullary carcinoma of the thyroid. Acta Pathol Microbiol Scand [A] 231:1-57, 1972.
31. Mendelsohn G et al. Calcitonin and histaminase in C-cell hyperplasia and thyroid carcinoma. A light microscopic and immunohistochemical study. Am J Pathol 92:35-43, 1978.
32. Bondeson L, Ljungberg O. Occult thyroid carcinoma at autopsy in Malmo, Sweden. Cancer 47:319-323, 1981.

33. White IL et al. Occult medullary carcinoma of thyroid: An usual clinical and pathologic presentation. Cancer 47:1364-1368, 1981.
34. Aldabagh SM, Trujillo YP, Taxy JB. Occult medullary thyroid carcinoma. Unusual histologic variant presenting with metastatic disease. Am J Clin Pathol 85:247-250, 1986.
35. Pearlman SJ, Lawson W, Biller HF. Occult medullary carcinoma of the thyroid presenting as neck and parapharyngeal metastases. Otolaryngol Head Neck Surg 99:509-512, 1988.
36. Lang W, Borrusch H, Bauer L. Occult carcinomas of the thyroid. Evaluation of 1020 sequential autopsies. Am J Clin Pathol 90:72-76, 1988.
37. Bergholm U. Clinical characteristics in sporadic and familial medullary thyroid carcinoma. Cancer 63:1196-1204, 1989.
38. Mizukami Y et al. Sporadic medullary microcarcinoma of the thyroid. Histopathology 21:375-377, 1992.
39. Furmanchuk AW, Roussak N, Ruchti C. Occult thyroid carcinomas in the region of Minsk, Belarus. An autopsy study of 215 patients. Histopathology 23:319-325, 1993.
40. Tschawrakow G, Welkow M. Uber das Grahms-Karizom der Schildddruse. Zentralbl Pathol 137:78-81, 1991.
41. Komatsu M, Kobayashi S, Ito N, Sugenoya A, Iida F. Ultrasonography in the diagnosis of malignant lymphoma of the thyroid. Nihon Geka Gakkai Zassi 95:187-191, 1994.
42. Burt A, Goudie RB. Diagnosis of primary thyroid carcinoma by immunohistological demonstration of thyroglobulin. Histopathology 3:279-286, 1979.
43. DeLellis RA et al. Calcitonin and carcinoembryonic antigen as tumor markers in medullary thyroid carcinoma. Amer J Clin Pathol 70:589-594, 1978.
44. De Micco C et al. Immunohistochemical study of thyroid peroxidase in normal, hyperplastic and neoplastic human thyroid tissues. Cancer 67:3036-3041, 1991.
45. Yamashita H et al. Immunohistological differentiation of benign thyroid follicular cell tumors from malignant ones: Usefulness of anti-peroxidase and JT-95 antibodies. Acta Pathol Jpn 43:46-49, 1993.
46. Hosoya T, Sakurai K. Histochemical response of papillary thyroid carcinomas to the monoclonal antibody (JT-95). Gann No Rinsho 37:721-724, 1991.
47. Takeyama H et al. Production of a novel monoclonal antibody, which can detect antigen of thyroid carcinoma. Cancer Res 56:1817-1822, 1996.
48. Pizzolo G, Sloane J, Beverly P. Differential diagnosis of malignant lymphoma and nonlymphoid tumors using monoclonal antileukocyte antibody. Cancer 46:2640-2647, 1980.
49. Faure P et al. Diagnostic features of primary malignant lymphoma of the thyroid with monoclonal antibodies. Cancer 61:1852-1861, 1988.
50. Miyauchi A. Genetics in medullary thyroid carcinoma. Pathol Clin Med 6:772-777, 1988.
51. Hill CS et al. Medullary (solid) carcinoma of the thyroid gland: An analysis of the M.D. Anderson Hospital experience with patients with the tumor, its special features and its histogenesis. Medicine 52:141-171, 1973.
52. Lawson W, Biller HF. Solitary thyroid nodule: Diagnosis and management of malignant disease. Am J Otolaryngol 4:43-73, 1983.
53. Saad MF et al. Medullary carcinoma of the thyroid. A study of the clinical features and prognostic factors in 161 patients. Medicine 63:319-342, 1984.
54. Seizmore GW. Medullary carcinoma of the thyroid gland. Semin Oncol 14:306-314, 1987.

55. Staunton MD, Greening WP. Clinical diagnosis of thyroid cancer. Br Med J 4:532-535,1973.
56. Souhami L, Simpson J, Carruthers JS. Malignant lymphoma of the thyroid gland. Int J Radiat Oncol Biol Phys 6:1143-1147, 1980.
57. Senga O, Kasuga Y, Yokozawa T. Malignant lymphoma of the thyroid. Endocr Surg 1:77-89, 1984.
58. Solbiati L et al. The thyroid gland with low uptake lesions: Evaluation by ultrasound. Radiology 155:187-191, 1985.
59. Maniwa Y et al. Thyroid malignant lymphoma. Gann No Rinsho 34:1654-1658, 1988.
60. Mann RB Jaffe ES, Berard CW. Malignant lymphomas: A conceptual understanding of morphologic diversity. Am J Pathol 94:105-175, 1979.
61. Isaacson PG, Wright DE. Extranodal malignant lymphoma arising from mucosa associated lymphoid tissue. Cancer 53:2515-2524, 1984.
62. Aozasa K et al. Intermediate lymphocytic lymphoma of the thyroid. Cancer 57:1762-1767, 1986.
63. Anscombe AM, Wright DH. Primary malignant lymphoma of the thyroid—a tumor of mucosa-associated lymphoid tissue. Histopathology 9:81-97, 1985.
64. Tani E, Skoog L. Fine needle aspiration cytology and immunocytochemistry in the diagnosis of lymphoid lesions of the thyroid gland. Acta Cytol 33:48-52, 1989.
65. Burke JS, Butler JJ, Fuller LM. Malignant lymphoma of the thyroid. A clinical pathologic study of 35 patients including ultrastructural observations. Cancer 39:1587-1602, 1977.
66. Maurer R et al. Non-Hodgkin's lymphomas of the thyroid. A clinicopathological review of 29 cases applying the Lukes-Collins classification and an immunoperoxidase method. Virchow Arch 383:293-317, 1979.
67. Holm LE, Blomgren H, Lowhagen T. Cancer risks in patients with chronic lymphocytic thyroiditis. N Engl J Med 312:601-604, 1985.
68. Santana V, Rose NR. Neoplastic lymphoproliferation in autoimmune diseases: An update review. Clin Immunol Immunopathol 63:205-213, 1992.
69. Matsuzuka F et al. Clinical aspect of primary thyroid lymphoma: Diagnosis and treatment based on our experience of 119 cases. Thyroid 3:93-99, 1993.
70. Aozasa K. Hashimoto's thyroiditis as a risk factor of thyroid lymphoma. Acta Pathol Jpn 40:459-467, 1990.
71. Kawamoto H. Exact confidence interval for binomial distribution with JMP calculator. SUGI-J '96/IDS conference, 1996 proceedings, pp 241-244.
72. Sugitani I et al. Clinicopathologic and immunohistochemical studies of papillary thyroid microcarcinoma presenting with cervical lymphadenopathy. World J Surg 22:731-737, 1998.
73. Ito T et al. Unique association of p53 mutations with undifferentiated but not with differentiated carcinomas of the thyroid gland. Cancer Res 52:1369-1371, 1992.
74. Fagin JA et al. High-prevalence of mutations of p53 gene in poorly differentiated human thyroid carcinoma. J Clin Invest 91:179-184, 1993.
75. Dobashi Y et al. Stepwise participation of p53 gene mutation during dedifferentiation of human thyroid carcinomas. Diagn Mol Pathol 3:9-14, 1994.
76. Battista S et al. A mutated p53 gene alters thyroid cell differentiation. Oncogene 11:2029-2037, 1995.
77. Maruta J, Kawamoto H. Mutant p53 protein, proliferating cell nuclear antigen, and nucleolar organizer regions in thyroid carcinoma. Jpn J Cancer Clin 41:853-857, 1995.

78. Ho YS et al. p53 gene mutation in thyroid carcinoma. Cancer Lett 103:57-63, 1996.
79. Hutter RV et al. Spindle and giant cell metaplasia in papillary carcinoma of the thyroid. Am J Surg 110:660-668, 1965.
80. Ibanez MI et al. Thyroid carcinoma—biologic behavior and mortality. Cancer 19:1039-1052, 1966.
81. Aldinger K et al. Anaplastic carcinoma of the thyroid. A review of 84 cases of spindle and giant cell carcinoma of the thyroid. Cancer 41:2267-2275, 1978.
82. Spires JR, Schwartz MR, Miller RH. Anaplastic thyroid carcinoma. Association with differentiated thyroid cancer. Arch Otolaryngol Head Neck Surg 114:40-44, 1988.
83. Harada T. Fatal thyroid carcinoma. Anaplastic transformation of adenocarcinoma. Cancer 39:2588-2596, 1977.
84. Kapp DS, Livolsi VA, Sanders MM. Anaplastic carcinoma following well-differentiated thyroid cancer: Etiological considerations. Yale J Biol Med 55:521-528, 1982.
85. Hazard JB. Small papillary carcinoma of the thyroid: A study with special reference to so-called nonencapsulated sclerosing tumor. Lab Invest 9:86-97, 1960.
86. Kameya T et al. Clinico-pathological study of small and microcarcinoma of the thyroid. Nihon Rinsho 35:2581-2588, 1977.
87. Aiyoshi Y et al. Metastasis of the well differentiated thyroid microcarcinoma to the regional lymph node. Endocr Surg 12:43-49, 1995.
88. Yagi Y, Yagi S, Saku T. The localization of cytoskeletal proteins and thyroglobulin in thyroid microcarcinoma in comparison with clinically manifested thyroid carcinoma. Cancer 56:1967-1971, 1985.
89. Klinck GH, Winship T. Occult sclerosing carcinoma of the thyroid. Cancer 8:701-706, 1955.
90. Sampson RJ et al. Metastasis from occult thyroid carcinoma. Cancer 25:803-811, 1970.
91. Yamashita H et al. Prognosis of minute carcinoma of the thyroid follow up study of 49 patients. Acta Pathol Jpn 36:1469-1475, 1986.
92. Bramley MD, Harrison BJ. Papillary microcarcinoma of the thyroid gland. Brit J Surg 83:1674-1683, 1996.
93. Chen KTK, Rosai J. Follicular variant of thyroid papillary carcinoma: A clinicopathologic study of six cases. Am J Surg Pathol 1:123-130, 1977.
94. Sakamoto A, Kasai N, Sugano H. Poorly differentiated carcinoma of the thyroid. A clinicopathological entity for a high-risk group of papillary and follicular carcinoma. Cancer 52:1849-1855, 1983.
95. Carcangiu ML, Zampi G, Rosai J. Poorly differentiated ("insular") thyroid carcinoma. Am J Surg Pathol 8:655-668, 1984.
96. Silverberg S, Vidone RA. Adenoma and carcinoma of the thyroid. Cancer 19:1053-1062, 1966.
97. Farid NR, Shi Y, Zou M. Molecular basis of thyroid cancer. Endocr Rev 15:202-232, 1994.
98. Morson BC. The evolution of colorectal carcinoma. Clin Radiol 35:425-431, 1984.
99. Enbald P et al. The adenoma-carcinoma sequence in rectal adenomas. Am J Clin Pathol 90:121-130, 1988.
100. Fearson ER, Vogelstein B. A genetic model for colorectal carcinoma. Cell 61:759-767, 1990.
101. Stanbridge EJ. Identifying tumor suppressor genes in human colorectal cancer. Science 247:12-14, 1990.

102. Bubenhofer R, Hedinger C. Schilddrusenmalignome vor und nach Einfuhrung der Jodsalzprophylaxe. Schweizerische Medizinische Wochenschrift. Schweiz Med Wochenschr 107:733-741, 1977.
103. Saint-Andre JP, Guyetant S. Hypercalcitoninemies non tumorales Anatomic pathologique. Ann Endocrinol 57:23-26, 1996.
104. Niccoli P et al. Les hypercalcitoninemies en dehors des cancers medullaires de la thyroide. Ann Endocrinol 57:15-21, 1996
105. Guyetant S et al. C-cell hyperplasia associated with chronic lymphocytic thyroiditis: A retrospective quantitative study of 112 cases. Hum Pathol 25:514-521, 1994.
106. Perry A, Molberg K, Albores-Saavedra J. Physiologic versus neoplastic C-cell hyperplasia of the thyroid: separation of distinct histologic and biologic entities. Cancer 77:750-756, 1996.
107. Yamashita H et al. RET gene mutation and multifocality of medullary thyroid carcinoma: Proceedings of the 17th International Cancer Congress, Rio de Janeiro, Brazil, August 1998.
108. Yamashita H et al. Thyroid carcinoma in benign thyroid diseases: An analysis from minute carcinoma. Acta Pathol Jpn 35:781-788, 1985.
109. Yamashita H et al. Thyroid cancer associated with adenomatous goiter: An analysis of the incidence and clinical factors. Surg Today 29:495-499, 1997.
110. International Union Against Cancer (UICC). In Hermanek P, Sobin LH, eds. TNM Classification of Malignant Tumors, 4th ed. Berlin: Springer-Verlag, 1992, pp 35-37.
111. Noguchi S et al. Small carcinomas of the thyroid—a long-term follow-up of 867 patients. Arch Surg 131:187-191, 1996.
112. Lin KD et al. Clinical presentations and predictive variable of thyroid microcarcinoma with distant metastasis. Int Surg 82:378-381, 1997.
113. Rodriguez JM et al. Papillary thyroid microcarcinoma: Clinical study and prognosis. Eur J Surg 163:255-259, 1997.
114. Yamashita H et al. Extracapsular invasion of nodal metastasis is an indicator of distant metastasis and poor prognosis of patients with thyroid papillary carcinoma. Cancer 80:2268-2272, 1997.
115. Concato J et al. Importance of events per independent variable in proportional hazards analysis. I. Background, goals, and general strategy. J Clin Epidemiol 48:1495-1501, 1995.
116. Peduzzi P et al. Importance of events per independent variable in proportional hazards regression analysis. II. Accuracy and precision of regression estimates. J Clin Epidemiol 48:1503-1510, 1995.
117. Cox DR, Oakes D. Analysis of Survival Data. London: Chapman & Hall, 1984.
118. Gilliland FD et al. Prognostic factors for thyroid carcinoma. A population-based study of 15,698 cases from the surveillance, epidemiology and end result (SEER) program 1973-1991. Cancer 79:564-573, 1997.
119. Schelfhout LJ et al. Multivariate analysis of survival in differentiated thyroid cancer: The prognostic significance of the age factor. Eur J Cancer Clin Oncol 24:331-337, 1988.
120. Akazaki K, Kajita A, Higo N. [An autopsy case of microscopic sized thyroid carcinoma characterized by generalized bone metastases.] Syujyutu 14:66-71, 1960.
121. Patchefsky AS, Keller IB, Mansfield CM. Solitary vertebral column metastasis from occult sclerosing carcinoma of the thyroid gland: report of a case. Am J Clin Pathol 53:596-601, 1970.

122. Levi E. Carcinoma of the thyroid with metastases to lungs. NY State J Med 75:1544-1546, 1975.
123. Boehm T, Rothouse L, Wartofsky L. Metastatic occult follicular thyroid carcinoma. JAMA 235:2420-2421, 1976.
124. Jancic-Zgurias M, Jankovic R. Occult papillary carcinoma of the thyroid gland revealed by cancer pericarditis. Pathol Res Pract 181:761-764, 1986.
125. Michie HR et al. Cerebral metastases from occult papillary carcinoma of the thyroid. Br J Surg 74:647, 1987.
126. Lin KD et al. Skull metastasis with brain invasion from thyroid papillary microcarcinoma. J Fromos Med Assoc 96:280-282, 1997.

CHAPTER

5

Illustrated Guide to Thyroid Tumors

GREGORY P. SADLER, M.D.
PATRICK A. TRESELER, M.D.
ORLO H. CLARK, M.D.

Palpable thyroid nodules are relatively common: they are found in about 4% of the United States population. The vast majority of thyroid tumors, however, are benign colloid nodules or follicular adenomas. Thyroid cancer is relatively rare, accounting for fewer than 1% of all malignancies, with an incidence of 40 new cases per 1,000,000 population. With accurate diagnosis, however, thyroid cancer is an eminently treatable condition; most patients are cured and others receive excellent palliation.

Assessment of thyroid tumors include (1) taking an accurate medical history with an appreciation of the risk factors for thyroid cancer, including previous exposure to head and neck radiation or family history of thyroid cancer, (2) physical examination, and (3) fine-needle aspiration cytology (FNAC) performed on the thyroid nodule and examined by an experienced cytopathologist.

The thyroid gland demonstrates a remarkably heterogeneous group of tumors with a wide variety of biologic behavior. Patients with thyroid nodules demonstrated to be benign on FNAC may be either observed, treated with thyroid hormone, or if causing obstructive or cosmetic problems, surgically excised (usually by thyroid lobectomy). Thyroid cancers should be surgically removed, usually when more than occult (less than 1 cm) by total thyroidectomy. Depending on the histologic type of thyroid cancer, further treatment of residual or metastatic disease with ^{131}I ablation may be possible, as may inhibition of thyroid cell growth by suppressing thyroid-stimulating hormone (TSH) with thyroxine (T_4). In patients with differentiated thyroid tumors of follicular or parafollicular origin, tumor-specific markers such as thyroglobulin (Tg), calcitonin, and carcinoembryonic antigen (CEA) aid in following patients progress postoperatively. When suspected, recurrent or metastatic thyroid disease may be assessed by ^{131}I, ultrasound, CT, or MRI scanning.

Management of Patients With Thyroid Nodules and Thyroid Cancer

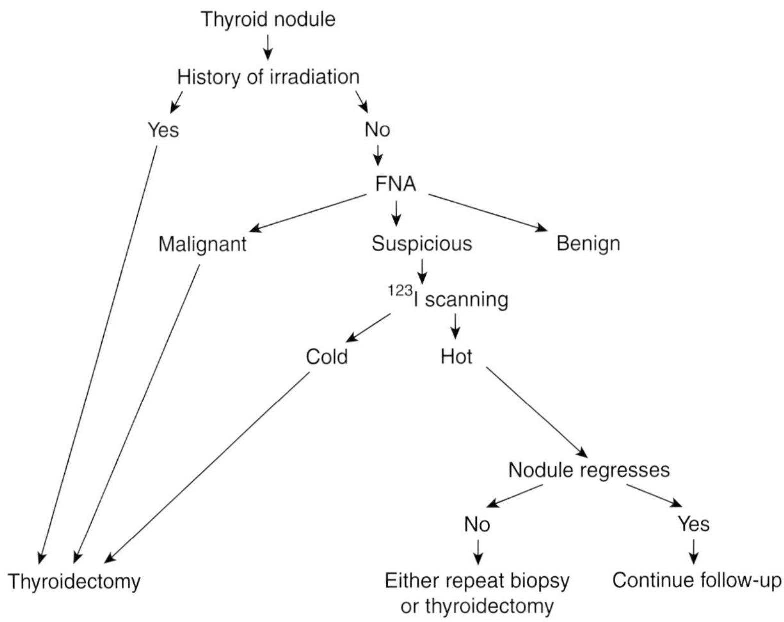

• FIGURE 5-1

Following accurate history taking and physical examination, the procedure of choice in evaluating thyroid nodules is FNAC. In most series, 75% of nodules are benign, 20% suspicious, and 5% malignant. Repeat FNAC is neccssary when the sample is nondiagnostic. False negative results are about 5% and false positive 1%. Significant medical history includes a history of exposure to head and neck irradiation or a family history of thyroid cancer.

Patient With Visible and Palpable Benign Thyroid Colloid Nodule

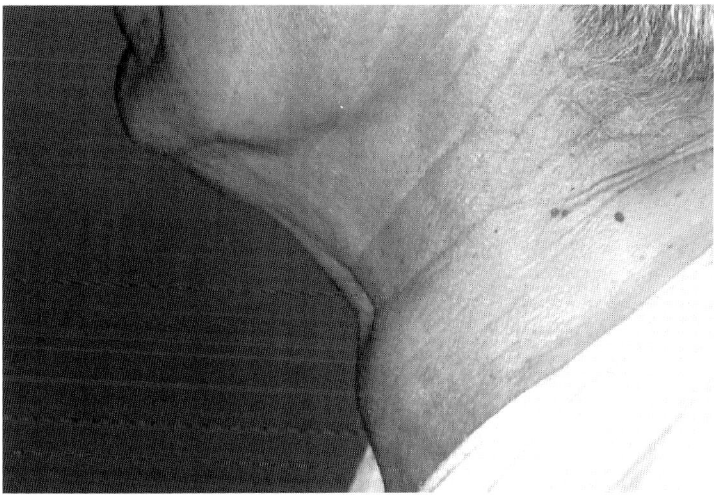

• FIGURE 5-2

Where FNAC shows thyroid nodules to be benign, ultrasonographic examination is performed to obtain a baseline reading of nodule size and a baseline serum Tg level is also determined. Patients may be treated with T_4 suppression therapy, maintaining TSH levels between 1.0 and 0.1 MIU/L, in an attempt to reduce the size of the nodule. Nodules that increase in size on this regimen, cause obstructive pressure symptoms that are cosmetically unacceptable, or nodules where Tg levels rise (despite T_4 treatment) should be surgically removed by thyroid lobectomy.

Massive Multinodular Goiter

A 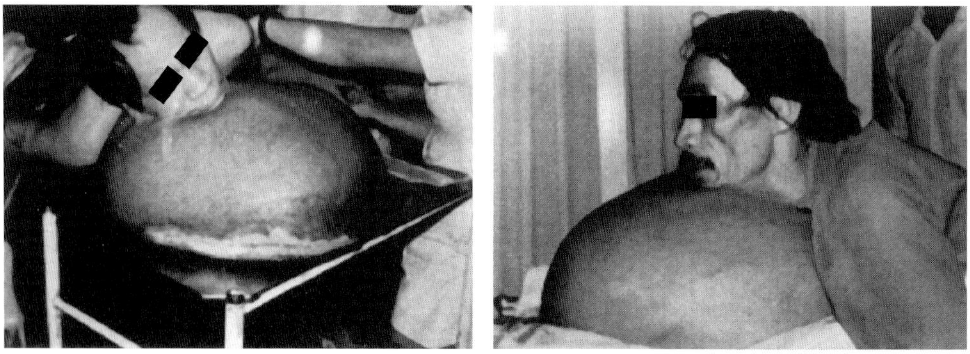 B

• FIGURE 5-3

Large nodular goiters may give rise to "obstructive" symptoms such as dyspnea or dysphagia; these symptoms may be accentuated if the goiter descends and becomes retrosternal. Examination often reveals an enlarged gland with nodules of differing size and firmness; one nodule may be predominant. A number of patients over 60 years of age in whom nodular goiter has been present for more than 17 years develop thyrotoxicosis (Plummer's disease). Goiters may be removed by subtotal or total thyroidectomy for pressure symptoms, cosmesis, or when malignancy is suspected.

Nodular Goiter

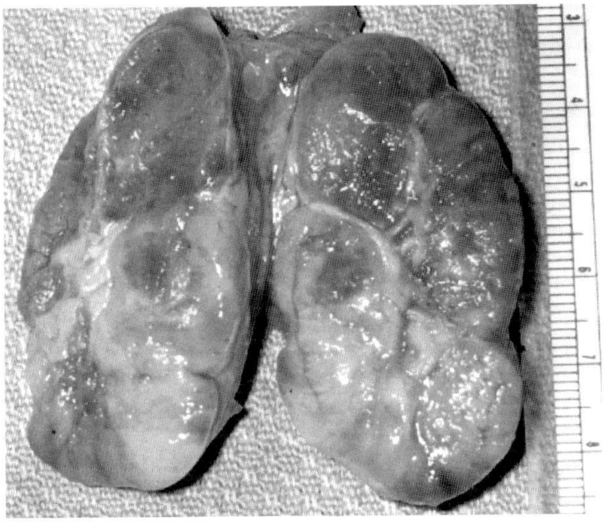

• **FIGURE 5-4** Illustration of nodular goiter.

Nodules vary in size and firmness; they are filled with a gelatinous, colloid-rich matrix, and areas of colloid may be seen between areas of normal thyroid tissue. Hemorrhage into colloid cysts or nodules may give rise to pain and sudden increase in the size of the nodule; this is usually determinable by FNAC of the nodule.

Thyroid Follicular Adenoma

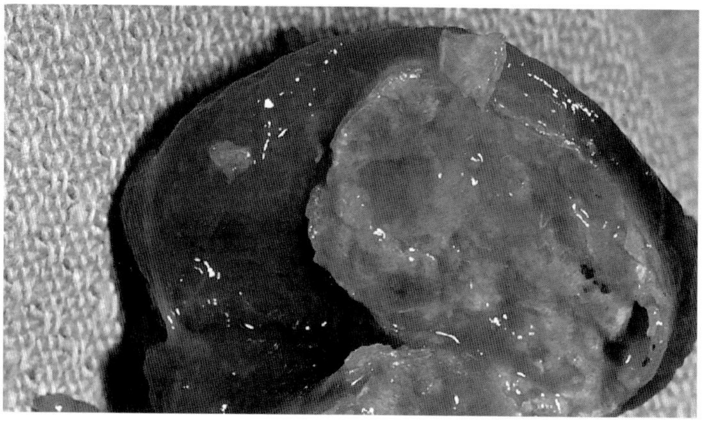

• FIGURE 5-5

Follicular adenoma is a benign thyroid tumor that may be located anywhere within the thyroid gland. It is indistinguishable on FNAC from follicular thyroid carcinoma; thus where FNAC demonstrates thyroid follicular cells, 80% of patients will have a benign follicular adenoma and 20% a follicular carcinoma. Scanning with ^{123}I may reveal whether a follicular neoplasm is "warm" or "hot" (with a low chance of malignancy) or "cold" (where the chance of malignancy is increased) and therefore may be of help in treatment planning. Thyroid lobectomy is sufficient treatment in patients with benign follicular thyroid neoplasms.

Histology of Benign Thyroid Follicular Adenoma

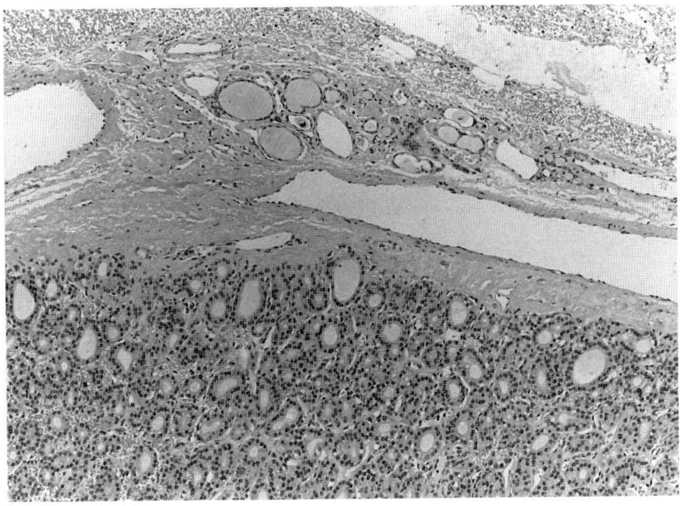

• FIGURE 5-6

The photomicrograph shows a proliferation of thyroid follicular epithelial cells surrounded by a relatively thin fibrous capsule, outside of which lies benign thyroid parenchyma. The adenoma is generally more cellular than the surrounding thyroid tissue, with cells arranged in macrofollicles or microfollicles. Mild cytologic atypia and even mitotic figures can be present, but by definition there is no invasion of tumor cells across the fibrous capsule or into vessels.

Criteria for Nodules at Risk of Malignancy

Forty percent of patients presenting with a thyroid nodule who have a history of head and neck irradiation will have a thyroid carcinoma located in the gland; 60% of these carcinomas will be in the nodule and 40% elsewhere in the gland. Thus FNAC of the nodule in these patients may be misleading. The thyroid cancer is usually papillary in type (85% to 90%), multifocal, and frequently involves local lymph nodes. Total thyroidectomy is generally recommended in these patients. Papillary cancer also occurs more frequently in patients with Cowden's syndrome, familial polyposis, and in individuals with other family members who have had thyroid cancer.

Thyroid Nodules at Risk for Cancer

HISTORY

Low-dose therapeutic or diagnostic head and neck irradiation
Family history of thyroid cancer
Multiple endocrine neoplasia, types 2A and 2B
Rapidly enlarging nodule
Symptoms of obstruction or hoarseness
Hoarseness
History of exposure to low-dose therapeutic radiation
New nodules in young (under 18) or older (over 65) individuals

PHYSICAL EXAMINATION

Solitary nodule
Hard
Fixed to surrounding structures
Palpable ipsilateral lymph nodes
Size (greater than 3 cm)

Incidence of Different Types of Thyroid Cancer

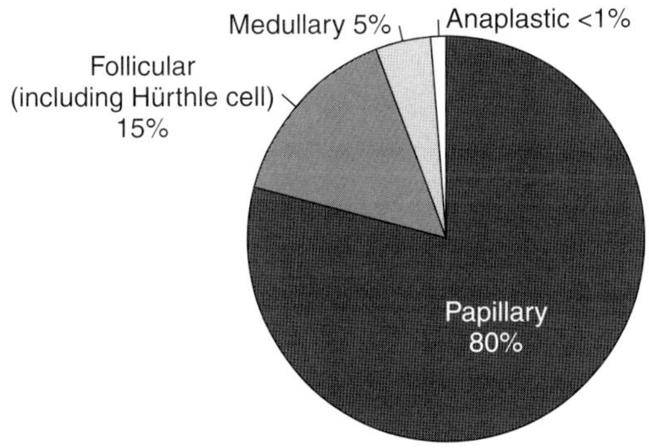

• FIGURE 5-7

The incidence of different types of thyroid cancer is outlined as shown above.

Radioiodine Scan of Cold Thyroid Nodule

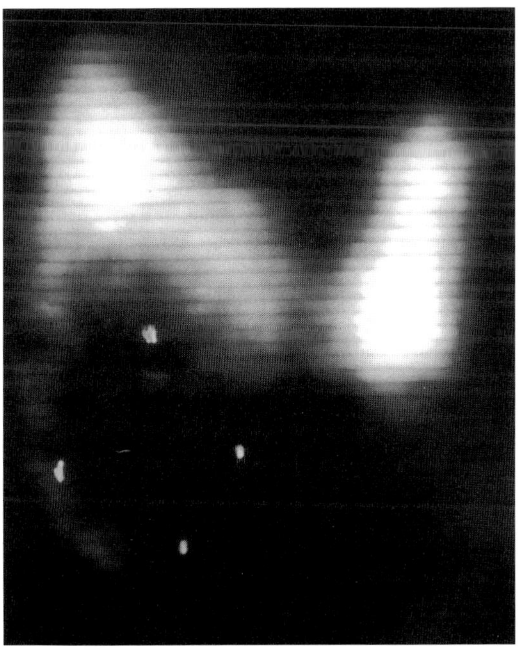

• FIGURE 5-8

Scanning thyroid nodules with ^{123}I or ^{99m}Tc is useful in assessing functional activity. Roughly 85% of nodules scanned in this way take up less iodine than the surrounding thyroid tissue. These "cold" lesions have a 10% to 25% chance of malignancy. Of the 5% of nodules that are "hot" on scanning, only about 1% will be malignant. Radioiodine scanning is no longer used for screening patients in medical centers where expert cytologic evaluation is available.

Papillary Thyroid Cancer

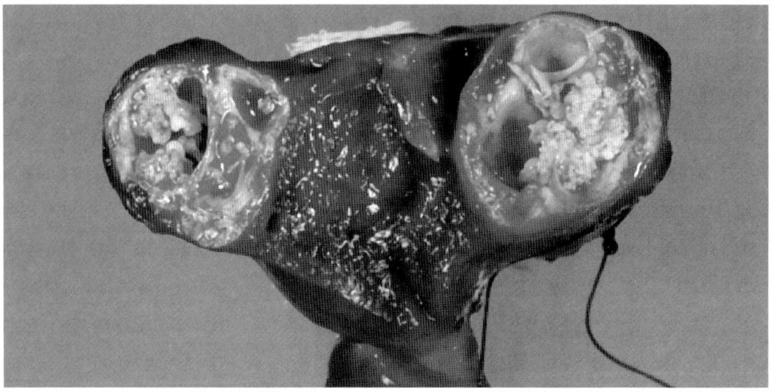

• FIGURE 5-9

The most common thyroid malignancy, papillary cancer is seen more commonly in women than in men (2 to 1) and young people (age groups 30 to 40 years of age), it is the predominant thyroid cancer of children (75%) and is commonly multifocal. Macroscopically tumors are usually hard and whitish and remain flat when sectioned with a blade. Patients tend to be euthyroid and present with a slow-growing mass in the neck. Cervical lymphadenopathy may be present, although distant metastases are uncommon. Diagnosis is suspected by history and examination and confirmed by FNAC. For best results, papillary carcinoma is treated by total or near-total thyroidectomy, followed by ^{131}I scanning and/or ablation for residual or metastatic disease. Low-risk patients are treated with enough T_4 to keep TSH levels at less than 1.0 MIU/L; high-risk patients should have TSH levels of less than 0.1 MIU/L. Disease progress can be monitored by following serum Tg levels (these should remain below 3 ng/ml on T_4).

Histologic Characteristics of Papillary Thyroid Cancer

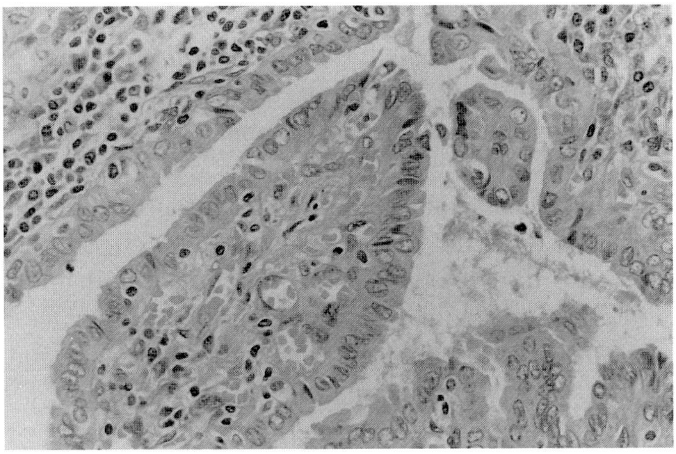

• FIGURE 5-10

Classically, papillary thyroid cancer exhibits papillary projections, although any pattern may be exhibited from mixed papillary/follicular structures to a pure follicular pattern. Cells are cuboidal to columnar and the nuclei are crowded and pseudostratified. Characteristic nuclear features establish the diagnosis. Three main tumor groups are recognized: (1) *occult* cancers (also known as papillary microcarcinomas), which are clinically nonpalpable and smaller than 1 cm in size with no evidence of local invasion into the thyroid capsule, and not associated with any lymph node metastases. These tumors are usually incidental surgical or histologic findings and associated with extremely low morbidity and mortality rates. (2) *Intrathyroidal* cancers are larger than 1 cm and are confined wholly within the thyroid gland but demonstrate local invasion. (3) *Extrathyroidal* cancers have invaded through the thyroid capsule to involve adjacent structures. Patients with these tumors have a poorer prognosis.

Cytology of Papillary Thyroid Cancer

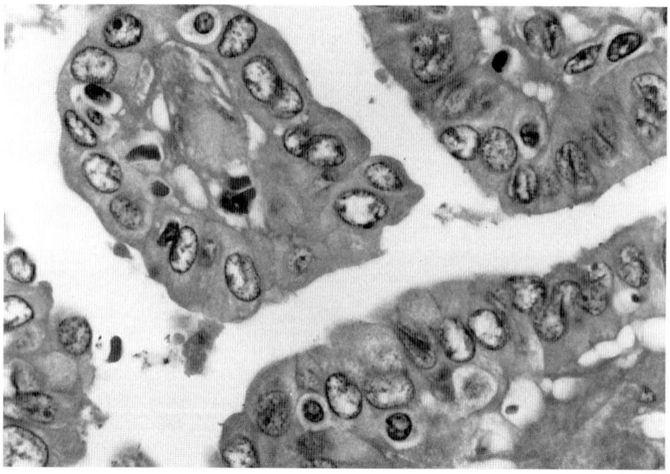

• **FIGURE 5-11**

Tumor cell nuclei typically show finely dispersed chromatin, small nucleoli, nuclear creases or grooves, and intranuclear cytoplasmic inclusions (nuclear pseudoinclusions). The characteristic nuclear chromatin clearing of papillary thyroid carcinoma ("Orphan Annie eye nuclei") is an artifact of formalin fixation and a useful histologic finding in patients with follicular variants of papillary thyroid cancer. This finding is not seen in unfixed FNAC preparations. At lower-power magnification, papillary structures may be observed in some cases.

Chest X-ray Evaluation for Metastasis From Papillary Thyroid Cancer

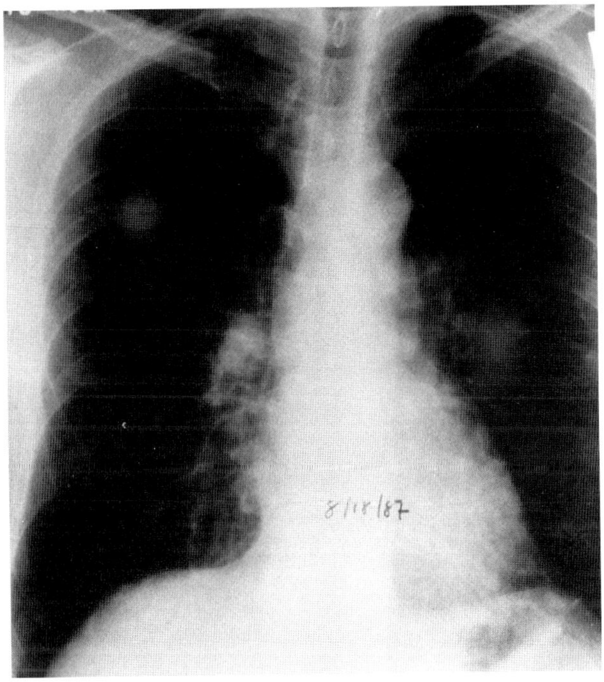

• FIGURE 5-12

Although distant metastases are uncommon at initial presentation (about 10%), up to 20% of all patients will eventually develop distant disease. Papillary thyroid cancer tends to metastasize to local cervical lymph nodes (the so-called lateral aberrant thyroid is, in fact, metastatic papillary thyroid cancer). Distant metastases disseminate to the lungs (the most common site in children) and bone; they may be detected and treated by ^{131}I scanning (which is more sensitive than plain chest x-ray films).

Survival Time Calculated by MACIS Scores

The MACIS scale is a sophisticated prognostic method for predicting survival of patients with papillary thyroid cancer; it was devised by Hay at the Mayo Clinic. The following patient details and tumor characteristics are assessed and allotted a score: *m*etastases, *a*ge at presentation, *c*ompleteness of original surgical resection, *i*nvasion, and *s*ize of original tumor. Scores are totaled to give a definitive MACIS score. Higher scores are associated with a poorer prognosis.[1] MACIS score = 3.1 (if age <40) *or* .08 × age (if age >40), +0.3 × tumor size (cm), +1 (if incompletely resected), +1 (if locally invasive), +3 (if distant metastases present).

Follicular Thyroid Cancer

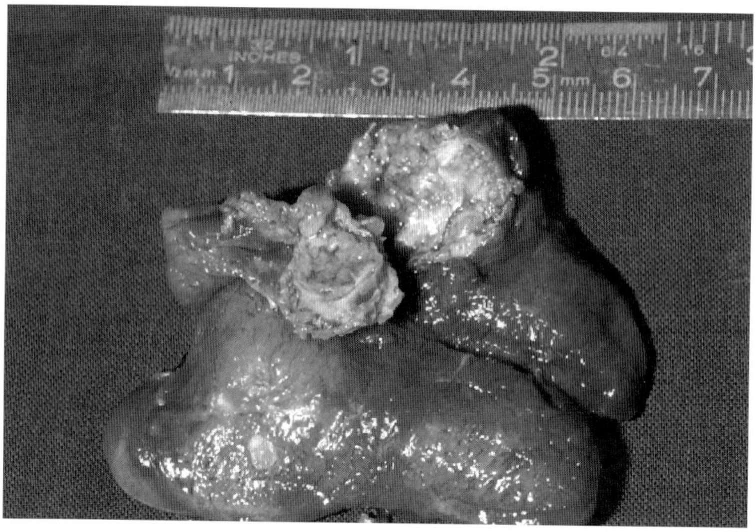

• FIGURE 5-13

Follicular thyroid cancer presents as a solitary nodule and usually occurs in patients about 10 years older than those with papillary thyroid cancer. The female/male ratio is 3:1. Rapid increase in size of one nodule in a multinodular thyroid gland is a common presentation. Distant metastases at presentation are more frequently seen than in papillary thyroid cancer, but cervical lymphadenopathy is relatively uncommon (about 10%) and is usually a late feature of the disease. The preliminary diagnosis is established by history taking and physical examination; FNAC indicates a follicular neoplasm. A definitive diagnosis is established only by demonstrating histologic evidence of capsular or vascular invasion. Patients with minimal capsular invasion can be treated by thyroid lobectomy, since their prognosis is excellent. The treatment of choice for all other patients is total thyroidectomy, followed by ^{131}I scanning and/or ablation for residual or metastatic disease. Patients with minimally invasive follicular thyroid cancer are treated with T_4 suppression to keep TSH levels below 1.0 MIU/L. Patients with extensive thyroid invasion should have TSH levels below 0.1 MIU/L. Disease progress can be monitored by following serum Tg levels (these should remain below 3 ng/ml on T_4 therapy).

Histology of Follicular Neoplasms

A

B

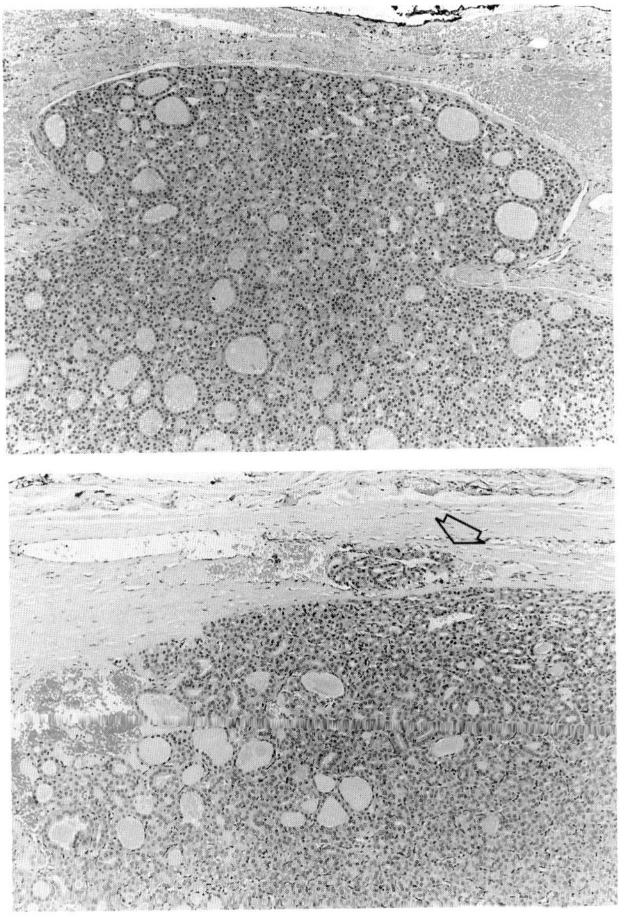

• FIGURE 5-14

Follicular carcinomas classically display a follicular pattern. However, as in papillary carcinoma, architectural patterns may vary. Follicles, although present, may be very small and devoid of colloid ("microfollicles"). Characteristically the tumor is surrounded by a tumor capsule in 90% of cases. Follicular carcinoma is differentiated histologically from benign thyroid follicular adenoma by demonstrating either (1) invasion of the tumor through the tumor capsule (Fig. 5-14, *A*) or (2) invasion of the tumor into capsular blood/lymphatic vessels (Fig. 5-14, *B*). If these invasive features are seen in only rare foci in what otherwise resembles a follicular adenoma, it is termed *minimally invasive*; if capsular or vascular invasion is widespread, it is termed *widely invasive*, and has a worse prognosis. Most cases of so-called insular thyroid carcinomas would fall into this latter group. Cytologic features of papillary thyroid are absent by definition; if present, such tumors are termed *follicular variant of papillary carcinoma*.

FNAC From Follicular Neoplasms

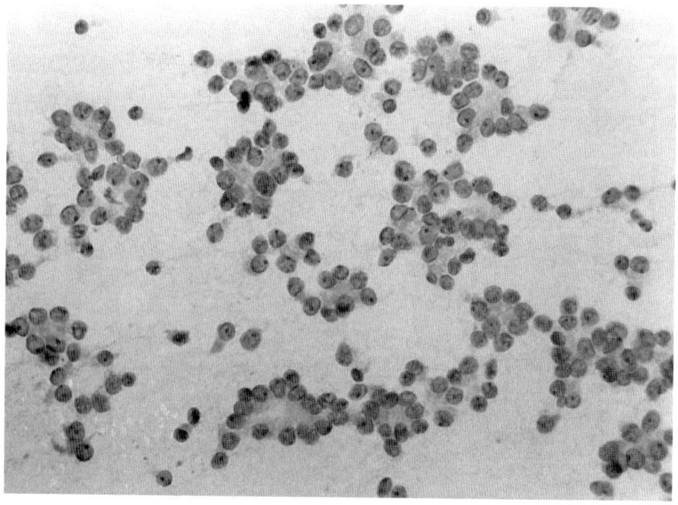

• FIGURE 5-15

Figure 5-15 shows thyroid follicular epithelial cells arranged in aggregates and occasional microfollicles in an FNA sample from a follicular neoplasm (which in this case proved to be a follicular carcinoma). Cell cytoplasm is often indistinct, and cell nuclei are generally round with fine to coarsely granular chromatin and occasional nucleoli. Nuclear features of papillary thyroid carcinoma, such as nuclear grooves and pseudoinclusions, are not seen. One cannot distinguish between benign follicular neoplasms (i.e., follicular adenomas) and malignant follicular neoplasms (i.e., follicular carcinomas) with certainty by FNA, because the architectural features of capsular and vascular invasion cannot be assessed. Although nuclear atypic such as irregular nuclear size, shape, hyperchromasia, and prominent nuclei are more common in follicular carcinoma than in follicular adenoma, such features cannot reliably distinguish benign from malignant follicular neoplasms. Complete excision of such lesions is required for definitive assessment.

X-ray Evaluation of the Pelvis for Metastatic Follicular Thyroid Cancer in Femur and Pelvic Bones

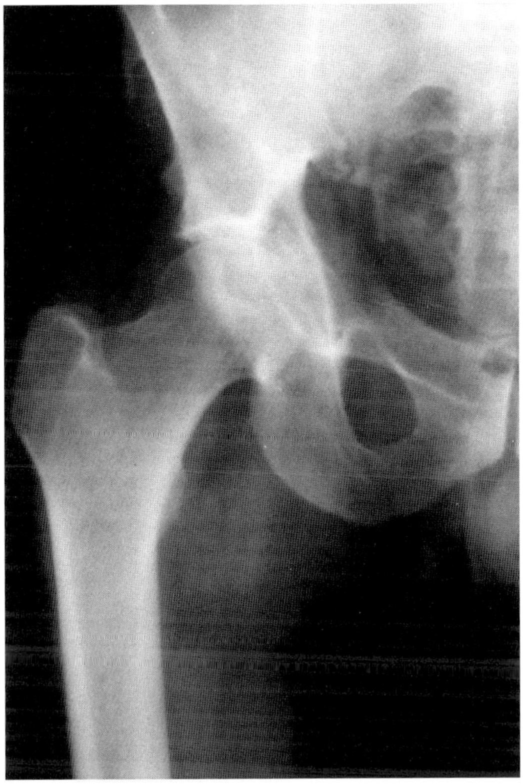

• FIGURE 5-16

Hematogenous metastatic spread to bone, lung, and liver is encountered more commonly in follicular carcinoma than in papillary thyroid carcinoma. Lymphatic metastatic spread tends to be a feature of advanced disease.

^{131}I Scanning for Widespread Metastatic Follicular Carcinoma

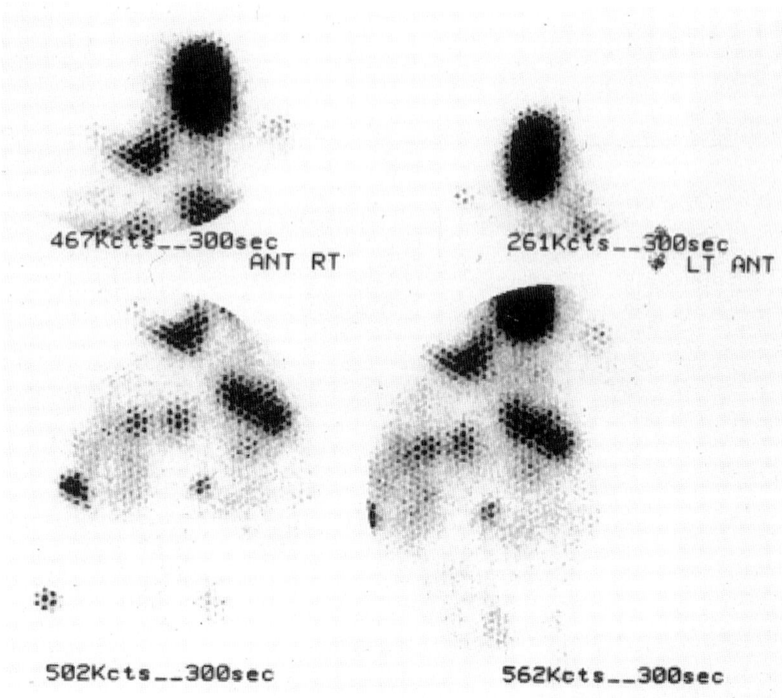

• FIGURE 5-17

Removal of all normal thyroid tissue by total thyroidectomy in patients with differentiated thyroid cancer (papillary and follicular) greatly facilitates postoperative scanning and treatment of metastatic disease by ^{131}I. Patients are allowed to become hypothyroid by replacing T_4 treatment with T_3 for 6 weeks and then removing all treatment completely for 2 weeks. TSH levels rise, facilitating ^{131}I uptake into any residual thyroid cells. With this technique, ^{131}I scanning can detect and treat metastases in about 75% of patients in whom metastatic disease is present. It is more effective in patients with follicular thyroid cancer than those with papillary cancer and less effective in patients with Hürthle cell cancer (only about 10% of these tumors concentrate ^{131}I).

Hürthle Cell Cancer

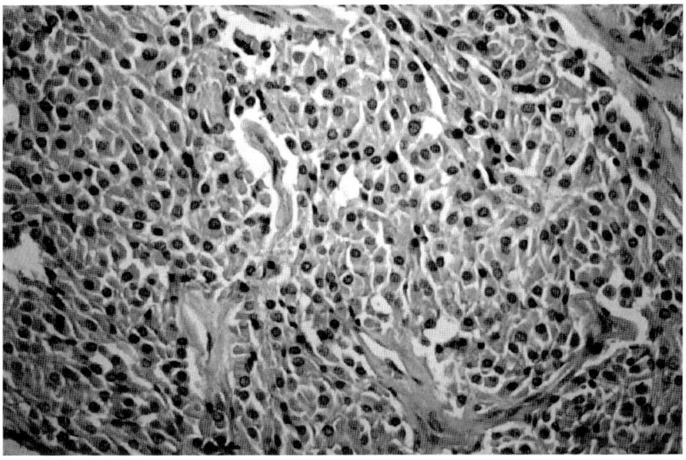

• FIGURE 5-18

Accounting for about 3% of all thyroid cancers, Hürthle cell tumors are derived from the oxyphilic cells of the thyroid gland and are classified as variants of follicular thyroid carcinoma. Tumors are composed of follicles or sheets of cells with abundant granular eosinophilic cytoplasm, the function of which is unknown. They differ from follicular thyroid cancer in that they are more likely to invade regional nodes and are more likely to be multifocal and bilateral. They are also less likely to concentrate ^{131}I. They carry a somewhat worse overall prognosis than do follicular thyroid cancers, although this difference is not apparent when cases are matched stage for stage with typical follicular carcinomas. Sestamibi scanning is usually positive in patients with metastatic Hürthle cell cancer.

FNAC From Hürthle Cell Tumor

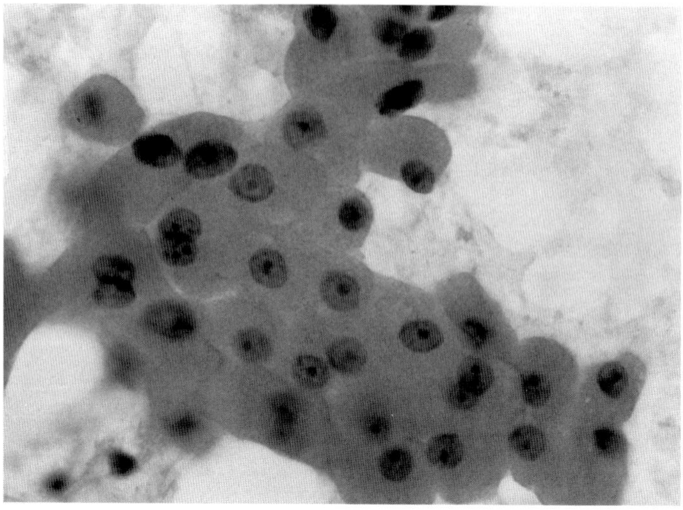

• FIGURE 5-19

This smear shows cells with abundant granular eosinophilic cytoplasm, present singly and in sheets. The nuclei are large and generally contain a single prominent nucleolus. Significant atypia may be seen in smears. As with follicular neoplasms (of which the World Health Organization considers Hürthle cell neoplasm to be a variant), tumor behavior cannot be reliably predicted by FNAC. Excision with histologic examination must be performed to look for capsular or vascular invasion to establish a diagnosis of malignancy. Nonneoplastic Hürthle cells can be seen in benign conditions such as Hashimoto's thyroiditis and nodular goiter.

Anaplastic Thyroid Cancer

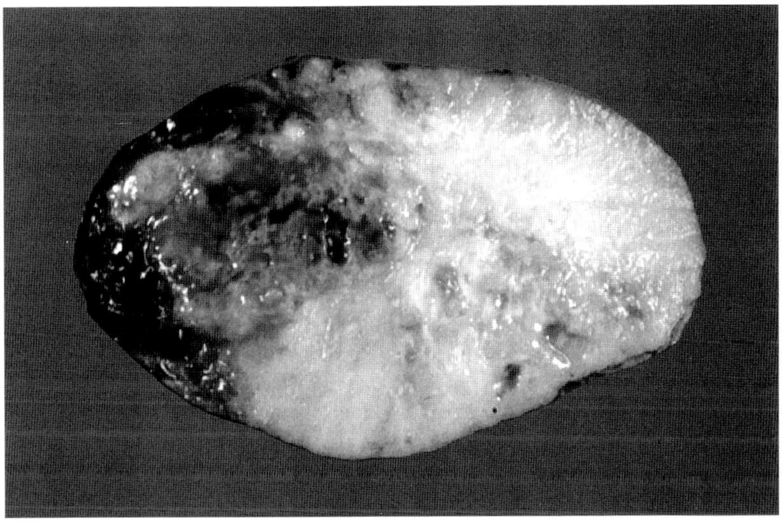

• FIGURE 5-20

About 1% of differentiated thyroid carcinomas dedifferentiate to anaplastic or undifferentiated cancer. Patients typically are elderly women in whom a long-standing neck lump has recently rapidly enlarged. Obstructive symptoms such as dysphagia and dyspnea are common. Hoarseness from recurrent laryngeal nerve invasion may also be present. Tumors are usually hard and frequently fixed to surrounding structures; overlying skin ulceration may be present. Diagnosis is usually confirmed by FNAC.

Anaplastic Thyroid Cancer Invading Through Overlying Skin

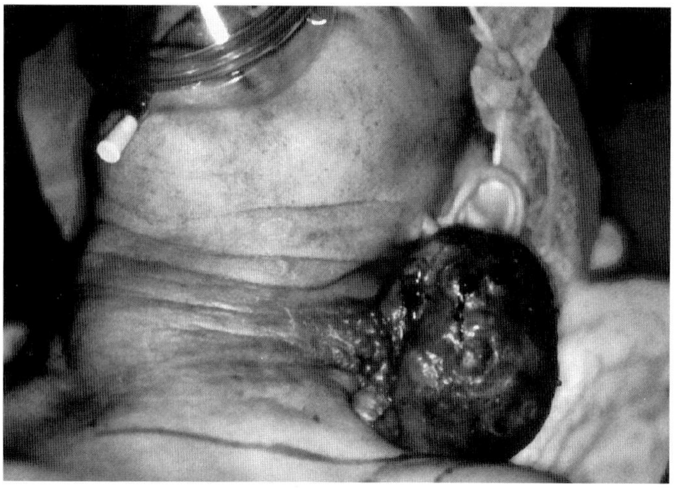

• FIGURE 5-21

These rapidly fatal tumors are one of the most aggressive carcinomas encountered. Invasion into surrounding structures or through overlying skin (as shown above) is common. Current treatment regimens employ a combination of biopsy together with radiotherapy, chemotherapy and surgical debulking, or total thyroidectomy if possible, although few patients survive beyond 6 months. The 5-year survival rate is less than 5%.

FNAC From Anaplastic Thyroid Cancer

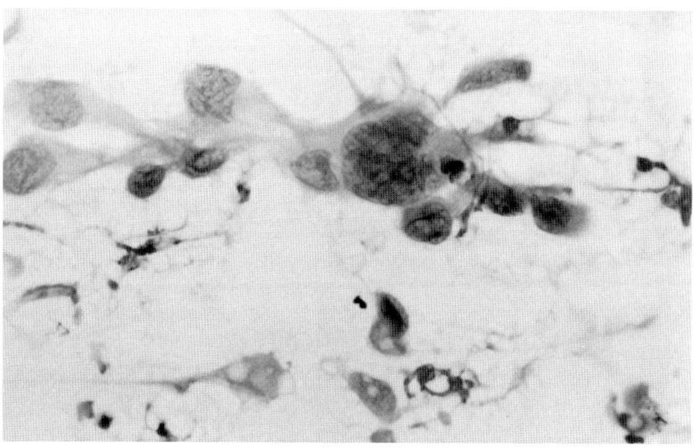

• FIGURE 5-22

Highly pleomorphic, cytologically malignant cells characterize this aggressive neoplasm. Many of the tumor cells are gigantic, with bizarre nuclear shapes and coarsely clumped nuclear chromatin. Spindle-shaped malignant cells resembling sarcoma cells are also frequently observed. Necrotic cellular debris and inflammatory cells may also be seen.

Thyroid Lymphoma

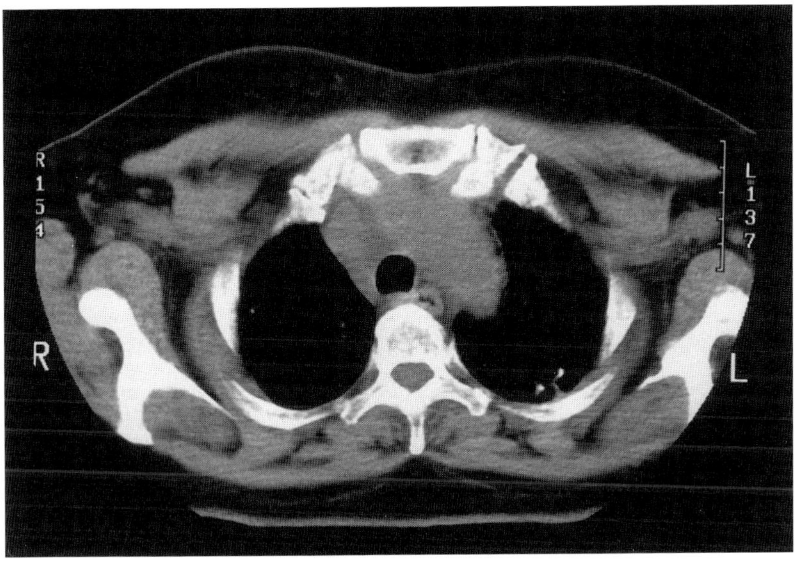

• FIGURE 5-23

Most thyroid lymphomas are of the non-Hodgkins' B-cell type, which frequently develop de novo from a background of chronic lymphocytic thyroiditis (Hashimoto's thyroiditis); patients therefore may have a preexisting goiter and may already be hypothyroid and receiving treatment with T_4. Presentation may mimic anaplastic thyroid carcinoma. Most commonly the patients are elderly women with a history of a rapidly enlarging neck mass. The diagnosis is tentatively established by FNAC and confirmed by open biopsy. Current treatment for large cell lymphomas is a combination of radiotherapy and chemotherapy cytoxin, hydroxyadriamycin, Oncovin, and prednisone (CHOP). Taxol has been recommended by some investigators. Thyroidectomy may be necessary to alleviate obstructive symptoms. Survival rates are about 50% at 5 years, although patients with only intrathyroidal disease fare far better than those with extrathyroidal disease (40% vs. 85%). Less aggressive therapy may be required for low-grade small cell B-cell lymphomas.

FNAC From Thyroid Lymphoma

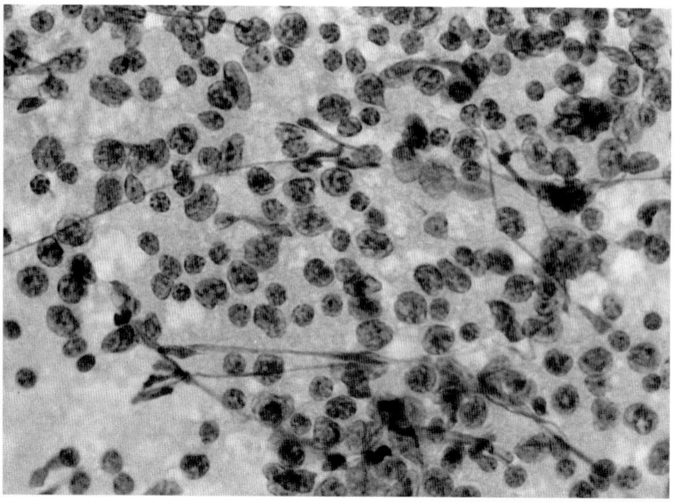

• FIGURE 5-24

Monotonous populations of large lymphoid cells with relatively open chromatin and distinct nucleoli, as seen in this smear, characterize cases of large cell lymphoma of the thyroid. The most frequently found type of thyroid lymphoma is large cell B-cell lymphoma. Lymphomas of small lymphocytes (most commonly B-cell lymphomas of mucosa-associated lymphoid tissue, or MALT lymphomas) also occur frequently but are difficult to distinguish from lymphocytic thyroiditis without surface study markers or standard histologic analysis of excisional biopsies. Many tumors previously classified as the small cell variant of anaplastic thyroid carcinoma have proved to be thyroid lymphomas after cell marker analysis.

Medullary Thyroid Cancer

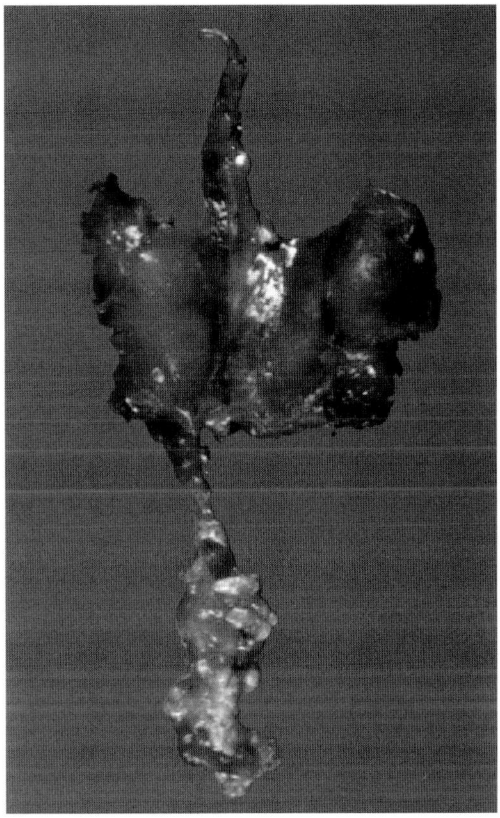

• FIGURE 5-25

About 5% of thyroid malignancies are medullary thyroid cancers (MTC). Most medullary thyroid cancers are sporadic (70%); the remainder are familial, as seen in MEN2A, MEN2B, or as familial MTC with no other associated endocrinopathies. There is a female/male ratio of 1.2:1, and patients with familial disease present at a younger age. Tumors present as neck masses that not infrequently are painful. Diagnosis is established by history, examination, FNAC, and demonstration raised serum levels of calcitonin and/or CEA.

The treatment is total thyroidectomy and central neck dissection, and disease progress may be monitored by serum calcitonin and/or CEA levels.

Histology of Medullary Thyroid Cancer

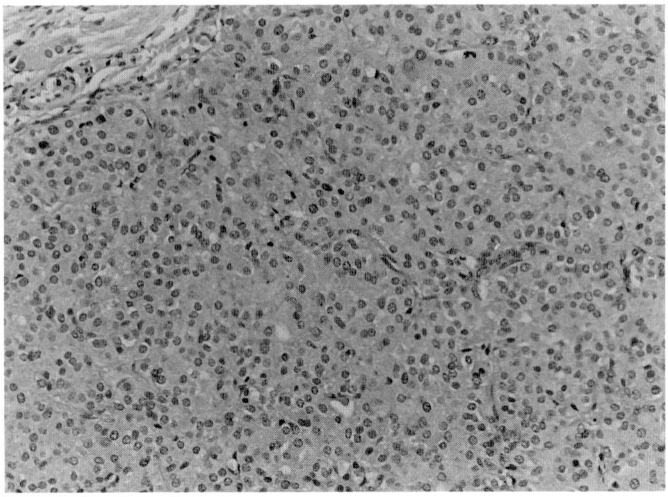

• FIGURE 5-26

Tumors are derived from the calcitonin-secreting parafollicular or C cells of the thyroid. Embryologically these cells originate from neuroectodermal tissue located in the ultimobranchial bodies, explaining why tumors are most commonly located laterally in the upper or mid thyroid. Microscopically tumors are markedly heterogeneous, with sheets or vague clusters of polygonal to spindle-shaped neoplastic cells separated by variable amounts of collagen and amyloid. Carcinoma is usually preceded by C-cell hyperplasia and tumors characteristically stain positively for CEA and calcitonin.

FNA for Medullary Thyroid Cancer

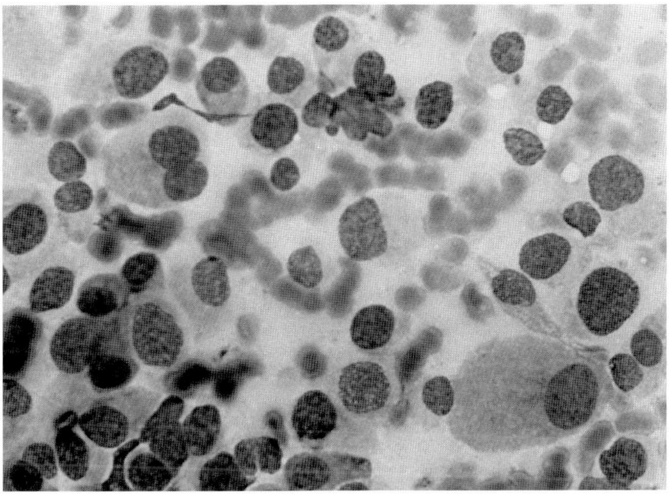

• FIGURE 5-27

The tumor cells of medullary thyroid carcinoma typically vary in size and shape and have cytoplasm that is pale and scant. Follicular or papillary structures are typically absent. Tumor cell nuclei have coarsely granular "salt and pepper" chromatin, characteristic of neuroendocrine tumors, and are often eccentrically placed. When the cells are uniformly small, they may mimic a small cell lymphoma, and when large with abundant cytoplasm may be mistaken for Hürthle cells. The cells of medullary carcinoma may also have a spindle shape, superficially mimicking sarcoma. Calcitonin-containing amyloid may be present in the background; as an aid to diagnosis, this may be identified by Congo red stain or anticalcitonin immunostains.

Typical Phenotype of MEN2B Patients

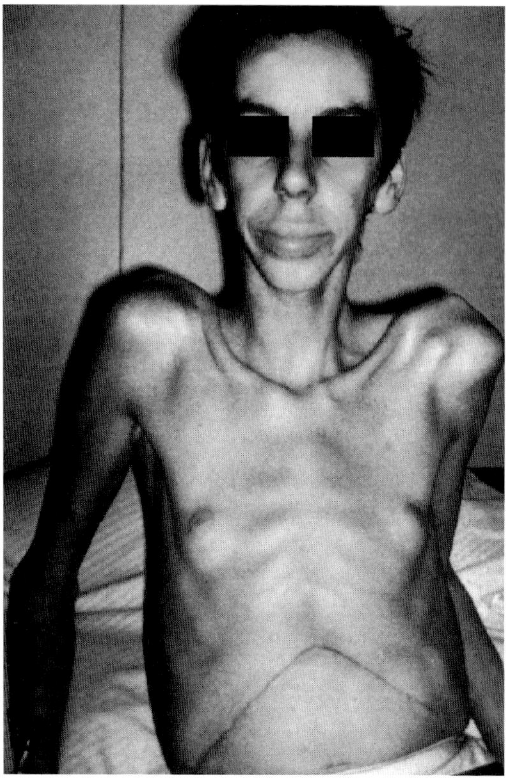

• FIGURE 5-28

Patients with MEN2B typically have Marfanoid features, ganglioneuromas, pheochromocytoma, and MTC. The "rooftop" incision in this patient is from previous surgery for pheochromocytoma. All patients presenting with MTC should have routine 24-hour urinalysis for catecholamines and metanephrines to assess the possible presence of a phenochromocytoma before they are subject to surgery.

Mucosal Ganglioneuromas and Scalloping of the Tongue in MEN2B

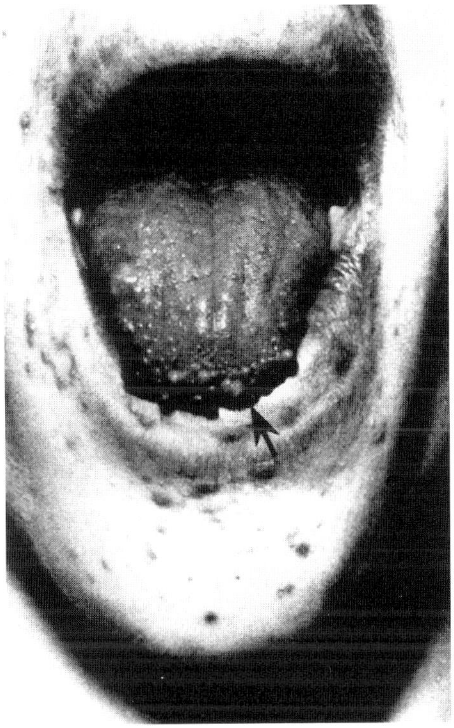

• FIGURE 5-29

Ganglioneuromas of the mucous membranes are seen in the mouth and conjunctiva. The gene for MEN2B and MEN2A has been mapped to chromosome 10, enabling physicians to screen relatives of affected individuals and offer the possibility of prophylactic thyroidectomy to family members carrying the gene before MTC develops. All new patients with MTC should also be screened for RET point mutations to rule out the possibility of familial disease.

MRI for Metastatic MTC in Neck Nodes

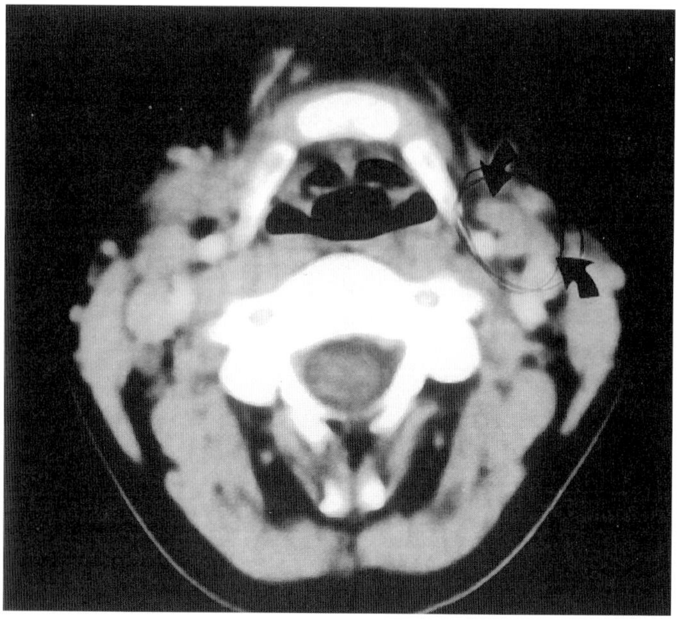

• FIGURE 5-30

Medullary thyroid cancer typically spreads to local lymph nodes in the neck and superior mediastinum; distant metastases to liver, bone, and lung are a late feature. Production of calcitonin by tumor deposits may lead to distressing symptoms, such as flushing and diarrhea, and thus recurrent or metastatic disease should be resected where possible. Table 5-1 summarizes the different types of thyroid cancer, and Table 5-2 summarizes currently known oncogenes and chromosomes implicated in thyroid and parathyroid tumor formation.

TABLE 5-1 Types of Thyroid Cancer

	Papillary	Follicular	Medullary	Anaplastic
Distribution (%)	84	10	5	1
Usual age at presentation	25-35	40-55	*	>60
Diagnosis by FNAC	Yes	No	Yes	Yes
Treatment with ^{131}I	Yes	Yes†	No‡	§
10-year survival rate (%)	85	80	50	0

*Patient 40 to 50 years old for nonfamilial medullary thyroid cancer.
Patient 20 to 30 years old for MEN2 or familial medullary thyroid cancer.
†Hürthle cell carcinomas generally do not take up ^{131}I.
‡About 10% positive on scanning.
§Anaplastic thyroid cancers do not usually take up ^{131}I, but most patients have associated differentiated thyroid cancer.

TABLE 5-2 Chromosomes and Oncogenes Associated With Parathyroid Tumor Formation

Tumor	Chromosomes Implicated	Oncogenes Implicated
Follicular adenoma	11q	*ras, gsp*
"Hot" follicular adenoma		*gsp*, TSH receptor
Papillary carcinoma	10q, 1q	RET/PTC (1, 2, 3) TRK-T1, *met, gsp*, RB
Follicular carcinoma	3p	*ras* (H, N, K), *met, gsp*, RB
Medullary carcinoma	10q	RET
Anaplastic carcinoma		p53, *ras* (H, N), RB

REFERENCE

1. Hay ID et al. Predicting outcome in papillary thyroid carcinoma; Development of a reliable prognostic scoring system in a cohort of 1779 patients surgically treated at one institution during 1940 through 1989. Surgery 114:1050-1057, 1993.

PART

II

IMAGING TOOLS AND TECHNOLOGY

CHAPTER 6

Nuclear Medicine

RALPH R. CAVALIERI, M.D.

To some degree, most carcinomas of thyroid origin retain the ability to concentrate iodide, although this property is usually demonstrable only when serum thyrotropin (TSH) levels are elevated. This fact led to the hope that radioactive iodine might be the "magic bullet" for the detection and treatment of thyroid cancer outside of the thyroid gland. Indeed, this hope has in large measure been realized in that the accumulated experience of nearly half a century has established the value of radioactive iodine as an adjunct in the treatment of thyroid cancer.

In this chapter we will review the changing role of radionuclide imaging in the evaluation of thyroid nodules; the value of radioiodine and other radionuclides in the detection and localization of metastatic disease in patients who have undergone initial surgery for differentiated thyroid cancer (DTC); the "stunning" of thyroid tissue by diagnostic amounts of ^{131}I; the potential applications of recombinant human TSH; and the use, benefits, and side effects of ^{131}I therapy for ablation of thyroid remnant tissue and for treatment of metastatic disease. The discussion will include such controversial areas as ^{131}I treatment of patients with elevated serum thyroglobulin levels and negative diagnostic ^{131}I scans.

RADIONUCLIDES AND IMAGING INSTRUMENTATION

The choice of a radioactive agent for in vivo studies depends on the clinical question to be addressed. Of the isotopes of iodine, ^{123}I is close to an ideal agent both for imaging and for assessing the function of the thyroid gland. This radionuclide emits gamma radiation at 159 Kev, an energy that produces high-resolution images using modern scintillation cameras. Because of its 13-hour physical half-life ($T_{1/2}$) and absence of beta emission, ^{123}I exposes the gland to relatively low radiation doses. The commonly administered activity of ^{123}I for imaging the thyroid ranges from 200 to 400 μCi (7.4 to 14.8 MBq), which gives the same radiation dose to the gland as 2 to 4 μCi (7.4 to 14.8 KBq) of ^{131}I, that is, 2.6 to 5.2 rads (cGy) (Table 6-1). Radioiodine is given orally, and imaging may be performed at any time between 5 hours and 24 hours after administration.

TABLE 6-1 Radionuclides Used for In Vivo Thyroid Studies

Radionuclide (chemical form)	Half-life	Gamma Energy (principal Mev)	Radiation Exposure to Thyroid (rad/mCi)	Usual Dose Range (mCi)	Use
^{123}I iodide	13 hours	0.159	13	0.1-0.4	Nearly ideal for uptake and imaging thyroid
^{131}I iodide	8 days	0.364	130	0.005-0.01 (uptake) 2-10 imaging	Mainly for imaging and treating thyroid cancer
^{99m}Tc pertechnetate	6 hours	0.14	0.13	2-5	Widely available; excellent for imaging thyroid gland

Radiation exposures (in rads/millicurie administered) for radioiodines were calculated using the following assumptions: thyroid gland weight = 20 g (normal adult); maximum uptake = 25% of dose; half-time of uptake = 5 hours; and biologic half-life in gland = 65 days. The radiation exposure to the gland in infants and children is several-fold higher than that in adults. The value for ^{123}I assumes no contamination with other radioiodines. Exposure calculations for radioiodines from Medical Internal Radiation Dose (MIRD), Dose Estimate Report No. 5 (J Nucl Med 16:857, 1975); those for ^{99m}Tc from MIRD Dose Estimate Report No. 8 (J Nucl Med 17:74, 1977).

^{99m}Tc in the form of pertechnetate (TcO_4^-) is concentrated by the thyroid gland and other organs that concentrate iodide (salivary glands, gastric mucosa). However, this agent does not undergo organification in the thyroid and is therefore not a true tracer of iodine metabolism. ^{99m}Tc has a $T_{1/2}$ of 6 hours and emits a medium-energy gamma (140 Kev) but no beta emission, so the radiation exposure to the thyroid is low (see Table 6-1). ^{99m}Tc is readily available in all nuclear medicine facilities and is relatively inexpensive, factors that account for its routine use for thyroid gland imaging. The quality of images and diagnostic value of ^{99m}Tc pertechnetate images are nearly equivalent to that using ^{123}I, although many nuclear physicians prefer ^{123}I images because of the lower background. ^{99m}Tc pertechnetate is administered intravenously in amounts ranging from 2 to 5 mCi (37 to 185 MBq), and imaging of the thyroid is begun within 10 minutes after injection.

It is worth noting that some follicular neoplasms (including adenomas and follicular carcinomas) may appear functional or even "hot" on a ^{99m}Tc pertechnetate image and "cold" on radioiodine image, presumably because such tumors are able to trap but do not organify iodine. This type of discordance between ^{99m}Tc and radioiodine images occurs infrequently and, when there is discordance, the lesion is usually benign.[1] Many groups still prefer ^{123}I over ^{99m}Tc for imaging of thyroid nodules.

^{131}I is the only radioiodine that is useful for therapy, by virtue of its energetic beta emission, which has an average path length in tissue of about 1 mm. The principal diagnostic use of ^{131}I is in whole-body scanning for functioning metastases from DTC, for which application the physical $T_{1/2}$ of 8 days permits scans to be obtained over a period of several days.

In virtually every modern nuclear medicine laboratory routine, thyroid imaging is done using a scintillation camera fitted with a pinhole collimator. The scintillation camera has largely replaced rectilinear scanners. The pinhole collimator provides a magnified image of the gland, with better resolution than either the conventional parallel-hole collimator or rectilinear scanner.[2] The pinhole technique also allows oblique views of the gland. Because of the geometry of the pinhole collimator, however, the apparent size of the target structure is highly dependent on its distance from the collimator aperture, and the image is distorted at the periphery of the field of view. For ^{123}I and ^{131}I images of the thyroid, a minimum of 30,000 counts ought to be obtained; for ^{99m}Tc at least 100,000 counts are recommended (or 10-minute acquisition time). When dealing with thyroid nodules it is important to correlate the image with the palpable lesion by placing radioactive spot markers on the skin overlying or adjacent to the nodule. Additional markers are placed on the thyroid cartilage and suprasternal notch. Anterior (pinhole) images are obtained both with and without the markers in place while the patient remains in the same supine position.

Whole-body scans are obtained using the scintillation camera with the patient on a special scanning table. This technique is employed in surveys for thyroid cancer, usually involving administration of ^{131}I. A high-energy collimator is required when using ^{131}I. Anatomic markers are helpful in correlating foci of radioiodine uptake with palpable abnormalities or radiographic lesions.

Single-photon emission computed tomography (SPECT) is available in most nuclear medicine laboratories, where it is used routinely for myocardial perfusion imaging. The technique provides three-dimensional images or tomographic "slices" through the organ of interest. The scintillation camera rotates around the patient, and the acquired data are computer processed to yield images of higher resolution than those provided by planar techniques. When used with radioiodine or ^{99m}Tc, SPECT is useful in defining substernal thyroid tissue and with ^{131}I in searching for distant metastases from thyroid carcinoma, such as in the lungs or liver.

EVALUATING THYROID NODULES

The terms "cold," "warm," and "hot" are commonly used to describe the function of a thyroid nodule as revealed by nuclear imaging. These descriptors refer to the amount of radionuclide detected in the lesion relative to that in surrounding normal thyroid tissue. Nearly all malignant lesions in the gland and most benign nodules concentrate less radioiodine than the normal gland and therefore appear "cold" on nuclear images. Typically a cold nodule must be at least 5 to 10 mm in diameter to be detected by scintigraphy (e.g., pinhole imaging), depending on its position and depth in the gland. A nodule that appears to have equal activity compared to adjacent paranodular tissue is defined as "warm" or isofunctional but may in fact be hypofunctional—(i.e., "cold"), because the image depicts the average activity in a given volume of gland and the palpable nodule represents a thicker portion of the gland.[2] The term "warm" is ambiguous because such a lesion may in fact be a cold nodule that is too small to be distinguishable from surrounding normal thyroid. A "hot" nodule is one that takes up relatively more radionuclide than adjacent tissue, and the normal thyroid tissue may be suppressed by the autonomously hyperfunctional nodule (low serum TSH). Nodules that function autonomously (i.e., independent of TSH) start out as warm and may eventually grow large enough to lead to hyperthyroidism with suppression of the normal gland. Clearly there is a continuum in the level of function as visualized by imaging.

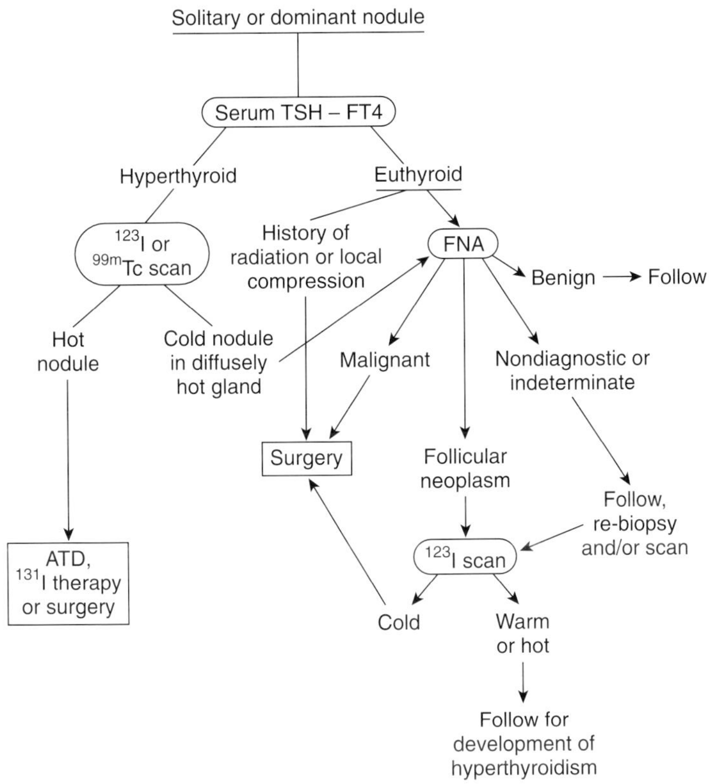

• **FIGURE 6-1** Diagnostic strategy for the workup of patients with a solitary thyroid nodule or a dominant nodule in a multinodular gland. *Serum TSH,* serum thyroid-stimulating hormone, measured by a sensitive assay; *FT4,* serum free thyroxine concentration; *FNA,* fine-needle aspiration biopsy; *ATD,* antithyroid drug (e.g., propylthiouracil). In patients with hyperthyroidism of Graves' disease and a coexisting cold nodule, thyroid malignancy should be ruled out before definitive therapy is initiated (e.g., ^{131}I therapy) for hyperthyroidism.

Fig. 6-1 presents a generally accepted algorithm outlining the respective roles of fine-needle aspiration (FNA) biopsy and nuclear imaging in the assessment of patients with a solitary thyroid nodule or a dominant nodule in a multinodular goiter.[3] This strategy is based in part on cost/benefit considerations.[4]

In these patients the initial assessment ought to include a thorough history, with specific reference to a history of radiation exposure, family history of thyroid cancer, symptoms of recent nodule growth or compression, symptoms of hyperthyroidism, physical examination, and laboratory tests of thyroid function, including measurement of serum TSH by a sufficiently sensitive assay to discriminate between euthyroid and hyperthyroid individuals. In the patient with a thyroid nodule and clinical and/or laboratory evidence of overt hyperthyroidism (suppressed TSH, high free T_4 and/or T_3), or subclinical

A 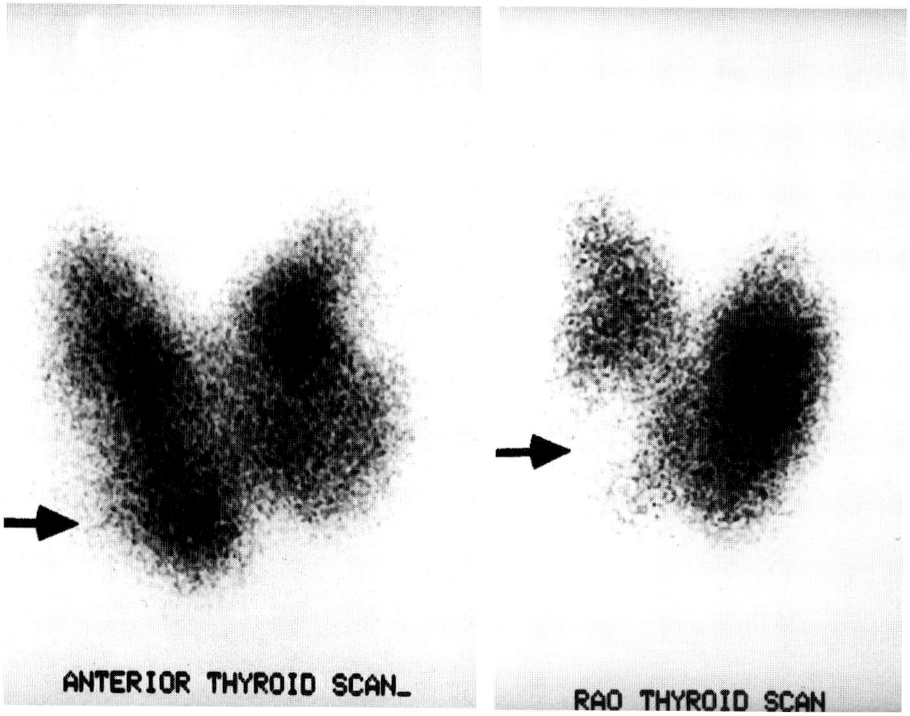 B

• **FIGURE 6-2** **A,** Anterior view. **B,** Right anterior oblique view (RAO) of thyroid pinhole images obtained 6 hours after administration of 300 μCi ^{123}I to a 56-year-old man with clinical and laboratory evidence of hyperthyroidism and a solitary thyroid nodule in the lower portion of the right lobe *(arrow)*. Only the RAO view shows the nodule to be nonfunctioning (cold). Following fine-needle aspiration, which revealed this nodule to be benign, the patient was successfully treated with ^{131}I.

hyperthyroidism (suppressed TSH alone), the approach is somewhat different from that in a euthyroid patient with a thyroid nodule. In the hyperthyroid patient with a thyroid nodule, nuclear imaging is indicated; either ^{99m}Tc pertechnetate or ^{123}I may be used. If the scan shows that the palpable nodule is hyperfunctioning (i.e., showing greater uptake of the radionuclide than the surrounding thyroid tissue), it is unlikely that the nodule is malignant. On occasion, a palpable nodule in a hyperthyroid patient is cold on nuclear scan, the remainder of the gland being hyperfunctional (Fig. 6-2). In such patients with a diffusely hyperactive gland containing a cold nodule, the possibility of malignancy in the nodule must be considered, and the diagnostic approach is the same as that for any cold nodule. Of course, the hyperthyroidism should be treated appropriately. Similarly, a dominant cold nodule in a toxic multinodular gland raises the possibility of coexisting malignancy.

It is axiomatic that two different thyroid disorders may coexist in the same patient.

In a euthyroid patient, on the other hand, the approach recommended by most specialists is to obtain cytologic specimens by FNA as the initial diagnostic test. If the FNA is nondiagnostic or shows a "follicular neoplasm," a nuclear scan is obtained, preferably using radioiodine ^{123}I. When FNA indicates a follicular neoplasm and the ^{123}I scan reveals a hyperfunctioning (warm or hot) nodule, the nodule is probably a benign adenoma. Exceptions to this generalization are rare, but they have been reported.[5,6]

FOLLOWING THYROIDECTOMY

Diagnostic scanning with radioiodine is recommended for patients who have recently undergone thyroid surgery for DTC and are candidates for radioiodine ablation of the residual normal thyroid tissue (remnant). The rationale for imaging before ablative therapy is to identify and quantify uptake in the thyroid remnant and to detect any functioning metastases in the neck or in more distant sites. This information helps to determine the amount of ^{131}I that is administered for therapy.

There are several biological factors that determine whether a particular metastatic lesion will be detected by radioiodine imaging. These include (1) the size of the tumor and its location (depth and proximity to organs that normally concentrate radioiodine, e.g., the stomach), (2) the ability of the tumor to concentrate and retain iodine, which is a function both of the degree of differentiation of the tumor and the circulating level of TSH, (3) the turnover of iodine in the tumor, that is, the biological half-life ($T_{1/2}$ biol) of radioiodine, which can vary from hours to days but is usually shorter than the $T_{1/2}$ biol of radioiodine in normal thyroid, and (4) the concentration of stable inorganic iodine in the circulation. Of the above biological factors, the serum TSH and the circulating stable iodide concentration can be influenced by steps taken in preparing the patient (see below).

There are also several physical and technical factors that affect the sensitivity of radioiodine scans. These include (1) the amount of ^{131}I administered (discussed below), (2) the time interval between ^{131}I administration and imaging, and (3) the type of imaging equipment. For scintillation cameras, the most widely used nuclear imaging devices in the United States, variables include the type of collimator (parallel-hole and sufficiently heavy for the high-energy photons of ^{131}I); duration of imaging (to achieve adequate counting statistics); completeness of whole-body and spot images; planar vs. single-photon emission tomography; computer processing of data; and quality control of film processing. Use of SPECT, which is frequently employed in nuclear medicine for myocardial imaging and other applications, increases the resolution and diagnostic accuracy of ^{131}I images, provided high-energy collimators are used.[7] Of equal importance to the biological and technical factors that influence diagnostic yield is the expertise of the physician who reads the images. The interpreter of the images must be experienced in reading scans containing low information density and be aware of the causes of false positive radioiodine scans.

Patient Preparation

In a patient who has had less than a total or near-total thyroidectomy (e.g., lobectomy or lobectomy plus isthmusectomy), the sensitivity of radioiodine imaging for detecting metastases is compromised. The main reasons for this are that a sizable thyroid remnant (e.g., an entire lobe) may make it impossible to obtain a serum TSH level sufficiently high to stimulate uptake in metastases, and the ^{131}I taken up by the remnant lobe tends to obscure abnormal foci of uptake within or near the thyroid bed.

To stimulate uptake of radioiodine by normal and malignant thyroid tissue, it is necessary to raise serum TSH levels above normal. The conventional approach involves discontinuation of thyroid hormone therapy to allow endogenous TSH to increase to supranormal levels (at least 30 mU/L); L-thyroxine (T_4) is discontinued for 5 to 6 weeks before imaging. To shorten the period of hypothyroidism, liothyronine (T_3) may be given (50 to 75 μg/day in divided doses) for 3 to 4 weeks following discontinuation of T_4. T_3 is discontinued 2 weeks before imaging. The serum TSH ought to be 30 mU/L or higher at the time the diagnostic dose of radioiodine is administered.[3] Patients should also have a serum thyroglobulin determination when hypothyroid in preparation for a radioiodine scan.

Pregnancy is a contraindication for the administration of ^{131}I for either diagnostic or therapeutic purposes. Therefore female patients capable of bearing children should undergo a pregnancy test, preferably by a quantitative serum human chorionic gonadotropin assay.

In times past, bovine TSH was administered to patients before imaging studies to stimulate uptake in metastases, but frequent hypersensitivity reactions, sometimes severe, led to the discontinuation of this practice in the 1970s. Recently, recombinant human TSH (rhTSH: Thyrogen, manufactured by Genzyme Corp., Cambridge, Mass.) has been developed, and, based on published results of clinical trials, is effective in stimulating uptake of ^{131}I by thyroid remnants and metastases in patients who remain euthyroid while receiving thyroid hormone therapy.[8,9] rhTSH is now available for routine use, and obviates the need to withdraw thyroid hormone for purposes of imaging and thus avoids the discomfort and sometimes serious medical and neuropsychiatric complications associated with hypothyroidism (e.g., salt and water retention, lethargy, depression).

When it is approved, the initial use of rhTSH will be in the diagnostic evaluation of patients following thyroidectomy for DTC primarily by demonstrating remnant thyroid tissue and/or metastatic tumor. In the follow-up of patients after ablative surgery, rhTSH will also allow serum Tg testing, as well as in diagnostic scanning, without discontinuing thyroid hormone therapy. Future applications of rhTSH might include preparation for ^{131}I therapy of DTC in patients in whom it is not possible to raise serum TSH sufficiently high or in whom it would be especially dangerous to withdraw thyroid hormone therapy.[10] Ramirez et al.[11] have discussed other potential applications of rhTSH in various thyroid conditions.

A low-iodine diet, followed for 7 to 10 days before administration of a diagnostic dose of radioiodine, has been shown to increase uptake of diagnostic as well as subsequent therapeutic doses of ^{131}I.[12] Simple low-iodine diets have been published.[13,14] It is even more important to avoid iodine-containing medications and radiographic contrast agents. Forced diuresis (e.g., by furosemide, 20 mg twice daily) has been shown to enhance clearance of iodide,[15] but I do not recommend this measure for routine diagnostic imaging.

A mild laxative (e.g., unflavored milk of magnesia) is advised to reduce interference in the scan caused by radioiodine in the large bowel. The laxative is given the evening before the first imaging session.

Imaging may be performed as early as 24 hours after administration of radioiodine, but better-quality scans are obtained after a longer interval, and some metastases appear only after 48 hours. Many recommend that imaging be done routinely both at 48 and 72 hours.

The Stunning Effect

The term "stunning" refers to the effect of diagnostic administration of ^{131}I on the uptake in thyroid tissue or metastases of subsequent therapeutic administration of ^{131}I. This phenomenon, which seems to involve a sublethal, presumably temporary suppression of iodine uptake, was noted decades ago.[16] It has received renewed attention in recent years.[17-20]

Jeevanram et al.[21] measured uptake of diagnostic and therapeutic amounts of ^{131}I by thyroid gland remnants in a series of 52 patients following thyroidectomy. They found that uptake of therapeutic ^{131}I was significantly reduced below the uptake of a "tracer" amount (5 mCi [185 MBq]) of ^{131}I. The degree of reduction was proportional to the estimated radiation dose but independent of the time interval (from 7 to 30 days) between the initial diagnostic administration and the subsequent therapy.[21] The degree of reduction was proportional to the calculated radiation dose delivered by the initial administration. Therefore quantitative estimates of ^{131}I uptake bear out the conclusions based on nonquantitative comparison of images that stunning is a real phenomenon. The question remains: How much ^{131}I can be administered for diagnostic imaging without causing significant impairment of the efficacy of a subsequent therapeutic dose of ^{131}I? The answer depends on the radiation dose delivered to the tissue by "diagnostic" ^{131}I, which in turn is a function of the fractional uptake of the ^{131}I, the volume of tissue, and the effective half-life of the radioiodine in the tissue.

Park et al.[18] retrospectively compared scans in 26 patients obtained following administration of 3, 5, or 10 mCi (111, 185, or 370 MBq) ^{131}I with scans performed after ^{131}I therapy. By visual inspection of the scans they found that uptake of the ^{131}I therapy in thyroid remnants or metastases was reduced significantly in 20 of the 26 cases. The effect occurred more frequently in the group given 10 mCi (370 MBq) for scanning than in the patients given 3 or 5 mCi (111 or 185 MBq). Thyroid remnant tissue seemed to be more vulnerable to stunning than metastases. In contrast, when scans were done using ^{123}I, which, unlike ^{131}I, has no beta emission, no such stunning phenomenon was found.

To avoid stunning, Park et al.[19] has proposed that ^{123}I be used for initial imaging in postthyroidectomy patients being evaluated for thyroid remnant ablation and in those with palpable cervical masses. These authors compared the diagnostic yield of ^{131}I and ^{123}I scans in postthyroidectomy preablation patients with DTC and in postablation patients, using the post-^{131}I therapy scan as the "gold standard." In the former group, diagnostic ^{131}I scans in 42 patients revealed 93% of the foci of uptake, and ^{123}I scans (using 0.3 mCi of ^{123}I) in 86 patients showed 90% of the foci revealed on post-therapy scans (the difference between ^{131}I and ^{123}I uptake was not significant). At 1-year after ablative surgery, follow-up ^{131}I scans revealed 92% of foci, whereas ^{123}I scans showed 69% (p = 0.079). The authors concluded that the diagnostic accuracy of ^{123}I was equal to that of ^{131}I for postoperative evaluation, but for follow-up ^{131}I appears to be superior to ^{123}I.[19]

The use of ^{123}I for imaging metastases has limitations. Because the physical half-life of ^{123}I is nearly 15 times shorter than that of ^{131}I, 10 mCi (370 MBq) of ^{123}I has about the same detection efficiency as 6.5 mCi (240 MBq) of ^{131}I when imaging is performed 24 hours after administration.[22] At later times following administration (i.e., 48 hours and later, when metastases are more likely to be seen), the counting rates from ^{123}I relative to ^{131}I fall off rapidly. The cost per millicurie of ^{123}I is several times that of ^{131}I. Finally, ^{123}I does not allow calculation of radiation dosimetry, which requires measurements over a period of several days.

Many centers now limit the quantity of ^{131}I for diagnostic imaging to 2 or 3 mCi (74 or 111 MBq) per administration, accepting a lower sensitivity to avoid the stunning effect. Clearly, higher amounts would detect more metastases. Waxman et al.[23] showed that scans performed with 10 mCi (370 MBq) of ^{131}I reveal more foci than with 2 mCi (74 MBq), and scans performed following ^{131}I therapy with 100 mCi or more show foci not detected with 10 mCi (370 MBq). Moreover, from their study using ^{131}I-filled phantoms and state-of-the-art imaging instruments (in 1986), Arnstein et al.[24] calculated that even with 30 mCi (1110 MBq) of ^{131}I, some potentially treatable lesions would be missed, depending on their size and depth. The question that has not yet been answered is whether treatment of metastases that are detected only with higher amounts of ^{131}I (and therefore concentrating relatively less of the ^{131}I) leads to improved outcome in terms of decreased recurrence rate or prolonged survival. In a follow-up study of two groups of patients, one with negative 2 mCi (74 MBq) scans and positive 10 mCi (370 MBq) scans, and the other group with positive 2 mCi (74 MBq) scans, Ramanna et al.[25] found no significant difference in the completeness of subsequent ablative therapy.

Maxon and Smith[26] have pointed out that, although ^{131}I administered in amounts greater than 2 mCi might uncover more lesions, this rarely alters management decisions. McDougall[20] compared diagnostic scans obtained from 48 to 72 hours after administration of 2 mCi (74 MBq)^{131}I with post- ^{131}I therapy scans in 147 patients and found evidence of stunning in only two patients (1.4%). Furthermore, the posttherapy scans revealed additional lesions not seen on the 2 mCi scan in only 12 cases (8%). It appears from this and other experience that significant stunning can be avoided while useful information may be obtained in the majority of postthyroidectomy patients by limiting the amount of ^{131}I for the diagnostic study to 2 mCi (74 MBq). When these lower amounts of ^{131}I are administered, it is particularly important to pay close attention to patient preparation and to optimize technical factors in the imaging procedure. Figs. 6-3 and 6-4 illustrate a patient whose diagnostic (2 mCi) scan shows one metastatic focus in the chest and whose post-^{131}I therapy scan shows two metastases.

Radioiodine Therapy Scans

It is generally accepted that scans should be performed within the first week to 10 days following therapeutic administration of ^{131}I. Such scans uncover

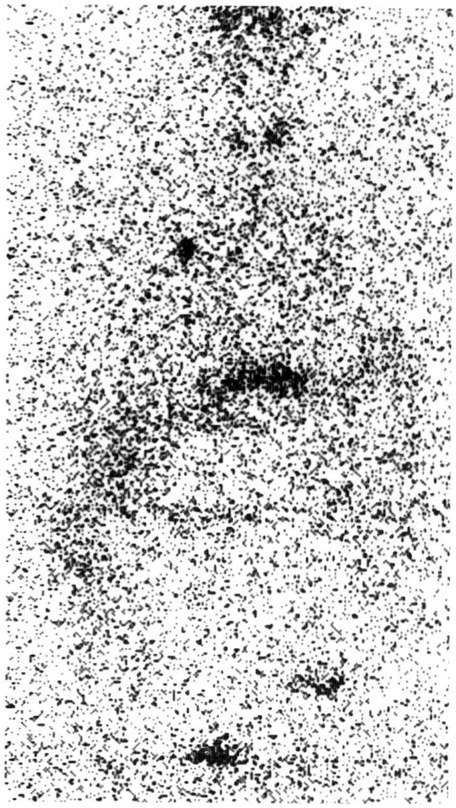

• **FIGURE 6-3** Whole-body scan (anterior view) at 48 hours after diagnostic administration (2 mCi) of ^{131}I in a 71-year-old man who had undergone a subtotoal thyroidectomy and postoperative ablation therapy (30 mCi ^{131}I) for follicular carcinoma 2 years before this scan. This diagnostic scan shows two small foci in the thyroid bed (probably remnant) and a third discrete focus of uptake in the right chest. The latter corresponded with a solitary 2 cm mass in the right lung seen on chest x-ray films. ^{131}I activity in the stomach, large bowel, and urinary bladder are not considered abnormal.

new, unsuspected metastases in 22% to 31% of patients and are therefore useful in staging patients and determining prognosis.[27,28] Sherman et al.[29] reported that 15% of the time posttherapy scans added significant information that could have changed management decisions.

The interpretation of radioiodine scans must take into account normal sites of uptake, which include salivary glands, gastric mucosa, and large bowel (Fig. 6-5). Normal secretions (nasal, salivary, sweat) and urine, which contain a high concentration of radioiodine, are potential sources of artifact. Sites at which sweat may pool (e.g., in braided hair) and saliva in the esophagus may cause confusion.[26,30,31] Uptake in breast tissue, which may be asymmetric, can be misinterpreted as lung or chest wall metastases. Radioiodine

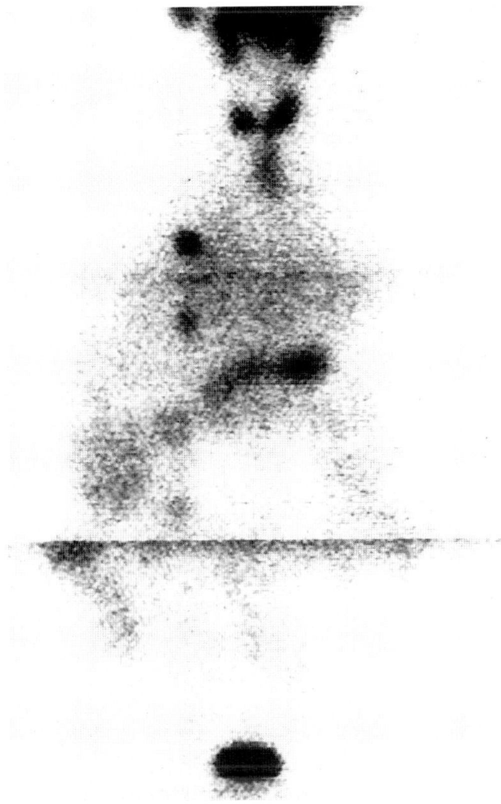

• **FIGURE 6-4** Post-^{131}I therapy scan in the same patient as in Fig. 6-3. This is an anterior whole-body scan obtained 4 days after administration of 200 mCi ^{131}I. In addition to the thyroid bed foci noted on the diagnostic scan (see Fig. 6-3), two foci are seen in the right lung. The vertical midline activity extending from the neck into the upper chest represents ^{131}I in saliva within the esophagus. The patient was given a drink of water and the scan was repeated; this focus of activity was no longer seen.

concentrates in glandular breast tissue, even in women who have ceased breast-feeding months previously.[32] The liver is often visualized on scans obtained following administration of large amounts of ^{131}I, particularly 3 to 7 days following therapy.[33,34] Radiolabeled thyroid hormone released into the blood from functioning thyroid tissue (normal or malignant) is concentrated in normal liver parenchyma. This diffuse pattern of hepatic uptake should not be confused with hepatic metastases, which would appear as focal regions of uptake.

Nonthyroid neoplasms, cysts, and inflammatory lesions can be confused with metastatic disease from thyroid carcinoma, because such lesions may concentrate radioiodine. These include primary lung carcinoma, gastric adenocarcinoma, teratoma-containing gastric mucosa, struma ovarii, spinal

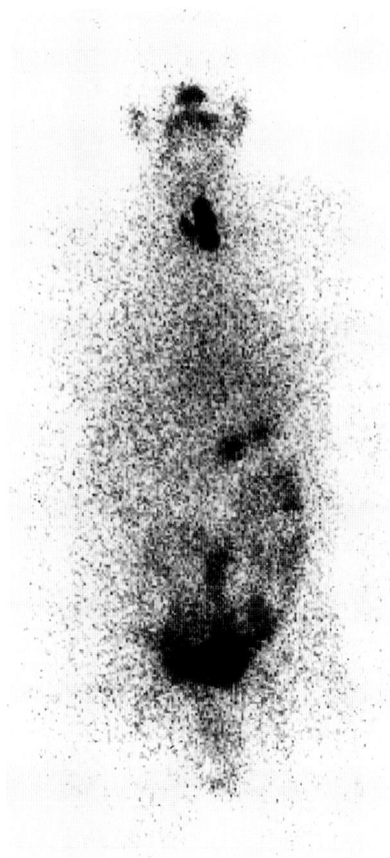

• **FIGURE 6-5** Whole-body scan (anterior) obtained 24 hours after administration of 2.5 mCi ^{123}I to a patient who had undergone near-total thyroidectomy for an invasive papillary carcinoma 6 weeks earlier. The scan shows a large focus of asymmetric activity in the lower neck, interpreted as thyroid remnant plus probable tumor in local lymph nodes. The activity in the head represents salivary gland uptake and nasal secretions, and that in the abdomen and pelvis is stomach (uptake by the parietal cells), bowel, and bladder contents (all normal sites of radioiodine accumulation).

cord meningioma, ovarian cystadenoma, Meckel's diverticulum, large renal cysts, chronic sinusitis, lymphoepithelial cyst in the parotid gland, scrotal hydrocele, inflammatory lung disease, and inflammatory skin lesions (e.g., psoriatic plaque).[26,35] Radioiodine uptake in normal or hyperplastic thymus gland (in adults) has been described.[36,37] The reader is referred to recent reviews for causes of artifacts and false positive radioiodine scans.[3,31]

It should be routine in nuclear medicine facilities to have an experienced person review images before the patient leaves the unit. If any possible artifacts are suspected, steps should be taken to remove the cause and the patient should undergo repeat imaging. If radioiodine uptake is seen in the midline of the neck or thorax, the possibility should be considered that this is saliva or nasal secretion in the pharynx or esophagus and the patient should be given something to eat or drink prior to repeat scanning. Lateral images of the skull often help to distinguish between surface and intracranial activity. Handkerchiefs that might contain secretions should be removed from pockets. Urine or sweat on the skin can usually be washed away, but it may be necessary to ask the patient to shower before a repeat imaging procedure is performed.

Other Radiopharmaceuticals

The sensitivity of ^{131}I scans for metastastic thyroid carcinoma is less than 100%. The frequency of false negative diagnostic scans has been reported to be as high as 35%.[38] Several other tumor-seeking radiolabeled agents are available for detecting and localizing radioiodine-negative metastases.

^{201}Thallium. The most extensive experience has been with thallium chloride (^{201}Tl) as an alternative radiopharmaceutical agent for detecting metastatic thyroid carcinoma. Thallium, a monovalent cation, is transported across the plasma membrane of cells by the same mechanism as potassium. Early studies indicated that ^{201}Tl yielded high sensitivity for thyroid carcinoma metastases.[39,40]

Hoefnagel et al.[41] retrospectively reviewed experience with ^{201}Tl and ^{131}I scanning in 301 patients with DTC. Among 226 patients with negative ^{131}I scan results (5 mCi, 185 MBq), 26 had positive ^{201}Tl scan results; of these, 23 were confirmed by biopsy. The authors reported a sensitivity of ^{131}I scanning of only 48%, but when both agents were used, sensitivity was 98%. One of the advantages of ^{201}Tl imaging is that it does not require withdrawal of thyroid hormone. Subsequent reports based on prospective studies have been less enthusiastic about the value of ^{201}Tl for use in DTC. Brendel et al.[42] analyzed data on 31 patients with DTC and found a sensitivity of ^{201}Tl imaging of only 45%, much lower than the 84% sensitivity of ^{131}I in their study. They noted that metastases in bone and liver were often missed by ^{201}Tl. Burman et al.[43] found good concordance between ^{131}I and ^{201}Tl in 17 patients; in three of these cases ^{201}Tl uncovered more extensive metastases (all confirmed histologically or by MRI). In another prospective study, Dadparvar et al.[44] reported a higher sensitivity with ^{131}I (80%) than with ^{201}Tl (60%). However, they found ^{201}Tl to be of value mainly in ^{131}I-negative patients in whom metastatic disease was suspected because of elevated serum thyroglobulin levels. Charkes et al.[45] reported that sensitivity of detection of metastases using ^{201}Tl is increased by the use of SPECT. One limitation of ^{201}Tl for imaging in this disease is its low specificity, since a large variety of neoplasms and inflammatory lesions concentrate ^{201}Tl. Furthermore, ^{201}Tl is of no value in assessing thyroid gland remnants.[46] Iida et al.[47] reported that in 149 postoperative patients, 65 of whom had evidence of recurrent tumor, ^{201}Tl scans gave a sensitivity of 78% and a specificity of 95%. In agreement with other reports, Iida et al. found that serum thyroglobulin correctly detected recurrent disease in more than half of ^{201}Tl negative cases. Van Sorge-Van Boxel et al.[48] confirmed the superiority of the combination of serum thyroglobulin and ^{201}Tl imaging over either one alone, but they found that serum thyroglobulin and ^{131}I scans together correctly diagnosed all patients with recurrent disease but did not necessarily localize all the metastases in every case. In such patients ^{201}Tl scans detected metastases that were missed with ^{131}I.

The published data indicate that ^{201}Tl can be useful in localizing metastases in selected patients, particularly when diagnostic ^{131}I scans yield negative results and metastases are suspected on the basis of elevated serum thyroglobulin levels or clinical evidence. In practice, for the detection of recurrent or persistent thyroid cancer, serum thyroglobulin used in conjunction with ^{131}I imaging has decreased the use of ^{201}Tl. Nevertheless, there are some patients with isolated metastases that do not take up ^{131}I (even when given in therapeutic amounts) and in whom localization by ^{201}Tl imaging might aid in planning surgical excision or directing external radiotherapy.

^{99m}Tc Sestamibi (MIBI). A cationic lipophilic agent that is concentrated in mitochondria-rich cells. Its uptake by cells is dependent on blood flow and integrity of plasma and mitochondrial membranes. Although it is used principally for imaging the myocardium, ^{99m}Tc MIBI has been shown to concentrate in normal and neoplastic thyroid tissue and in a variety of other cancers.[49] The precise role of this agent in assessing patients with thyroid cancer is still under study. Available evidence indicates that, like ^{201}Tl, ^{99m}Tc MIBI may be useful in localizing recurrent thyroid carcinoma in ^{131}I-negative patients in whom there is other evidence of recurrence.[50-53] Because of the 6-hour half-life of ^{99m}Tc, allowing the administration of 20 to 25 mCi (740 to 925 MBq), and its more suitable photon energy for imaging, ^{99m}Tc MIBI produces images of higher quality than with ^{201}Tl. ^{99m}Tc MIBI concentrates especially well in Hürthle cell tumors, which typically take up radioiodine poorly.[51] Therefore this is the agent of choice for imaging patients with suspected metastases from Hürthle cell carcinoma. Imaging with ^{99m}Tc MIBI, as with ^{201}Tl, does not require an elevated serum TSH. On the other hand, both ^{201}Tl and ^{99m}Tc MIBI have the disadvantage of high uptake in the myocardium and, in the case of ^{99m}Tc MIBI, in the liver and intestinal tract, so thyroid cancer metastases in or near these organs could easily be missed.

Other agents that have been shown to concentrate in at least some metastatic DTC tumors include ^{99m}Tc tetrofosmin,[54] which, like MIBI, is employed for myocardial perfusion imaging; ^{111}Indium-labeled octreotide,[55] and; ^{99m}Tc dimercaptosuccinic acid in the pentavalent form (DMSA[V]).[56]

^{67}Gallium (^{67}Ga) is taken up in a variety of neoplasms and in sites of chronic inflammation (e.g., granuloma). Some thyroid cancers, particularly poorly differentiated or undifferentiated carcinoma and lymphoma, concentrate ^{67}Ga, but because most well-differentiated thyroid cancers take up little or no ^{67}Ga, this agent has little use in patients with DTC.[57]

Nuclear bone scanning (using ^{99m}Tc diphosphonates) does not detect bone metastases from thyroid carcinoma with sufficient sensitivity to recommend this technique for routine surveillance of patients with this disease.[58,59] Alam et al.[60] reported that the combination of ^{201}Tl and ^{99m}Tc diphosphonate scans appears to improve detection of bone metastases. In their study of 27 patients with 77 bone lesions, when individual bone lesions were counted, only 75% of the lesions were seen on diphosphonate scans, but 93.5% were detected by the combination of ^{201}Tl and ^{99m}Tc diphosphonate scanning. It would be of interest to see these findings confirmed in a larger group of patients.

^{18}FDG PET Scanning. Malignant tumors typically have a high rate of glycolysis and actively take up glucose (and its nonmetabolized radiolabeled analog, ^{18}F-fluorodeoxyglucose; ^{18}FDG). ^{18}F is a positron-emitting radionuclide with a half-life of 110 minutes. ^{18}FDG is concentrated by a variety of neoplasms including thyroid carcinoma.[61,62,63] Positron-emission tomography (PET) requires specialized equipment that is not widely available. Recent studies indicate that ^{18}FDG-PET and ^{131}I scans are complementary in diagnosing metastatic thyroid cancer. ^{131}I-negative tumors are more often positive with ^{18}FDG, and ^{18}FDG-negative tumors tend to be positive with ^{131}I. This is most likely a result of the fact that ^{18}FDG uptake is highest in poorly differentiated thyroid cancer.[63] In general, PET images have higher resolution than conventional scans including SPECT images. ^{18}FDG-PET scans show low background in the chest and liver, giving this agent a relative advantage over ^{201}Tl and ^{99m}Tc sestamibi. Sisson[64] has presented preliminary evidence that ^{18}FDG uptake by thyroid tumor is enhanced when serum TSH levels are elevated.

^{131}I THERAPY

The terms *ablation* and *ablative ^{131}I therapy* will be used here to mean ^{131}I therapy that is intended to destroy residual normal thyroid tissue (thyroid remnant) that often remains following surgery for DTC. The term *^{131}I therapy* will be used to denote therapy that is intended to destroy residual, recurrent, or metastatic thyroid carcinoma, whether or not remnant thyroid tissue is present.

Ablative ^{131}I Therapy of Thyroid Gland Remnants

The rationale for postoperative ablation with ^{131}I is fourfold: (1) The diagnostic utility of serum thyroglobulin testing is increased when all normal thyroid tissue is eliminated; (2) the sensitivity of follow-up diagnostic radioiodine scanning is increased because serum TSH levels can rise to levels sufficiently high to stimulate radioiodine uptake in metastases; (3) any uptake subsequently seen in the thyroid bed is an indication of locally recurrent tumor; and (4) the ablative therapy might destroy microscopic tumor deposits in the thyroid remnant or in regional lymph nodes. (Micrometastases have been detected in ipsilateral lymph nodes in 75% to 90% of patients with papillary carcinoma.[74,75])

Available data indicate that ablative therapy is probably not necessary in all patients with DTC. In young adults (under age 40) who have undergone adequate surgery for a small (less than 1.5 cm), noninvasive, well-differentiated thyroid carcinoma, without regional or distant metastases, ablation would probably not improve on an already excellent prognosis. Data from several large series indicate that among patients with moderate to high risk of recurrence, as determined at the time of surgery, postoperative ablation decreases the rate of recurrence and prolongs survival.[65-68] There is still controversy regarding where to draw the line,[69-71] but the trend is in favor of ablative therapy for nearly all patients except those with occult tumors and the best prognosis.

Dosimetric Considerations

The radiation dose necessary to destroy thyroid remnant tissue has been estimated at a minimal 30,000 rads (300 Gy).[72,73] The radiation dose delivered to the target can be computed from three parameters: the mass (volume) of tissue, the fractional uptake of radioiodine (usually measured at 24 hours), and the effective half-life ($T_{1/2}$ eff) of radioiodine in the tissue. In the case of thyroid remnant, the approximate volume of thyroid tissue left behind can be provided by the surgeon's estimate or by ultrasonographic examination. The 24-hour radioiodine uptake in the neck can be measured, and the $T_{1/2}$ eff can be estimated over a period of 5 to 7 days following a diagnostic administration of ^{131}I.[72] A simple formula is used to calculate the amount of ^{131}I that must be administered to achieve ablation in a single treatment with a high likelihood of success.[28,72] Because there is a wide range of uptake and effective half-life from one individual to another, the actual radiation dose delivered to the remnant does not correlate with the administered amount of ^{131}I.[72] Maxon et al.[73,76] have shown that the dosimetric approach has the advantage of avoiding the administration of larger amounts of ^{131}I than are required for ablation. Nevertheless, many institutions choose to give a standard amount of ^{131}I for ablation (e.g., 29.9 mCi [1.1 GBq]), which, with some exceptions, is the largest quantity that can be administered to outpatients. Other centers give an arbitrary amount (e.g., 100 mCi [3.7 GBq]) for ablation, which currently requires that the patient be hospitalized for 1 to 3 days to avoid excessive radiation exposure to family and the public. Success of ablation is assessed by follow-up radioiodine scans (at 9 to 12 months). The goal is to reduce uptake in the thyroid bed at 24 or 48 hours to less than 0.2% to 0.3%.[77,78] For 80% of patients, a single "outpatient" dose of ^{131}I (i.e., 29.9 mCi [1.1 GBq]) is sufficient to ablate the remnant.[69,77] Large remnants require higher amounts of ^{131}I and tend to require repeat administrations. Of course, when necessary, repeated doses of ^{131}I should be administered until the goal is achieved.

Patient Preparation

We recommend that ablation be deferred for 6 to 8 weeks after thyroid surgery to allow for complete healing and subsidence of edema. During the postoperative period, the patient is maintained euthyroid on T_3, 0.025 mg two or three times a day, and this is discontinued at least 14 days before administration of ^{131}I to allow serum TSH to rise to at least 30 mU/L. A low-iodine diet is followed for 2 weeks before and for 2 to 3 days after ^{131}I administration. Medications containing iodine and radiographic contrast dyes (which contain iodine) are avoided for at least 1 month before ablation.

We recommend administration of a diagnostic amount (2 mCi) of ^{131}I for measurement of the percentage of uptake in the thyroid bed at 24 hours and a whole-body scan with pinhole imaging of the neck at 48 hours after ^{131}I. In addition, when functioning thyroid remnant is seen and uptake is greater than 0.3%, some recommend measuring ^{131}I in the neck every 2 to 3 days for a week to estimate the $T_{1/2}$ eff. Alternatively, if dosimetry is not performed, one may perform diagnostic imaging using ^{123}I (0.3 to 1.0 mCi), as described above.

Ablative therapy is preceded by obtaining informed consent from the patient and by issuing instructions to the patient and family regarding precautions to avoid excessive radiation exposure to family and public. As previously mentioned, serum TSH and thyroglobulin determinations and a quantitative pregnancy test are done before ^{131}I administration, which is given by mouth. Thyroid hormone therapy (L-T_4 or a combination of L-T_4 and T_3)[72] is begun 24 hours following the administration of the ablative therapy to minimize the time during which the patient is hypothyroid and to hasten the decline in serum TSH, thus slowing release of ^{131}I from the thyroid. A posttherapy whole-body scan is usually performed within 7 to 10 days later to detect any regional or distant metastases that may have been missed by the diagnostic scan.

Follow-Up

Patients are maintained on thyroid hormone therapy, usually L-T_4, in doses in sufficient to suppress serum TSH to levels commensurate with the risk of recurrence. Serum thyroglobulin is monitored every 3 months for the first year, or until thyroglobulin becomes less than 2 to 3 ng/ml while the patient is receiving thyroid hormone. At 6 to 12 months after ablative surgery, thyroid hormone is withdrawn for whole-body scan and serum thyroglobulin testing if the following conditions are met: a whole-body scan is negative for metastases (assuming TSH levels are higher than 30 mU/L and excess iodine intake has been avoided before the scan is performed), the neck uptake is less than 0.3% (at 24 or 48 hours), serum thyroglobulin is less than 10 ng/ml, and there is no clinical evidence of recurrent tumor. (Because the sensitivity of thyroglobulin assays varies from one laboratory to another, the cutoff level above which the test indicates the presence of functioning will also vary.) Then there is no need to repeat a whole-body scan for at least 1 year. In patients with a low risk of recurrence, routine whole-body scan is probably unnecessary after the first negative follow-up whole-body scan, as long as there is no evidence of recurrent tumor by clinical examination, chest x-ray evaluation, and serum thyroglobulin testing.

In patients who have persistent thyroid bed activity (more than 0.3% uptake of administered ^{131}I), repeat ablative therapy is advisable.

^{131}I Therapy of Metastatic Differential Thyroid Cancer

Indications for ^{131}I therapy include persistent or recurrent tumor in the neck that is not surgically resectable or demonstrable on diagnostic ^{131}I scan; distant metastases shown by ^{131}I whole-body scan; and evidence of the tumor's presence when the diagnostic ^{131}I scan is negative. Such evidence is an elevated serum thyroglobulin level (in a postablation patient without serum anti-thyroglobulin antibodies), a positive result to biopsy, or a positive radiographic, CT, MRI, or nuclear scan using a radiolabeled agent other than radioiodine.

Dosimetric Considerations

One can compute the radiation dose (in rads) that will be delivered to a tumor from a given administered quantity of ^{131}I by estimating the following three parameters: the mass of the tumor, the percent of ^{131}I uptake, and the $T_{1/2}$ eff of ^{131}I in the tumor.

$$\text{Rads per mCi } ^{131}\text{I given} = \frac{T\tfrac{1}{2} \text{ eff (days)} \times \% \text{ uptake} \times 150}{\text{Tumor mass (g)}}$$

The same formula allows one to calculate the amount of ^{131}I that must be administered to deliver a given radiation dose to the tumor.[72]

Maxon et al.[12] have determined that 98% of metastases respond to a radiation dose of 8000 rads or higher, whereas only 20% responded to a dose less than 8000 rads. Others have reported similar results.[79] Hurley and Becker[72] recommend ^{131}I treatment for metastases if one can achieve a radiation dose greater than 5000 rads. These authors suggest that doses in the range of 5000 to 30,000 rads may not always cure the disease but may cause a sufficient response to relieve symptoms and prolong useful life. In the case of very small metastases (micrometastases), for example, 0.1 mm in diameter (approximately the size of a thyroid follicle), because the range of beta particles from ^{131}I is 1 mm, about half of the energy of the beta emission from ^{131}I within the lesion will be deposited outside the lesion.[80] Consequently, dosimetry calculations using standard formulas (S factors) will overestimate the radiation exposure to micrometastases.[81]

An alternative approach to ^{131}I treatment of metastatic DTC is the one originally employed by Benua et al.[82] and Leeper.[83] The maximum amount of ^{131}I is given that will not cause significant untoward effects. The major complications to be avoided are bone marrow suppression and pulmonary fibrosis. Whole-body retention (determined from urinary ^{131}I excretion) and blood concentration of ^{131}I are measured over a period of several days following administration of a diagnostic amount of ^{131}I. From these data the therapeutic amount of ^{131}I is calculated that will give less than 200 rads to the blood and less than 120 mCi ^{131}I retained in the whole body at 48 hours (less than 80 mCi if diffuse pulmonary metastases are present). Using this regimen, metastases regressed and survival was enhanced in the majority of patients under age 40; patients older than 40 did not respond as well.[83]

Many centers follow a simple rule in deciding on the amount of ^{131}I. For suspected or known tumor in the thyroid bed or in cervical lymph nodes, a fixed dose of 150 mCi (5.55 GBq) is given (in a normal-sized adult). For distant metastases (lung, mediastinum, bone), 150 to 200 mCi is administered. A dose of 200 mCi (7.4 GBq) is unlikely to result in serious complications; however, limiting any one therapeutic administration to 200 mCi may undertreat some patients. It is important to give an adequate dose of ^{131}I for the initial treatment, as a smaller amount may merely stun the tumor, blunting uptake of subsequent treatment doses without preventing tumor progression. As emphasized by Hurley and Becker[72] and Maxon and Smith,[26] in patients with life-threatening disease, it is critical to treat them with the maximal tolerable amount of ^{131}I initially. This can best be done using one or another dosimetric approaches.

Using Lithium

Tumors that respond to ^{131}I therapy tend to exhibit longer ^{131}I retention times than those tumors that do not respond.[76,84] The effectiveness of ^{131}I is enhanced in some cases by administration of lithium (Li^+) chloride as an adjunct ^{131}I therapy. Li^+ inhibits the release of radioiodine from the thyroid gland and from thyroid cancers by a mechanism that is not clearly understood, but Li^+ does not inhibit uptake of radioiodide, so the net effect is to increase the accumulation of radioiodine.[85] Clinical experience indicates that those tumors that have the shortest $T_{1/2}$ eff show the greatest effect of Li^+.[86] The agent is administered for 2 or 3 days before ^{131}I therapy and continued for 5 days after therapy. Serum levels ought to be monitored during administration of Li^+. It is recommended that the use of Li^+ be considered in patients with particularly short $T_{1/2}$ eff based on estimates using diagnostic ^{131}I.

Elevated Serum Thyroglobulin and Negative Diagnostic ^{131}I Scans

In one large series, about 10% of patients who had been treated by thyroidectomy and ^{131}I ablation developed elevated serum thyroglobulin without ^{131}I scan positivity or other evidence of recurrent tumor.[87] The frequency of this combination of findings depends on several factors, not the least of which is the threshold value used to define an abnormally elevated thyroglobulin level. Some authors recommend a threshold level above 10 ng/ml while the patient is undergoing thyroid hormone suppression therapy and 40 ng/ml when off thyroid hormone therapy.[38,39] Unfortunately, the assay for serum thyroglobulin is not standardized and uniform, with the result that various laboratories obtain different values for the same specimen.

There are several possible reasons for a rise in serum thyroglobulin throughout in a patient who has undergone thyroidectomy and ^{131}I ablation: (1) Multiple, widely dispersed functioning metastases are present, but are too small to be detected by diagnostic ^{131}I scan; (2) metastases produce thyroglobulin but do not take up sufficient ^{131}I to be detected on a diagnostic scan; (3) the patient has received excess iodine (e.g., in an x-ray contrast agent), or serum TSH levels are too low for detection of tumor by ^{131}I scanning; (4) the source of thyroglobulin is normal thyroid tissue that has not been ablated; and (5) the thyroglobulin result is false positive (which may be caused by serum antithyroglobulin antibodies).

Explanations 1 and 2 would seem to account for most cases. In three separate series, from 70% to 94% of patients with elevated serum thyroglobulin levels and negative ^{131}I scans had evidence of local or distant tumor on post-^{131}I therapy scans.[88-90] Following treatment with large amounts (150 to 300 mCi) of ^{131}I, serum thyroglobulin levels fell in nearly all patients, reaching less than 5 ng/ml in half of them.[90] Schlumberger et al.[91] treat thyroglobulin-positive, scan-negative patients with a fixed amount of 100 mCi ^{131}I; the treatment is repeated every 4 to 6 months until the posttherapy scan yields negative results. Serum thyroglobulin decreased to levels below 40 ng/ml (off thyroid hormone) in most of the patients. Pulmonary micronodules, as revealed by CT, disappeared in seven of eight patients treated by this technique. Sisson et al.[80] reported that after ^{131}I treatment, radiographically visible pulmonary metastases decreased in size in seven of nine patients and disappeared in the other two patients. These authors recommend ^{131}I therapy for patients with similar conditions but raised the question as to whether the risks associated with large single and cumulative doses of ^{131}I might exceed the benefits. Long-term data on survival in patients treated "blindly" with ^{131}I are not yet available, but it seems likely that at least some of these patients are helped by ^{131}I therapy.

The question of blind treatment with ^{131}I of patients with positive thyroglobulin and negative diagnostic ^{131}I scans is still controversial. McDougall[78] argued that patients who die of DTC die from gross disease involving vital organs, not from elevated serum thyroglobulin levels. He added that serum thyroglobulin levels may vary widely, depending on the level of circulating TSH, the threshold level of thyroglobulin above which one treats blindly with ^{131}I is arbitrary, and one cannot know the appropriate amount of ^{131}I to prescribe for therapy when the results of the diagnostic scan are negative. The end point of therapy is not defined, and the risks associated with large cumulative doses of ^{131}I may not be worth the uncertain benefits of treatment in this group of patients, many of whom have an excellent prognosis.

The pros and cons of blind ^{131}I therapy have been discussed by others.[88,92] Our own approach is the following: prior to ^{131}I therapy, a thorough search to find the source of the thyroglobulin is conducted, using various imaging modalities, including ultrasonography of the neck, MRI of the neck and mediastinum, and/or nuclear scanning ^{201}Tl or ^{99m}Tc MIBI. Isolated metastatic lesions that are found to be accessible (e.g., in the neck) are resected, following which the patient is treated with ^{131}I. Fig. 6-6 illustrates the post-^{131}I therapy seen in a patient whose diagnostic ^{131}I scan was negative.

Complications of ^{131}I Therapy

Acute and Subacute Complications

Radiation Thyroiditis. This may occur in patients who have a large amount of thyroid remnant following administration of ^{131}I for ablation. This is encountered only rarely in patients who have had a total or near-total thyroidectomy. The symptoms may include diffuse neck pain, with radiation to jaws or ears, and tenderness in the region of the thyroid. Symptoms are transient and usually respond to anti-inflammatory drugs. Rarely, corticosteroids are necessary. The radiation-induced thyroiditis may cause transient hyperthyroidism, which can be ameliorated with beta-adrenergic blocking drugs. Patients with large metastases of functioning follicular thyroid carcinoma may exhibit thyrotoxicosis, which could be exacerbated by ^{131}I therapy due to the radiation-induced release of thyroid hormone from the metastases. In such patients, pretreatment with antithyroid drugs prior to ^{131}I therapy may minimize or prevent this complication.[26]

Sialadenitis. This occurs in 10% to 30% of patients following administration of more than 100 mCi of ^{131}I and is manifested by swelling and tenderness in the salivary glands, unpleasant taste, and dry mouth. These symptoms usually begin on the second day and resolve after 3 days. In a minority of patients, particularly those who have received multiple therapies and large cumulative doses of ^{131}I, salivary gland soreness and swelling may persist for a year or more. The acute and chronic effects of ^{131}I on the salivary glands can be minimized or prevented altogether by increasing salivary flow by having the patient suck on lemon drops and encouraging fluid intake beginning on the day of therapy.[93,94]

Nausea. The most common gastrointestinal symptom of ^{131}I therapy is nausea, which may begin within 2 hours and last for a day or two following

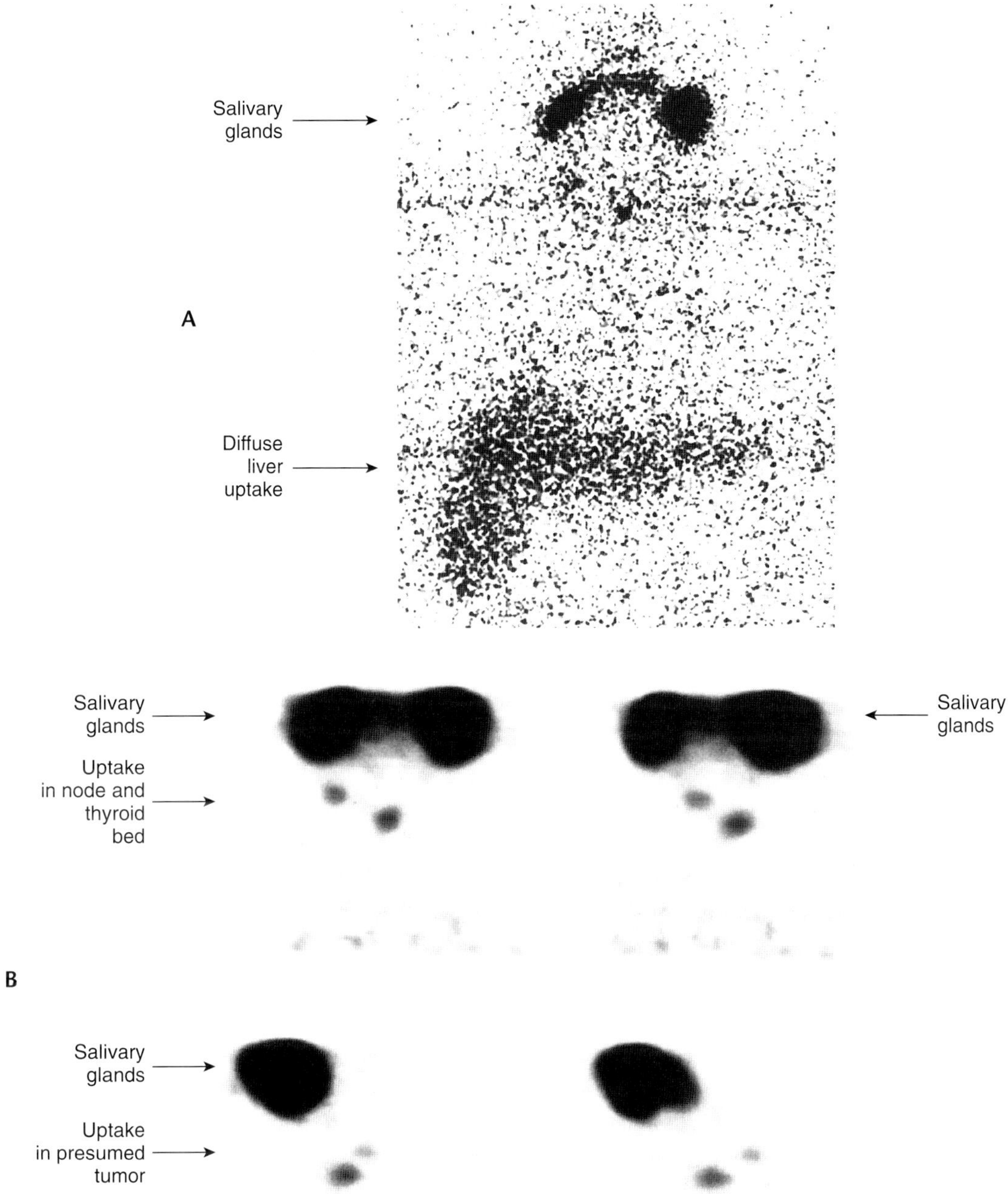

• **FIGURE 6-6** **A,** This 46-year-old patient underwent a total thyroidectomy and ^{131}I ablation 1 year previously for an invasive papillary carcinoma. The diagnostic (2 mCi) ^{131}I scan was negative, but ^{131}I therapy (200 mCi) was given because of persistently elevated serum thyroglobulin. This posttherapy planar whole-body scan shows two small foci of uptake in the neck—one discrete focus in the midline and one indistinct focus in a right cervical node plus intense salivary gland uptake and diffuse hepatic activity (normal). **B,** SPECT reprojection images of the neck showing the two cervical foci of uptake much more distinctly.

administration of ^{131}I. It is important to prevent and treat nausea especially to avoid vomiting of the ^{131}I. The patient is told to eat no solid food from midnight the day of the therapy until 2 hours after therapy to speed absorption of the ^{131}I and minimize retention in the stomach. A standing order is written for antiemetics, either by intramuscular injection or by rectum, to be given at the first hint of nausea.

Radiation-Induced Edema or Hemorrhage. In metastatic cancer, radiation-induced edema or hemorrhage may cause pain and should be treated with analgesics. When brain or spinal cord metastases are present, the radiation effect may lead to serious neurologic consequences. When central nervous system metastases are known or suspected by clinical findings, diagnostic ^{131}I scanning, or MRI, pretreatment with high doses of corticosteroids is advised to prevent the acute swelling that often follows ^{131}I therapy.[26]

Long-Term Effects

Gonadal Function. Gonadal function may be depressed by ^{131}I therapy in a dose-dependent fashion. For each millicurie of ^{131}I administered, testes receive about 0.08 rads and ovaries 0.14 rads. (Metastasis in the pelvis will increase exposure to gonads.) A temporary rise in serum follicle-stimulating hormone occurs, depending on the amount of ^{131}I given for therapy.[95] A dose-dependent decline in sperm count and reduction in sperm motility has been described.[95,96] These effects are usually reversible after about a year.[97] The effects on ovarian endocrine function have been less well studied. Overall rates of infertility, miscarriages, premature births, and congenital abnormalities in women previously treated with ^{131}I do not differ significantly from control values.[94-101]

Bone Marrow Suppression. A dose-dependent pancytopenia occurs following ^{131}I therapy, with the nadir in white cell and platelet counts at 4 to 6 weeks. Recovery is the rule, and no long-term depression of bone marrow function has been seen when the radiation exposure to the blood (and marrow) is kept to a maximum of 200 rads (cGy) and when the whole-body ^{131}I content is not more than 120 mCi per administration.[83] Nevertheless, when spine metastases are treated with ^{131}I, especially when combined external radiation therapy is considered, monitoring of blood counts is advised at appropriate intervals.[97]

Leukemia. Many studies have shown no increase in the incidence of leukemia following either diagnostic or therapeutic amounts of ^{131}I.[102-104]

Nevertheless, leukemia has been reported in patients treated for thyroid cancer with ^{131}I and should be a concern when the cumulative ^{131}I dose exceeds 800 mCi.[105]

Solid Tumors. Carcinoma of the urinary bladder has been reported following ^{131}I therapy,[94] and the relative risk of colorectal cancer is increased in a dose-dependent fashion.[104] Radiation exposure to the bladder is decreased by encouraging fluids and frequent voiding for 2 to 3 days after ^{131}I therapy. The liberal use of laxatives, so that the patient has one to two bowel movements per day, will miminize the radiation exposure to the colon.[26]

Pulmonary Fibrosis. This is a potential complication when large amounts of ^{131}I are used to treat patients with diffuse or widespread multiple pulmonary metastases. This untoward effect is largely avoided by limiting the amount of ^{131}I administered in these cases, such that a maximum of 80 mCi is retained in the body at 48 hours after administration.[106]

CONCLUSION: RADIATION SAFETY

^{131}I for therapeutic use is usually supplied in liquid form and should be stored in a cool, dark place (to avoid oxidation of the iodide) and dispensed in a fume hood. Precautions should be taken to limit exposure of technologists by inhalation of volatile ^{131}I and by avoiding direct contact with the isotope. The administration of more than 30 mCi (1110 MBq) of ^{131}I therapy to a patient with thyroid carcinoma usually requires hospitalization of the patient, who is confined to a private room with a shower and toilet to avoid radiation exposure to other patients, hospital personnel, and the public. The United States Nuclear Regulatory Commission has recently issued Regulatory Guide 8.39 pertaining to the release of patients administered radioactive materials. The aim of these guidelines is to minimize radiation exposure to members of the family and the general public. In some instances more than 30 mmCi ^{131}I may be administered to outpatients.

Nursing staff members are instructed by nuclear medicine and/or radiation safety staff in radiation precautions, specifically to limit close contact with the patient, to perform only essential nursing functions, and to avoid contamination by saliva and excreta. The patient's urine following therapy is ordinarily not collected. Radiation safety personnel monitor the radiation emanating from the patient at intervals following therapy to determine when the patient can be discharged from the hospital.[107] Before discharge, written instructions are given to the patient to safeguard the family, particularly young children, both from external exposure and ingested ^{131}I activity. The Society of Nuclear Medicine has prepared a pamphlet for patients who receive radioiodine therapy.[108]

REFERENCES

1. Kusic Z et al. Comparison of Tc-99m and iodine-123 imaging of thyroid nodules: Correlation with pathologic findings. J Nucl Med 31:393-399, 1990.
2. Cavalieri RR, McDougall IR. In vivo isotopic tests and imaging. In Braverman LE, Utiger RD, eds. The Thyroid. A Fundamental and Clinical Text, 7th ed. Philadelphia: Lippincott, 1996, pp 352-376.
3. Singer PA et al. Treatment guidelines for patients with thyroid nodules and well-differentiated thyroid cancer. Arch Intern Med 156:2165-2172, 1996.
4. Van Herle AJ et al. The thyroid nodule. Ann Int Med 96:221-232, 1982.
5. Nagai GR et al. Scintigraphic hot nodules and thyroid cancer. Clin Nucl Med 12: 123-127, 1987.
6. Sandler MP, Fellmeth B, Salhany KE, Patton JA. Thyroid carcinoma masquerading as a solitary benign hyperfunctioning nodule. Clin Nucl Med 13:410-415, 1988.
7. Cavalieri RR, Gerard SK. Unpublished observation.
8. Meier CA et al. Diagnostic use of recombinant human thyrotropin in patients with thyroid carcinoma (Phase I/II study). J Clin Endocrinol Metab 78:188-196, 1994.
9. Ladenson P et al. Comparison of administration of recombinant human thyrotropin with withdrawal of thyroid hormone for radioactive iodine scanning in patients with thyroid carcinoma. N Engl J Med 337:888-896, 1997.
10. Rudavsky AZ, Freeman LM. Treatment of scan-negative thyroglobulin-positive metastatic thyroid cancer using radioiodine ^{131}I and recombinant human thyroid stimulating hormone. J Clin Endocrinol Metab 82:11-14, 1997.
11. Ramirez L et al. Recombinant human thyrotropin is a potent stimulator of thyroid function in normal subjects. J Clin Endocrinol Metab 82:2836-2839, 1997.
12. Maxon HR et al. A low iodine diet in ^{131}I ablation of thyroid remnants. Clin Nucl Med 8:123-126, 1983.
13. Lakshmanan M et al. A simplified low iodine diet in I-131 scanning and therapy of thyroid cancer. Clin Nucl Med 13:866-868, 1988.
14. Cavalieri RR. Nuclear imaging in the management of thyroid carcinoma. Thyroid 6:485-492, 1996.
15. Seabold JE et al. Diuretic-enhanced I-131 clearance after ablation therapy for differentiated thyroid cancer. Radiology 187:839-842, 1993.
16. Rawson RW, Rall JE, Peacock W. Limitations in the treatment of cancer of the thyroid with radioactive iodine. J Clin Endocrinol Metab 11:1128-1142, 1951.
17. Park HM. Stunned thyroid after high-dose I-131 imaging. Clin Nucl Med 17:501-502, 1992.
18. Park HM et al. Influence of diagnostic radioiodines on the uptake of ablative dose of iodine-131. Thyroid 4:49-54, 1994.
19. Park H, Park Y, Zhou X. Detection of thyroid remnant/metastases without stunning: An ongoing dilemma. Thyroid 7:277-280, 1997.
20. McDougall I. 74 MBq radioiodine ^{131}I does not prevent uptake of therapeutic doses of ^{131}I (i.e., does not cause stunning in differentiated thyroid cancer). Nucl Med Commun 18:505-512, 1997.

21. Jeevanram RK et al. Influence of initial large dose on subsequent uptake of therapeutic radioiodine in thyroid cancer patients. Nucl Med Biol 13:277-279, 1986.
22. Maxon HR et al. High-activity I-123 for the diagnostic evaluation of patients with thyroid cancer. J Nucl Med 34:42P, 1993.
23. Waxman A et al. The significance of I-131 scan dose in patients with thyroid cancer: Determination of ablation. Concise communication. J Nucl Med 22:861-865, 1981.
24. Arnstein NB, Carey JE, Spaulding SA, Sisson JC. Determination of iodine-131 diagnostic dose for imaging metastatic thyroid cancer. J Nucl Med 27:1764-1769, 1986.
25. Ramanna L et al. Treatment rationale in thyroid carcinoma: Effect of scan dose. Clin Nucl Med 10:687-689, 1985.
26. Maxon HRI, Smith HS. Radioiodine-131 in the diagnosis and treatment of metastatic well differentiated thyroid cancer. Endocrinol Metab Clin North Am 19:685-719, 1990.
27. Spies WG et al. Value of post-therapy whole-body I-131 imaging in the evaluation of patients with thyroid carcinoma having undergone high-dose I-131 therapy. Clin Nucl Med 14:793-800, 1989.
28. Reynolds JC. Per cent ^{131}I uptake and post-therapy scans: Their role in the management of thyroid cancer. Thyroid 7:281-284, 1997.
29. Sherman SI et al. Clinical utility of post-treatment radioiodine scans in the management of patients with thyroid carcinoma. J Clin Endocrinol Metab 78:629-634, 1994.
30. Bakheet S, Hammami MM. Spurious lung metastases on radioiodine thyroid and whole body imaging. Clin Nucl Med 18:307-312, 1993.
31. McDougall IR. Whole-body scintigraphy with radioiodine-131: A comprehensive list of false-positives with some examples. Clin Nucl Med 20:869-875, 1995.
32. Hammami MM, Bakheet S. Radioiodine breast uptake in nonbreastfeeding women: Clinical and scintigraphic characteristics. J Nucl Med 37:26-31, 1996.
33. Maayan ML et al. Hepatic visualization after I-131 in patients with thyroid carcinoma. N Engl J Med 295:1258-1259, 1976.
34. Rosenbaum RC, Johnston GS, Valente WA. Frequency of hepatic visualization during I-131 imaging for metastatic thyroid carcinoma. Clin Nucl Med 13:657-660, 1988.
35. Bakheet SM, Hammami MM. False-positive radioiodine whole-body scan in thyroid cancer patients due to unrelated pathology. Clin Nucl Med 19:325-329, 1994.
36. Mishigishi T et al. Visualization of the thymus with therapeutic doses of radioiodine in patients with thyroid cancer. Eur J Nucl Med 20:75-79, 1993.
37. Veronikis IE, Simpkin PH, Braverman LE. Uptake of I-131 in the anterior mediastinum in thyroidectomized patients with differentiated thyroid cancer. J Invest Med 43:226A, 1995.
38. Schlumberger M et al. Iodine-131 and external radiation in the treatment of local and metastatic thyroid cancer. In Falk SA, ed. Thyroid Disease, 2nd ed. Philadelphia: Lippincott-Raven, 1997, pp 601-617.
39. Tonami N, Hisada K. Tl-201 scintigraphy in postoperative detection of thyroid cancer: A comparative study with I-131. Radiology 136:461-464, 1980.
40. Nemec J et al. The rational use of Tl-201 scintigraphy in the evaluation of differentiated thyroid cancer. Eur J Nucl Med 9:261-264, 1984.
41. Hoefnagel CA et al. Role of Thallium-201 total-body scintigraphy in follow-up of thyroid carcinoma. J Nucl Med 27:1854-1857, 1986.
42. Brendel AJ et al. Thallium-201 imaging in the follow-up of differentiated thyroid carcinoma. J Nucl Med 29:1515-1520, 1988.
43. Burman KD, Anderson JH, Wartofsky L, et al. Management of patients with thyroid carcinoma: Application of Thallium-201 scintigraphy and magnetic resonance imaging. J Nucl Med 31:1958-1964, 1990.

44. Dadparvar S et al. The role of iodine-131 and thallium-201 imaging and serum thyroglobulin in the management of differentiated thyroid carcinoma. Cancer 71:3767-3773, 1993.
45. Charkes ND, Vitti RA, Brooks K. Thallium-201 SPECT increases detectability of thyroid cancer metastases. J Nucl Med 31:147-153, 1990.
46. Ramanna L, Waxman A, Braunstein G. Thallium-201 Scintigraphy in differentiated thyroid cancer: Comparison with radioiodine scintigraphy and serum thyroglobulin determinations. J Nucl Med 32:441-446, 1991.
47. Iida Y, Hidaka A, Hatabu H, Kasagi K, Konishi J. Follow-up study of postoperative patients with thyroid cancer by thallium-201 scintigraphy and serum thyroglobulin measurement. J Nucl Med 32:2098-2100, 1991.
48. Van Sorge-Van Boxel RAJ, Van Eck-Smit BLF, Goslings BM. Comparison of serum thyroglobulin, I-131 and Tl-201 scintigraphy in the post-operative follow-up of differentiated thyroid cancer. Nucl Med Commun 14:365-372, 1993.
49. Zak IT, Seabold JE, Gurll NJ. Tc-99m MIBI scintigraphic detection of metastatic insular thyroid carcinoma. Clin Nucl Med 20:31-36, 1995.
50. Sundram FX, Goh ASW, Ang ES. Role of technetium-99m sestamibi in localization of thyroid cancer metastases. Ann Acad Med (Singapore) 22:557-559, 1993.
51. Yen TC et al. The role of technetium-99m sestamibi whole-body scans in diagnosis of metastatic Hurthle cell carcinoma of the thyroid gland after total thyroidectomy: A comparison with iodine-131 and thallium-201 whole-body scans. Eur J Nucl Med 21:980-983, 1994.
52. Dadparvar S, Chevres A, Tulchinsky M, Krishna-Badrinath L, Khan A, Slizofski W. Clinical utility of technetium-99m methoxyisobutylisonitrile imaging in differentiated thyroid carcinoma: Comparison with thallium-201 and iodine-131 Na scintigraphy, and serum thyroglobulin quantitation. Eur J Nucl Med 22:1330-1338, 1995.
53. Nemec J et al. Positive thyroid cancer scintigraphy using technetium-99m methoxyisobutylisonitrile. Eur J Nucl Med 23:69-71, 1996.
54. Klain M et al. Technetium-99m-tetrofosmin imaging of differentiated mixed thyroid cancer. J Nucl Med 36:2248-2251, 1995.
55. Baudin E et al. Octreotide scintigraphy in patient with differentiated thyroid carcinoma: contribution for patients with negative radioiodine scan. J Clin Endocrinol Metab 81:2541-2544, 1996.
56. Yen TC et al. Comparative radionuclide imaging of metastatic insular carcinoma of the thyroid: Value of technetium-99m (V)DMSA. J Nucl Med 37:78-80, 1996.
57. Higashi T et al. Clinical evaluation of 67Ga in the diagnosis of anaplastic carcinoma and lymphoma of the thyroid. Radiology 141:491-497, 1981.
58. Castillo LA et al. Bone scans in bone metastases from functioning thyroid carcinoma. Clin Nucl Med 5:200-209, 1980.
59. DeGroot LJ, Reilly M. Use of isotope bone scans and skeletal survey x-rays in the follow-up of patients with thyroid carcinoma. J Endocrinol Invest 7:175-179, 1984.
60. Alam S et al. Value of combined technetium-99m hydroxy methylene diphosphonate and thallium-201 imaging in detecting bone metastases from thyroid carcinoma. Thyroid 7:705-712, 1997.
61. Scott GC, Meier DA, Dickinson CZ. Cervical lymph node metastases of thyroid papillary carcinoma imaged with fluorine-18-FDG, technetium-99m-pertechnetate, and iodine-131-sodium iodide. J Nucl Med 36:1843-1845, 1995.

62. Sisson JC. Selection of the optimal scanning agent for thyroid cancer. Thyroid 7:295-302, 1997.
63. Grunwald F et al. Fluorine-18 fluorodeoxyglucose positron emission tomography in the follow-up of differentiated thyroid cancer. Eur J Nucl Med 23:312-319, 1996.
64. Sisson JC et al. Uptake of 18-fluoro-2-deoxy-D-glucose by thyroid cancer: Implications for diagnosis and therapy. J Clin Endocrinol Metab 77:1090-1094, 1993.
65. Krishnamurthy GT, Blahd WH. Radioiodine I-131 therapy in the management of thyroid cancer. Cancer 40:195-202, 1977.
66. DeGroot LJ et al. Natural history, treatment, and course of papillary thyroid carcinoma. J Clin Endocrinol Metab 71:414-424, 1990.
67. Samaan NA et al. The results of various modalities of treatment of well-differentiated thyroid carcinoma: A retrospective review of 1599 patients. J Clin Endocrinol Metab 75:714-720, 1992.
68. Mazzaferri EL, Jhiang SM. Long term impact of initial surgical and medical therapy on papillary and follicular thyroid cancer. Am J Med 97:418-428, 1994.
69. Snyder J, Gorman C, Scanlon P. Thyroid remnant ablation: Questionable pursuit of an ill-defined goal. J Nucl Med 24:659-665, 1983.
70. Hay ID. Papillary thyroid carcinoma. Endocrinol Metab Clin North Am 19:545-576, 1990.
71. Mazzaferri EL. Treating differentiated thyroid carcinoma: Where do we draw the line? Mayo Clin Proc 66:105-111, 1991.
72. Hurley JR, Becker DV. Treatment of thyroid carcinoma with radioiodine. In Gottschalk A, Hoffer PB, Potchen EJ, eds. Diagnostic Nuclear Medicine, 2nd ed. Baltimore: Williams & Wilkins, 1988, pp 792-814.
73. Maxon HRI et al. Radioiodine-131 therapy for well-differentiated thyroid cancer—a quantitative radiation dosimetric approach; outcome and validation in 85 patients. J Nucl Med 33:1132-1136, 1992.
74. Sampson RJ et al. Metastases from occult thyroid cancer. Cancer 25:803-808, 1970.
75. Noguchi S, Noguchi A, Murakami N. Papillary carcinoma of the thyroid. I. Developing pattern of metastases. Cancer 26:1053-1060, 1970.
76. Maxon HR et al. Relation between effective radiation dose and outcome of radioiodine therapy for thyroid cancer. N Engl J Med 309:937-941, 1983.
77. DeGroot LJ, Reilly M. Comparison of 30 and 50 mCi doses of iodine-131 for thyroid ablation. Ann Intern Med 96:51-53, 1982.
78. McDougall IR. ^{131}I treatment of ^{131}I negative whole body scan, and positive thyroglobulin in differentiated thyroid carcinoma: What is being treated? Thyroid 7:669-672, 1997.
79. Kimming B, Hermann HJ. Measurement of dose during radioiodine treatment of thyroid cancer. Acta Endocrinol 252 (Suppl):72-79, 1983.
80. Sisson J et al. 131-I treatment of micronodular pulmonary metastases from papillary thyroid carcinoma. Cancer 78:2184-2192, 1996.
81. Maxon HR, Thomas SR, Samaratunga RC. Dosimetric considerations in the radioiodine treatment of macrometastases and micrometastases from differentiated thyroid cancer. Thyroid 7:183-187, 1997.
82. Benua RS et al. The relation of radiation dosimetry to results and complications in the treatment of metastatic thyroid cancer. Am J Roentgenol 87:171-182, 1962.
83. Leeper RD. The effect of ^{131}I therapy on survival of patients with metastatic papillary or follicular thyroid carcinoma. J Clin Endocrinol Metab 36:1143-1152, 1973.

84. O'Connell ME et al. Radiation dose assessment in radioiodine therapy. Dose-response relationships in differentiated thyroid cancer using quantitative scanning and PET. Radiother Oncol 28:16-26, 1993.
85. Gershengorn MC, Izumi M, Robbins J. Use of lithium as an adjunct to radioiodine therapy of thyroid carcinoma. J Clin Endocrinol Metab 42:105-111, 1976.
86. Reynolds JC, Robbins J. The changing role of radioiodine in the management of differentiated thyroid cancer. Semin Nucl Med 27:152-164, 1997.
87. Pacini F et al. Therapeutic doses of iodine-131 reveal undiagnosed metastases in thyroid cancer patients with detectable serum thyroglobulin levels. J Nucl Med 28:1888-1891, 1987.
88. Mazzaferri EL. Treating high thyroglobulin with radioiodine: A magic bullet or a shot in the dark? [Editorial]. J Clin Endocrinol Metab 80:1485-1487, 1995.
89. Ronga G et al. Can I-131 whole-body scan be replaced by thyroglobulin measurement in the post-surgical follow-up of differentiated thyroid carcinoma? J Nucl Med 31:1766-1771, 1990.
90. Pineda JD et al. Iodine-131 therapy for thyroid cancer patients with elevated thyroglobulin and negative diagnostic scan. J Clin Endocrinol Metab 80:1488-1492, 1995.
91. Schlumberger M et al. Detection and treatment of lung metastases of differentiated thyroid carcinoma in patients with normal chest x-rays. J Nucl Med 29:1790-1794, 1988.
92. Clark OH, Hoelting T. Management of patients with differentiated thyroid cancer who have positive serum thyroglobulin levels and negative radioiodine scans. Thyroid 4:501-505, 1994.
93. Allweiss P et al. Sialadenitis following I-131 therapy for thyroid carcinoma: concise communication. J Nucl Med 25:755-758, 1984.
94. Edmonds CJ, Smith T. The long-term hazards of the treatment of thyroid cancer with radioiodine. Br J Radiol 59:45-51, 1986.
95. Pacini F et al. Testicular function in patients with differentiated thyroid carcinoma treated with radioiodine. J Nucl Med 35:1418-1422, 1994.
96. Handlesman DJ, Turtle JR. Testicular damage after radioiodine (I-131) therapy for thyroid cancer. Clin Endocrinol 118:465-472, 1983.
97. Sweeney DC, Johnston GS. Radioiodine therapy for thyroid cancer. Endocrinol Metab Clin North Am 24:803-839, 1995.
98. Sarkar SD et al. Subsequent fertility and birth histories of children and adolescents treated with ^{131}I for thyroid cancer. J Nucl Med 17:460-464, 1976.
99. Casara D et al. Pregnancy after high therapeutic doses of iodine-131 in differentiated thyroid cancer: potential risks and recommendations. Eur J Nucl Med 20:192-194, 1993.
100. Dottorini ME et al. Assessment of female fertility and carcinogenesis after iodine-131 therapy for differentiated thyroid carcinoma. J Nucl Med 36:21-27, 1995.
101. Schlumberger M et al. Exposure to radioactive iodine (131-I) for scintigraphy or therapy does not preclude pregnancy in thyroid cancer patients. J Nucl Med 37:606-612, 1996.
102. Beierwaltes WH. The treatment of thyroid carcinoma with radioactive iodine. Semin Nucl Med 8:79-94, 1978.
103. Hall P et al. Leukemia incidence after iodine-131 exposure. Lancet 340:1-4, 1992.
104. de Vathaire F et al. Leukemias and cancers following iodine-131 administration for thyroid cancer. Br J Cancer 75:734-739, 1997.

105. Brincker H, Hansen HS, Anderson AP. Induction of leukemia by 131-I treatment of thyroid carcinoma. Br J Cancer 28:232-237, 1973.
106. Leeper RD, Shimaoka K. Treatment of metastatic thyroid cancer. Clin Endocrinol Metab 9:383-404, 1980.
107. Culver CM, Dworkin HJ. Radiation safety considerations for post-iodine-131 thyroid cancer therapy. J Nucl Med 33:1402-1405, 1992.
108. Guidelines for patients receiving radioiodine treatment. Soc Nuclear Medicine, 1850 Samuel Morse Dr., Reston, Virginia, 1991.

CHAPTER

7

Magnetic Resonance Imaging

CHARLES B. HIGGINS, M.D.

A number of imaging techniques have been used to evaluate thyroid carcinoma. The traditional approach has usually employed ultrasonography and radionuclide techniques for guiding management of thyroid diseases. In recent years, magnetic resonance imaging (MRI) has been shown to have value in thyroid disease.[1-6] However, its role has generally been limited to specific indications: preoperative staging of aggressive malignancies and postoperative evaluation for recurrence of thyroid cancer.

In this chapter we will review the current applications and results achieved with MRI for the evaluation of thyroid cancer. It should be emphasized at the outset that MRI continues to be a rapidly evolving technology, and there is much less experience with the use of this modality when compared with other diagnostic procedures for thyroid diseases. Consequently, conclusions regarding the value and eventual role of MRI for the evaluation of thyroid cancer must remain speculative at this time.

MRI TECHNIQUES

MRI of the thyroid involves a protocol that consists of transaxial images of both the neck and at least the upper thorax. The tomograms extend from the hyoid bone to the base of the heart in most instances. For MRI of the thorax, electrocardiographic gating or peripheral gating of image acquisition is done to mitigate signal loss associated with cardiac motion. A radiofrequency receiver, coil shaped to closely encompass the thorax (chest or torso coil), is used. Transaxial images 5 to 10 mm thick are initiated at the cervicothoracic junction and extend caudally. A single multislice sequence extends to at least the base of the heart. T1-weighted spin-echo images of the thorax are acquired. Subsequently the neck portion of the study is carried out employing a neck coil. A series of sagittal images of the neck are used to prescribe the position of 5 mm thick transaxial images starting at the level of the hyoid bone. T1-weighted spin-echo and T2-weighted fast spin-echo images are acquired, followed by T1-weighted spin-echo images after administration of magnetic resonance contrast medium (gadolinium chelate). In some but not all patients, T1-weighted spin-echo images of the thorax are also acquired after a contrast medium is administered. Fat saturation is usually applied for the T1-weighted images after contrast medium.

The specific imaging protocol is shown in the box. Most papers describing the use of MRI in thyroid disease have used the same or a very similar protocol.

Magnetic Resonance Imaging Protocol

Chest

Torso coil
SE, TR = RR, TE 20 msec, 5 mm slice thickness
+/– SE, TR = RR, TE = 20 msec, after gadolinium chelate with fat saturation

Neck

Neck coil
SE, TR = 600 msec, TE = minimum, 5 mm slice thickness
FSE, TR = 3500 msec, TE = 85 to 102 msec, 5 mm slice thickness
SE, TR = 600 msec, TE = minimum, 5 mm slice thickness after gadolinium chelate with fat saturation
SE, spin-echo; *FSE,* fast spin-echo

TR = repitition time
TE = echo time
RR = R to R interval of electrocardiogram

THYROID NODULES

Thyroid nodules are shown on magnetic resonance images as discrete, well-demarcated regions of high signal intensity on T2-weighted spin-echo images (Fig. 7-1). Nodules may be similar, slightly lower, or higher in signal intensity when compared with the normal thyroid gland on T1-weighted spin-echo images. Foci of high signal intensity on T1-weighted images have been attributed to hemorrhage into solid nodules or colloid cysts.

MRI features of adenoma and adenomatous hyperplasia have been described.[3,4] Benign and malignant nodules are not distinguishable from each other by signal intensity characteristics. Suggestive but not definitive features of benign adenoma are distinct margin, regular contour, and pseudocapsule. Homogeneous high intensity on T2-weighted images is characteristic of benign cyst or cystic involution of an adenoma. Adenomas are enhanced to a greater extent than normal thyroid tissue, whereas cysts display no enhancement on gadolinium-enhanced T1-weighted spin-echo images.

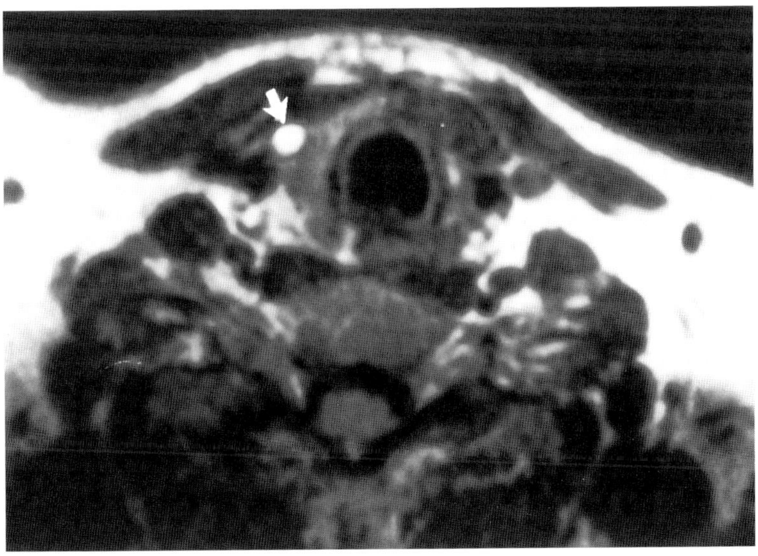

• **FIGURE 7-1** Spin-echo MR image shows a discrete, sharply marginated, high signal intensity nodule *(arrow)* in the right lobe of the thyroid.

STAGING OF THYROID CARCINOMA

The magnetic resonance signal characteristics of thyroid carcinoma are not consistently distinctive in comparison with other thyroid masses or goiters. On T1-weighted spin-echo images, carcinoma has been found to be isotense, slightly hypointense, and slightly hyperintense when compared with normal thyroid gland. On T2-weighted images, the signal intensity is heterogeneous and mostly hyperintense when compared with normal thyroid tissue. MRI can be used to stage the malignant tumor by displaying extraglandular extension, airway (Fig. 7-2) or esophageal invasion, muscular invasion (Fig. 7-3), vascular invasion, and cervical lymphadenopathy.[3] MRI is more effective than ultrasonography for retrotracheal and mediastinal extension of tumors. Invasion of muscle is recognized by increased signal intensity of the muscle on T2-weighted images. Because of this sign, MRI may be the most sensitive technique for determining muscle invasion.

The outcome of patients with thyroid carcinoma is strongly influenced by the presence of nodal metastasis. Lymph nodes can be readily recognized in the neck using magnetic resonance; the nodes usually have low to medium intensity on T1-weighted spin-echo images and high intensity on T2-weighted images. Signal intensity characteristics cannot usually be relied on to discriminate malignant from inflammatory or hyperplastic nodal enlargement. An exception is the unique appearance of some nodal metastases caused by papillary thyroid carcinoma. In some instances, enlarged cystic lymph nodes with high signal intensity on T1-weighted spin-echo images may be pathognomic of metastatic papillary carcinoma (Fig. 7-4). These nodules also have homogeneous high signal intensity on T2-weighted images.

The distinctive features of malignant lymphadenopathy are based mainly on size criteria.[7] Size criteria are somewhat unreliable, since adjustment of the cutoff value reciprocally alters sensitivity and specificity. New size cutoffs have been established based on extensive pathologic analysis of more than 2700 lymph nodes in head and neck malignancies.[8] The study concluded that nodes with a minimum diameter greater than 11 mm for high jugular nodes and 10 mm for other nodes are likely metastases. The sensitivity and specificity of these size criteria were 89% and 73%, respectively. The results of a multicenter study revealing that 46% of metastatic nodes were less than 1 cm in diameter are problematic for reliance on size criteria.[9]

Other indicators of lymph node metastases are central necrosis of nodes and extracapsular spread. Necrosis of lymph nodes is indicated by high signal intensity of the necrotic region on T2-weighted spin-echo images and lack of enhancement of the necrotic region on T1-weighted images after administration of gadolinium chelates. Consequently, enlarged nodes displaying heterogeneous enhancement by gadolinium chelates on T1-weighted

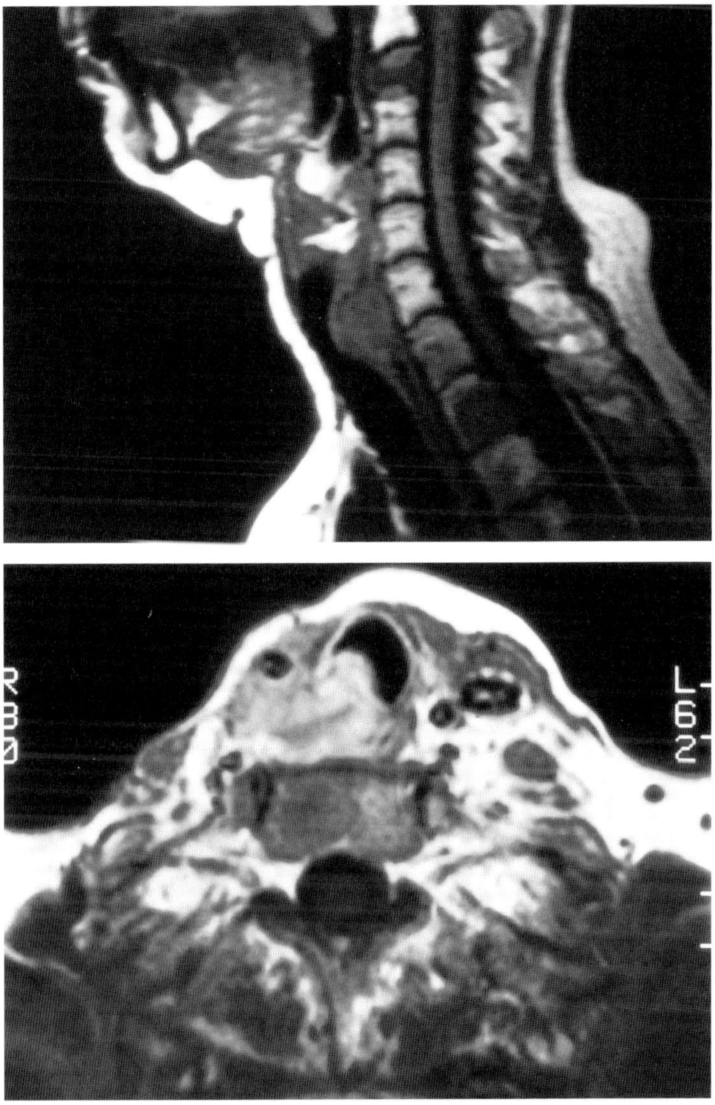

A

B

• **FIGURE 7-2** **A,** Sagittal T1-weighted and **B,** transaxial T1-weighted images after gadolinium chelate MR images of the neck demonstrate recurrence of thyroid cancer in the trachea. There are also metastases in the cervical vertebrae as indicated by replacement of the fatty marrow.

images are more likely to harbor metastatic tumor because of regions of tumor necrosis. Gadolinium-enhanced, fat-suppressed T1-weighted images have been reported to enable improved recognition of nodal necrosis.[10] However, in a large series of cases, 74% of metastatic cervical nodes contained necrosis or cystic areas on pathologic examination, but necrosis was recognized in only 32% of metastatic nodes on imaging studies.[10]

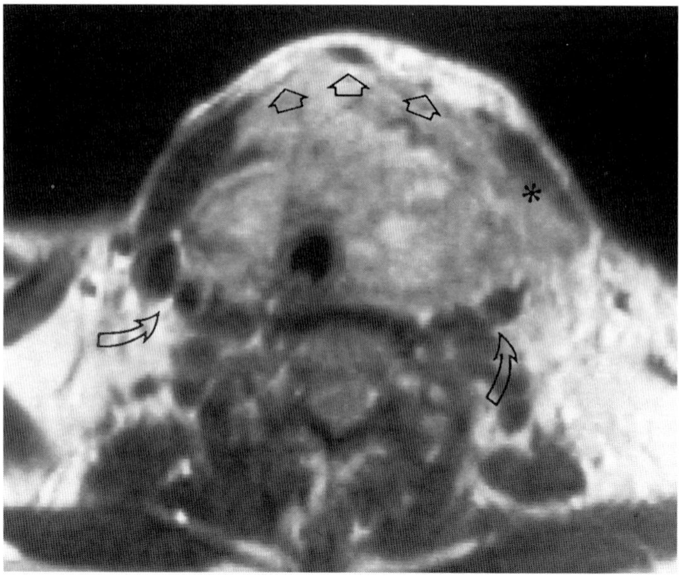

• **FIGURE 7-3** T2-weighted transaxial image shows extensive thyroid malignant tumor with invasion of strap muscles *(open arrows)* and left sternocleidomastoid *(asterisk)* muscles. The neurovascular bundles are displaced posterolaterally by the large tumor *(curved open arrows)*.

Extracapsular extension of lymph node metastasis is a clear indicator of malignant lymphadenopathy. The spread of the tumor beyond the capsule of the node is indicated by an irregular nodal margin and obliteration of the surrounding fat plane. The alteration in the nodal-fat boundary may be most readily shown on T1-weighted spin-echo images. Another feature of metastatic nodes is greater sphericity of metastatic nodes. A maximum longitudinal (L) to transaxial (T) ratio of less than 2 has been reported to be characteristic of metastatic nodes.[11] One study concluded that an L/T ratio of less than 2 was a more accurate sign of lymphadenopathy than size criteria or necrosis.[11]

A new group of magnetic resonance contrast media have been introduced with the potential to characterize metastatic lymph nodes.[12,13] Dextran-coated ultrasmall supraparamagnetic iron oxide (USPIO) particles are accumulated in different portions of the reticuloendothelial system, depending on the particle size of the media. The formulation of USPIO particles with a particle size of less than 20 nm is taken up by macrophages in lymph nodes after intravenous administration. At 24 to 36 hours after administration, the iron oxide particles cause depression or vitiation of signal of normal nodes on T2-weighted spin-echo images. Because tumor cells do not have phagocytic capability, part or all of metastatic nodes remain high intensity on post-contrast T2-weighted images.

A
B

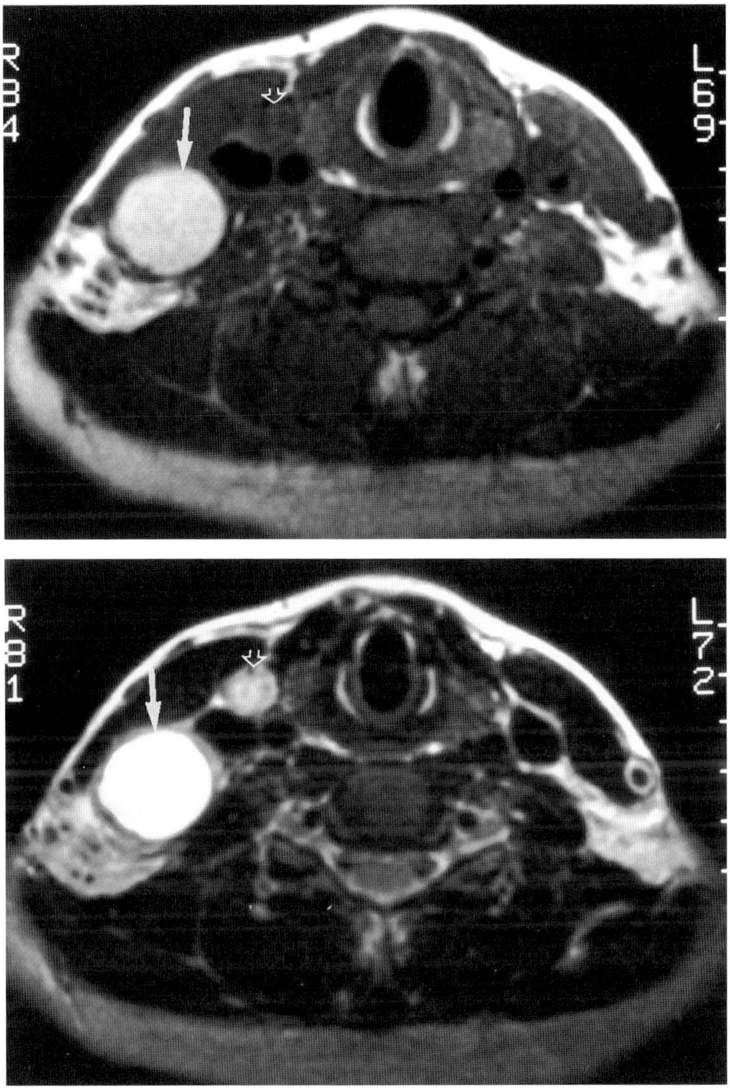

• **FIGURE 7-4** **A,** T1- and **B,** T2-weighted transaxial images in a patient with metastatic papillary thyroid cancer. The cystic metastasis to the right lymph nodes *(arrow)* shows high signal intensity on both sequences. The recurrent tumor in the carotid sheath bed *(open arrows)* has low intensity on T1-weighted and high intensity on T2-weighted images.

POSTOPERATIVE EVALUATION

After total thyroidectomy, the thyroid bed usually displays a rim of low-signal-intensity tissue surrounding the trachea (Fig. 7-5, *A*). This consists of scar tissue that has low intensity on T1- and T2-weighted images.

A

B

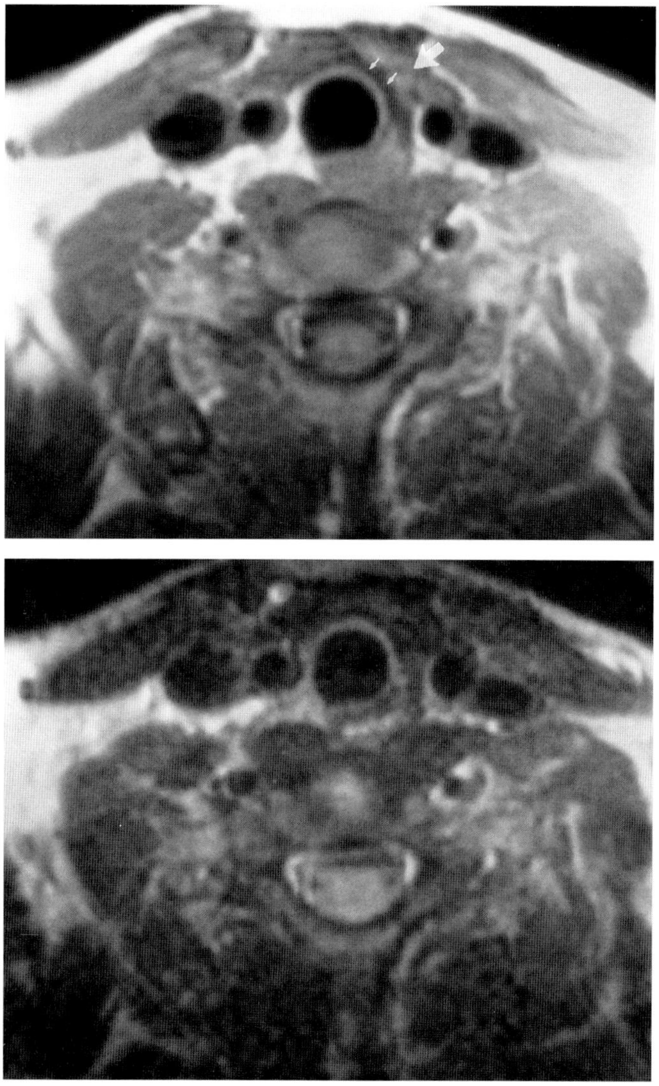

• **FIGURE 7-5** **A,** T1- and **B,** T2-weighted images of the neck after total thyroidectomy. There is a rim of low signal intensity caused by normal scar tissue *(small arrows)* in the thyroid bed. There is also thickening and distortion of the strap muscles *(large arrow)*. Both the scar tissue and muscle demonstrate low signal on the T2-weighted image.

Occasionally, muscle thickening and distortion can simulate a mass, but this tissue displays low intensity on T2-weighted images (Fig. 7-5, *B*).

MRI is effective for the identification of recurrence in the thyroid bed and in cervical and thoracic lymph nodes after surgery.[3,6] It is particularly useful for postoperative monitoring of patients with tumors that do not avidly accumulate radioiodine. About 50% of papillary and nearly 70% of follicular carcinomas accumulate sufficient ^{131}I for scintigraphic imaging and ablation with radioiodine. Papillary carcinoma has been divided into pure papillary, mixed papillary-follicular, and predominantly follicular with minor papillary component. The degree of differentation toward follicular components determines the avidity of ^{131}I uptake and elevation of serum thyroglobulin. Hürthle cell tumor is a variant of follicular carcinoma with low probability of ^{131}I uptake and cannot be imaged with the radioiodine scan. Therefore the utility of postoperative monitoring with MRI is greater for patients with Hürthle cell, medullary, and anaplastic carcinomas. It also should have value for some papillary and fewer follicular carcinomas, depending on their affinity for radioiodine. MRI may also be indicated to determine the site and to monitor the size of the recurrence signaled by rising serum thyroglobulin (papillary, follicular, and Hürthle cell carcinoma) or thyrocalcitonin (medullary carcinoma) levels.

MRI is especially useful for distinguishing between scar tissue in the thyroid bed and distortion of muscle in the thyroid bed from recurrent tumor. The rationale for the use of MRI for this purpose is the empiric observation and experimental measurement of distinctly different T2 relaxation times of nonfibrous tumors relative to fibrous tissues and tumors.[14,15] Fibrous tissue has a short T2 relaxation time, consequently, low signal intensity on T2-weighted images (see Fig. 7-5, *B*). Thyroid carcinoma has a much longer T2 relaxation time and consequently displays high signal on T2-weighted spin-echo images (Figs. 7-6 through 7-9). Scar tissue has a signal similar to or lower than skeletal muscle, whereas the tumor shows much higher signal than muscle does.

A report from our hospital showed the accuracy of using magnetic resonance signal characteristics to distinguish between tumor recurrence and postoperative fibrosis.[2] Local tumor recurrence was characterized as substantially higher signal intensity than skeletal muscles on T2-weighted images, whereas scar tissue had a low or similar signal intensity when compared with muscle (Fig. 7-10). A more recent report[6] showed similar results and documented improved accuracy in comparison with thallium scans for detecting recurrent tumors.

Gadolinium chelates produce substantial enhancement of recurrent tumor on T-weighted spin-echo images (see Fig. 7-7). Frequently, fat-saturated (suppressed) T1-weighted images are used to accentuate the enhancement of the tumor tissue. Six months after surgery, scar tissue in the thyroid bed does not show prominent enhancement with gadolinium chelates.

As discussed above, magnetic resonance is also effective for identifying lymph node metastases. The likelihood that lymph nodes recognized on

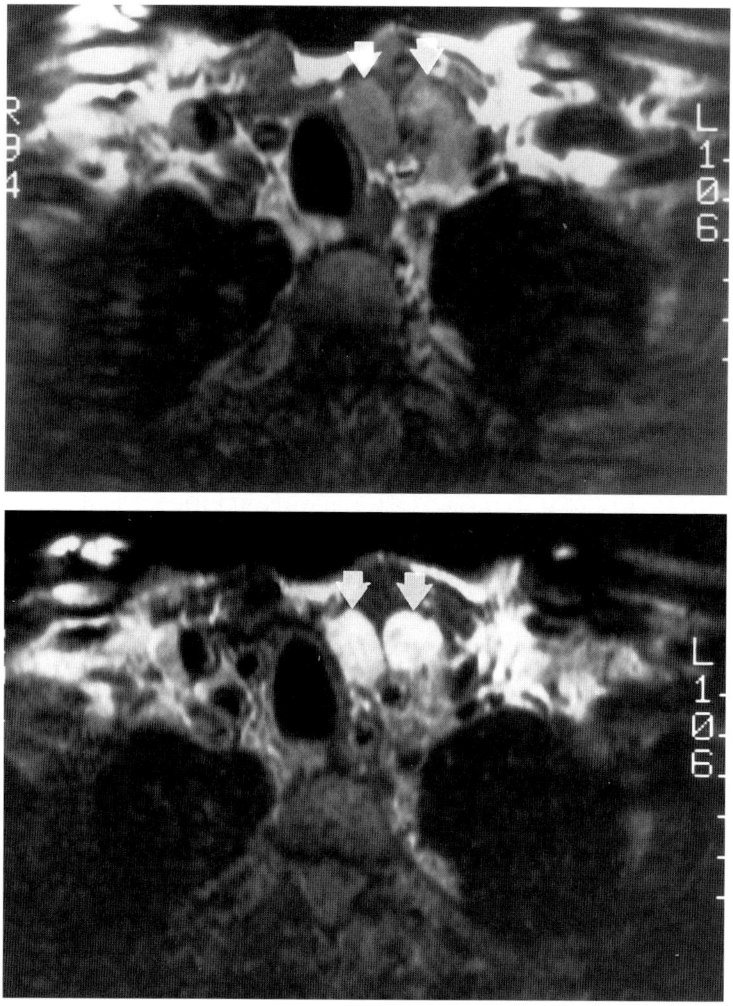

A

B

• **FIGURE 7-6** **A,** T1- and **B,** T2-weighted images below the cervicothoracic junction show two masses *(arrows)* on the left side. These masses have high signal intensity on the T2-weighted images.

magnetic resonance images harbor metastatic tumor is based on the criteria described earlier: short axis diameter greater than 1 cm; increased sphericity (L/T ratio < 2); nonhomogeneous enhancement with magnetic resonance contrast media; nonhomogeneous enhancement on T2-weighted images; and extranodal extension. It should be noted that both benign and metastatic nodes may show substantial homogeneous enhancement after administration of gadolinium chelates. The recognition of enhanced nodes is usually facilitated by using fat-saturated T1-weighted images.

A

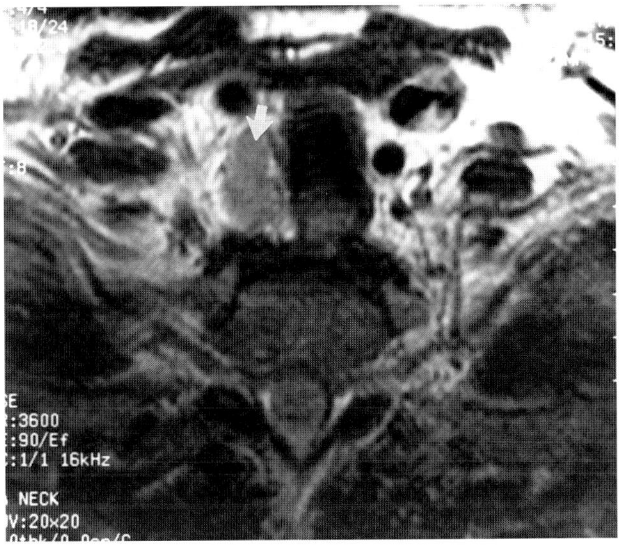

B

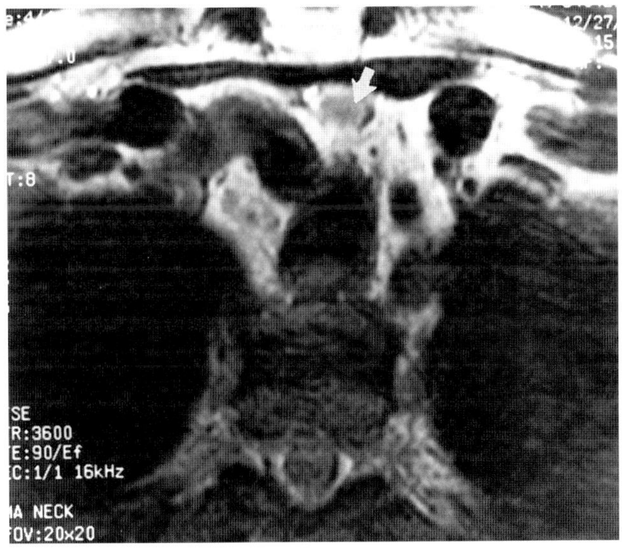

• **FIGURE 7-7** T2-weighted fast spin-echo images at **A**, the cervicothoracic junction and **B**, the superior mediastinum demonstrate two sites of recurrent tumor *(arrow)*. The tumor displays signal intensity higher than that of skeletal muscle.

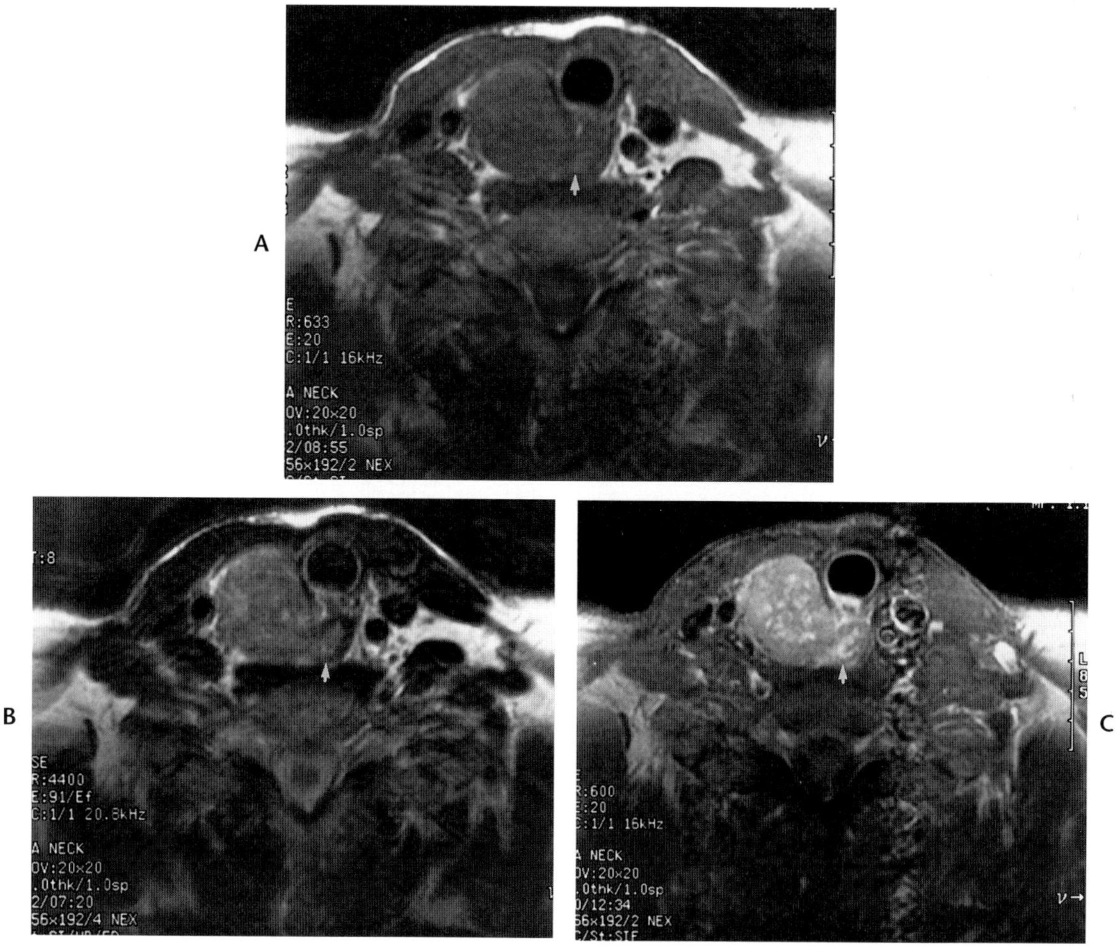

• **FIGURE 7-8** **A,** T1-weighted, **B,** T2-weighted, and **C,** contrast-enhanced T1-weighted images obtained 9 months later in the same patient as shown in Fig. 7-7. The recurrent tumor on the right side of the neck has increased in size. The tumor shows marked enhancement with gadolinium chelate. The tumor abuts and cannot be clearly separated from the esophagus *(arrow)*.

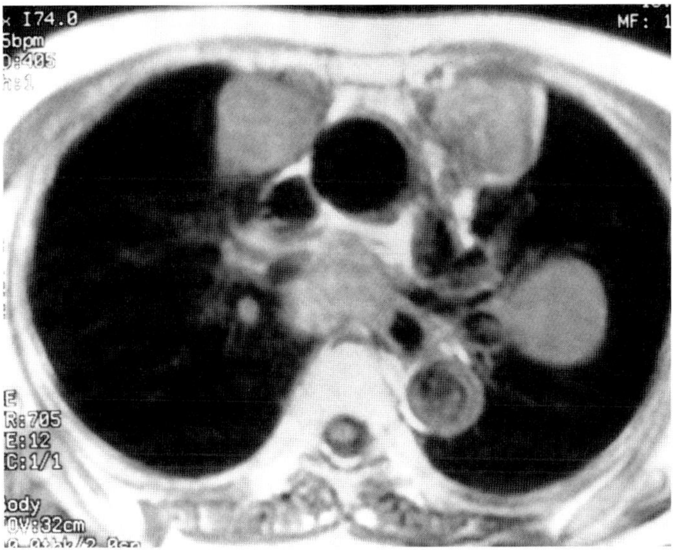

• **FIGURE 7-9** ECG-gated short echo-time (12 msec) image of the chest demonstrates multiple metastatic masses in the lungs and mediastinum.

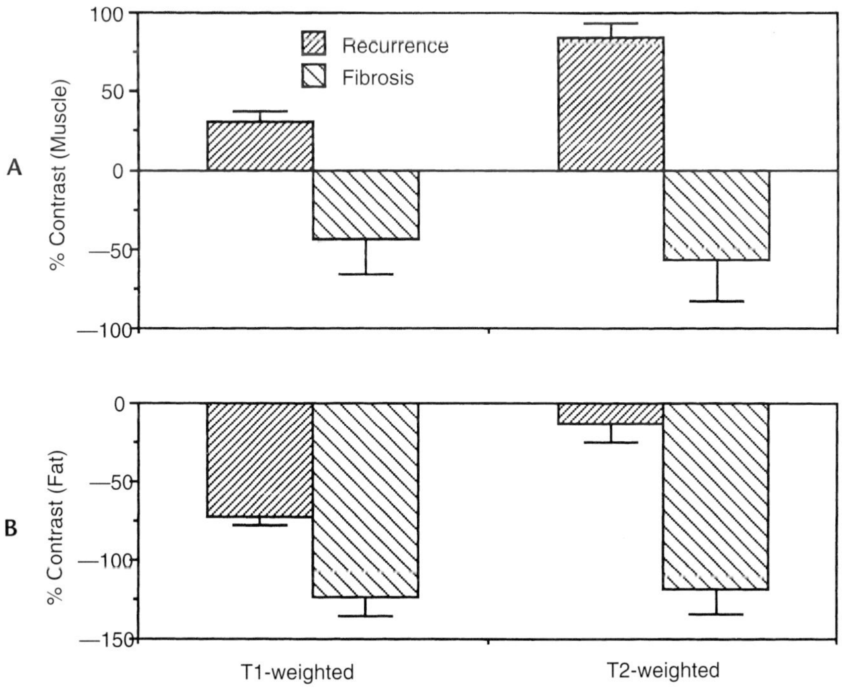

• **FIGURE 7-10** Block diagram shows the percentage contrast of the scan (fibrosis) in the thyroid bed and recurrent thyroid cancer on T1- and T2-weighted images. **A,** Percentage contrast vs. muscle; **B,** Percentage contrast vs. fat.

CONCLUSION

The use of magnetic resonance imaging is indicated in some cases for preoperative staging of thyroid carcinoma. It is most advantageous for the evaluation of patients in whom there is clinical concern for recurrence in the neck and mediastinum. Differentiation of recurrent tumor from scar tissue is usually possible using T2-weighted spin-echo images and gadolinium-enhanced T1-weighted images.

REFERENCES

1. Higgins CB et al. MR imaging of the thyroid. Am J Roentgenol 147:1255-1261, 1986.
2. Auffermann W et al. Recurrent thyroid carcinoma: Characteristics on MR images. Radiology 168:753-757, 1988.
3. Higgins CB, Auffermann W. MR imaging of thyroid and parathyroid glands: A review of current status. Am J Roentgenol 151:1095-1106, 1988.
4. Nøma S et al. Thyroid gland: MR imaging. Radiology 164:495-499, 1987.
5. Nøma S et al. Thyroid masses: MR imaging and pathologic correlation. Radiology 168:759-764, 1988.
6. Ohnishi T et al. Detection of recurrent thyroid cancer: MR versus thallium-201 scintigraphy. Am J Neuroradiol 14:1050-1057, 1993.
7. Anzai Y, Brunberg JA, Lufkin RB. Imaging of nodal metastases in the head and neck. J Magn Reson Imaging 7:774-783, 1997.
8. Van den Brekel MWM et al. Cervical lymph node metastases: Assessment of radiological criteria. Radiology 177:379-384, 1990.
9. Don D et al. Evaluation of cervical lymph node metastases in squamous cell carcinoma of head and neck. Laryngoscope 105:669-674, 1995.
10. Barakos JA, Dillon WP, Chuo WM: Orbit, skull base, and pharynx: Contrast enhanced fat suppression MR imaging. Radiology 179:191-198, 1991.
11. Steinkamp HJ et al. Enlarged cervical lymph nodes at helical CT. Radiology 191:795-798, 1994.
12. Weissleder R et al. Ultrasmall superparamagnetic iron oxide: Characterization of a new class of contrast agents for MR imaging. Radiology 175:489-493, 1990.
13. Anzai Y et al. Initial clinical experience with dextran coated superparamagnetic iron oxide for detection of lymph node metastases in patients with head and neck cancer. Radiology 192:709-715, 1994.
14. Glazer HS et al. Radiation fibrosis: Differentiation from recurrent tumor by MRI. Radiology 156:721-726, 1985.
15. Sundaram M, McGuire MH, Schajowicz F. Soft tissue masses: Histologic basis for decreased signal (short T2) in T2-weighted MR images. Am J Roentgenol 148:1247-1250, 1987.

CHAPTER

8

Ultrasonography

TSUKASA MURAKAMI, M.D.

About three decades have passed since ultrasonography was introduced into medical practice for patients with thyroid nodules.[1-4] Continued progress in ultrasonic diagnostic equipment permits detailed visualization of thyroid nodules. Ultrasonography is superior to palpation or radionuclide scintigraphy for detecting thyroid nodules.[5-7] Since it is difficult to determine by ultrasonography whether a thyroid nodule is benign or malignant, ultrasonography has primarily been used for detecting multinodularity and for differentiating cystic nodules from solid ones.[8] Ultrasonography is also used selectively rather than routinely in the United States because of the expense.[9,10]

Today, ultrasonography using high-resolution equipment is a sensitive means for morphologic evaluation of thyroid nodules. Okamoto et al.[11] and Lin et al.[12] believe that ultrasonography, as well as fine-needle aspiration (FNA) cytology should be used in the initial examination of most patients with thyroid nodules. The merits of ultrasonography in thyroid diseases include:

- Measurement of the thyroid volume or the diameter of nodules
- Detection of occult nodules
- Characterization of nodules

- Evaluation of metastatic lymph nodes or invasion into surrounding tissues in patients with invasive thyroid cancer
- Follow-up examination for patients with thyroid cancer or benign thyroid nodules after thyroidectomy
- Evaluation of vascularity using color Doppler ultrasonography
- Guidance for FNA or ethanol injection therapy for thyroid nodules

Ultrasonic examination of the thyroid is performed in a supine or sitting position with the patient's neck hyperextended. FNA can be performed in the same position following ultrasonic examination, if FNA is indicated. Transducers with high frequencies are employed because the thyroid lies superficially in the anterior neck, which enables detailed observation and characterization of the nodules. We use the digital ultrasound system LOGIQ 500 (GE Yokogawa Medical Systems, Ltd., Tokyo, Japan) equipped with a linear-array probe with frequencies of 6 to 13 MHz (LA39). Spatial resolution of the system is about 2 mm.

Ultrasonography is a safe and informative technique, but there are some limitations. Large or protruded nodules are more difficult to examine thoroughly by ultrasonography. It is also more difficult to examine nodules in obese patients, those who cannot hyperextend their necks, and those in whom contact of a probe with their neck is incomplete because of previous radical neck operations.

ULTRASONIC APPEARANCE OF THYROID CANCERS

Differentiation of Papillary Thyroid Cancers From Benign Thyroid Nodules

We have previously reported that irregular nodules, ill-defined nodules, nodules that are hypoechogenic, or have heterogeneous internal echoes or calcifications are more likely to be papillary thyroid cancers than benign nodules.[13,14] Other investigators have also reported that the absence of cystic degenerative changes or the absence of a halo is a sign suggestive of thyroid cancer.[8,15,16] Despite these reports, differentiating thyroid cancers from benign thyroid nodules is difficult on the basis of ultrasonography, because these ultrasonic findings are not specific for thyroid cancer.[8,16] Ultrasound identification of invasion into the surrounding tissues of the nodule is the sole specific ultrasonic sign of thyroid cancer but is rarely seen (Fig. 8-1).[17]

Recently we reevaluated the accuracy of ultrasonic findings in determining whether a thyroid nodule is benign or malignant. Between October 1996 and March 1997, 292 patients (264 women and 28 men, aged 20 to 82 years,

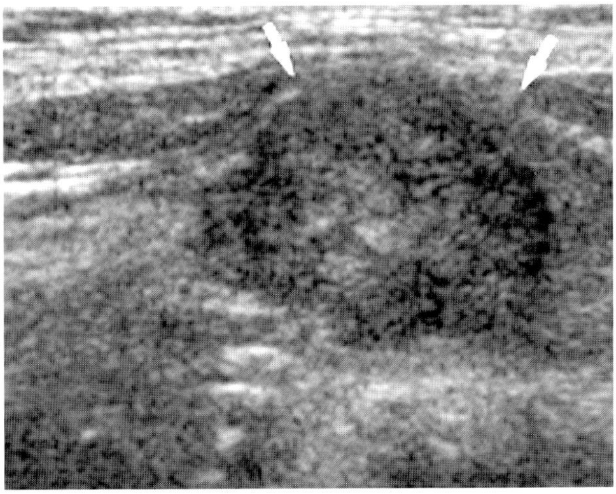

• **FIGURE 8-1** Longitudinal scan of a papillary thyroid cancer. Capsule of the thyroid is interrupted *(arrows)*, suggesting invasive growth of the nodule beyond the capsule.

median 53 years) with thyroid nodules had ultrasonic examinations prior to thyroidectomy. A solitary nodule was observed in 150 patients and multiple nodules were demonstrated in the remaining 142 patients. Among these 292 patients, 104 of the nodules were papillary thyroid cancer histologically. There were also 243 other nodules and those were benign. Ultrasonic appearances of this entire group of 347 nodules were analyzed by multivariate regression analysis using JMP programs for Macintosh (SAS Institute, Cary, N.C.).

As shown in Table 8-1, ultrasonic appearances of the nodule, such as the presence of calcification, irregular shape, absence of cystic elements, absence of halo, and hypoechogenic internal echo, were significant signs of papillary thyroid cancer (Figs. 8-2 through 8-6). When a nodule had a calculated probability of cancer using the estimated parameters over 0.5, the sensitivity, specificity, and positive predictive value of ultrasonography for thyroid cancer were 76.0%, 92.2%, and 80.6%, respectively. Ultrasonography helps to identify suspicious thyroid nodules that should be further examined by FNA.

Microcarcinomas and Intraglandular Disseminated Papillary Thyroid Cancers

In experienced hands, high-resolution ultrasonography can detect occult thyroid nodules. Although management of occult nonpalpable nodules

TABLE 8-1 Multivariate Analysis of Ultrasonic Findings of Thyroid Nodules*

	Estimate	SE	*p* Value
Calcification	1.744	0.386	0.000
Irregular shape	1.338	0.377	0.000
Solid nodule	1.291	0.400	0.001
Absence of halo	1.106	0.407	0.007
Hypoechogenicity	0.945	0.422	0.025
Intercept	–3.849	0.408	0.000

*Presence of these findings is indicative of papillary thyroid cancer.
SE, standard error.

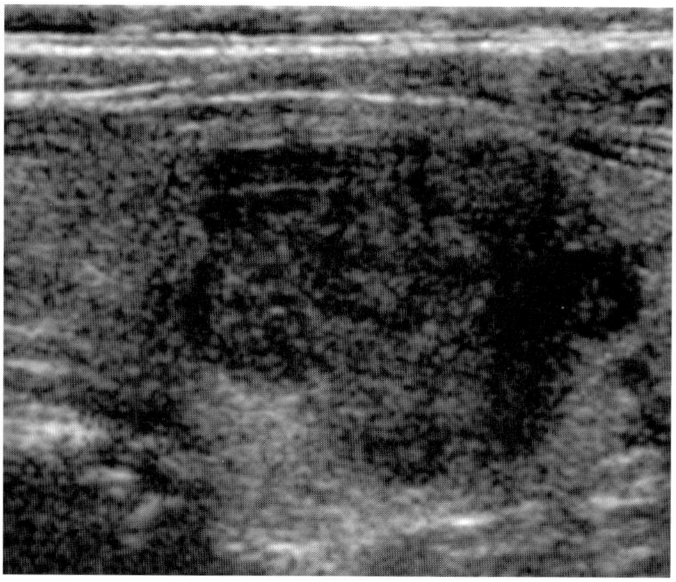

• **FIGURE 8-2** Longitudinal scan of a papillary thyroid cancer, showing an irregularly shaped hypoechogenic nodule.

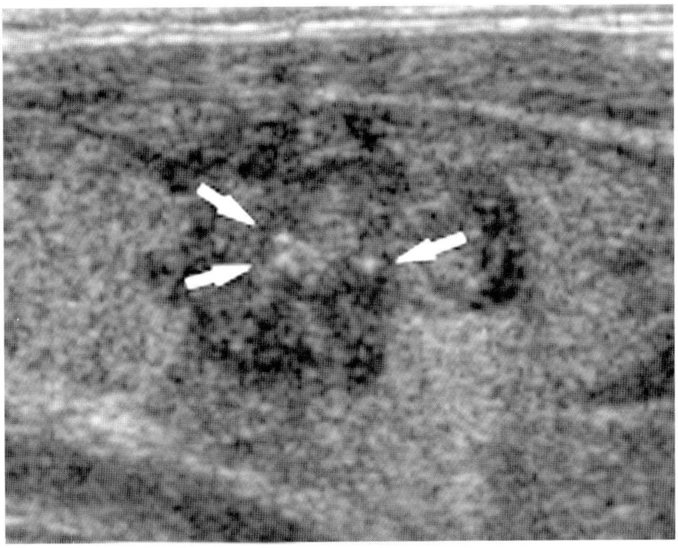

• **FIGURE 8-3** Longitudinal scan of a papillary thyroid cancer, showing an irregularly shaped nodule that has hypoechogenic heterogeneous internal echo and calcifications *(arrows)*.

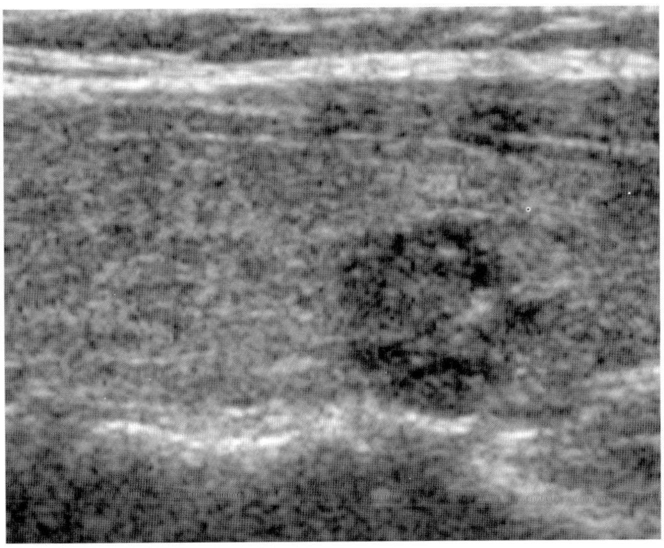

• **FIGURE 8-4** Longitudinal scan of a papillary thyroid cancer. Diameter of the nodule is smaller than those of nodules shown in Figs. 8-1 through 8-3. However, irregular shape, hypoechogenicity, and the presence of calcification indicate that the nodule is malignant.

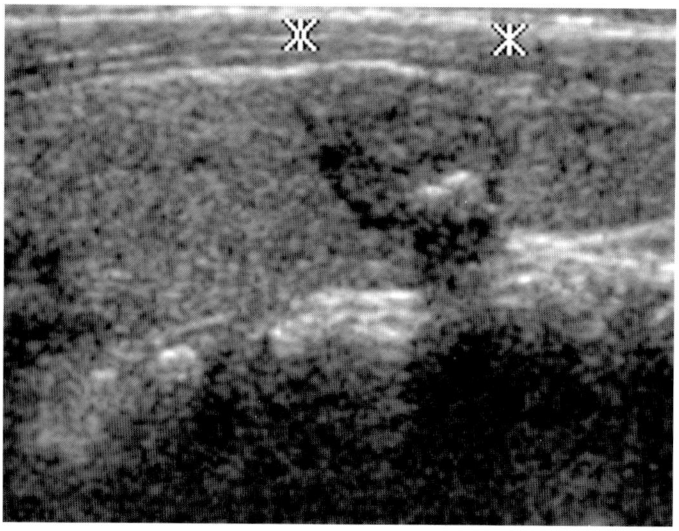

• **FIGURE 8-5** Longitudinal scan of a papillary thyroid cancer. Although the nodule has a halo and an isoechogenic internal echo, the irregular shape of the nodule suggests papillary thyroid cancer. Coarse calcifications can also be seen.

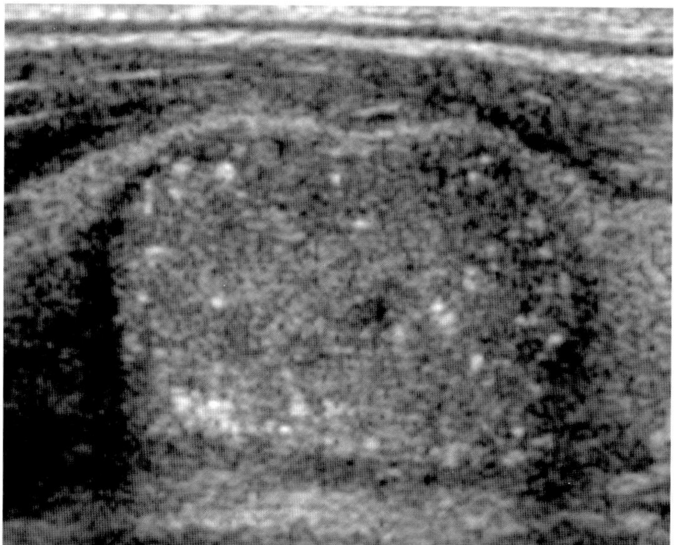

• **FIGURE 8-6** Longitudinal scan of a papillary thyroid cancer. Note the multiple fine echogenic dots, which are highly suggestive of papillary thyroid cancer.

TABLE 8-2 Incidence of Ultrasonic Findings in Papillary Thyroid Cancers

	Nodule Diameter		
	10 mm or Less (%)	Greater Than 10 mm (%)	*p* value
Solid nodule	43 (93.5)	42 (72.4)	0.009
Absence of halo	37 (80.4)	48 (82.8)	NS
Hypoechogenicity	36 (78.3)	46 (79.3)	NS
Irregular shape	35 (76.1)	46 (79.3)	NS
Heterogeneity	33 (71.7)	43 (74.1)	NS
Ill demarcation	29 (63.0)	26 (44.8)	NS
Calcification	23 (50.0)	34 (58.6)	NS
TOTAL THYROID PATIENTS	46	58	

*Findings are divided by the diameter of the nodules. Solid nodules without any cystic changes are more frequent in microcarcinomas than in cancers greater than 10 mm in diameter ($p = 0.009$ by Fisher's exact test).
NS, not significant.

detected incidentally is controversial,[18] we believe an accurate cytologic diagnosis should be made. Among our patients, 46 of the 104 papillary thyroid cancers mentioned earlier were 10 mm or less; the remaining 58 cancers were larger than 10 mm. Ultrasonic appearances were compared between these two groups. There were no significant differences in the ultrasonic appearances, except for the incidence of cystic change between microcarcinomas and overt cancers (Table 8-2). An irregularly shaped hypoechogenic, solid nodule is the typical feature of thyroid microcarcinomas as seen on ultrasonography (Fig. 8-7). Preoperative detection of intraglandular dissemination of papillary thyroid cancer is very important when selecting the extent of thyroidectomy. Ultrasonography with FNA cytologic confirmation of other thyroid nodules is necessary for more accurate preoperative evaluation in patients with papillary thyroid cancers.

Papillary Thyroid Cancers in Multinodular Goiter

The incidence of concomitant thyroid cancer in multinodular goiters is relatively high.[19] It is therefore probably important to detect these cancers both for recommending thyroidectomy and to select the extent of thyroidectomy. Ultrasonography in multinodular goiter demonstrates complex features

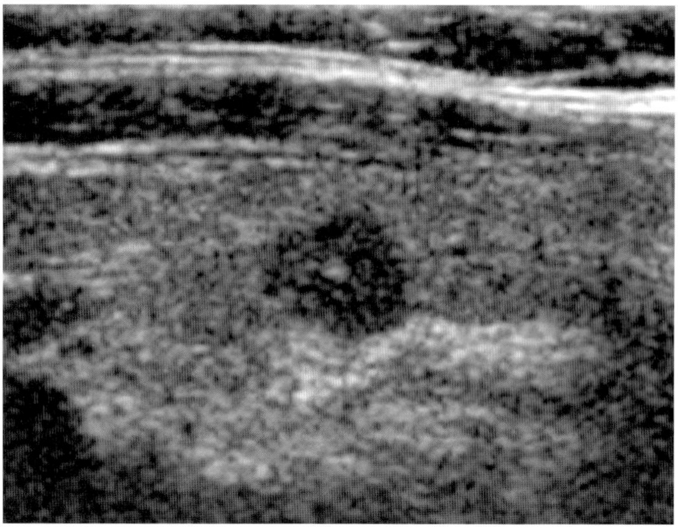

• **FIGURE 8-7** Longitudinal scan of a typical microcarcinoma. The diameter of the nodule is 6 mm.

reflecting various pathologic processes, such as hyperplastic, degenerative, and cystic changes. Differentiation between thyroid cancers and adenomatous nodules is therefore sometimes difficult. Among 121 patients with multinodular goiter, 41 were found to have concomitant thyroid cancers. Twenty-one (51.2%) of these 41 patients were correctly diagnosed preoperatively by ultrasonography as having concomitant thyroid cancers.

Rare Variant of Papillary Thyroid Cancer

Cystic papillary thyroid cancer is hard to diagnose on the basis of palpation or FNA, since epithelial cells degenerate in the cyst, making the diagnosis of thyroid cancer more difficult. A solid element with multiple punctate echogenic dots protruding into the cyst suggests a cystic papillary thyroid cancer (Fig. 8-8).[20] Invasive growth of a solid element is also a sign of a cancerous nodule (Fig. 8-9).

Diffuse sclerosing papillary thyroid cancers often demonstrate diffuse enlargement of one or both thyroid lobes. Multiple high echogenic dots in a diffusely enlarged gland are an ultrasonic clue to this diagnosis.[21]

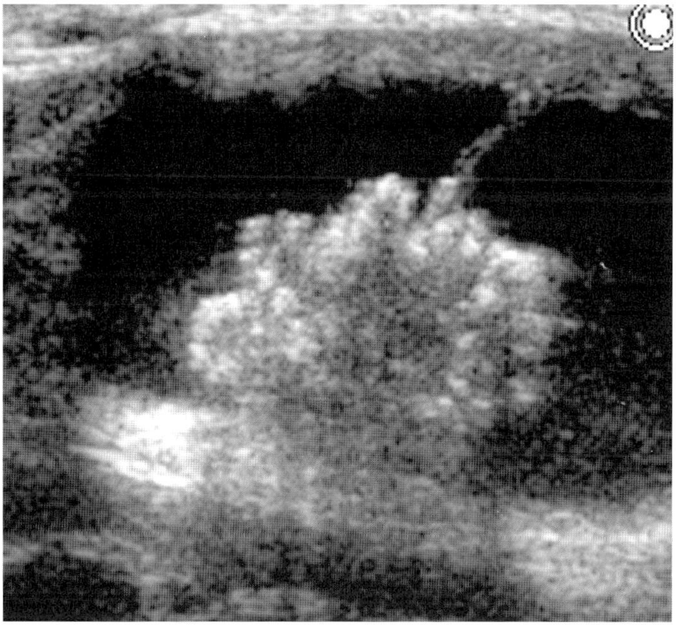

• **FIGURE 8-8** Longitudinal scan of a cystic papillary thyroid cancer. Multiple punctate echogenic dots in a solid element protruding into the cyst are characteristic.

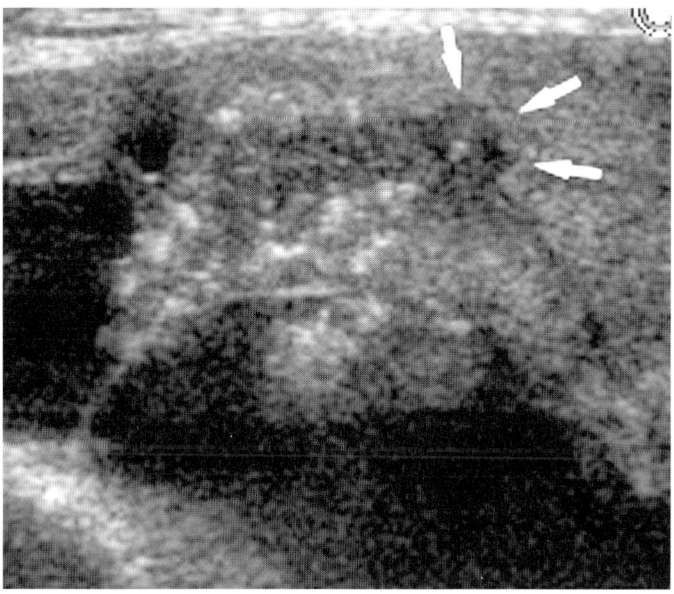

• **FIGURE 8-9** Ultrasonogram of another cystic papillary thyroid cancer. Irregular margin of the solid element *(arrows)* is also suggestive of a cancerous nodule.

Other Thyroid Cancers

It is difficult to differentiate follicular cancers from benign follicular neoplasms by ultrasonography since follicular cancers usually lack the distinctive ultrasonic findings that are seen in papillary cancers. In large nodules with benign ultrasonic features, absence of cystic degeneration is suggestive of follicular cancers but is not definitive. Medullary thyroid cancers are usually hypoechogenic by ultrasonography. Medullary thyroid cancers may be calcified, but cystic change and a halo around the tumor is usually not observed.[22] Anaplastic thyroid cancers present as a large irregular invasive mass. Ultrasonography usually offers little help evaluating anaplastic thyroid cancers. Malignant lymphomas of the thyroid, by contrast, have a characteristic ultrasonic appearance. The involved lobe is diffusely enlarged and hypoechogenic. Differences in size and internal echogenicity between both lobes help suggest this diagnosis (Fig. 8-10). There is currently minimal information regarding ultrasonic features in metastatic cancers to the thyroid in these rare cancers.[23]

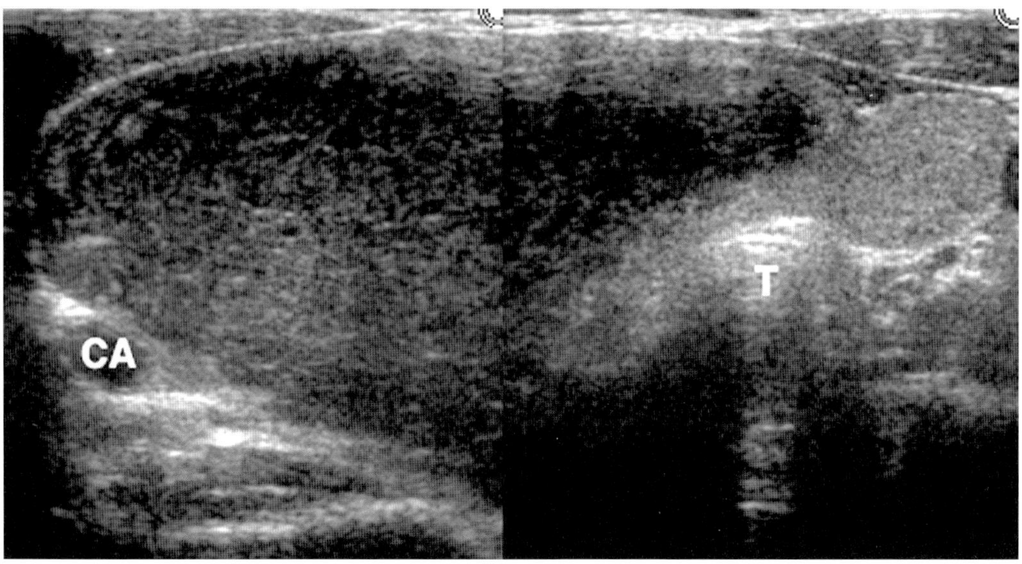

• **FIGURE 8-10** Transverse scan of malignant lymphoma of the thyroid. Right lobe and isthmus of the thyroid are diffusely swollen and hypoechogenic. The left lobe does not seem to be involved. (*CA*, common carotid artery; *T*, trachea.)

EVALUATION OF LYMPH NODE METASTASES

Ultrasonic identification of lymph nodes greater than 9 mm in thickness,[24] those with a longitudinal-transverse diameter ratio less than 2.0,[25] or those without a central echogenic line,[26] suggests a metastatic thyroid cancer in the lymph nodes. A central echogenic line is also present in some metastatic lymph nodes.[27] Ahuja et al.[28] reported that punctate calcifications in lymph nodes or hyperechogenic lymph nodes suggest metastatic papillary thyroid cancer. We agree with these observations, but these ultrasonic findings are rarely observed in microscopic lymph node metastases. Ultrasonography is effective in detecting enlarged lymph nodes, but it is often difficult to differentiate small metastatic lymph nodes from benign nodes.[29] A combination of FNA with ultrasonography, we believe, helps make a correct diagnosis (Figs. 8-11 and 8-12).[30,31]

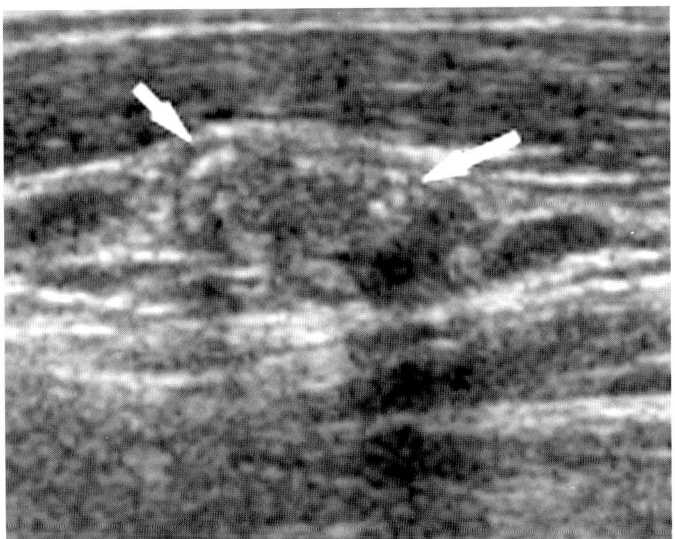

• **FIGURE 8-11** Longitudinal scan of a metastatic lymph node from papillary thyroid cancer. An echogenic lymph node with punctate calcifications *(arrows)* is suggestive of metastatic papillary thyroid cancer.

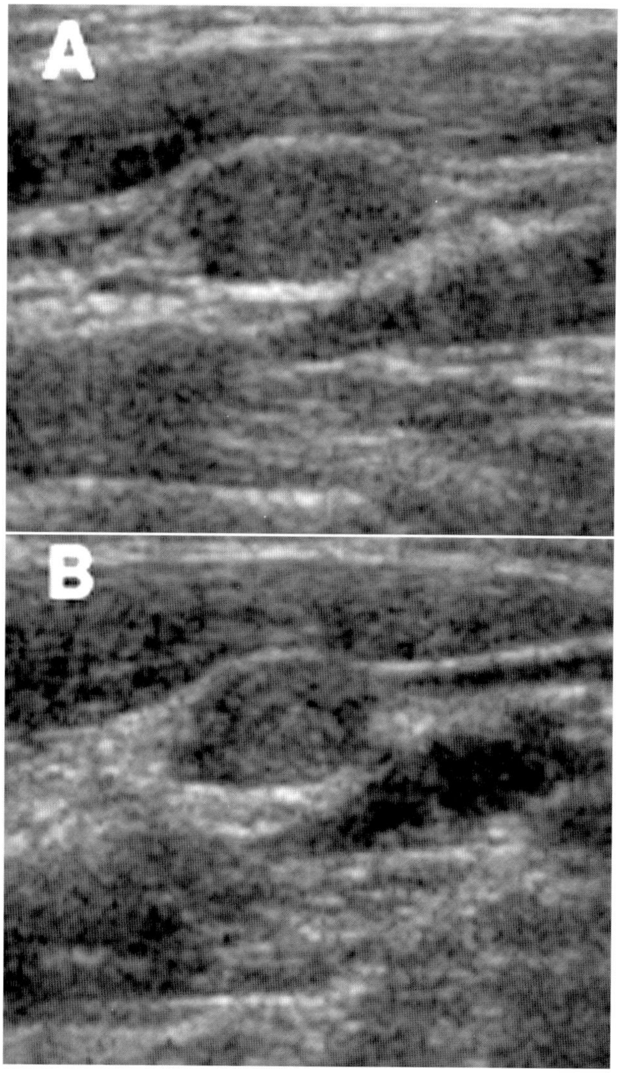

• **FIGURE 8-12** **A,** Longitudinal scan and **B,** transverse scan of a metastatic lymph node from papillary thyroid cancer. The lymph node is echogenic, with a longitudinal-transverse ratio of 1.3.

COLOR DOPPLER ULTRASONOGRAPHY

Visualization of the vascularity of thyroid nodules is possible using color Doppler ultrasonography (Fig. 8-13). Increased blood flow is observed in most hyperfunctioning nodules.[32,33] Color Doppler ultrasonography, however, does not seem to be able to differentiate between benign and malignant

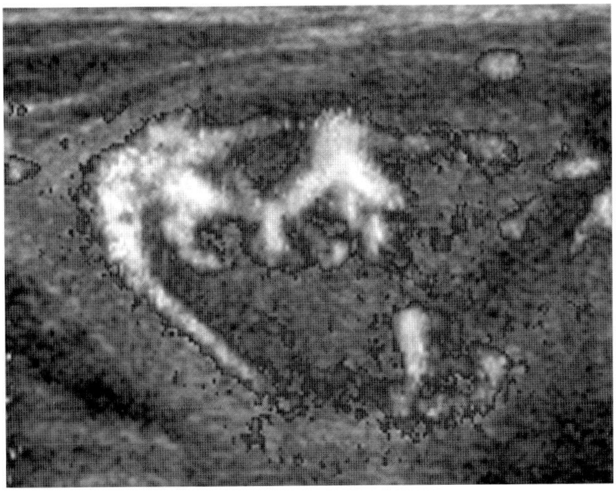

• **FIGURE 8-13** Color Doppler imaging of a follicular adenoma. Blood flow in the nodule as well as around the nodule is demonstrated. Increased blood flow is observed more frequently in follicular adenomas than in papillary thyroid cancers.

TABLE 8-3 Color Doppler Ultrasonography of Follicular Adenomas and Papillary Thyroid Cancers*

	Number of Follicular Adenomas (%)	Number of Papillary Thyroid Cancers (%)
Number in which blood flow was not increased	4 (23.5)	21 (72.5)
Increased peripheral blood flow	4 (23.5)	5 (17.2)
Increased internal blood flow	9 (53.0)	3 (10.3)
TOTAL	17 (100)	29 (100)

*Differentiating cancer from adenoma is difficult, whereas vascularity is significantly different between the adenoma and cancer ($p = 0.002$ by Pearson's test).

thyroid nodules.[34] Shimamoto et al.[35] reported that blood flow depends on the size of the nodule rather than on the histologic structure.

We studied the vascularity of 29 papillary thyroid cancers and 17 follicular adenomas using power-mode Doppler ultrasonography. This equipment can detect subtle vascular changes within thyroid nodules. Follicular adenomas were more vascular than papillary thyroid cancers (Table 8-3). Overall, the contribution of color Doppler ultrasonography is small for differentiating between thyroid cancers and benign thyroid nodules.

ASPIRATION CYTOLOGY AND ULTRASONOGRAPHY

FNA is an established technique for preoperative evaluation of thyroid nodules.[36-39] An expert cytologist, plus adequate samples obtained from the correct nodule, are essential for accurate cytologic diagnosis. Ultrasonic guidance for FNA can reduce false cytologic results caused by geographic sampling errors, inadequate samples from cystic nodules, or bloody aspirates.[40] Rosen et al.[41] have reported that FNA under ultrasonic guidance enables cytologic diagnosis in 60% of patients in whom results of conventional FNA were nondiagnostic. Barely palpable or questionable nodules (small nodules and nodules in a diffusely swollen gland), dominant nodules in a multinodular goiter, nodules with cystic components, and small lymph nodes adjacent to a thyroid nodule require ultrasonic guidance for FNA.

We routinely use ultrasonic examination with an LA39 probe before FNA. When FNA under ultrasonic guidance is indicated, aspiration is performed at the same time. A 22-gauge needle attached to a 5 ml disposable syringe is inserted into the nodule. The sampling site is confirmed by viewing the needle tip on an ultrasonographic monitoring display using a 7.5 MHz probe (I739) (Fig. 8-14).[42] We do not use syringe holders for suction. Usually a single aspiration for each nodule is done. In 2 recent months, we performed 201 FNAs under ultrasonic guidance. Benign, malignant, and suspicious cytologic findings were observed in 129, 27, and 6 FNAs, respectively. Inadequate specimens were obtained in 39 FNAs (19.4%). In 75% of the patients in whom the initial sample was inadequate, an adequate specimen was obtained at a second FNA. Repeat aspirations may improve efficacy of FNA.

CONCLUSION

Ultrasonography is an important examination for evaluating patients with thyroid diseases. Ultrasonography helps to detect and characterize thyroid nodules. Ultrasonography is also a useful tool for follow-up examination of patients with benign thyroid nodules or after thyroidectomy. Ultrasonic examination must be performed before FNA, since decisions regarding the

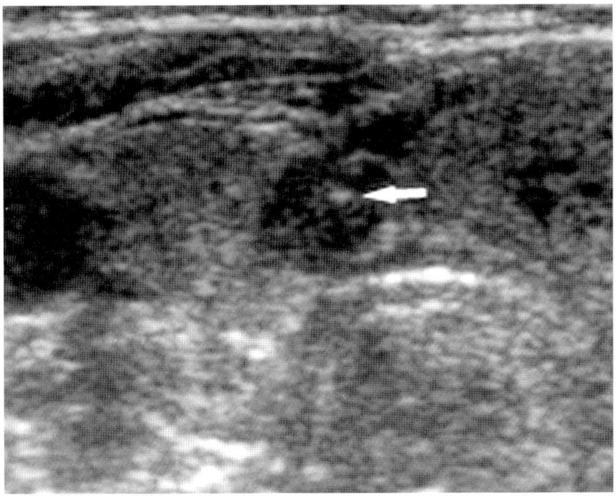

• **FIGURE 8 14** Fine-needle aspiration cytology under ultrasonic guidance. Needle tip demonstrated as an echogenic dot in the nodule *(arrow)* enables confirmation of correct sampling site.

proper sampling site may lead to more accurate cytologic results. Ultrasonic guidance also contributes to correct sampling in FNA, especially in patients with multinodular goiters. Ultrasonography is advocated as a first-choice examination for patients with any type of thyroid disease.

REFERENCES

1. Fujimoto Y et al. Ultrasound scanning of the thyroid gland as a new diagnostic approach. Ultrasonics 5:177-180, 1967.
2. Blum M, Weiss B, Hernberg J. Evaluation of thyroid nodules by A-mode echography. Radiology 101:651-656, 1971.
3. Blum M et al. Clinical applications of thyroid echography. N Engl J Med 287:1164-1169, 1972.
4. Rosen IB, Walfish PG, Miskin M. The use of B mode ultrasonography in changing indications for thyroid operations. Surg Gynecol Obstet 139:193-197, 1974.
5. Ikekubo K et al. Evaluation of radionuclide imaging and echography in the diagnosis of thyroid nodules. Clin Nucl Med 11:145-149, 1986.
6. Brander A et al. Clinical versus ultrasound examination of the thyroid gland in common clinical practice. J Clin Ultrasound 20:37-42, 1992.
7. Tan GH, Gharib H, Reading CC. Solitary thyroid nodule. Comparison between palpation and ultrasonography. Arch Intern Med 155:2418-2423, 1995.
8. Solbiati L et al. The thyroid gland with low uptake lesions: Evaluation by ultrasound. Radiology 155:187-191, 1985.
9. Ross DS. Evaluation of the thyroid nodule. J Nucl Med 32:2181-2192, 1991.
10. Giuffrida D, Gharib H. Controversies in the management of cold, hot, and occult thyroid nodules. Am J Med 99:642-650, 1995.

11. Okamoto T et al. Test performances of three diagnostic procedures in evaluating thyroid nodules: Physical examination, ultrasonography and fine needle aspiration cytology. Endocrine J 41:243-247, 1994.
12. Lin JD et al. Thyroid ultrasonography with fine-needle aspiration cytology for the diagnosis of thyroid cancer. J Clin Ultrasound 25:111-118, 1997.
13. Murakami T et al. Ultrasonographic diagnosis of solitary thyroid nodule. Jpn J Med Ultrasonics 14:126-133, 1987.
14. Murakami T et al. Ultrasonographic diagnosis of nodular goiter. Jpn J Med Ultrasonics 15:264-272, 1988.
15. Watters DAK et al. Role of ultrasound in the management of thyroid nodules. Am J Surg 164:654-657, 1992.
16. Brkljacic B et al. Ultrasonic evaluation of benign and malignant nodules in echographically multinodular thyroids. J Clin Ultrasound 22:71-76, 1994.
17. Solbiati L, Cioffi V, Ballarati E. Ultrasonography of the neck. Radiol Clin North Am 30:941-954, 1992.
18. Tan GH, Gharib H. Thyroid incidentalomas: Management approaches to nonpalpable nodules discovered incidentally on thyroid imaging. Ann Intern Med 126:226-231, 1997.
19. Yamashita H et al. Thyroid cancer associated with adenomatous goiter: An analysis of the incidence and clinical factors. Surg Today 27:495-499, 1997.
20. Hatabu H et al. Cystic papillary carcinoma of the thyroid gland: A new sonographic sign. Clin Radiol 43:121-124, 1991.
21. Fujimoto Y et al. Diffuse sclerosing variant of papillary carcinoma of the thyroid. Cancer 66:2306-2312, 1990.
22. Gorman B et al. Medullary thyroid carcinoma: Role of high-resolution US. Radiology 162:147-150, 1987.
23. Murakami T et al. Identification of metastatic carcinoma in the thyroid by determination of thyroglobulin level in aspirates and ultrasonic findings. Intern Med 32:46-49, 1993.
24. Sakai F et al. Ultrasonic evaluation of cervical metastatic lymphadenopathy. J Ultrasound Med 7:305-310, 1988.
25. Vassallo P et al. Differentiation of benign from malignant superficial lymphadenopathy: The role of high-resolution US. Radiology 183:215-220, 1992.
26. Rubaltelli L et al. Sonography of abnormal lymph nodes in vitro: Correlation of sonographic and histologic findings. Am J Roentgenol 155:1241-1244, 1990.
27. Evans RM, Ahuja A, Metreweli C. The linear echogenic hilus in cervical lymphadenopathy. A sign of benignity or malignancy? Clin Radiol 47:262-264, 1993.
28. Ahuja AT et al. Metastatic cervical nodes in papillary carcinoma of the thyroid: Ultrasound and histological correlation. Clin Radiol 50:229-231, 1995.
29. Hajek PC et al. Lymph nodes of the neck: Evaluation with US. Radiology 158:739-742, 1986.
30. Sutton RT et al. US-guided biopsy of neck masses in postoperative management of patients with thyroid cancer. Radiology 168:769-772, 1988.
31. Brekel MWM et al. Lymph node staging in patients with clinically negative neck examinations by ultrasound and ultrasound-guided aspiration cytology. Am J Surg 162:362-366, 1991.
32. Fobbe F et al. Appearance of thyroid diseases using color-coded duplex sonography. Eur J Radiol 9:29-31, 1989.

33. Becker D et al. Thyroid autonomy with color-coded image-directed Doppler sonography: Internal hypervascularization for the recognition of autonomous adenomas. J Clin Ultrasound 25:63-69, 1997.
34. Clark KJ, Cronan JJ, Scola FH. Color Doppler sonography: Anatomic and physiologic assessment of the thyroid. J Clin Ultrasound 23:215-223, 1995.
35. Shimamoto K et al. Thyroid nodules: Evaluation with color Doppler ultrasonography. J Ultrasound Med 12:673-678, 1993.
36. Altavilla G, Pascale M, Nenci I. Fine needle aspiration cytology of thyroid gland diseases. Acta Cytol 34:251-256, 1990.
37. Rosa GLL et al. Evaluation of the fine needle aspiration biopsy in the preoperative selection of cold thyroid nodules. Cancer 67:2137-2141, 1991.
38. Gharib H, Goellner JR. Fine-needle aspiration biopsy of the thyroid: An appraisal. Ann Intern Med 118:282-289, 1993.
39. Gharib H. Fine-needle aspiration biopsy of thyroid nodules: Advantages, limitations, and effect. Mayo Clin Proc 69:44-49, 1994.
40. Rizzatto G et al. Aspiration biopsy of superficial lesions: Ultrasonic guidance with a linear-array probe. Am J Roentgenol 148:623-625, 1987.
41. Rosen IB et al. Ultrasound-guided fine-needle aspiration biopsy in the management of thyroid disease. Am J Surg 166:346-349, 1993.
42. Yokozawa T et al. Accurate and simple method of diagnosing thyroid nodules by the modified technique of ultrasound-guided fine needle aspiration biopsy. Thyroid 5:141-145, 1995.

PART

III

DECISION MAKING: SELECTING A SURGICAL APPROACH

CHAPTER 9

Total Thyroidectomy

GREGORY P. SADLER, M.D.
ORLO H. CLARK, M.D.

Carcinoma of the thyroid gland is a term encompassing a wide spectrum of different histologic types. Several types of primary thyroid carcinoma are recognized, although approximately 90% to 95% of thyroid carcinomas are *differentiated* tumors of follicular cell origin giving rise to papillary, follicular, or Hürthle cell carcinoma. These tumors are collectively referred to as *differentiated thyroid cancer* (DTC).

Patients with well-differentiated thyroid cancer may have an indolent course, often lasting many years. This feature of the disease, combined with the fact that the incidence of clinical thyroid cancer is relatively low (about 40 new cases per 1,000,000 of the population per year) and mortality from the condition is rare (1400 deaths per year in the United States), has resulted in continued debate surrounding the optimal choice of surgical treatment for DTC.[1] In essence, the debate centers around this key question: Should total thyroidectomy be the treatment of choice for patients with DTC and if so, why?

This question has not been satisfactorily answered in the past 30 years because of three important observations: (1) about 85% of patients with DTC do well, regardless of the extent of the thyroidectomy performed; (2) in inexperienced surgical hands, the more extensive the thyroidectomy, the higher the morbidity rate; and (3) as yet, no prospective, randomized trial comparing different methods of treatment has been performed. One should remember, however, that although DTC usually acts in a benign manner, it results in more deaths than any other endocrine tumor (excluding cancer of the ovary).[2,3]

Essentially, three schools of thought have emerged in the past two decades, each advocating a different philosophy in the management of DTC and providing data and considered reasoning to support their viewpoint. These three surgical approaches are (1) partial thyroidectomy (usually hemithyroidectomy with isthmusectomy); (2) routine near-total thyroidectomy (total lobectomy on the side of the dominant tumor and subtotal resection on the other side), with total thyroidectomy in high-risk patients; and (3) total thyroidectomy. Continued debate centers around whether the cited advantages of total thyroidectomy outweigh the increased complication rate that may be encountered with the procedure. These advantages include removal of multifocal disease, decreased incidence of local recurrence, reduced risk of anaplasia in any residual tissue, facilitation of diagnosing unsuspected metastatic disease by radioiodine scanning or treatment with ^{131}I, and greater sensitivity of blood thyroglobulin levels to predict recurrent or persistent disease. It is also easiest to perform a total thyroidectomy at the initial operation when there is no scar tissue.

THE CONSERVATIVE VIEWPOINT

Expert opinion in the United States and Europe would agree that the most minimal procedure for thyroid carcinoma should be a total thyroid lobectomy and isthmusectomy with removal of any ipsilateral lymph nodes in the central neck.[4,5] Anything less than total thyroid lobectomy results in an increased incidence of recurrence and halves long-term survival rates.[6] Proponents of a more conservative approach to thyroid surgery argue that the risk for complications, such as permanent hypoparathyroidism or recurrent laryngeal nerve damage arising from thyroid lobectomy and isthmusectomy for unilateral well-differentiated thyroid carcinoma, are lower than those for total thyroidectomy.[7-9] However, the complication rates quoted vary considerably. One study reports a complication rate of 69% following total thyroidectomy, with 9% of patients experiencing permanent hypocalcemia.[10] This seems remarkably excessive when compared with rates of 1% to 3% for permanent hypocalcemia and 1% for permanent recurrent laryngeal nerve damage quoted by authors experienced in total thyroidectomy, including our group.[11-13] Indeed, this argument appears to question the operative technique of total thyroidectomy by surgeons in these centers rather than whether total thyroidectomy is the best procedure for the patient.

That total and completion thyroidectomy can be routinely practiced with minimal morbidity and mortality has been previously reported by the authors in a series of articles. These included 146 patients undergoing total thyroidectomy for thyroid carcinoma between 1987 and 1992 and 160 patients between 1977 and 1984. There were no patients with permanent dysfunction of the recurrent laryngeal nerve, and only three of 306 patients developed permanent hypoparathyroidism.[14-16] In 1994, Reeve et al.[17] demonstrated that trainee surgeons taught the technique of total thyroidectomy in a specialized endocrine unit were subsequently able to perform the operation in a general hospital setting with low morbidity and mortality. The argument that a less than total thyroidectomy should be practiced because the majority of general surgeons in the community may be incapable of performing total thyroidectomy without significant morbidity is therefore flawed. A more sound argument would be that those surgeons wanting to practice thyroid surgery should first be taught how to do a safe total thyroid lobectomy, then a safe total thyroidectomy in a specialized unit that is focused on the care of patients with thyroid disorders.

Surgeons favoring subtotal/near-total thyroidectomy maintain that concomitant microscopic, multicentric disease is of no clinical significance as a source of recurrent or metastatic disease. Therefore reoperation for recurrent disease in the thyroid remnant is rare, anaplastic transformation in the thyroid remnant is so rare that it is of little or no consequence, toxicity from ^{131}I ablation of the thyroid remnant is nonexistent, and following ^{131}I ablation, thyroglobulin levels may still be followed.[18-23] We would suggest, however, that leaving thyroid tissue is recommended for such reasons as protecting the parathyroid gland or recurrent laryngeal nerve. Although one can ablate normal thyroid tissue with ^{131}I, this treatment does not ablate coexisting thyroid tumors, so that a subsequent treatment dose with ^{131}I must be used, thus increasing the total dose given.

The strongest argument in favor of a more conservative approach to thyroid surgery was provided by Hay et al.[53] at the Mayo Clinic. They developed a postoperative prognostic scale for risk of dying from papillary cancer. Called the AGES score, it takes into account such factors as *a*ge, pathologic tumor grade, *e*xtent of disease, and *s*ize of tumor. Two groups of patients were identified using this system: low-risk (young patients, well-differentiated tumors, no local invasion or distant metastases, and small primary lesions) and high-risk (older patients, poorly differentiated tumors, locally invasive tumors, distant metastases, and large primary lesions [>4cm]) patients. Of the two groups, 85% (of 860 patients) were in the low-risk group and the cancer risk mortality in this group was 2% at 25 years following bilateral thyroid resection, compared with 1% mortality after unilateral lobectomy. Thus in 85% of patients with papillary thyroid cancer, the extent of the original thyroid surgery had little bearing on the mortality rates.[24] The AGES classification, however, is primarily a postoperative classification, since invasion, grade, and distant metastases are often unknown until the thyroidectomy is performed or thereafter.

A different picture emerged in patients categorized in the high-risk category. Cancer risk mortality at 25 years in this group was 65% following unilateral lobectomy and 35% following bilateral thyroidectomy, suggesting a clear advantage in patients who underwent a bilateral procedure. Total thyroidectomy, however, conferred no survival advantage over subtotal/near-total thyroidectomy in these patients. However, less radioiodine can be used in patients undergoing total thyroidectomy, since one does not have to ablate the thyroid remnant before ablating the tumor.

The debate regarding the optimal treatment for patients with DTC has therefore continued. Advocates of total thyroidectomy state that the advantages conferred by total thyroidectomy, as outlined above, should make it the treatment of choice for patients with DTC and that in experienced hands complication rates are low. Proponents of a more conservative approach to surgery, however, counter that if little or no long-term survival advantage is conferred on patients by performing total thyroidectomy as opposed to subtotal/near-total thyroidectomy, why subject them to the increased risk of morbidity associated with the procedure?

ARGUMENT FOR TOTAL THYROIDECTOMY

We firmly advocate the use of total thyroidectomy (when it can be performed safely) for patients with DTC, believing that the procedure confers distinct advantages in patient management over and above lesser procedures. This view is shared by other authors.[13,24-29] Numerous reports have now been published confirming that total thyroidectomy in experienced hands can be performed with minimal morbidity (less than 3%) and no higher mortality than occurs with subtotal procedures. Furthermore, it has been demonstrated that the technique of total thyroidectomy can be performed safely and efficiently by general surgeons following appropriate training by experienced endocrine surgeons. It has also been recommended for patients with benign thyroid problems.[30]

Surgeons who do not feel comfortable performing a total thyroidectomy should perform a total lobectomy and isthmusectomy, and if necessary, the second lobe can be removed at a subsequent operation. We recommend near-total thyroidectomy when it lessens the risk of hypoparathyroidism or nerve injury. When the parathyroid glands and recurrent laryngeal nerves are situated off the thyroid gland, we see no reason to leave thyroid tissue. Total thyroidectomy should be the procedure of choice for thyroid cancer for the following reasons when it can be performed with minimal morbidity.

Reduced Incidence of Local Recurrence and Anaplastic Change. Coexisting, contralateral, intraglandular, papillary thyroid carcinoma has been shown to be present in 30% to 87.5% of patients with clinical papillary thyroid cancer at the time of the initial operation.[31,32] Whether this is of clinical significance is not clear, since autopsy studies demonstrate that nonclinically detectable papillary thyroid cancer is present in up to 28% of patients dying of nonthyroidal disease.[33] Clearly documented, however, is that recurrent thyroid carcinoma is more common in patients who undergo any procedure less than total thyroidectomy.[6] Furthermore, 50% of all patients who develop local recurrence in the neck subsequently die from it.[25,34]

Total thyroidectomy removes all intrathyroidal tumor foci, an important fact in the management of patients who have previously received head and neck irradiation, have familial DTC, or who fall into the high-risk category by virtue of their age (over 40 years of age). Although the risk of anaplastic change in the residual thyroid remnant is low (1%), its occurrence in patients is almost invariably fatal.[25,34-36] By removing all possible intrathyroidal foci of tumor, the potential risk of anaplastic change in the remaining thyroid remnant is eliminated.

Facilitation of ^{131}I Scanning. Metastatic DTC can be detected and treated by radioactive iodine in about 75% of patients.[37] Screening and treatment are greatly facilitated by removal of all normal thyroid tissue (which effectively competes for iodine uptake); This is probably the most compelling of arguments in favor of total thyroidectomy for DTC.[25,38]

Screening with radioactive iodine (^{131}I) is a much more sensitive test of metastatic disease than are chest x-ray evaluation or CT scanning, but, ^{131}I scanning is less sensitive than serum thyroglobulin determination.[37] Micrometastases in the chest are detectable by radioiodine scanning even when chest x-ray evaluation shows no evidence of disease. About 75% of these patients have been successfully treated after receiving ablative doses of ^{131}I for micrometastases, especially when total thyroidectomy has been performed. Unfortunately, the success rate of treating pulmonary macrometastases with ^{131}I is less than 10%, so early detection is most important.[39,40]

Mazzaferri and Young[6] reported a 6.4% recurrence rate in 110 patients who had undergone treatment with total thyroidectomy and adjunctive therapy (^{131}I and thyroid hormone suppression of TSH), compared with an 11%

rate in patients who had undergone total thyroidectomy alone. This finding was supported by Samaan et al,[41] who recorded fewer recurrences following treatment with ^{131}I but no evidence of increased survival. These success rates may underestimate the benefits of ^{131}I ablation in these retrospective studies, because patients at higher risk and with more extensive tumors were more likely to have received ^{131}I ablation therapy.

Radioactive iodine scanning and treatment follows a fairly standard protocol. Following initial or completion total thyroidectomy, patients are prescribed triiodothyronine (T_3) in the postoperative period because its duration of action (approximately 1 day) is shorter than that of thyroxine (T_4) (approximately 1 week). The T_3 is discontinued for 2 weeks before scanning, and the patient is given a low-iodine diet to enhance ^{131}I uptake into any metastases or remaining normal thyroid tissue. In most medical centers a screening dose of roughly 2 mCi of ^{131}I is then administered and the uptake is measured at 24 hours. The uptake in most patients should be less than 1% after total thyroidectomy, with no hot spots in the neck or elsewhere (remnant normal thyroid or local or distant metastases). The most frequent cause of a hot spot in the neck following initial screening is residual thyroid tissue present in the thyroid bed. Studies by Massin et al.[42] suggest that the more extensive the original thyroidectomy, the lower the failure rate of treatment. Utiger[43] is also an advocate of treating patients with DTC with total or near-total thyroidectomy and postoperative radioactive iodine ablation. We generally recommend treatment with 30 to 50 mCi for patients considered to be at low risk and 100 to 150 mCi for patients considered to be at high risk with DTC.

Accurate Postoperative Monitoring of Thyroglobulin Levels. Thyroglobulin (Tg) is a unique tumor marker that is produced only by normal and neoplastic thyroid tissue. Once all thyroid tissue has been removed, thyroglobulin levels should effectively fall to low levels (less than 3 ng/ml). By monitoring thyroglobulin levels (which should remain below 3 ng/ml), disease progress can be followed. When blood Tg levels increase, recurrent disease must be present and appropriate screening with ^{131}I should be performed.[44] The best time to determine serum Tg is when the patient is hypothyroid just before scanning with ^{131}I, since TSH is the best stimulus for Tg production.[37]

Patients who have serum Tg levels that increase into the abnormal range when they are rendered hypothyroid for scanning and have no evidence of ^{131}I uptake should probably be treated with about 100 mCi of ^{131}I, since in about one third of these patients uptake can be demonstrated after the treatment dose and subsequent Tg levels are less than 3 ng/ml.[37]

TOTAL THYROIDECTOMY IN MEDULLARY THYROID CANCER

Medullary thyroid cancer (MTC) accounts for about 5% of thyroid cancers. Tumors are of C-cell origin; thus radioiodine and TSH suppression therapy are frequently unhelpful.[45] The high incidence of multicentricity in patients with familial MTC and the more aggressive behavior of tumors in these patients, especially in patients with MEN2B and sporadic MTC, is why most surgeons argue that the optimal surgical treatment is total thyroidectomy. This should be combined with a meticulous central compartment nodal clearance from carotid sheath to trachea and from the innominate vein to the thyroid cartilage (these nodes are frequently involved early in the disease process and should routinely be cleared along with paratracheal nodes).[46-48]

Screening of patients with familial MTC for RET point mutations on chromosome 10 has replaced provocation testing with pentagastrin or calcium-stimulated calcitonin levels to make the diagnosis.[49] This program has enabled young patients at risk of developing MTC and who are RET positive to undergo total thyroidectomy before medullary thyroid cancers develop from the C-cell hyperplasia. Reports demonstrate that in experienced hands, children tolerate this procedure remarkably well with a low incidence of morbidity and virtually no mortality.[50,51] They are subsequently at no risk of dying from MTC.

TOTAL THYROIDECTOMY IN MINIMAL AND MINIMALLY INVASIVE THYROID CANCER

Minimal (or *occult/microcarcinoma*) tumors originally included papillary cancers up to 15 mm in diameter but now are defined as papillary carcinomas of 10 mm or less in size with no evidence of local invasiveness through the thyroid capsule and not associated with lymph node metastases.[52] They are usually nonpalpable and are thus usually incidental findings at surgical, histologic, or autopsy examination. Studies have demonstrated occult papillary thyroid cancer to be present in 28% of thyroid glands removed at autopsy.[31] The recurrence rate for patients with tumors 10 mm or less following removal is about 6%, and the mortality rate is about 0.4%.[53]

A similar scenario exists with minimally invasive follicular tumors, in which there is evidence of minimal invasion through the tumor capsule at one or more spots. When there is invasion into but not through the capsule these are classified as *atypical adenomas,* although there are rare documented reports of metastases occurring, and they should not be regarded as low-grade carcinomas.

There have been documented instances of deaths with occult carcinoma of the thyroid.[20,54,55] Consensus among authors, however, suggests that in patients found to have a minimally invasive follicular thyroid cancer or a minimal papillary thyroid carcinoma in a thyroid specimen removed for other reasons, unilateral thyroid lobectomy and isthmusectomy is usually sufficient surgical treatment, unless there is angioinvasion or the tumor is at the margins of resection. Similarly, in rare cases of encapsulated papillary thyroid carcinoma, total lobectomy is all that is needed. This view is supported by a study demonstrating no difference in survival among patients who had been treated for occult carcinoma of the thyroid by either total thyroidectomy or thyroid lobectomy, whether or not lymphatic spread was present.[56]

However, we recommend obtaining a serum thyroglobulin level in patients with minimally invasive follicular carcinoma or occult papillary thyroid cancer. If it is elevated, a bone scan should be considered with a completion total thyroidectomy so that radioiodine can be used to scan and treat (if possible) metastatic disease.

CONCLUSION

In experienced hands, total thyroidectomy is associated with a low rate of morbidity and virtually negligible mortality. The operation is usually not difficult to accomplish safely, but surgeons must be trained in the field. Use of parathyroid autotransplantation when parathyroid glands cannot be maintained on a vascular pedicle appears to have reduced the rate of permanent hypocalcemia. With meticulous dissection, the rate of recurrent laryngeal nerve damage should be only about 1%. For patients with recurrent laryngeal nerve damage on one side, or where parathyroid glands are situated very anteriorly on the thyroid gland and their status is questionable, total thyroidectomy may not be considered the most appropriate surgical option: near-total thyroidectomy should be used in these patients to decrease the risk of complications. The remnant thyroid tissue can then be ablated with ^{131}I.

However, we think that when technically possible, as is almost always the case, there are several compelling arguments for the treatment of differentiated thyroid carcinoma by total thyroidectomy. These reasons include removal of multifocal disease, decreasing the incidence of local recurrence, reducing the risk of anaplasia in any residual tissue, improving the sensitivity of blood thyroglobulin levels to predict recurrent or persistent disease, and, most important, facilitating the diagnosis of unsuspected metastatic disease by radioiodine scanning or treatment with ^{131}I, thus reducing incidence of distant recurrence.

REFERENCES

1. Cancer Statistics 1995. New York: American Cancer Society, 1995.
2. Foster JS. Morbidity and mortality after thyroidectomy. Surg Gynecol Obstet 146:423-429, 1978.
3. Robbins J et al. Thyroid carcinoma: A lethal endocrine neoplasm. Ann Intern Med 115:133-147, 1991.
4. Solomon BL, Wartofsky L, Burman KD. Current trends in the management of well differentiated papillary thyroid carcinoma. J Clin Endocrinol Metab 81:333-339, 1996.
5. Baldet L et al. The management of differentiated thyroid cancer in Europe in 1988. Results of an international survey. Acta Endocrinol 120:547-558, 1989.
6. Mazzaferri EL, Young RL. Papillary thyroid carcinoma: A 10-year follow-up report of the impact of therapy in 576 patients. Am J Med 70:511-518, 1981.
7. Cady B. Surgery of thyroid cancer. World J Surg 5:3-5, 1976.
8. Farrar SB, Cooperman M, James AG. Surgical management of papillary and follicular carcinoma of the thyroid. Ann Surg 192:701-704, 1980.
9. Schroder DM, Chambors A, France CJ. Operative strategy for thyroid cancer: Is total thyroidectomy worth the price? Cancer 58:2320-2328, 1986.
10. Flynn MB et al. Local complications after surgical resection for thyroid carcinoma. Am J Surg 168:404-407, 1994.
11. Attie JN, Khafif RA. Preservation of the parathyroid glands during total thyroidectomy: Improved techniques using microsurgery. Am J Surg 130:399-403, 1975.
12. Thompson NW, Nishiyama RH, Harness JK. Thyroid carcinoma: Current controversies. Curr Probl Surg 15:1-10, 1978.
13. Lennquist S. Surgical strategy in thyroid carcinoma. A clinical review. Acta Chir Scand 152:321-338, 1986.
14. Clark OH et al. Thyroid cancer: The case for total thyroidectomy. Eur J Cancer Clin Oncol 24:305-310, 1988.
15. Grossman RF et al. The case for total thyroidectomy revisited. In Johnson JT, Didlokar MS, eds. Head and Neck Cancer, vol 3. Amsterdam: Excerpta Medica, 1993, pp 879-883.
16. Levin KE et al. Reoperative thyroid surgery. Surgery 111:604-609, 1992.
17. Reeve TS et al. Can total thyroidectomy be performed as safely by general surgeons in provincial centers as by surgeons in specialized endocrine surgical units? Making the case for surgical training. Arch Surg 129:834-836, 1994.
18. Tollefsen HR, Shah JP, Huvos AG. Papillary carcinoma of the thyroid. Recurrence in the gland after initial treatment. Am J Surg 124:468-472, 1972.
19. Rossi RL et al. Current results of conservative treatment for differentiated thyroid carcinoma. World J Surg 10:612-622, 1986.
20. McConahey WM, Hay ID, Woolner LB. Papillary thyroid cancer treated at the Mayo Clinic, 1946 through 1970: Initial manifestations, pathological findings, therapy and outcome. Mayo Clin Proc 61:978-996, 1986.
21. Beahrs OH. Surgical treatment for thyroid cancer. Br J Surg 71:976-979, 1984.

22. Beierwaltes WH et al. An analysis of ablation of thyroid remnants with ^{131}I in 511 patients from 1947-1984: Experience at University of Michigan. J Nucl Med 25:1287-1293, 1984.
23. Mazzaferri RL. Papillary and follicular thyroid cancer: Selective therapy. Compr Ther 7:6-14, 1981.
24. Orsenigo E et al. Total thyroidectomy in the treatment of thyroid cancer. Eur J Surg Oncol 21:478-481, 1995.
25. Mazzaferri EL et al. Papillary thyroid carcinoma: The impact of therapy in 576 patients. Medicine 56:171-196, 1977.
26. Jacobs JK, Aland JW, Ballenger JF. Total thyroidectomy: A review of 213 patients. Ann Surg 197:542-549, 1983.
27. Loré JM. An Atlas of Head and Neck Surgery, 3rd ed. Philadelphia: WB Saunders, 1988, p 737.
28. Reeve TS, Delbridge L. Thyroid cancers of follicular cell origin. Proc Surg 19:78-88, 1988.
29. Harness JK et al. Deaths due to differentiated thyroid cancer: A 46-year perspective. World J Surg 12:623-628, 1988.
30. Reeve TS et al. Total thyroidectomy. The preferred option for multinodular goiter. Ann Surg 206:782-786, 1987.
31. Hirabayashi RN, Lindsay S. Carcinoma of the thyroid gland: A statistical study of 390 patients. J Clin Endocrinol Metab 21:1596-1610, 1961.
32. Russel WO et al. Thyroid Carcinoma: Classification, intraglandular dissemination and clinicopathological study based upon whole organ section of 80 glands. Cancer 16:1425-1432, 1963.
33. Sampson RJ. Prevalence and significance of occult thyroid cancer. In DeGroot LJ, Frohman LA, Kaplan EL, Refetoff S, eds. Radiation-associated thyroid carcinoma. New York: Gruhne & Statton, 1977, p 137.
34. Silverberg SG, Hutter RVP, Foote FW. Fatal carcinoma of the thyroid: Histology, metastases and causes of death. Cancer 25:792-794, 1970.
35. Tollefsen HR, DeCosse JJ, Hutter RVP. Papillary carcinoma of the thyroid: A clinical and pathological study of 70 fatal cases. Cancer 17:1035-1039, 1964.
36. Wychulis AR, Beahers OH, Woolner LB. Papillary carcinoma associated with anaplastic carcinoma in the thyroid gland. Surg Gynecol Obstet 120:28, 1965.
37. Clark OH, Hoelting T. Management of patients with differentiated thyroid cancer who have positive serum thyroglobulin levels and negative radioiodine scans. Thyroid 4:501-505, 1994.
38. Varma VM, Beierwaltes WH, Nofal MM. Treatment of thyroid cancer: Death rates after surgery and after surgery followed by sodium iodide ^{131}I. JAMA 214:1437-1441, 1970.
39. Schlumberger M et al. Long-term results of treatment of 283 patients with lung and bone metastases from differentiated thyroid carcinoma. J Clin Endocrinol Metab 63:960-965, 1986.
40. Casara D et al. Differential features of pulmonary metastases in differentiated thyroid cancer: Natural history and multivariate anaylsis of prognostic variables. J Nucl Med 34:1626-1631, 1993.
41. Samaan WA et al. Impact of therapy for differentiated carcinoma of the thyroid: An analysis of 706 cases. J Clin Endocrinol Metab 56:1131-1138, 1983.

42. Massin JP et al. Pulmonary metastases in differentiated thyroid carcinoma. Study of 58 cases with implications for primary tumor treatment. Cancer 53:982-992, 1984.
43. Utiger RD. Treatment of thyroid cancer. N Engl J Med 337:928-930, 1997.
44. Ozata M et al. Serum thyroglobulin in the follow-up of patients with treated differentiated thyroid cancer. J Clin Endocrinol Metab 75:98-105, 1994.
45. Soh EY, Clark OH. Surgical considerations and approach to thyroid cancer. Endocrinol Metab Clin North Am 25:115-139, 1996.
46. Duh QY et al. Medullary thyroid carcinoma. The need for early diagnosis and total thyroidectomy. Arch Surg 124:1206-1210, 1989
47. Delius RE, Thompson NW. Early total thyroidectomy in patients with multiple endocrine neoplasia IIB syndrome. Surg Gynecol Obstet 169:442-444, 1989.
48. Dunn JM, Farndon JR. Medullary thyroid carcinoma. Br J Surg 80:6-9, 1993.
49. Wells SA et al. Predictive DNA testing and prophylactic thyroidectomy in patients at risk for multiple endocrine neoplasia type 2A. Ann Surg 220:237-250, 1994.
50. Stael AP et al. Total thyroidectomy in the treatment of thyroid carcinoma in childhood. Br J Surg 82:1083-1085, 1995.
51. Harness JK et al. Differentiated thyroid carcinoma in children and adolescents. World J Surg 16:547-553, 1992.
52. Hedinger C, Williams ED, Sobin LH, eds. Histological typing of thyroid tumors, 2nd ed. No.11. In International Classification of Tumors, World Health Organization. New York: Springer-Verlag, 1988, pp 9-10.
53. Hay ID et al. Papillary thyroid microcarcinoma: A study of 543 cases observed in a 50 year period. Surgery 112:1139-1147, 1992.
54. Allo MD, Christianson W, Koivunen D. Not all "occult" papillary carcinomas are minimal. Surgery 104:971-976, 1988
55. Salvadori B et al. "Occult" papillary carcinoma of the thyroid: A questionable entity. Eur J Cancer 29A:1817-1820, 1993.
56. Hubert JP et al. Occult papillary thyroid carcinoma of the thyroid. Arch Surg 115:394-399, 1980.

CHAPTER

10

Partial Thyroidectomy

IRVING B. ROSEN, M.D.

Most thyroid malignancy is well differentiated, characterized by papillary and follicular carcinoma, but most frequently a mixed histologic picture of both is found. The incidence of thyroid cancer in the United States[1] has been reported to be approximately 13,000 new cases annually; approximately 1400 people die of the disease each year. This accounts for only 1% of all malignancies, so thyroid cancer is viewed as rare, both in the United States and worldwide. Current reviews of thyroid cancer[2] concur with the reported frequency but note a remarkable increase in its occurrence: approximately twofold to fivefold between 1935 and 1975. The reports note that this cannot be fully accounted for by either radiation exposure or radioactive fallout, although how this can be precisely assessed is puzzling.[2]

It is widely appreciated that the outlook of thyroid cancer, in contrast with all other malignancies, has a far superior survival rate. Despite the reported low incidence of thyroid cancer, the pool of surviving patients is a large one, which emphasizes the need for awareness of problems. This is often dismissed because of the focus on other malignancies that occur more frequently and that presently have a dismal outlook. Innovations in thyroid cancer management are limited, but the topic itself has continually stimulated polemic differences in management among interested physicians. As a result, conservative and less conservative policies that are implicitly conflictual have been recognized. Even at the brink of the modern era of thyroid cancer treatment, directly opposing points of view are articulated in cancer textbooks between contributing authors and editors.[3,4] The topic of thyroid cancer surgery is popular at surgical meetings, mainly because of the controversy associated with its treatment policies. Medical thyroidologists, who are stereotypically viewed as "conservative," have actually supported an aggressive stance in treatment management.[2,5] Regardless of the advocates the surgeon elects to heed, it is important to understand the rationales behind the various approaches. This chapter will highlight the case for a conservative approach.

NATURAL HISTORY

Advocates of the conservative approach for management of thyroid malignancy rely heavily on studies of the natural history of thyroid cancer, which they feel support a less extensive approach in therapy. Stratification of risk based on age has been well established and is widely accepted.[6] This has been followed by an enumerative risk-factor formula, i.e., AGES (age, grade, extent, size; see Chapter 9), devised by the Mayo Clinic group,[7] which has earned serious consideration, although its formulation has not led to a dynamic alteration in cancer therapeutics. Various other formulas and staging systems have been devised; these include not only AGES,[7-9] but also the European Organization for Research on Treatment of Cancer (EORTC) scheme, and these classifications: TNM, AMES, MACIS (metastases, age, completeness of surgery, invasion of cancer, and size), clinical class, Ohio, Memoris Sloan-Kettering, and SAG.[2,6,10,11] Brierley et al.[10] studied the virtues of the various classifications by analyzing their material using the criteria of various formulas. They concluded, "There was no statistically significant difference in the predictive abilities of TNM, AGES, MACIS, AMES, or EORTC."[10] They also stated, "The adoption of a single staging system is optimal and should be sought." In a sense, the zeal for staging systems has been a substitute for static treatment policies.

Along with risk factor system elaboration, the role of molecular biologic inquiry has been unparalleled in scope and intensity of investigation. Thyroid neoplasia does not have a limited number of involved oncogenes but rather, a plethora of oncogenetic factors, tumor suppressor genes, and growth factors.[12-14] The bibliography cited herein is worth consulting for current review. The hoped-for application of molecular biologic investigation can be appreciated in this statement from Jossart and Grossman[13];

"Current strategies for determining the optimal type of operation and postoperative therapy in these groups of thyroid cancer are unreliable. The molecular events occurring in these tumors must be determined to develop a prognostic biomarker that can optimize therapy and thus outcome." Despite what might be viewed as voluminous and valuable in the area of molecular biologic investigation into thyroid neoplasia, clinical beliefs and perceived results are still the major influences in treatment selection.

Rossi and Cady[6] separated their patients with differentiated thyroid carcinoma into three risk groups for outcome, which they subsequently reduced to two for the sake of simplicity. Patients were divided into a high-risk group consisting of men over 40 and women over 50 years of age, and a low-risk group consisting of all younger patients. Patients in the low-risk group had a recurrence rate of 5% and a mortality rate of 1%, compared with patients in the high-risk group, with recurrence of 20% and mortality of 15%.[6,15] It was felt that these simplified risk groups superseded prognostic effects of primary disease extension, pathologic type, and therapy. Even when incurable neck disease was encountered, Cady[6] found that only 11% of patients in the low–risk group died, compared with 79% in the high-risk group.

Hay et al.[7,8] reported on a multifactorial analysis of more than 14,200 patient-years of experience using an AGES classification; later they shifted to a MACIS scheme. Of 14 possible variables studied, only patient age, tumor grade, extent, metastases, and size were significantly important in predicting death from papillary cancer. The prognostic score was calculated as PS = 0.05 × Age in years (if age 40 or over) +1 (if grade 2), or +3 (if grade 3 or 4), +1 (if extrathyroid), or +3 (if distant spread) + 0.2 × Tumor size. Eighty-six percent of their patients were in the low-risk group, with scores of 3.99 or less, and had a 20-year mortality rate of only 1%, in contrast to the very high-risk group, who had a staging score of 5 to 5.99, with 92% mortality. Patients with a score of 4 or more were all considered to be in the high-risk group. They noted that for patients at minimal risk, no improvement in survival was demonstrated when patients underwent more than an ipsilateral lobectomy. However, in a subgroup with an AGES score of 4 or more, survival after bilateral resection (ipsilateral lobectomy and partial contralateral lobectomy) was higher than after ipsilateral lobectomy alone. In neither the minimal nor the higher-risk subgroup was survival significantly improved by performance of a total thyroidectomy when compared with their lesser bilateral procedure. In their series of 52 patients, with a local recurrence followed for as long as 41 years, no patient with tumor recurrence limited to the thyroid remnant died of thyroid cancer.

Fujimoto et al.[16] acknowledged the importance of prognostic factors that emerged in retrospective studies of thyroidectomy patients, mainly carried out by the American authors cited previously.[6-8,15] Reporting on his experience at the Tokyo Women's Medical College Hospital, Fujimoto et al[16] found the ratio of low-risk to high-risk population was 93 to 7, and the cancer-related deaths, with an average 9-year patient follow-up, showed 0% mortality rate for low-risk and 29% mortality rate for high-risk groups, respectively. They noted that if low-risk cancer at initial operation is definitely identified, distant metastases will hardly ever present clinically. Therefore unnecessarily extensive surgery could be avoided, with implicit avoidance of surgical complication. They further noted that in iodine-rich countries, the ratio of low- to high-risk carcinoma was 90 to 10, whereas in iodine-deficient areas, the ratio of high-risk cancer appears to be higher. They described a subtotal thyroidectomy to include the resection of a lobe, isthmus, and a medial third of the contralateral lobe, although it is still grouped under hemithyroidectomy classifications for the sake of analysis. In the study of their low-risk patient population, 2 of 273 patients had recurrences in the thyroid remnant following hemithyroidectomy after being monitored for 5 to 13 years. They concluded that leaving a sizable thyroid portion permitted low-risk patients to enjoy a good outcome without thyroid replacement therapy, permitting a much easier regimen to observe.

Shah et al.[17] undertook the study of 146 patients by matched-pair analysis with 73 patients aged 45 years or older who were matched in each arm for significant prognostic factors. One group underwent lobectomy, the other group total thyroidectomy. The 20-year survival rate in the lobectomy group was 82%, compared with 73% in the total thyroidectomy group with an insignificant p value. They also concluded that low-risk patients undergoing lobectomy are as likely to do well as those undergoing total thyroidectomy.

Shaha et al.[11] did a retrospective review of more than 1000 patients with differentiated cancer of the thyroid by both univariate and multivariate techniques, and Kaplan-Meier survival curves were plotted. Criteria for the low-risk group included age younger than 45, tumors smaller than 4 cm, low-grade histology, and absence of metastases or extrathyroidal invasion. Analysis of their data showed statistical differences for local recurrence between *partial* lobectomy and *total* lobectomy to be 27% vs. 4%. There was no statistical difference in local recurrence between total lobectomy and total thyroidectomy patients (4% vs. 1%), nor was there any difference in overall failure rates between total lobectomy and total thyroidectomy patients. They felt that surgical treatment should be individualized based on risk-group analysis as well as intraoperative findings and that *partial* lobectomy was not an acceptable procedure for cancer.

The authors responsible for the American Cancer Society National Cancer Database 1995[1] on thyroid cancer noted that survivors in well-differentiated thyroid cancer were reported at a 97% rate for 5 years and noted that "total thyroidectomy with or without nodal metastasis had no 5-year survival advantage over ipsilateral lobectomy in patients . . . regardless of stage." Despite this fact, they also reported that lobectomy and isthmusectomy were performed in only 34.2% and 41.6% of papillary and follicular cancer patients, respectively, while total thyroidectomy with or without lymph node removal was performed in the remainder.

Farrar et al.[18] reported on 25 years' experience treating 155 patients with papillary and follicular carcinoma of the thyroid. Multicentricity was noted in 26%. Twenty-nine patients underwent total thyroidectomy, and 126 patients underwent partial thyroidectomy. Follow-up ranged from 1 to 25 years, with a mean of 10 years. Node surgery was also performed in appropriate situations. Cure rates were statistically identical between the two groups (92.6% total, 90.4% partial), with and without nodal involvement. Tumor recurrence was also similar between the two groups studied, as well as node-positive and node-negative disease. Morbidity was far less for the partial group than for the total group. They concluded that "total thyroidectomy is not indicated in the treatment of papillary and follicular thyroid cancer."

Multicentricity[2] of malignant deposits within the thyroid has been reported in 21% to 46% of papillary cancer cases. This appears to be a particularly critical feature of cancer that evokes the need for a total thyroidectomy solution. Multicentricity can include occult micropapillary cancer (OMP) as a cause, but not exclusively so. A study has shown that OMP can be found in 16.7% of patients with benign thyroid disease who are undergoing surgery.[19] Other frequencies of OMP have been cited as 2% to 36% of thyroid glands, and such occurrences have been noted in 9% to 13% of autopsy series.[2] OMP is considered to be a different biologic entity from clinical disease and papillary microcarcinoma.[2] The biologic implication of OMP is usually considered to be inconsequential, but infrequent reports have linked OMP with uncontrolled tumor growth, even though it is viewed particularly by pathologists as "almost a normal finding."[19] In a frequently quoted study, Tollefsen and DeCosse[20] noted that 36 (30%) of 118 patients with papillary cancer were multicentric. However, clinical disease developed in only seven (4%) of 164 patients who had undergone a unilateral lobectomy, suggesting that clinical tumor recurrence was infrequent when compared with the presumed total frequency of residual contralateral tumor. The very favorable outlook of this disease is so reassuring to these authors that they view the occurrence of multicentric contralateral cancer as inconsequential and sufficiently curable by partial thyroidectomy for the index lesion alone.[18,20]

ARGUMENT FOR PARTIAL THYROIDECTOMY

Selecting a conservative approach does not necessarily mean performing a hemithyroidectomy or partial thyroidectomy only. Rather, it refers to performing less than a true total thyroidectomy, as described by its great protagonists, Clark and Siperstein,[21] as exemplified in the regimens advocated by authors who do not identify themselves as totalists.[6-9,15,20] Variations in surgical policy, all of which can be viewed as conservative, require consideration.

Rossi and Cady noted that "the extent of thyroid gland resection, the extent of lymph node resection and the number of lymph node metastases involved had no bearing on patient survival" and that "there may be a higher risk of local recurrence in patients treated by thyroid lobectomy but a recurrence in the remnant thyroid tissue never caused a death."[6,15] Patients in the low-risk age group with a small tumor and without major capsular involvement of follicular cancer can be treated by a total lobectomy. Where subtotal lobectomy is performed for benign disease and an occult malignancy is found on final pathologic analysis, no further operation is performed. Of 57 patients treated in this fashion, no patient had recurrent cancer or died of disease, and none of the 20 patients with occult carcinoma had recurrent disease. For a high-risk patient, total lobectomy on the side of the cancer and contralateral subtotal or near-total lobectomy on the contralateral side are advocated by Cady.[15]

Fujimoto et al.[16] noted, "Hemithyroidectomy is a method of operation applicable for a patient with low-risk papillary cancer that is macroscopically localized in one thyroid lobe." In addition to this, they advocated a modified radical neck dissection on the side of the tumor with removal of ipsilateral or bilateral peritracheal and prelaryngeal nodes; this procedure was carried out in 85% of their low-risk patients. They described primary tumor recurrences in 2 of 273 patients monitored for 5 to 13 years and feel that ultrasonography and careful intraoperative palpation can usually detect significant bilateral involvement. If intrathyroidal metastatic lesions are in close proximity to surgical margins, the remaining contralateral lobe is removed. Of their 344 low-risk patients who underwent hemithyroidectomy, 0.6% showed local recurrence, 0.6% recurrence in the contralateral lobe, 2.9% recurrence in ipsilateral nodes, and 0.9% recurrence in contralateral nodes. Not one of their patients died of thyroid cancer. Their high-risk patients underwent a total thyroidectomy.

On analysis by Hay and Grant,[7-9] patients with minimal risk (AGES score of 3.99 or less) showed no improvement in survival when patients underwent more than ipsilateral lobectomy although in high-risk patients (10% of the patients in their series), survival after bilateral resection was much higher than after ipsilateral lobectomy alone. However, they supported the use of a bilateral resection (but not a total thyroidectomy) consisting of ipsilateral total lobectomy with a contralateral subtotal or near-total lobectomy. They pointed out that "to base a surgical strategy solely on survival data would ignore the problems associated with local recurrence. The increased risk of reoperation, the patient's mental anguish, and the considerable time and expense of repeat evaluation and operation are a few of these considerations." They did demonstrate that unilateral resection was associated with an increased frequency of local recurrence compared with their form of bilateral resection, even in low-risk patients.

Shah et al.[17] supported the selective use of total thyroidectomy, but, they felt, patients with a primary tumor of 4 cm or less without gross disease of the contralateral lobe or evidence of distant metastases can be treated appropriately with total lobectomy only.

Shaha et al.[11] felt that a minimal operation for solitary thyroid nodule should be ipsilateral lobectomy and isthmusectomy and condemn a partial lobectomy for cancer because of an increased local recurrence rate. They felt they could not demonstrate any long-term survival difference between total thyroidectomy and lobectomy. Four low-risk patients in their series died; two of them had been treated before 1960. Histologic blocks in two of these patients also revealed poor differentiation, which by implication should have disqualified these patients from the low-risk category.

Even Clark and Siperstein[21] noted that a procedure less than lobectomy for any thyroid nodule that might be malignant is contraindicated, except for small tumors less than 1.5 cm in diameter situated in the isthmus or on the anterior surface of the thyroid. They conceded that lobectomy and isthmusectomy are acceptable for encapsulated or sclerosing papillary thyroid cancer of less than 1.5 cm in diameter or for microinvasive follicular carcinoma. They noted that the unilateral procedure may be appropriate for unreliable or noncompliant patients who wish to avoid taking thyroid hormone; such patients would therefore avoid the risk for myxedema after a total thyroidectomy.

Although small thyroid malignancies are usually viewed as inconsequential, other reports on the adverse aspects of small thyroid cancer[18,22] indicate that even such small malignancies deserve careful clinical evaluation to ensure that they will indeed lend themselves to an abbreviated procedure, as is commonly observed. Furthermore, the recent recognition of aggressive variants and types of papillary carcinoma may also discourage the application of a strict unilateral approach.[23] Tall cell and insular cell cancer[2,23] were shown in one series to incur a 25% recurrence rate, which implies the need for effective surgical treatment that usually entails the notion of a total procedure.

SURGERY FOR METASTATIC CERVICAL NODAL DISEASE

Metastatic cervical nodal disease occurs in up to 90% of patients with papillary thyroid carcinoma; its relevance as a risk factor for failure has been stressed by Clark and Siperstein[21] and Noguchi and Murakami.[24] Both groups advocate modified radical neck dissection for established metastatic cervical lymphadenopathy in preference to a "berry-picking procedure." It provides both an effective cosmetic and oncologic result. In the past, nodal disease was considered to be a harbinger of poor outcome, so that radical neck dissection was seriously advised, even in cases in which the extent of thyroidectomy was limited.[4] George Crile, Jr.[3] was among the first to oppose the use of routine radical neck dissection in nodal disease, and since that time there has been even further minimalization of the role of nodal metastases in overall planning. Nevertheless, Noguchi and Murakami[24] in accordance with their Japanese confreres, advocate the use of modified radical neck dissection, even with limited resection of the thyroid, to be advisable and necessary for enhanced cancer control; they feel this treatment philosophy might reflect differences in national behavior of thyroid malignancy.

Rossi and Cady[6] described the use of modified neck dissection in low-risk patients when nodes are preoperatively palpated avoiding the submandibular space, but he recognized the need for sacrifice of the sternocleidomastoid muscle if it is involved by massive disease. If nodes are palpable only during operation, a limited lymph node dissection is performed through the thyroidectomy collar incision. Where no node metastasis is palpable intraoperatively, no node dissection is carried out, since they feel that no proof exists that a "prophylactic" node dissection improves survival. They felt that lymph node metastasis did not affect survival and indeed actually appeared to improve it, which turned out to be more a reflection of the age of involved patients than of the nodal disease. Even recurrent lymph node metastases, which were more frequent in patients with initially positive nodes than in those with negative nodes, did not affect long-term survival. While palpable nodal metastases were less frequently encountered in the high-risk group, the notion of modified neck dissection in this group was liberalized in the approach of Rossi and Cady. Although the influence of nodal disease on outcome is still debatable, it does appear to be an important part of the problem of thyroid cancer management,[25] making it difficult to understand why this topic is frequently ignored by clinicians involved in thyroid cancer management.

POSTOPERATIVE MANAGEMENT

Radioiodine Therapy

The need for postsurgical radiotherapy with ^{131}I (radioactive iodine) may be controversial, but its use is now receiving increasing support, especially among endocrinologists.[2,5] Radioactive iodine is really ideal in a patient who has had a total thyroidectomy, and radioactive iodine can be administered 6 weeks after surgery to a patient who has been given liothyronine for 4 weeks. It can also be given in patients with a thyroid remnant.

Fujimoto et al.[16] felt that the excellent prognosis for most patients with low-risk papillary carcinoma precludes the use of any adjuvant therapy with radioiodine.

Cady[15] felt that there is little evidence that the use of radioactive iodine in low-risk patients is of any benefit in survival, although he thought that it could be used in low-risk patients with nodal disease as an option to surgery, although he preferred surgical excision. He advocated radioactive iodine for high-risk patients with resectable local disease, recurrent local disease, and distant metastasis to lungs, bones, and other sites. He suggested a dose of 30 mCi as appropriate for treatment and noted high curability in low-risk patients with pulmonary metastases.

Shaha et al.[11] noted, "We definitely question the need for radioactive iodine tracer scanning in each and every patient with low-risk thyroid cancer." Furthermore, the repeated radioactive iodine diagnostic scans that require the hypothyroid state should be avoided in low-risk patients because of the interference with well-being by the induction of the myxedematous state, although this may be reasonable in the high-risk patient.[15] Recombinant TSH can now be used with radioactive iodine to scan for recurrent or persistent thyroid cancer.

Levothyroxine Therapy

Long-term suppression of serum thyrotropin by T_4 is viewed as standard postoperative practice, particularly by endocrinologists, because it is thought to inhibit cancer recurrence and facilitate patient survival.[2] Cady[15] questioned the value of thyroid hormone administration in his patients, and his studies have indicated that long-term medication compliance is faulty, which Cady felt is avoided by partial thyroidectomy.

Fujimoto et al.[16] felt that suppression therapy may not be associated with improved survival rates, since low-risk patients have such a favorable prognosis, regardless of treatment. Most patients undergoing partial thyroidectomy are euthyroid, so lifelong administration of thyroid hormone is unnecessary. In a series of 150 patients who underwent surgery, Fujimoto et al. found euthyroidism in 63%, a frequency of latent hypothyroidism in 21%, hypothyroidism in 16%, the latter two of which required thyroid replacement. Fujimoto et al.[16] also described poor drug compliance by patients and a lack of postoperative tumor recurrence rate or mortality usually linked with suppressed serum thyrotropine levels, as opposed to nonsuppressed thyrotropine levels. Their adoption of a no-thyroid-hormone-replacement policy for the last 30 years has been viewed by the group as satisfactory, with good long-term results, but others would disagree with this practice.

COMPLICATIONS AND RESULTS

Morbidity in the form of hypoparathyroidism and recurrent nerve injury and the need to avoid this, particularly in good-risk patients with an excellent outcome, are cited by those who advocate a lesser procedure. They also cite the aggravation of morbidity that might occur if total thyroidectomy became absolute policy and it were done by the less-experienced surgeon.

Flynn et al.[26] reported on 91 patients with thyroid cancer over a 36-year period who had undergone surgery by multiple surgeons. Permanent hypoparathyroidism occurred in 9% of the total thyroidectomy group, whereas temporary hypocalcemia occurred in 42% of the total thyroidectomy group. Tracheostomy was necessary in four patients who were undergoing total thyroidectomy, three after subtotal thyroidectomy and one after lobectomy. One recurrent laryngeal nerve injury occurred after a total thyroidectomy.

Rossi and Cady[6] reported complications of conservative therapy to include bleeding, 0.6%, permanent cord palsy, 0.3%, hypoparathyroidism (transient), 1.3%, thoracic duct fistula, 0.3%, unilateral superior laryngeal nerve palsy, 0.3%, and operative death, 0.3%.

Edis[27] noted that recurrent nerve paralysis rarely occurs, although transient weakness does, presumably as a result of edema of the nerve and indicated the contribution of endotracheal intubation to cord palsy and reported the paralysis percentage as being 1%, although in secondary surgical procedures this figure may approximate 10%. Permanent hypoparathyroidism should be less than 5%, and authors are cited as describing frequencies of 0% and 2%. Hay et al.[7] described permanent unilateral vocal cord palsy in 2% and permanent hypocalcemia 5%, occurring almost exclusively in total thyroidectomy patients.

Clark and Siperstein[21] noted that many authors have reported complication rates in total thyroidectomy to be less than 2% and that their hypoparathyroidism rate was 0.6%. LaQuagli et al.,[28] in reporting on their results of management of thyroid cancer in children, noted that the use of total or subtotal thyroidectomy or radical neck dissection in children does not prevent recurrence and is associated with an increased risk of complications and that these procedures should be avoided in pediatric patients. In 49 patients, there were 15 cases of permanent hypocalcemia, 14 of permanent recurrent nerve palsy, one of facial nerve palsy, and one of tracheal stenosis.

Farrar et al.[18] described total thyroidectomy as showing a 21% frequency of hypoparathyroidism, 3.4% frequency of recurrent nerve injury as compared with partial thyroidectomy, which showed a frequency of hypoparathyroidism of 1.6%, and recurrent nerve injury of 0.8%.

Although total thyroidectomy can be carried out with exceptionally low morbidity, as evidenced by reported experiences, there is no question that unilateral procedure avoids the possibility of a transient or permanent hypoparathyroidism of any serious degree.

CONCLUSION

Authorities who find themselves within the conservative camp are not always in total agreement on all aspects of cancer treatment, but they do agree on the benefits of avoiding a total thyroidectomy. To their mind, risk factor analysis has demonstrated a low- and high-risk group in well-differentiated thyroid cancer behavior, with most patients falling in the low-risk group. They have stressed that the abundant low-risk group has an excellent outcome and that less than a total thyroidectomy is sufficient to produce this excellent result. The obvious feeling behind the conservative policy is the avoidance of undue morbidity or dysfunction, unnecessary treatment, surgical and otherwise, and deformity in a group of patients that is predominantly young and female and appears to be predestined for an excellent result following treatment. The variations in the conservative camp may be appreciated when one recognizes that a hemithyroidectomy may be combined with a routine modified neck dissection.[16] Others will use a bilateral thyroidectomy but avoid a total approach in the name of morbidity avoidance.[7,8,9] Perhaps the most committed conservative orientation may be seen in those who favor partial thyroidectomy in well-differentiated carcinoma,[6,7,11,21] avoidance of postoperative radioactive iodine ablation,[15,16] and postoperative thyroid suppression,[15,16] (Table 10-1).

While metastatic nodal disease is a well-established fact, it does not usually receive a great deal of attention. The differences between activist and nonactivist advocates in this area are minimal.[15,16,21,29] The conservative orientation has obvious advantages and some disadvantages as listed in Table 10-2, but

TABLE 10-1 Comparison of Stereotypical Approaches to Well-Differentiated Thyroid Cancer

	Conservative Approach	Comprehensive Approach
Extent of surgery	Hemithyroidectomy[6,11,17,18,20] Ipsilateral lobectomy + partial contralateral lobectomy[7]	Total thyroidectomy[21]
+ Lateral neck nodes palpated preoperatively	Modified neck dissection[26]	Modified neck dissection[21,29]
+ Lateral neck nodes found at operation	Limited neck dissection[6,15]	Modified neck dissection[21,29]
0 Palpable nodes	Ignore[6,15]	Limited neck dissection (sampling)[29]
Radioactive iodine (postoperative)	No[6,15,16]	Yes[2]
TSH suppression	No[6,15,16]	Yes[2]

TABLE 10-2 Pros and Cons of a Conservative Approach to Well-Differentiated Thyroid Cancer

Advantages	Disadvantages
High cure rate	Increased local recurrence rate
Avoidance of postoperative hypoparathyroidism	Cannot use serum thyroglobulin as marker for recurrence
Simplifies need for postoperative adjuvant treatments (e.g., radioactive iodine, thyroxine)	Cannot use radioactive iodine as effectively
Minimizes opportunity for recurrent nerve injury	Delay in detection by radioactive iodine of systemic cancer
Less operative time required	

should not be taken to mean neglect of surgical intervention in patients with thyroid nodular disease who have appropriate indications for surgical treatment (Fig. 10-1). The good outcome of this malignancy permits this variation in therapeutic approach whose varied advocates all aspire to serve the betterment of patient welfare. I favor a near-total thyroidectomy, appropriate node

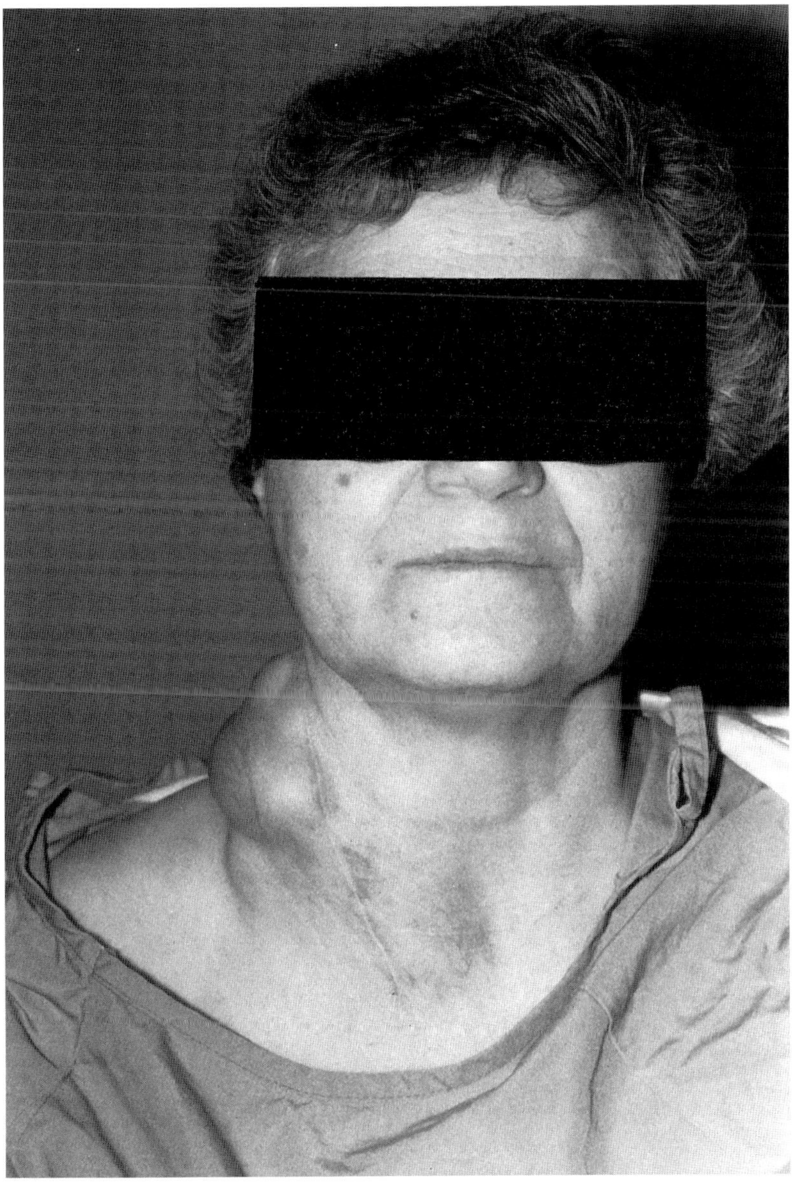

• **FIGURE 10-1** A patient who was followed for 20 years with thyroid mass and presented with extensive neck metastases. Early thyroidectomy for appropriate indications might have prevented tumor progression.

sampling and dissection, postoperative adjuvant radioiodine ablation, and suppression of thyroid-stimulating hormone by thyroxine intake. The concept of a perfect cure for cancer is still worthwhile, even when applied to a cancer with such a fortunate outlook as low-risk, well-differentiated thyroid malignancy.

REFERENCES

1. Hundahl S, Fleming I, Shah J. Thyroid Cancer in National Cancer Database 1995. Atlanta: American Cancer Society, 1995.
2. Ain K. Papillary thyroid carcinoma: Etiology, assessment and therapy. Endocrin Metab Clin North Am 24:711-716, 1995.
3. Crile G Jr. Surgical treatment of malignant tumors of the thyroid gland. In Pack G, Ariel I, eds. Treatment of Cancer and Allied Diseases: Tumors of the Head and Neck, vol. 3, 2nd ed. New York: Harper & Brothers, 1959.
4. Pack G, Ariel I. Tumors of the thyroid gland. In Pack G, Ariel I, eds. Treatment of Cancer and Allied Diseases: Tumors of the Head and Neck, vol. 3, 2nd ed. New York: Harper & Brothers, 1959.
5. Solomon B, Wartofsky L, Berman K. Management of differentiated thyroid carcinoma: Results of a survey of ATA members. American Thyroid Association Conference, Tampa, Fla., 1993.
6. Rossi R, Cady B. Differentiated carcinoma of thyroid gland. In Rossi R, Cady B, eds. Surgery of the Thyroid and Parathyroid Glands, 3rd ed. Philadelphia: WB Saunders, 1991, pp 139-150.
7. Hay I et al. Ipsilateral lobectomy versus bilateral lobar resection of papillary thyroid carcinoma. Surgery 102:1088-1095, 1987.
8. Hay I. Prognostic factors in thyroid carcinoma. In Oppenheimer E, ed. Thyroid Today. Deerfield, Ill: Flint Laboratories vol. 12, 1989, pp 1-9.
9. Grant C et al. Local recurrence in papillary thyroid carcinoma: Is extent of surgical resection important? Surgery 104:954-961, 1988.
10. Brierley J et al. A comparison of different staging systems, predictability of patient outcome, thyroid carcinoma as an example. Cancer 79:2414-2423, 1997.
11. Shaha A, Shah J, Loree T. Low risk differentiated thyroid carcinoma. Ann Surg Oncol 4:328-333, 1997.
12. Farid N, Zou M, Shi Y. Genetics of follicular thyroid cancer. Endocrin Metab Clin North Am 24:865-884, 1995.
13. Jossart G, Grossman R. Thyroid oncogenesis. In Clark O, Duh Q, eds. Textbook of Endocrine Surgery. Philadelphia: WB Saunders, 1997, pp 237-242.
14. Hosal S et al. Immunohistochemical localization of P53 in human thyroid neoplasm. Endocr Pathol 8:21-28, 1997.
15. Cady B. Predictors of thyroid tumor aggressiveness. In Clark O, Duh Q, eds. Textbook of Endocrine Surgery. Philadelphia: WB Saunders, 1997, pp 197-204.
16. Fujimoto Y, Obara T, Yamashita T. Hemithyroidectomy and regional node dissection. In Clark O, Duh Q, eds. Textbook of Endocrine Surgery. Philadelphia: WB Saunders, 1997, pp 82-89.
17. Shah J et al. Lobectomy versus total thyroidectomy for differentiated carcinoma of the thyroid. Am J Surg 166:331-335, 1993.

18. Farrar W, Cooperman N, James A. Surgical management of papillary and follicular carcinoma of the thyroid. Ann Surg 192:701-704, 1980.
19. Fink A et al. Occult micropapillary carcinoma associated with benign follicular thyroid disease and unrelated thyroid neoplasm. Mod Pathol 8:816-820, 1996.
20. Tollefsen H, DeCosse J. Papillary carcinoma of the thyroid. Am J Surg 106:728-734, 1963.
21. Clark O, Siperstein A. Commentary. Surgery of thyroid gland. In Rossi R, Cady B, eds. Surgery of the Thyroid and Parathyroid Glands, 3rd ed. Toronto: WB Saunders, 1991, pp 207-214.
22. Rosen IB, Azadian A, Walfish P. Adverse aspects of small thyroid cancer and need for treatment. Head Neck 17:373-376, 1995.
23. van den Brekel M et al. Prognostic features in tall cell papillary carcinoma and insular thyroid carcinoma. Laryngoscope 107:254-259, 1997.
24. Noguchi S, Murakami N. The value of lymph node dissection in patients with differentiated thyroid cancer. Surg Clin North Am 67:251-261, 1997.
25. Mazzaferri E, Jhiang S. Long term impact of initial surgical and medical therapy in papillary and follicular thyroid cancer. Am J Med 97:418-428, 1995.
26. Flynn M et al. Local complications after surgical resection for thyroid carcinoma. Am J Surg 168:404-407, 1994.
27. Edis A. Prevention and management of complications associated with thyroid and parathyroid surgery. Surg Clin North Am 50:83-92, 1979.
28. LaQuagli A et al. Recurrence and morbidity in differentiated thyroid carcinoma in children. Surgery 104:1149-1156, 1988.
29. McHenry CR, Rosen IB, Walfish PG. Prospective management of nodal metastases in differentiated thyroid cancer. Am J Surg 162:353-356, 1991

CHAPTER 11

Surgical Options

SHIRO NOGUCHI, M.D., Ph.D.

There is no standard therapy for differentiated nonmedullary thyroid cancer because of its heterogeneity and because most tumors have a natural history requiring long-term follow-up before the effectiveness of any single or combined therapies can be determined. During the long follow-up period, there have been technologic developments in diagnosis, such as the introduction of fine-needle aspiration (FNA) biopsy and changes in the general awareness of the disease. These and other features created difficulty in interpreting the results of prolonged follow-up studies. Two opposing opinions remain regarding the optimum treatment for patients with thyroid cancer. Some experts consider the disease to be an indolent, frequently localized tumor that can easily be controlled by conservative methods,[1-8] whereas others consider it a potentially lethal disease that warrants aggressive therapy.[9-12]

In patients with papillary cancer, many small, often microscopic metastatic cancer foci can be found in apparently normal thyroid tissue, away from the major cancer foci, and also in the regional lymph nodes.[13,14] Some investigators pay more attention to these intraglandular foci of cancer, whereas others are more concerned about the regional lymph nodes.[14-18]

PATIENT CHARACTERISTICS

At the Noguchi Thyroid Clinic from 1946 to 1996, 5099 patients were treated for papillary cancer of the thyroid. When patients who underwent noncurative surgery and whose primary tumor was less than 10 mm in diameter were excluded, there were 3733 patients. There were 2966 patients operated on between 1946 and 1991. Noncurative surgery was performed in 124 patients, including 30 open biopsies, 81 subtotal thyroidectomies, and 13 total thyroidectomies. Ninety-eight patients had unresectable thyroid cancer invading the carotid artery and/or trachea. Metastases were also present in the mediastinum in four patients, in the lung in 10, in the bone in two, and at other sites in 10 patients (remote metastasis). They were included in the noncurative group. Before 1965, 94% of patients who underwent noncurative surgery had incomplete resection of the neck tumor, whereas after 1965, the proportion of incomplete resection decreased to between 78% and 71%. The 5- and 10-year survival rates for incomplete resection and distant metastasis groups were 72.6% and 76.9%, and 61.4% and 61.3%, respectively. The figures were not significant.

Seven hundred sixty-six patients (25.8%) had one or more benign conditions diagnosed either before or at the time of thyroid surgery. Chronic thyroiditis was present in 212 patients (7.1%); most of them underwent operation on suspicion of the presence of concomitant thyroid cancer. Eighty-three (5.5%) had Graves' disease. In 24 patients, the cancer diagnosis was established before surgery; in eight patients the nodules were diagnosed as benign nodules before surgery, and in 51 patients thyroid cancer was found during surgery; 506 (17.1%) had benign nodular thyroid disease.

In 514 patients (17.3%), the tumor diagnosed as benign preoperatively was cancerous. However, 468 of them (91%) had no adhesion or invasion of the surrounding tissues. In the remaining 252 patients, benign tumors were found as well as cancer.

In the present series the female/male ratio was 9.8:1. This extreme female predominance was within the range (8.8:1 to 13:1) previously reported from Japan,[17,19-21] but considerably different from those reported from the United States[11,22-24] and Europe,[25-27] which were 1.4:1 to 2.8:1 and 2.9:1 to 3.8:1, respectively. The median age of patients in both men and women was 45; the mean age was 46.1 and 45.2, respectively. The age was almost comparable with that in the series from the Mayo Clinic[22] and that of the Rocky Mountain Cancer System Data.[23] However, when closely examined, there has been a shift to an older population in recent years (Fig. 11-1).

The primary tumor involved only one lobe of the thyroid in 77.1% of patients, one lobe and the isthmus in 9.1%, and both lobes in 13.8%. Hay[28] reported 71% of papillary cancers involved one lobe. Multiple foci of

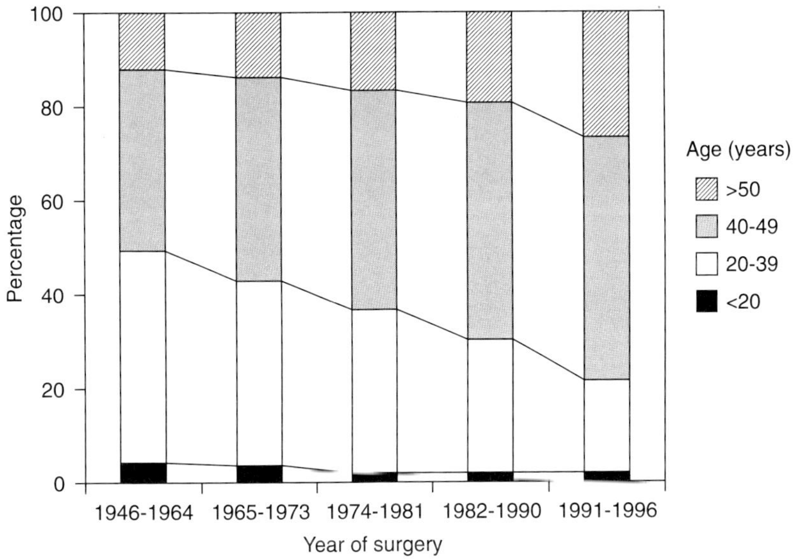

• **FIGURE 11-1** Age of patients in relation to calendar years.

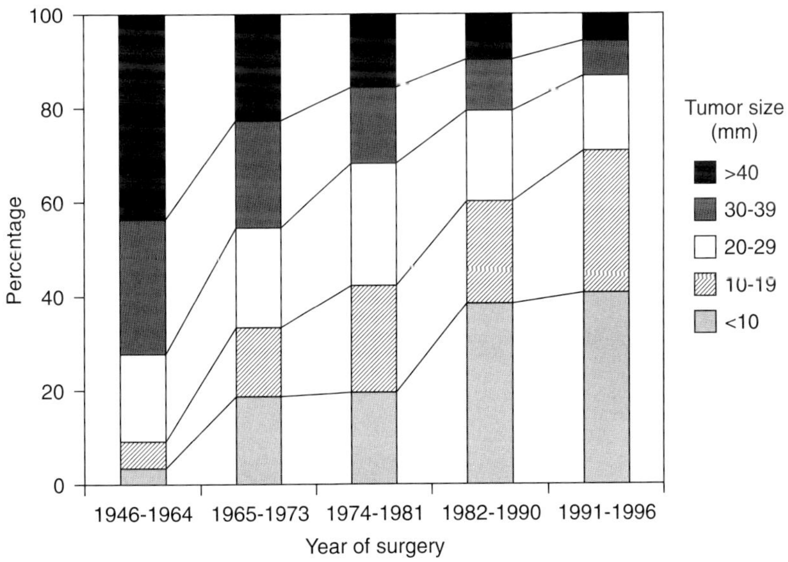

• **FIGURE 11-2** Change of tumor size with calendar years.

papillary cancer were 17.4% in our series; this figure is less than the 26% reported by Hay. The mean size of the primary tumor was 27.1 mm. Closer observation of the size revealed a gradual decrease over the past 50 years from a mean maximum diameter of 33.2 mm to 24.3 mm in the years from 1946 to 1964 and from 1983 to 1991, respectively (Fig. 11-2).

Invasion/adhesion of the primary tumor into the surrounding tissue occurred in 30.7% of patients; invasion/adhesion to the recurrent laryngeal nerve occurred in 663 patients (22.4%). However, resection of the recurrent laryngeal nerve was necessitated in 159 patients (5.4%); this is because our policy is to try to preserve the recurrent laryngeal nerve when hoarseness was not evident before surgery. A similar practice, with satisfactory results, was reported by Nishida et al.[29] The incidence of recurrent laryngeal nerve involvement decreased from the 27.5% that we previously reported to 22.4% ($p < 0.0001$).[16] Invasion or adhesion to the esophagus was observed in 376 patients (12.7%) who underwent potentially curative surgeries. One patient eventually developed esophageal diverticulitis, which lead to death.

OPERATIVE PROCEDURES

Thyroidectomy

Total thyroidectomy was performed in 75 (2.5%), subtotal thyroidectomy in 1233 (41.6%), lobectomy in 1217 (41.0%), and partial lobectomy in 441 (14.9%) patients. Our routine method of subtotal thyroidectomy, which many would consider to be near-total thyroidectomy, is to leave behind about 1 or 2 g of the upper pole of the unaffected lobe with the parathyroid gland in situ. When intraglandular dissemination is present on the contralateral upper pole, we try to leave behind 1 or 1 1/2 g of the upper pole on the side with less tumor. Lobectomy is almost always accompanied by isthmusectomy. Although we are aware that total thyroidectomy is a safe procedure when it is performed by skilled, well-experienced surgeons,[9,30] we still try to avoid performing total thyroidectomy, because calcitonin has been reported by some investigators to have a role in preventing osteoporosis.[31,32] The 441 patients who underwent partial lobectomy require a special explanation, since partial lobectomy is considered inadequate for thyroid cancer. Eighty-five patients had concomitant benign disease; in 20 patients the tumor was invasive or adherent to adjacent structures. In 78 of these patients modified radical neck dissection was performed, and 69 underwent partial node dissection at the central compartment. The remaining 294 were operated on for benign tumor. The average tumor size of patients having partial lobectomy was smaller (median diameter of 20 mm, compared with 24 mm for the entire series).

Lymph Node Excision

Among the entire group of patients, modified radical neck dissection was performed in 72.1%, partial node excision (central compartment dissection)

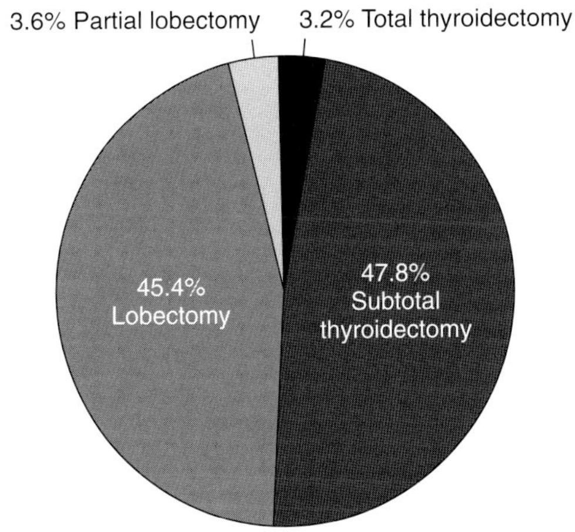

• **FIGURE 11-3** Types of thyroidectomy in 2139 patients who underwent modified radical neck dissection.

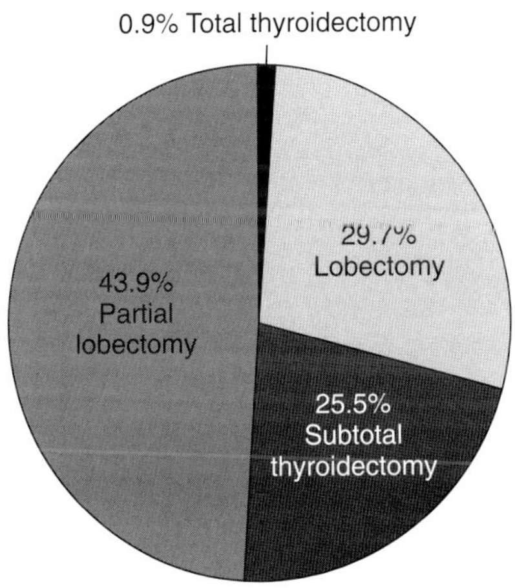

• **FIGURE 11-4** Types of thyroidectomy in 827 patients who underwent partial node excision or no node excision.

in 8.5%, and no lymph node excision in 19.4%. Types of thyroidectomy and lymph node excision are well correlated, as shown in Figs. 11-3 and 11-4. Patients who underwent total thyroidectomy and partial node excision or no node excision were those who had multinodular adenomatous goiter. Seventy-eight patients underwent partial lobectomy and modified radical neck dissection; 73 of these patients were operated on before 1972 with less than 25 mm in maximum diameter. In the remaining five patients, the reason for choosing this procedure is not known.

The modified radical neck dissection encompassed dissection of the fat and lymph nodes around the trachea (central compartment) and those

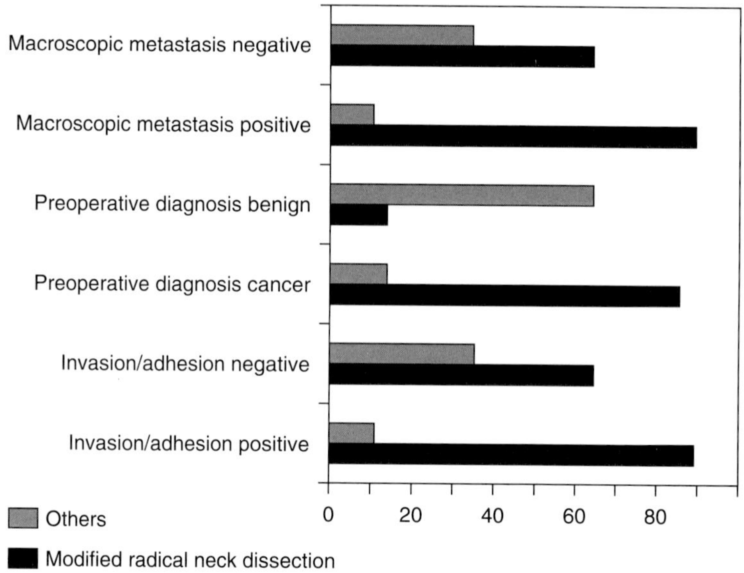

• **FIGURE 11-5** Types of lymph node excision performed in different groups of patients.

around the jugular vein extending from the carotid artery to the trapezius muscle and from the subclavian vein to the hypoglossal nerve (lateral compartment). Patients who underwent modified radical neck dissection had macroscopic metastasis or invasion/adhesion to surrounding tissues. Fourteen percent of patients whose preoperative diagnosis of benign disease underwent this procedure, whereas 86% were operated on for diagnosed or suspected cancer. Further analysis was performed by dividing the patients into two groups, those who were treated with modified radical neck dissection and those who were not, because of the small number of patients who were treated with the central compartment excision. Modified radical neck dissections were primarily performed because of gross nodal metastasis, preoperative diagnosis of cancer, and invasion of cancer to surrounding tissues (Fig. 11-5).

Complications related to the modified radical neck dissection are listed in Table 11-1. Recurrent laryngeal nerve dissection was necessary in 6.7% of the modified radical neck dissection group, in contrast to 1.9% of the patients in other groups. We do not consider recurrent laryngeal nerve dissection to be a complication of modified radical neck dissection, but rather consider it a manifestation of invasiveness of the primary tumor. We always identify the nerve and avoid careless injury of it. Transient accessory nerve palsy can occur when nodal metastasis adheres to the nerve and separation

TABLE 11-1 Complications Associated With Modified Radical Neck Dissection (N = 2139)

Accessory nerve palsy, transient	11
Accessory nerve palsy, permanent	4
Horner's syndrome, transient	6
Horner's syndrome, permanent	11
Chylous leakage	5
TOTAL	37

is difficult. There has been no permanent paralysis of the accessory nerve since 1968. Horner's syndrome occurred in 17 patients; in 11 it was permanent. It can easily occur when a tape is looped around the carotid artery, because sympathetic trunks are located right behind the artery. It can be either transient or permanent, depending on the gravity of the injury. Chylous leakage can be avoided, unless the involved node is located right on the thoracic duct. However, careful examination to locate leakage is essential.

Recurrence From Remnant Thyroid

Total thyroidectomy was performed on an extremely small proportion of patients in our series because of our policy of avoiding hypoparathyroidism, and avoiding calcitonin deficiency, which can be a potential cause of osteoporosis in the future. We usually pay special attention to recurrence from the remnant thyroid, which was seen in 90 patients. Among them, 78 were easily treated by a second operation, and 12 patients were lost. Lung metastasis was a cause of death in six of these patients, mediastinum metastasis in three, in one patient the recurrent tumor was found on the posterior side of the mesopharyngeal region, and two who died had large and heavily invasive tumors at presentation. One died 19 years after the initial surgery, and the other died 4.5 years after the initial surgery, with huge nodal metastases.

SURGICAL MANAGEMENT OF LYMPH NODE METASTASIS

Thirty-nine percent of these patients were judged to have enlarged lymph nodes before or during surgery. Of those patients, 51.5% had up to 10 histologically positive nodes, 38.4% had more than 11 positive nodes, and

6.1% who had enlarged nodes were found to be histopathologically negative. Among patients who were judged not to have metastasis preoperatively or intraoperatively, 67.2% had up to 10 and 11.3% had more than 11 positive nodes; 21.4% had no histologically positive nodes. These figures were essentially identical to our previous report.[14] Nodal metastases were present in 92.0% of men and 85.5% of women patients; the difference was statistically significant (p < 0.004). Similar observations were made by others.[25,27] Tubiana et al.[33] noted that when clinically palpable nodal metastasis was present, the risk ratio of disease-specific death increased 1.44 times. Sellers et al.[34] reported that palpable nodal metastases, particularly in older patients, indicated a poorer prognosis. Similar observations were made by others.[18,35,36] Recently Simon and Goretzki[37] indicated a high rate of nodal recurrence and suggested the usefulness of modified radical neck dissection. Scheumann et al.[38] reported improvement of the recurrence rate and survival rate after modified radical neck dissection. However, their indications for nodal dissection criteria were not clearly stated. Although many had failed to find improved survival rates after modified radical neck dissection,[10,22,39-42] we were able to demonstrate the beneficial effect of modified radical neck dissection on survival in patients with papillary cancer of the thyroid with clinically evident nodal metastases (Fig. 11-6) and also in patients with extrathyroidal invasion. Multivariate analysis also revealed risk factors (Table 11-2).

There are several possible reasons why previous studies have failed to demonstrate any benefit of modified radical neck dissection. This procedure

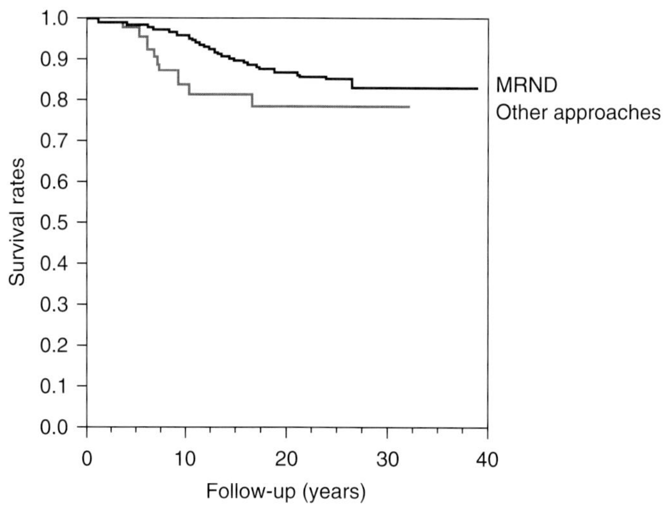

• **FIGURE 11-6** Survival rates of patients over 40 years of age with metastases of any size.

has often been applied exclusively for the treatment of advanced disease. The reported percentage of patients with papillary cancer of the thyroid who underwent radical or modified radical neck dissection ranged from 12.3% to 30% in institutions where the procedure is reserved only for patients with gross nodal metastasis.[10,35,42-44] Patients having a more extensive disease generally tended to undergo more extensive surgery. If one simply compares the recurrence rate in a group of patients who underwent modified radical neck dissection with that in another group of patients who underwent less extensive node excision or who did not receive node excision, a difference in survival rates may or may not be found, depending on other criteria, such as extent of disease and patient age (Fig. 11-7).

TABLE 11-2 Multivariate Analysis of Risk Factors for Recurrence

Factors	*p* Value
Sex	0.0001
Age	0.0001
Calendar year of surgery	0.0001
Diameter	0.0004
Invasion	0.0029
MRND*	0.0020
Gross nodal metastasis	0.0001

* Modified radical neck dissection.

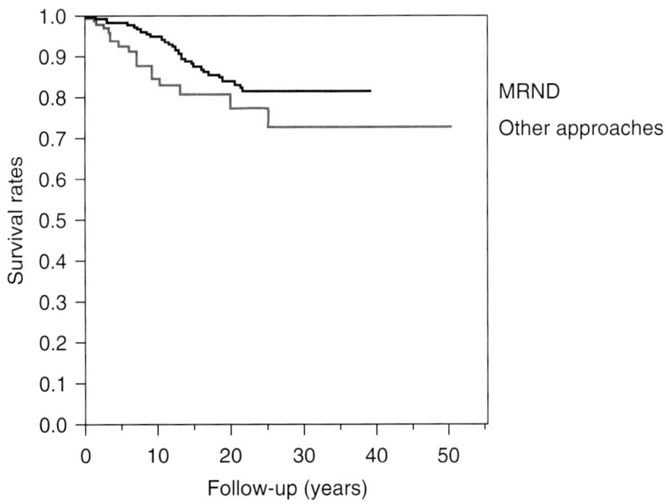

• **FIGURE 11-7** Survival rates of patients whose tumors had extrathyroidal invasion.

Recurrence in cervical nodes can be treated easily and successfully by a second operation. Recurrence in the lymph node seems to have less influence on survival than recurrence at other sites.[10,39] Moreover, even though microscopic nodal metastases are very common,[14,16] it is evident that many metastases remain dormant and do not grow to clinical disease.[45] Because of the indolent nature of papillary cancer, the probability of differences in the disease-specific survival rates among groups given different treatment is small, and therefore analysis of a large number of cases is necessary before any significant difference in the results of various treatments will be evident.[46]

Patient Indications

Just as not all patients benefit from total thyroidectomy,[8,30] not all patients benefit from modified radical neck dissection. There are numbers of studies concerning risk factors with univariate and/or multivariate analyses (Table 11-3). However, except for age and the size of the primary tumor, when it is specifically mentioned, there is no agreement among authors as to which factors are related to postoperative outcome. In our cohort we searched for patients who benefited from modified radical neck dissection with univariate and multivariate analyses. Age and the size of the primary tumor were significant risk factors. Preoperative diagnosis was one of the risk factors by univariate analysis in this series, which includes many patients whose diagnosis was based mainly on physical examination. In the past, patients with less advanced cancer were likely to be misdiagnosed as having benign nodules. However, in recent years the accuracy of preoperative diagnosis has been greatly improved by routine use of FNA cytology and other diagnostic modalities (Fig. 11-8). Moreover, prognosis was correlated with the size of the primary tumor, extrathyroidal invasion, and the presence of gross nodal metastasis. The presence of nodal metastases, including very small ones, is also one of the risk factors, particularly in patients over 40 years of age (Fig. 11-9).

The presence of microscopic metastasis, however, will not be useful for the purpose of deciding the operative strategy, unless nodal sampling is routinely performed at the correct sites.[57] Gender as a prognostic factor continues to be debated. As shown in Table 11-1, in our series, of the patients operated on between 1965 and 1988, women had fewer recurrences and better survival rate.[56] In the present series, when patients between 1946 and

TABLE 11-3 Risk Factors Associated With Modified Radical Neck Dissection

Author	Year	Age	Gender	GNM	Diameter	Grade	Metastasis	Invasion	Total	Method of Analysis
Russell MA et al.[13]	1975	Yes	Yes	N/M	N/M	N/M	N/M	No	N/M	Univariate
Byar DP et al.[47]	1979	Yes	Yes	N/M	Yes	N/M	Yes	N/M	N/M	Multivariate
Fourquet A et al.[48]	1983	Yes	Yes	N/M	N/M	N/M	N/M	N/M	N/M	Multivariate
Carcangiu ML et al.[41]	1985	Yes	No	Yes	Yes	N/M	Yes	Yes	No	Univariate
Tubiana M et al.[33]	1985	Yes	Yes	Yes	N/M	Yes	N/M	N/M	N/M	Multivariate
Tenvall J et al.[49]	1985	Yes	No	N/M	N/M	No	N/M	Yes	N/M	Multivariate
Hannequin P et al.[50]	1986	Yes	Yes	N/M	N/M	Yes	Yes	Yes	N/M	Multivariate
Bacourt F et al.[51]	1986	Yes	No	Yes	N/M	Yes	N/M	N/M	N/M	Multivariate
Kerr DJ et al.[52]	1986	Yes	No	Yes	N/M	N/M	Yes	Yes	N/M	Multivariate
Simpson WJ et al.[35]	1987	Yes	No	Yes	Yes	N/M	Yes	Yes	N/M	Multivariate
Cady B and Rossi R[53]	1988	Yes	No	N/M	Yes	N/M	N/M	No	No	Univariate
Brooks JR et al.[54]	1988	Yes	Yes	No	N/M	N/M	N/M	N/M	No	Univariate
Thoresen SO et al.[55]	1989	Yes	No	N/M	N/M	No	N/M	No	N/M	Multivariate
Hay ID.[28]	1990	Yes	Yes	N/M	Yes	Yes	Yes	Yes	No	Univariate
Jensen MH et al.[23]	1990	Yes	Yes	Yes	N/M	N/M	Yes	N/M	N/M	Univariate
Sellers M et al.[34]	1992	Yes	N/M	Yes	Yes	N/M	Yes	N/M	N/M	Univariate
Rösler H et al.[25]	1992	Yes	N/M	Yes	Yes	N/M	N/M	Yes	Yes	Univariate
Noguchi S et al.[56]	1994	Yes	Yes	Yes	Yes	N/M	N/M	Yes	No	Multivariate
Scheumann GF et al.[38]	1994	Yes	Yes	Yes	N/M	N/M	Yes	Yes	N/M	Multivariate

When univariate and multivariate analyses were described, the result of multivariate analysis was taken. *GNM*, gross nodal metastasis, *Grade*, histologic grade; *N/M*, not specifically mentioned.

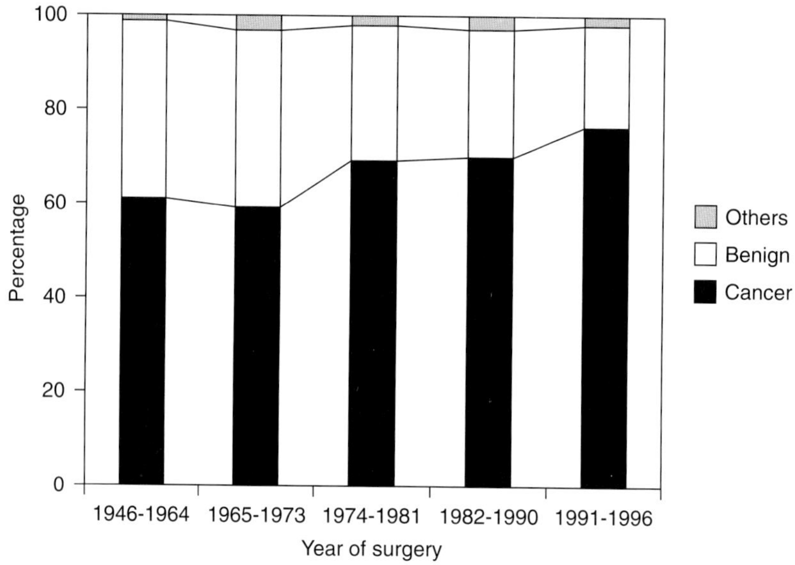

• **FIGURE 11-8** Improvement of diagnosis with calendar years.

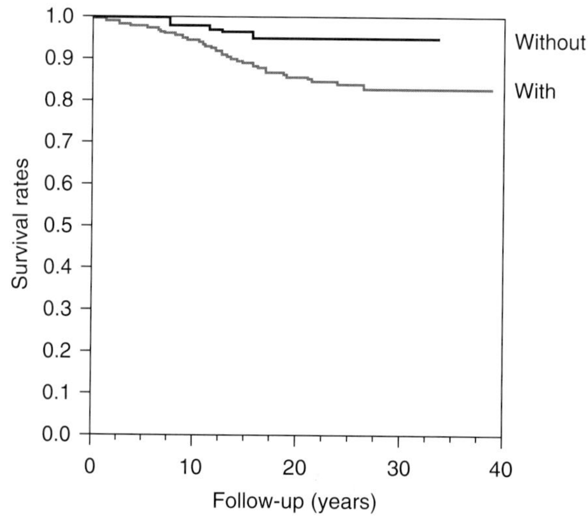

• **FIGURE 11-9** Survival rates of patients over 60 years of age, with and without metastases (n = 1539; log-rank $p < 0.0042$; Wilcoxon $p < 0.012$).

1991 (whole cohort) were analyzed, there was a difference between the sexes. However, when we analyzed only those who underwent operations after 1971, there was no statistically significant difference between the two sexes. The prognostic factors could differ from one population to another, as indicated by Hannequin et al.[50]

TABLE 11-4 Subset of Patients Who Benefit From Modified Radical Neck Dissection

Type of Patient	Percentage of Patients
With gross metastasis	39.1
Preoperative cancer diagnosis	71.8
With microscopic metastasis	67.6
Extrathyroidal invasion	30.7
Women over 60 years of age	15.8

Modified Radical Neck Dissection

Subsets of patients who benefited from modified radical neck dissection are summarized in Table 11-4 The size of the primary tumor is ostensibly not related to the benefit of modified radical neck dissection. However, this does not mean that there is a lack of relationship between the size of the primary tumor and nodal metastasis; on the contrary, as the size of the primary tumor increases, the incidence of metastasis increased, as did the numbers of metastases in each patient. Modified radical neck dissection was performed more frequently in patients with larger tumors ($p < 0.0001$). This may explain why patients with larger tumors seemingly did not benefit from modified radical neck dissection.

Of 575 patients who did not undergo lymph node excision, 25 died. Determining factors in the patients' outcomes were the age at operation, (54.6 vs. 42.8 years [$p < 0.0001$]); calendar year of operation (1967 ± 3 vs. 1974 ± 1 [$p < 0.002$]); and the size of the primary tumor (33.4 ± 15.1 mm vs. 24.8 ± 15.0 mm [$p < 0.006$]). Invasion of the primary tumor in this subset of patients did not appear to adversely influence survival, presumably because patients with invasive tumors were usually treated by modified radical neck dissection.

Of 386 patients who experienced recurrence and/or died of the disease, recurrence-free duration ranged from 6 weeks to 43 years 4 months (Fig. 11-10). One hundred sixty-seven patients (43%) had recurrence within 5 years; 95 patients (25%) had recurrence at 5 to 10 years; 60 patients (16%) at 10 to 15 years; 45 patients (12%) at 15 to 20 years; and 18 patients (5%) more than 20 years after initial thyroidectomy. Recurrence in the lung was seen in 101 patients (3.4%) and recurrence in bone was seen in 31 patients (1.0%). These incidences of remote recurrence seem to be almost comparable to that reported by Hay,[28] but much lower than the results reported by Carcangiu et al.[41]

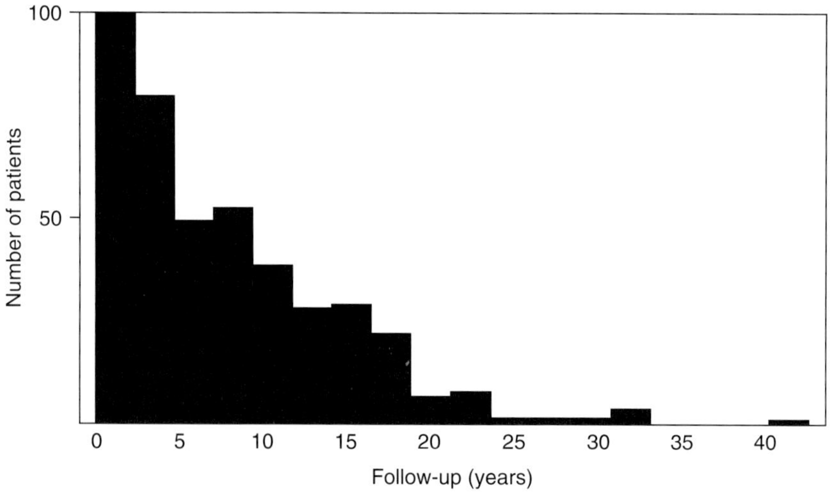

• **FIGURE 11-10** Duration before the first recurrence of cancer.

EVALUATING OUTCOME

In 1979, Byar and the European Organization for Research on Treatment of Cancer (EORTC)[47] made a scoring system for predicting the outcome of patients with thyroid cancer using a Weibull survival model. In 1983, Fourquet et al.[48] of the Curie Institute first used Cox's regression hazard model for prediction of the outcome of thyroid cancer. These early European studies include all types of thyroid cancer including anaplastic. In the United States, Cady.[58] at the Lahey Clinic proposed a unique and simple risk group definition called *AMES* (age, metastases, extent, and size). The concept and proposed risk factor scoring systems are precisely reviewed elsewhere.[28]

As seen in Table 11-3, gross nodal metastasis is recognized as one of the risk factors by many experts. However, nodal metastases are not included as risk factors in AMES, AGES (age, grade, extent, and size), or MACIS (metastases, age, completeness of surgery, invasion of cancer, and size) classification (see the box). In 1994, we proposed a new system that included a factor of gross nodal metastasis.[55] Our classification was based on age, sex, gross nodal metastasis, and in older women, the size of the primary tumor (Fig. 11-11). It was pertinent only to patients who underwent potentially curative surgery and classified patients into three groups. Patients in our excellent (low-risk) group had survival similar to that of the AMES low-risk group. In the AMES system, 89% of patients were in the low-risk group. Sixty-nine percent of our patients were in the excellent group by our classification system. The

AMES Differentiated Cancer Risk Group Definitions

Low-risk group

A. All younger patients without distant metastasis (men, <41; women, <51 years)

B. All older patients with:

1. Intrathyroidal papillary cancer or minor tumor capsular involvement follicular cancer and
2. Primary cancer <5 cm in diameter and
3. No distant metastasis

High-risk group

A. All patients with distant metastasis

B. All older patients with:

1. Extrathyroidal papillary cancer or major tumor capsular involvement follicular cancer and
2. Primary cancer 5 cm in diameter or larger, regardless of extent of disease

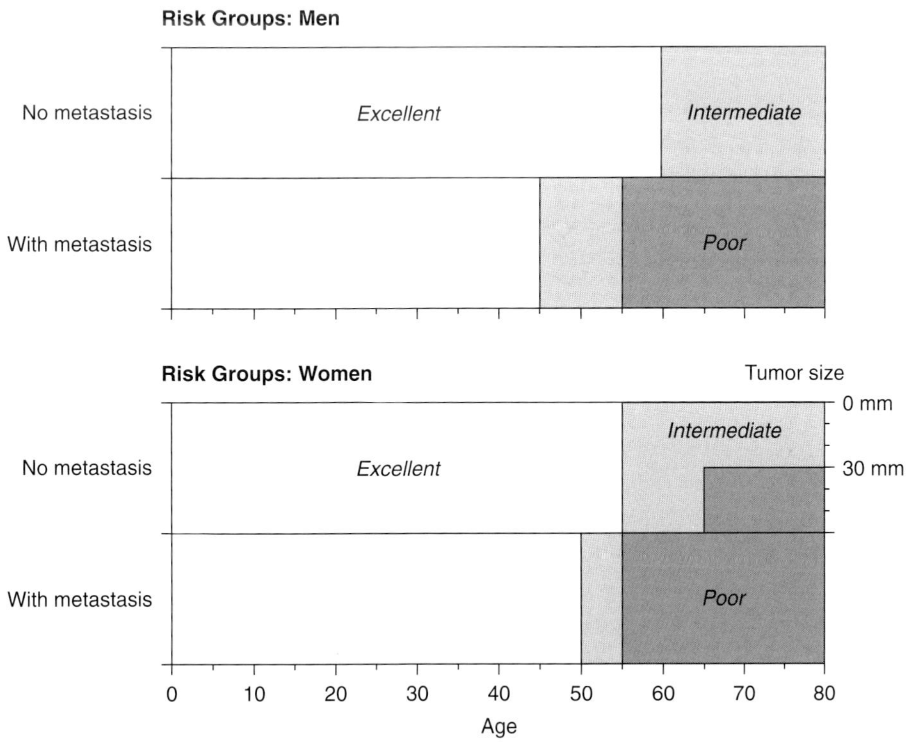

• **FIGURE 11-11** Risk groups: Noguchi Thyroid Clinic.

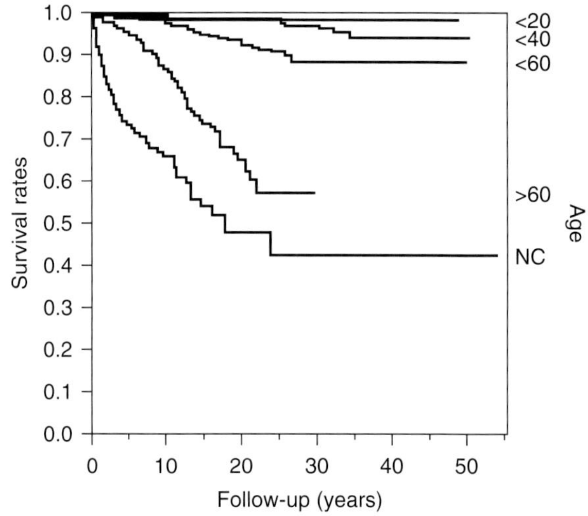

• **FIGURE 11-12** Survival rates of patients by age groups and noncurative (*NC*) surgery.

10-year death rates of AGES and AMES were 2.0% and 1.8%; using our classification, it was 1.6% for men and 0.7% for women.

CONCLUSION

Survival rates by age group and noncurative surgery are illustrated in Fig. 11-12. Older patients had more aggressive and unresectable thyroid cancers than younger patients.

Patients who will benefit from modified radical neck dissection are those with gross nodal metastasis, those with extrathyroidal invasion, and women over 60 years of age whose diagnosis of cancer can be established by physical examination alone. Total thyroidectomy is usually unnecessary unless the cancer is involved in most parts of both lobes. Such patients will represent at most 10% of papillary cancer cases; the remaining 90% may not benefit from total thyroidectomy.

REFERENCES

1. Starnes HF et al. Surgery for thyroid carcinoma. Cancer 55:1376-1381, 1985.
2. Christensen SB, Ljungberg O, Tibblin S. Surgical treatment of thyroid carcinoma in a defined population: 1960 to 1977. Evaluation of the results after a conservative surgical approach. Am J Surg 146:349-354, 1983.

3. Crile G Jr. Changing end results in patients with papillary carcinoma of the thyroid. Surg Gynecol Obstet 121:460-468, 1971.
4. Cady B et al. Risk factor analysis in differentiated thyroid cancer. Cancer 43:810-820, 1979.
5. Wanebo HJ, Andrews W, Kaiser DL. Thyroid cancer: Some basic considerations. Cancer J Clin 33:87-97, 1983.
6. Farrar WB, Cooperman M, James AG. Surgical management of papillary and follicular carcinoma of the thyroid. Ann Surg 192:701-704, 1980.
7. Fujimoto Y, Obara T, Yamashita T. Papillary thyroid carcinoma: Rationale for hemithyroidectomy and regional node dissection. In Clark OH, Duh Q-Y, eds. Textbook of Endocrine Surgery, 1st ed. Philadelphia:WB Saunders, 1997, pp 82-89.
8. Shaha AR, Shah JP, Loree TR. Low-risk differentiated thyroid cancer: The need for selective treatment. Ann Surg Oncol 4:328-333, 1997.
9. Clark OH. Total thyroidectomy: The treatment of choice for patients with differentiated thyroid cancer. Ann Surg 196:361-370, 1982.
10. DeGroot LJ, Kaplan EL, McCormick M, et al. Natural history, treatment, and course of papillary thyroid carcinoma. J Clin Endocrinol Metab 71:414-424, 1990.
11. Samaan NA, Schultz PN, Hickey RC, et al. The results of various modalities of treatment of well-differentiated thyroid carcinomas: A retrospective review of 1599 patients. J Clin Endocrinol Metab 75:714-720, 1992.
12. Thompson NW. Total thyroidectomy in the treatment of thyroid carcinoma. In Thompson NW, Vinik AI, eds. Endocrine Surgery Update. New York:Grune & Stratton, 1983, pp 71-84.
13. Russell MA, Gilbert EF, Jaeschke WF. Prognostic features of thyroid cancer: A long-term follow-up of 68 cases. Cancer 36:553-559, 1975.
14. Noguchi S, Noguchi A, Murakami N. Papillary carcinoma of the thyroid. I. Developing pattern of metastasis. Cancer 26:1053-1060, 1970.
15. Hughes CJ et al. Impact of lymph node metastasis in differentiated carcinoma of the thyroid: A matched-pair analysis. Head Neck 18:127-132, 1996.
16. Noguchi S, Murakami N. The value of lymph-node dissection in patients with differentiated thyroid cancer. Surg Clin North Am 67:251-261, 1987.
17. Noguchi M et al. Bilateral cervical lymph node metastases in well-differentiated thyroid cancer. Arch Surg 125:804-806, 1990.
18. Noguchi M et al. Papillary thyroid cancer and its surgical management. J Surg Oncol 49:140-146, 1992.
19. Ito J et al. Factors affecting the prognosis of patients with carcinoma of the thyroid. Surg Gynecol Obstet 150:539-544, 1980.
20. Harada T et al. Prognosis of thyroid carcinoma. Int Adv Surg Oncol 4:83-110, 1981.
21. Ozaki O et al. Modified neck dissection for patients with nonadvanced, differentiated carcinoma of the thyroid. World J Surg 12:825-829, 1988.
22. McConahey WM et al. Papillary thyroid cancer treated at the Mayo Clinic, 1946 through 1970: Initial manifestations, pathologic findings, therapy, and outcome. Mayo Clin Proc 61:978-996, 1986.
23. Jensen MH, Davis RK, Derrick L. Thyroid cancer: A computer-assisted review of 5287 cases. Otolaryngol Head Neck Surg 102:51-65, 1990.
24. Gilliland FD et al. Prognostic factors for thyroid carcinoma: A population-based study of 15,698 cases from the surveillance, epidemiology and end results (SEER) program 1973-1991. Cancer 79:564-573, 1997.

25. Ahuja S, Ernst H, Lenz K. Papillary thyroid carcinoma: Occurrence and types of lymph node metastases. J Endocrinol Invest 14:543-549, 1991.
26. Rösler H et al. Langzeitverläufe beim differenzierten Schilddrüsenkarzinom. Schweiz Med Wochenschr 122:1843-1857, 1992.
27. Tisell LE et al. Improved survival of patients with papillary thyroid cancer after surgical microdissection. World J Surg 10:854-859, 1996.
28. Hay ID. Papillary thyroid carcinoma. Endocrinol Metab Clin North Am 19:545-576, 1990.
29. Nishida T et al. Preservation of recurrent laryngeal nerve invaded by differentiated thyroid cancer. Ann Surg 226:85-91, 1997.
30. Attie JN et al. Feasibility of total thyroidectomy in the treatment of thyroid carcinoma: Postoperative radioactive iodine evaluation of 140 cases. Am J Surg 138:555-560, 1979.
31. McDermott MT, Kidd GS, Blue P. Reduced bone mineral content in totally thyroidectomized patients: Possible effect of calcitonin deficiency. J Clin Endocrinol Metab 56:936-939, 1983.
32. Gonzalez DC et al. Bone mass in totally thyroidectomized patients: Role of calcitonin deficiency and exogenous thyroid treatment. Acta Endocrinol 124:521-525, 1991.
33. Tubiana M et al. Long-term results and prognostic factors in patients with differentiated thyroid carcinoma. Cancer 55:794-804, 1985.
34. Sellers M et al. Prognostic significance of cervical lymph node metastases in differentiated thyroid cancer. Am J Surg 164:578-581, 1992.
35. Simpson WJ et al. Papillary and follicular thyroid cancer. Prognostic factors in 1578 patients. Am J Med 83:479-488, 1987.
36. Akslen LA, Myking AO. Differentiated thyroid carcinomas: The relevance of various pathological features for tumour classification and prediction of tumour progress. Virchows Arch A Pathol Anat Histopathol 421:17-23, 1992.
37. Simon D, Goretzki PE. Incidence of regional recurrence guiding radicality in differentiated thyroid carcinoma. World J Surg 20:860-866, 1996.
38. Scheumann GF et al. Prognostic significance and surgical management of locoregional lymph node metastases in papillary thyroid cancer. World J Surg 18:559-567, 1994.
39. Mazzaferri EL, Young RL. Papillary thyroid carcinoma: A 10 year follow-up report of the impact of therapy in 576 patients. Am J Med 70:511-518, 1981.
40. Cunningham MP et al. Survival discriminants for differentiated thyroid cancer. Am J Surg 160:344-347, 1990.
41. Carcangiu ML et al. Papillary carcinoma of the thyroid. A clinicopathologic study of 241 cases treated at the University of Florence, Italy. Cancer 55:805-828, 1985.
42. Proye C et al. Récidives ganglionaires cervicales des cancers thyroïdiens opérés: De l'inutilité du curage ganglionaire de principe (carcinomes médullaires exclus). Chirurgie 118:448-453, 1992.
43. Cady B. Surgery of thyroid cancer. World J Surg 5:3-14, 1981.
44. Rossi RL, Cady B, Silverman ML, et al. Current results of conservative surgery for differentiated thyroid carcinoma. World J Surg 10:612-622, 1986.
45. Noguchi S, Noguchi A, Murakami N. Papillary carcinoma of the thyroid. II. Value of prophylactic lymph node excision. Cancer 26:1061-1064, 1970.
46. Udelsman R, Lakatos E, Ladenson P. Optimal surgery for papillary thyroid carcinoma. World J Surg 20:88-93, 1996.
47. Byar DP et al. A prognostic index for thyroid carcinoma. A study of the EORTC Thyroid Cancer Cooperative Group. Eur J Cancer 15:1033-1041, 1979.

48. Fourquet A, Asselain B, Joly J. Cancer du la thyroide: Analyse multidimentionelle des facteurs prognostique. Ann Endocrinol 44:121-126, 1983.
49. Tenvall J et al. Prognostic factors of papillary, follicular and medullary carcinomas of the thyroid gland. Retrospective multivariate analysis of 216 patients with a median follow-up of 11 years. Acta Radiol Oncol 24:17-24, 1985.
50. Hannequin P, Liehn JC, Delisle MJ. Multifactorial analysis of survival in thyroid cancer. Pitfalls of applying the results of published studies to another population. Cancer 58:1749-1755, 1986.
51. Bacourt F et al. Multifactorial study of prognostic factors in differentiated thyroid carcinoma and a re-evaluation of the importance of age. Br J Surg 73:274-277, 1986.
52. Kerr DJ et al. Prognostic factors in thyroid tumours. Br J Cancer 54:475-582, 1986.
53. Cady B, Rossi R. An expanded view of risk-group definition in differentiated thyroid carcinoma. Surgery 104:947-953, 1988.
54. Brooks JR et al. Surgical therapy for thyroid carcinoma: A review of 1249 solitary thyroid nodules. Surgery 104:940-946, 1988.
55. Thoresen SO et al. Survival and prognostic factors in differentiated thyroid cancer—a multivariate analysis of 1,055 cases. Br J Cancer 59:231-235, 1989.
56. Noguchi S, Murakami N, Kawamoto H. Classification of papillary cancer of the thyroid based on prognosis. World J Surg 18:552-557, 1994.
57. Rosen IB, Maitland A. Changing the operative strategy for thyroid cancer by node sampling. Am J Surg 146:504-508, 1983.
58. Cady B. Predictors of thyroid tumor aggressiveness. In Clark OH, Duh Q-Y, eds. Textbook of Endocrine Surgery, 1st ed. Philadelphia: WB Saunders, 1997, pp 197-204.

PART

IV

MANAGEMENT

CHAPTER

12

Medullary Thyroid Carcinoma

JEFFREY F. MOLEY, M.D.

Medullary thyroid carcinomas (MTCs) arise from thyroid C cells. These tumors are relatively rare, constituting only 5% to 9% of all thyroid cancers seen in the United States. C cells, also called *parafollicular cells,* are derived from the neural crest and are considered to be part of the amine precursor uptake and decarboxylation (APUD) group of neuroendocrine cells. C cells compose only 1% of the total thyroid mass and are dispersed throughout the gland, with the highest concentration in the upper poles. The C cells are so named because of their unique ability to secrete the hormone calcitonin. Although calcitonin has been shown to be integral in calcium homeostasis in other vertebrate species, its role in humans is unclear. Calcitonin is a specific tumor marker for MTC. It is extremely useful in the screening of individuals predisposed to the hereditary forms of the disease, and in the follow-up of patients who have been treated. C cells are also capable of secreting other hormones, including carcinoembryonic antigen (CEA), histaminase, neuron-specific enolase, calcitonin gene related peptide, somatostatin, thyroglobulin, thyrotropin-stimulating hormone (TSH), adrenocortical-stimulating hormone, gastrin-related peptide, serotonin, chromogranin, and substance P.[1]

MTC was first described in the German literature as a malignant goiter with amyloid stroma.[2] MTC was considered to be a variant of anaplastic thyroid carcinoma until 1959 when Hazard et al.[3] recognized it as a unique entity. MTCs are well-demarcated, firm, gray-white tumors that may have a gritty consistency as a result of calcification (Fig. 12-1). Calcifications may be present on x-ray examination. Microscopically, the tumors are composed of uniform polygonal cells with finely granular eosinophilic cytoplasm and central nuclei. Varying numbers of spindle cells are present in nearly all tumors. The presence of amyloid is considered a distinctive feature of MTC, although it may not be found in all cases. The amyloid is thought to be formed from calcitonin or procalcitonin mole-

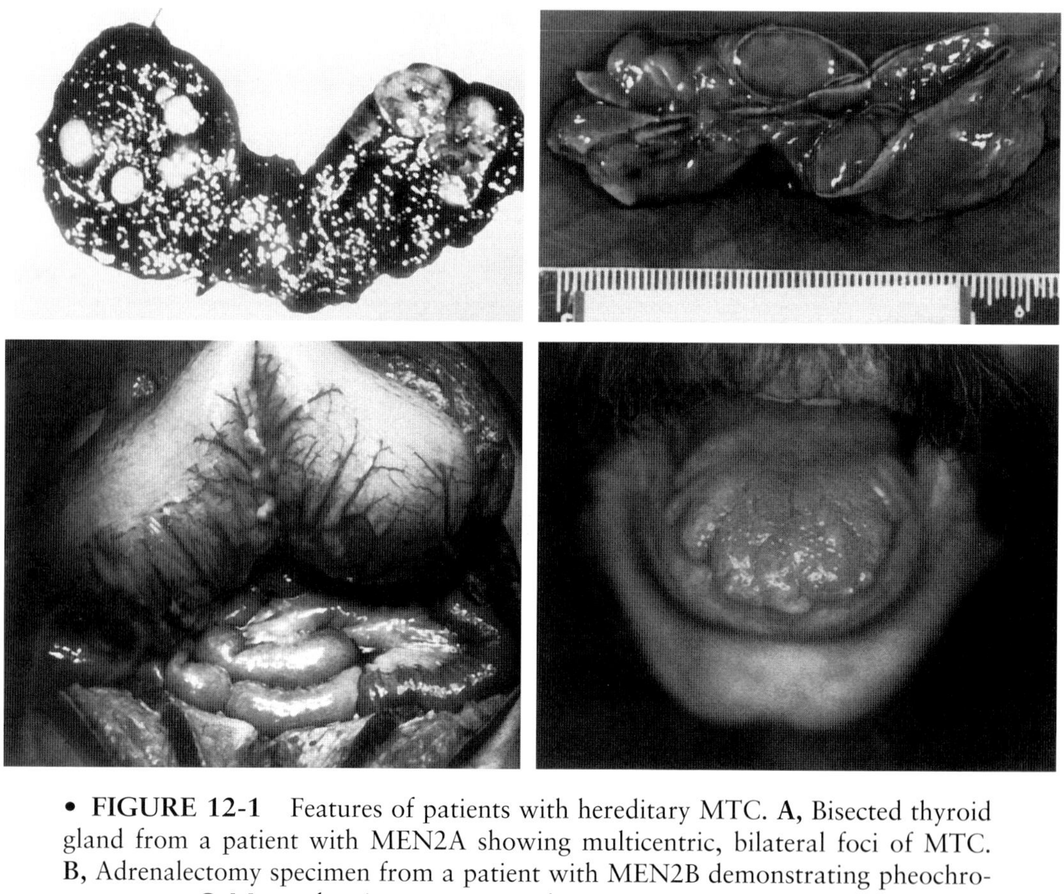

• **FIGURE 12-1** Features of patients with hereditary MTC. **A,** Bisected thyroid gland from a patient with MEN2A showing multicentric, bilateral foci of MTC. **B,** Adrenalectomy specimen from a patient with MEN2B demonstrating pheochromocytoma. **C,** Megacolon in a patient with MEN2B. **D,** Midface and tongue of patient with MEN2B showing characteristic tongue notching secondary to plexiform neuromas. (**A** courtesy Dr. SA Wells; **B, C,** and **D** courtesy Dr. R Thompson. From Moley JF. Medullary thyroid cancer. In Clark OH, Duh Q-Y, eds. Textbook of Endocrine Surgery. Philadelphia: WB Saunders, 1997.)

cules. In sporadic tumors, approximately 68% are solitary and unilateral, and 20% to 32% are bilateral or multifocal. In familial forms, 94% are bilateral or multifocal; only 6% are solitary. Histologically, the tumors have been classified according to dominant histologic patterns. These patterns include classic, amyloid-rich, insular, trabecular, and epithelial. Classic variants are the most common (48.9%), followed by amyloid-rich variants (38.3%).[4] C-cell hyperplasia is associated with MTC, particularly in the familial forms. It has been suggested that C-cell hyperplasia is a precursor lesion to MTC.[5,6,7]

Most cases of sporadic MTC and cases of hereditary MTC not detected by genetic screening present as a neck mass detected on physical examination. Diagnosis is made by biopsy (fine-needle aspiration [FNA] cytology) and measurement of stimulated calcitonin levels. Cervical nodal metastases are present in 25% to 63% of patients, depending on the reported series.[3,8-11] MTC spreads within the central compartment to perithyroidal and peritracheal lymph nodes (level VI nodes) (Fig. 12-2). The central compartment includes tissue on the trachea, extending to the carotid sheath, and from the hyoid bone to the innominate vein. Within this compartment, spread is commonly bilateral. Upper mediastinal nodes (level VII nodes) are also frequently involved. Further lymphatic spread can also occur to the lateral neck compartment, including jugular (levels II, III, and IV nodes), posterior triangle (level V nodes), and supraclavicular nodes.[12-14] Spread to the lower tracheobronchial lymph nodes is equivalent prognostically to the presence of distant metastasis.[15]

Primary MTC and tumor in lymph node metastases may involve adjacent structures by direct invasion or compression. Structures most commonly affected include the trachea, recurrent laryngeal nerve, jugular veins, and carotid arteries. Invasion of these structures may result in stridor, upper airway obstruction, hoarseness, dysphagia, and bleeding or arterial stenosis or occlusion. MTC in the thyroid or in cervical metastases may cause pain.

Distant metastases most often occur in the liver, lungs, and bone and may be an early event, associated with small primary tumors.[16] In a study from a Swedish registry,[17] it was noted that MTC patients with a palpable mass in the neck had distant metastatic disease in 20% of cases, regardless of heritability. Occult remote micrometastases are most likely the cause of most cases of persistent hypercalcitoninemia after extensive lymph node dissection.[18] Patients with MTC, especially those with a large tumor burden, often have diarrhea. Occasional patients with MTC may have Cushing's syndrome secondary to adrenocorticotropic hormone (ACTH) secretion by the tumor.

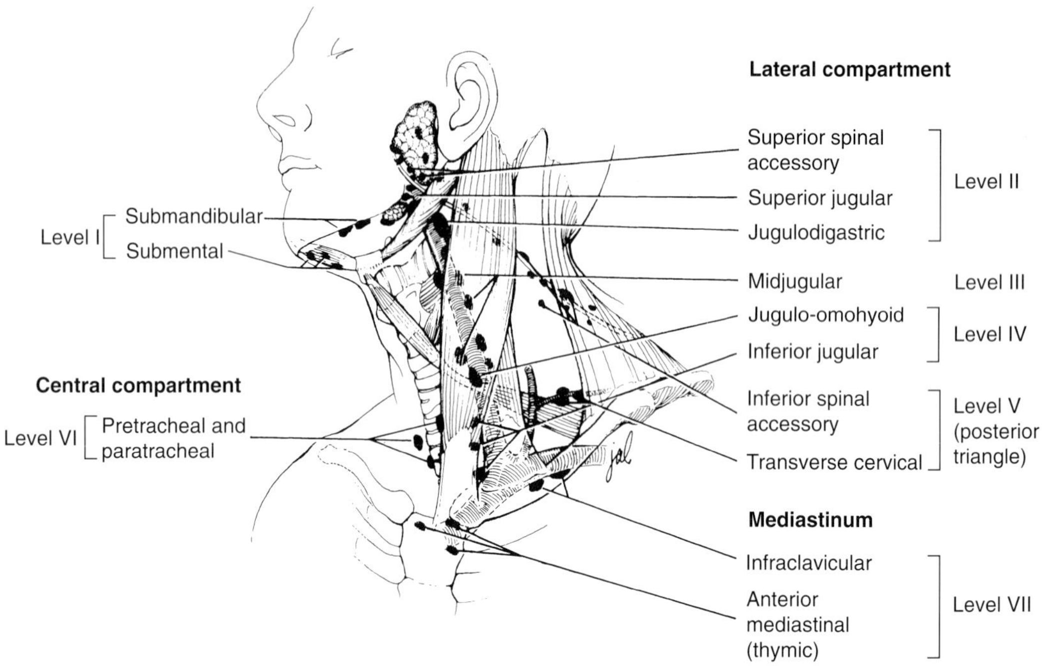

• **FIGURE 12-2** Anatomic landmarks and lymph node compartments in the neck and upper mediastinum encountered in surgical reinterventions in MTC. The central compartment is delimited inferiorly by the innominate vein, superiorly by the hyoid bone, laterally by the carotid sheath, and dorsally by the prevertebral fascia. It comprises lymphatic and soft tissues around the esophagus as well as pretracheal and paratracheal lymph nodes that drain the thyroid bed (level VI). The submandibular nodal group (level I) is subsumed in the central compartment by some classifications. The lateral compartments span the area between the carotid sheath, the sternocleidomastoid muscle, and the trapezius muscle. The inferior border is defined by the subclavian vein, and the hypoglossal nerve determines the superior boundary. The lymph node chain adjacent to the jugular vein is divided cranially to caudally in superior jugular nodes (level II), midjugular nodes (level III), and inferior jugular nodes (level IV). Lymph nodes situated in the posterior triangle between the dorsolateral sternocleidomastoid muscle, the trapezius muscle, and the subclavian vein are classified as level V nodes. Mediastinal lymphatic tissue is referred to as level VII lymph nodes. (From Musholt TJ, Moley JF. Management of recurrent medullary thyroid carcinoma after total thyroidectomy. Probl Gen Surg 14:89, 1997.)

MULTIPLE ENDOCRINE NEOPLASIA TYPE 2

Approximately 25% of MTCs occur in a hereditary clinical setting, and the genetic defect may be passed on to the offspring of affected patients in an autosomal dominant fashion. All patients with MTC should be queried about any family history of thyroid, parathyroid, or adrenal disorders. In patients affected by the hereditary forms, there is near-complete penetrance of MTC; essentially all persons who inherit the disease allele develop MTC. Other features of the syndromes are variably expressed, with incomplete penetrance. These features are summarized in Table 12-1. In multiple endocrine neoplasia (MEN) type 2A, approximately 42% of affected patients develop pheochromocytomas, whereas hyperparathyroidism is present in about 25% to 35%.[19] In MEN2B, about half develop pheochromocytomas, and all individuals develop neural gangliomas, particularly in the mucosa of the digestive tract, conjunctiva, lips, and tongue. MEN2B patients also have megacolon, marfanoid habitus, skeletal abnormalities, and markedly enlarged peripheral nerves (see Fig. 12-1). MEN2B patients

TABLE 12-1 Clinical Features of Sporadic MTC, MEN2A, MEN2B, and FMTC

Clinical Setting	Features of MTC	Inheritance Pattern	Associated Abnormalities	Genetic Defect
Sporadic MTC	Unifocal	None	None	Somatic RET mutations in 20%-80% of tumors
MEN2A	Multifocal, bilateral	Autosomal dominant	Pheochromocytomas, hyperparathyroidism	Germline missense mutations in extracellular cysteine codons of RET
MEN2B	Multifocal, bilateral	Autosomal dominant	Pheochromocytomas, mucosal neuromas, megacolon, skeletal abnormalities	Germline missense mutation in tyrosine kinase domain of RET
FMTC	Multifocal, bilateral	Autosomal dominant	None	Germline missense mutations in extracellular or intracellular cysteine codons of RET

do not develop hyperparathyroidism. Familial non-MEN medullary thyroid carcinoma (FMTC) is characterized by the development of MTC without any other endocrinopathies.[20]

MOLECULAR GENETICS

Clonality

Baylin et al.[21] initially demonstrated the clonality of MTCs. They examined the expression of glucose-6-phosphate dehydrogenase (G6PD) isoforms in a pheochromocytoma and an MTC from a patient with MEN2A who was heterozygous for the type A and type B G6PD isoforms. Patients who have heterozygous for the G6PD gene, which resides on the X chromosome, are mosaics, with some populations of cells expressing the maternal G6PD allele and some expressing the paternal allele. Analysis of blood from the patient described by Baylin et al. showed expression of both G6PD isoforms, whereas the tumors demonstrated expression of only one isoform, supporting the conclusion that the tumors are of clonal origin.

RET Gene Mutations in MEN2

The gene for MEN2A was localized to the pericentromeric region of chromosome 10 (10q11.2) in 1987.[22,23] Studies by Lairmore et al.[24] and Norum et al.[25] demonstrated that the predisposition gene for MEN2B and FMTC mapped to the same region as for MEN2A. The critical region for MEN2A was narrowed to a 480 kb segment near the centromere of human chromosome 10.[26,27] The RET proto-oncogene resides within this critical region, making it an obvious candidate gene for the MEN2 diseases. The RET proto-oncogene codes for a receptor tyrosine kinase and was originally found to be a dominant transforming gene activated by the replacement of the 5′ region with a portion of a zinc finger-like gene in T-cell leukemia cell lines.[28] The RET proto-oncogene encodes a protein with three domains: a cysteine-rich extracellular receptor domain, a hydrophobic transmembrane domain, and an intracellular tyrosine kinase catalytic domain (Fig. 12-3). The RET gene consists of at least 20 exons[29] and is expressed as five major mRNA species.[30,31]

In 1993, point mutations associated with MEN2A and FMTC were identified in exons 10 and 11 of RET, which encode the juxtamembrane portion of the extracellular receptor domain (Table 12-2).[32,33] These mutations result in a nonconservative substitution of one of five cysteine residues (codons

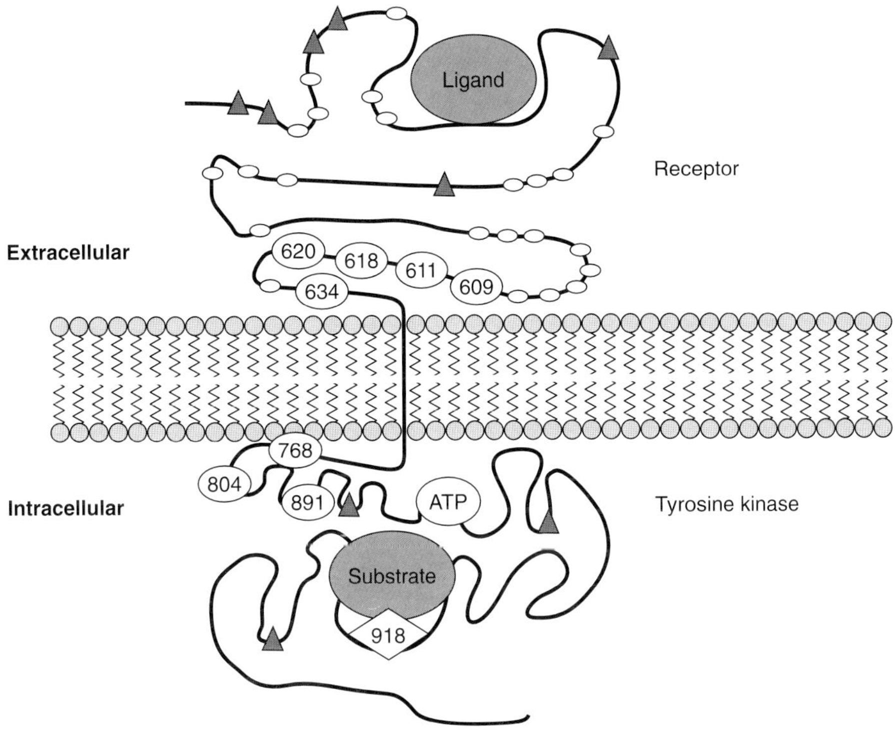

• **FIGURE 12-3** Diagram of RET gene product. Small ovals: Location of extracellular cysteine residues. Large ovals: Locations of germline mutations found in MEN2A and FMTC. Diamond: Location of germline codon 918 mutation found in the majority of MEN2B patients (codon 883 mutations have also been reported in a small number of patients with MEN2B). Triangles: Location of mutations in hereditary Hirschsprung's disease. As mentioned in the text, the RET gene product is thought to form a dimer that is complexed with glial-derived neurotrophic factor-alpha and/or neurturin. The RET gene product is divided into the intracellular, transmembrane, and extracellular domains.

609, 611, 618, 620, and 634) (see Fig. 12-3). Mutations associated with FMTC have also been described at codons 768 (Glu to Asp) in exon 13 and 804 (Val to Leu or Met) in exon 14 in the intracellular domain.[34,35] Several of these mutations have been shown to result in "gain of function" in the RET protein product with increased intrinsic tyrosine kinase activity and/or alterations of substrate recognition and transforming capability.[36]

In almost all cases of MEN2B, the RET proto-oncogene mutation is a missense methionine to threonine (ATG to ACG) change at codon 918 in exon 16.[37,38] This codon is positioned within the tyrosine kinase catalytic

TABLE 12-2 RET Mutations in Hereditary MTC

Syndrome	Missense Germline Mutations in the RET Proto-oncogene	
	Exon	Codon*
MEN2A, FMTC	10	609
		611
		618
		620
	11	634
FMTC	13	768
	14	804
	15	891
MEN2B	16	918
		883

*Some families with MEN2A and FMTC have the same RET mutation.

core of the intracellular domain and probably participates in the formation of the putative substrate recognition region. Recently two families with MEN2B have been described that have a codon 883 mutation in the tyrosine kinase domain of RET.[39]

Somatic mutations in the RET proto-oncogene have also been found in sporadic MTCs.[32,34,40] Most commonly these mutations involve codon 918, the codon mutated in MEN2B. Somatic mutations have also been found in other regions of the extracellular and intracellular domains. Missense, deletions, and insertion mutations have been described.

The RET gene product is expressed in a limited number of cell types in the normal individual, including the thyroid C cells, the adrenal medulla, and parts of the brain. The gene is important in the embryonic development of the enteric nervous system and the kidneys.[41] Glial derived growth factor (GDNF) and neurturin are ligands to the receptor domain of the RET gene product.[42-44] GDNF is a 32 kDa protein dimer which was first purified from glial cell lines and is a potent neurotrophic survival factor for motor neurons. There is compelling evidence that GDNF transduces a signal in RET.[45-48] A glycophosphatidylinositol-linked protein called *glial-derived neurotrophic factor receptor-alpha* (GDNFRα) is a cofactor in the signaling heterodimeric complex with RET. Current evidence suggests that GDNF binds directly to GDNFRα and indirectly with RET.

Dominant Oncogenes

Transforming genes whose protein products have a positive or dominant effect on cell growth and proliferative capacity are referred to as dominant oncogenes. The dominant acting oncogenes can be classified in three categories based on their function. In the first category are the molecules that act as growth factors or growth factor receptors. Oncogenes that act by this pathway may stimulate cell proliferation and transformation by causing inappropriate stimulation of signal transduction pathways. Activated RET in MTC is an example of this type of oncogene. The second category includes the second messengers and signal transduction molecules themselves, which act in the cytoplasm and the inner surface of the cell membrane. This group of molecules includes the ras gene products. The third category of dominant oncogenes includes genes that encode nuclear proteins and transcription factors, which are involved in controlling gene expression.

The role of RET in the development of MTCs is beginning to be understood. The subsequent molecular events that result in tumor progression, however, are only beginning to be investigated. In other types of cancer, including lung, colon, and breast cancer, multiple genetic abnormalities are found in tumor cells; it is likely that these tumors arise after multiple defects in different genes have occurred. Genetic analysis of MTCs has not been exhaustive, and very few abnormalities, aside from RET mutations, have been reported.

Absence of amplification of N-myc, c-myc, and Erb B2 has been reported in MTCs and pheochromocytomas.[49] Roncalli et al.[50] reported that N-myc expression in greater than 10% of tumor cells, as detected by immunohistochemistry, was associated with poorer survival, sporadic disease, and male sex. They found no evidence of gene amplification and did not determine the basis for the overexpression. Our group reported absence of mutation of the H-ras, N-ras, and K-ras genes in a series of pheochromocytomas and MTCs analyzed by direct sequencing.[51] Likewise, examination of nerve growth factor and nerve growth factor receptor (p75) showed no abnormality at the DNA or RNA levels.[49]

Tumor Suppressor Genes

There have been several studies evaluating loss of heterozygosity (LOH) at tumor suppressor loci in MTCs and pheochromocytomas, which are summarized in Table 12-3. The cumulative data indicate a higher than background incidence of LOH in pheochromocytomas on chromosome arms 1p, 3p, 17p, and 22q.[22, 52-58] In MTCs, the reports by Moley et al.[53] and Mulligan

TABLE 12-3 Loss of Heterozygosity in Pheochromocytomas and Medullary Thyroid Cancers

Report	Chromosomal Arms Tested	LOH in Pheochromocytomas (No. LOH/No. informative)	LOH in MTCs (No. LOH/No. informative)
Khosla et al., 1991[52]	1p, 2p, 3p, 5q, 10q, 13q, 16p, 17p, 17q, 22q	1p-13/31, 2p-1/34, 3p-4/24, 10q-1/22, 17p-7/27, 22q-5/18	1p-1/11, 22-1/7
Moley et al., 1992[53]	1p, 1q	1p-12/18 (9/9 from MEN2A and 2B patients)	1p-3/24
Yang et al., 1990[54]	1p	1p-5/8	
Mathew et al., 1987[22]	1p, 1q, 5,6,7, 11,12	1p-4/6	1p-3/8
Shin et al., 1993[55]	1p, 22q	1p-12/22, 22q-8/20	
Mulligan et al., 1993[56]	1-22, both arms	1p-15/25, 3p-10/18, 3q-9/15, 5q-1/7, 6q-1/7, 8p-1/8, 11p-3/19, 11q-2/23, 13-2/17, 17p-3/20, 17q-1/20, 22-8/20	1p-7/28, 3p-1/19, 3q-2/14, 7p-1/17, 10p-1/18, 10q-1/25, 11p-1/16, 13-2/22, 15-1/9, 21-1/8, 22-4/22
Dou et al., 1994[57]	2-23	3q-13/13 F, 6/8 S, 21q-4/6 F, 2/7 S, 22q-7/13 F, 1/10 S, 11q-2/6 F, 3/7 S	3q-2/7 F, 1/8 S, 22q-4/15 F, 2/8 S
Herfarth et al., 1997[58]	17p	17p-4/22	17p-0/14

F, familial (MEN2A and 2B); *LOH,* loss of heterozygosity; *S,* sporadic.
Table lists reports, chromosomal arms tested, and number of informative tumors with LOH. If arm tested is not listed in LOH column, it indicates that LOH was not found.

et al.[56] suggest a significant incidence of 1p LOH; however, evaluation of other chromosomal arms yielded no consistent findings. Lack of significant LOH on 10q, at the RET locus, supports the hypothesis that the RET proto-oncogene acts as a dominant oncogene, as opposed to a tumor suppressor gene. Our group has found no evidence of p53 mutations in exons 4 through 10 by single strand confirmation polymorphus (SSCP) analysis performed on 20 MTCs and 20 pheochromocytomas.[58]

There have been no reports of the involvement of DNA repair genes (MLH1, MSH2) in development or progression of pheochromocytomas or MTCs, and replication error repeats have not been a consistent finding in these tumors.[58]

CLINICAL MANAGEMENT OF MEDULLARY THYROID CANCER

Depending on the clinical setting, the presentation of MTC may vary considerably. Sporadic MTC is unilateral and unifocal in most cases, whereas MTC in the MEN2 syndromes is usually bilateral and multifocal (see Table 12-1). In FMTC, the tumors are indolent and appear later in life, whereas MTC in MEN2B usually presents in infancy or early childhood with gross evidence of cancer present in children as young as 6 months of age. These patients may die of widespread metastatic MTC at an early age, underscoring the importance of early diagnosis and treatment in this particular population.[59,60] The virulence of sporadic MTC can vary, and the disease can present in any age group, although the peak incidence is in the fifth and sixth decades of life.[4]

The prognosis of MTC is associated with disease stage at the time of diagnosis. Numerous studies of patients with MEN2A who are treated for MTC have demonstrated a direct correlation between early diagnosis and cure of the disease.[61-66] Clearly, early diagnosis and treatment are of significant importance in patients with the hereditary forms of MTC. Patients with MEN2A and FMTC have a normal outward appearance. In these patients, the diagnosis of MTC was initially made through screening efforts (measurement of calcitonin levels or RET gene mutation testing), undertaken because of other affected family members, or by detection of a thyroid nodule on physical examination. More than 50% of patients with MEN2B have normal parents, and the diagnosis is not usually made until a mass is discovered in the neck. Occasionally the diagnosis is made earlier by an astute clinician, who notes the characteristic phenotype. As mentioned, MEN2B patients have a "marfanoid" habitus, with long axial skeletal features, soft tissue hypergnathism of the midface, and hyperflexible joints. They also typically have neuromata of the lips, conjunctiva, and gastrointestinal tract.[67,68]

All patients with sporadic MTC, and most index cases of MEN2A, MEN2B, and FMTC present with a thyroid nodule. Cervical lymphadenopathy is present in more than 50% of patients. Respiratory complaints, hoarseness, and dysphagia can be seen in about 13% of patients. Approximately 12% of patients with sporadic MTC will present with evidence of distant metastatic disease.[4]

MTC does not concentrate iodine and appears as a cold nodule on thyroid scintigraphy scans. Plain x-ray films may show areas of calcifications in the neck. FNA is a sensitive means for establishing the diagnosis of MTC, especially if immunocytochemical staining for calcitonin is performed.

Thyroid C cells and MTC cells secrete calcitonin, which has been an invaluable marker for the presence of disease in screening and follow-up settings. Peripheral serum levels of this hormone are measured by radioimmunoassay. Over 30% of patients with MTC will have normal basal levels of calcitonin; therefore provocative calcitonin stimulation tests are routinely performed. The gastric hormone pentagastrin stimulates calcitonin secretion and is widely used (with or without additional calcium infusion) as a secretagogue in provocative calcitonin stimulation tests. The development of immunoradiometric assays increases detection to less than 3 pg/ml and therefore greatly improves the sensitivity and specificity of the provocative calcitonin stimulation test.

Our protocol for testing is as follows; after an intravenous infusion of calcium gluconate (2 mg/kg over 1 minute) followed by pentagastrin (0.5 mg/kg over 5 seconds), blood samples are obtained before and at 1, 2, 3, and 5 minutes after the infusion. Peak plasma calcitonin values generally occur at 1 to 2 minutes.[69] Wells et al.[62] showed that preoperative stimulated calcitonin levels of less than 1000 pg/ml were associated with MTC confined to the thyroid gland in more than 95% of patients with MEN2A and FMTC. Approximately half of the patients with stimulated calcitonin levels before 1000 pg/ml had only microscopic evidence of disease, whereas all patients with levels above 10,000 pg/ml had macroscopic evidence of disease, with about 17% of these having evidence of distant metastatic MTC. Clinical and pathologic studies have shown that MEN2 patients with MTC had an earlier stage of disease and a higher cure rate if the thyroid neoplasms were diagnosed biochemically rather than clinically with a palpable thyroid mass.[70]

Routine stimulated calcitonin testing, however, has several disadvantages. First, the test is very uncomfortable; patients often complain of nausea, diaphoresis, agitation, and urinary urgency. Historically, members of MEN2 kindreds at risk for inheriting the disease were screened at early ages, usually about 5 years of age, and required annual testing until the age of 45. It is understandable, therefore, why compliance was often poor, especially among adolescents and young children. Second, because the disease is inherited in an autosomal dominant fashion, 50% of at-risk patients will never develop the disease and would be spared the expense and inconvenience of routine scheduled testing if a definitive genetic test were applied. Third, calcitonin testing detects only the presence of existing disease, and requires either C-cell hyperplasia or MTC to produce elevations of plasma calcitonin levels. Routine genetic testing, as will be discussed, identifies RET mutation carriers earlier and more reliably than biochemical testing, and it obviates the need for continued testing in individuals found to be unaffected.

Stimulated calcitonin testing remains extremely important, however, in the follow-up of patients treated for MTC.

SURGICAL TREATMENT

Patients With Medullary Thyroid Cancer

Recommended surgical treatment of MTC is influenced by several factors. First of all, the clinical course of MTC is usually more aggressive than that of differentiated thyroid cancer, with higher recurrence and mortality rates. Second, MTC cells do not take up radioactive iodine, and radiation therapy and chemotherapy are ineffective. Third, MTC is multicentric in 90% of patients with the hereditary forms of the disease, and in 20% to 32% of patients with the sporadic form. Fourth, as previously mentioned, more than 50% of patients who present with palpable disease already have nodal metastases. Finally, the ability to measure postoperative stimulated calcitonin levels has allowed assessment of the adequacy of surgical extirpation.

Thorough surgical extirpation is the only curative treatment for MTC. Total thyroidectomy is the appropriate treatment for the primary tumor, accompanied by a central node dissection. In this operation, all thyroid tissue and all nodal tissue from the level of the hyoid bone superiorly to the innominate vessels inferiorly is removed. After the parathyroid glands are identified, central nodal tissue on the anterior surface of the trachea is removed, exposing the superior surface of the innominate vein behind the sternal notch. Fatty and nodal tissue between the carotid sheaths and the trachea is removed, including paratracheal nodes along the recurrent nerves. On the right, the junction of the innominate and right carotid arteries is exposed, and on the left, nodal tissue is removed to a comparable level behind the head of the left clavicle. A systematic approach to the removal of all nodal tissue in the central neck has been reported to decrease recurrence and improve survival rates when compared retrospectively with procedures where only grossly involved nodes were removed.[71]

At our institution, total parathyroidectomy with autotransplantation is performed at the same time as total thyroidectomy for MTC. This is done for several reasons. First, the parathyroid glands are closely associated with perithyroidal lymph nodes, and preservation of these glands risks leaving nodal metastases. Second, the vascular supply to a parathyroid gland may be interrupted by dissection and excision of perithyroidal and central nodes. Third, patients with MEN2A are at risk of developing hyperparathyroidism, which may be more easily diagnosed and treated if the parathyroids are in the forearm rather than in a previously operated neck. Parathyroid glands are therefore removed, placed in cold saline solution, and autotransplanted at the time of thyroidectomy for MTC.

Frozen-section biopsy is performed to confirm the presence of parathyroid tissue, and then one or two glands are sliced into 1 × 3 mm fragments. The fragments are placed into intramuscular pockets (two to three fragments per pocket) in the muscle of the nondominant forearm (in patients with MEN2A), or the sternocleidomastoid muscle (in patients with sporadic MTC, FMTC, and MEN2B). Each pocket is closed with a 4-0 silk suture. Remaining parathyroid tissue is viably frozen and stored.[72] The autografts generally function well within 4 to 6 weeks, at which time patients can be taken off of calcium supplementation.

In a recent series of thyroidectomies performed in 13 patients with hereditary MTC identified by genetic screening, total thyroidectomy and central node dissection with parathyroidectomy and parathyroid autografting were performed in all patients. All patients were normocalcemic after stopping calcium supplementation 8 weeks postoperatively.[73] In other series, the percentage of patients requiring calcium supplementation following parathyroidectomy with parathyroid autografting has ranged from 0% to 18%.[74] Other experts in this field attempt to preserve the glands with vascular supply intact during thyroidectomy for MTC and perform autotransplantation selectively when a parathyroid gland appears to be devascularized.[71,75]

The decision to perform a more extensive lateral node dissection is based on the clinical suspicion that the jugular nodes may be involved with tumor. Certainly patients with palpable adenopathy in the anterior or posterior jugular chain should undergo ipsilateral functional or modified radical neck dissection (see Fig. 12-2). In patients without such gross evidence of nodal involvement, the indications for removal of lateral nodes are less clear. We have found ipsilateral jugular nodal metastases to be present in more than 50% of patients with palpable primary MTC; therefore we perform an ipsilateral modified radical or functional neck dissection in all patients with palpable MTC. This operation entails removal of the jugular chain of nodes, which includes nodes anterior to and posterolateral to the jugular vein, from the level of the facial vein to the subclavian vessels, and laterally to the cervical plexus or, in some cases, to the spinal accessory nerve. Unless invaded by tumor, the jugular vein and sternocleidomastoid muscle are left intact.

Preventative Surgery for MEN2A Gene Carriers

Individuals with MEN2A and FMTC are virtually certain to develop MTC at some point in their lives (usually before age 30). Therefore at-risk family members who are found to have inherited the RET gene mutation are candidates for thyroidectomy, regardless of their stimulated plasma calcitonin levels. To test a patient for the presence of a mutation in RET, peripheral blood is drawn and the lymphocyte pellet is separated. Lymphocytes have nuclei, as opposed to red blood cells, and DNA is extracted by proteinase digestion and phenol extraction. Regions of the RET proto-oncogene are amplified by polymerase chain reaction, and mutations are detected by one of several techniques. These include direct DNA sequencing, analysis of restriction sites introduced or deleted by a mutation, or by gel shift analysis (denaturing gradient gel electrophoresis or single-strand conformation polymorphism analysis).[40,73,75]

Wells et al.[73] at Washington University in St. Louis studied 132 individuals from seven different kindreds, all affected by MEN2A. Of the 132 individuals, 48 had an established diagnosis of MEN2A and 58 were at 50% risk for inheriting the disease but had no clinical evidence of endocrine neoplasia. Twenty-six unaffected spouses of MEN2A kindred members served as control subjects. All individuals were evaluated by both direct and indirect genetic testing for the presence of RET gene mutations. In patients at 50% risk for disease (having an affected parent or sibling), calcium-pentagastrin–stimulated calcitonin levels were also obtained. Via polymerase chain reaction and sequence-based direct mutation analysis of genomic DNA from the 58 individuals at 50% risk for MEN2A, 21 individuals were identified who had inherited a RET mutation, associated with disease. The other 37 family members had two normal RET alleles. All 26 unaffected control subjects had normal RET alleles. After meeting with genetic counselors, who informed them of the pattern of disease inheritance and the basis for the genetic tests, total thyroidectomy was offered to all 21 individuals who were found to have inherited a RET mutation. The patients ranged in age from 6 to 21 years (mean age, 13.2 years). In 12 of the 21 patients (mean age, 12 years), the stimulated plasma calcitonin levels were within normal limits. In the remaining nine patients (mean age, 15.1 years; range, 8-20 years), the stimulated plasma calcitonin levels were elevated.

Of the 12 genetically positive individuals with normal stimulated plasma calcitonin levels, six patients (or their parents) decided not to undergo an immediate thyroidectomy for reasons of convenience of timing, or because they preferred to wait until calcitonin levels were elevated. Of the nine family members with elevated stimulated plasma calcitonin levels, two wished to delay thyroidectomy for several months for personal reasons. In the remaining 13 individuals (six with normal plasma calcitonin levels and seven with elevated levels), total thyroidectomy, lymph node dissection, and parathyroid autotransplantation were performed. Following thyroidectomy and parathyroid autotransplantation, patients were placed on thyroid, calcium, and vitamin D supplementation. Approximately 8 weeks after the operation, the oral calcium and vitamin D were discontinued. Two weeks after the oral calcium and vitamin D replacement were stopped, the serum calcium concentration was within the normal range in each patient. Of the seven patients whose preoperative plasma calcitonin levels were elevated, each had microscopic evidence of MTC on histologic examination. Two of the seven had macroscopic disease. Of the six patients with normal preoperative plasma calcitonin levels, either macroscopic MTC (n = 1), microscopic MTC (n = 2), or C-cell hyperplasia only (n = 3) was evident. A total of 212 lymph nodes were resected from the central zone of the neck (14.5 per patient) and on histologic examination, none contained metastases. In each of the 13 patients the stimulated plasma calcitonin levels were normal after total thyroidectomy.

In a similar study from The Netherlands, Lips et al.[75] identified 14 young members of families affected by MEN2A who had normal calcitonin test results but who were found to be MEN2A gene carriers by DNA testing. Thyroidectomy was performed in 8 of these 14, and foci of MTC were identified in all eight.

Skinner et al.[76] at Washington University in St. Louis subsequently evaluated thyroidectomy for MTC in 49 children with MEN2A and MEN2B. In this series, 14 children underwent a prophylactic thyroidectomy based on genetic testing. The average age of the children at the time of surgery was 10.5 years. Postoperative calcitonin levels were all undetectable, and there was no evidence of recurrent MTC in a mean follow-up of 1.3 years. To date, our group at Washington University has performed 63 thyroidectomies in at-risk kindred members found to have RET gene mutations. Lymph node metastases were identified in three patients. Postoperative calcitonin levels were normal in all patients except for one 6-year-old girl with MEN2B.

The fact that carcinoma was found in the glands of most of these young patients with normal stimulated calcitonin test results indicates that the operation was therapeutic, not prophylactic. There is some urgency, therefore, to applying this genetic test to other at-risk individuals and performing thyroidectomy on those who test positive genetically. The ideal age for performance of thyroidectomy in those patients found to be genetically positive has not been determined unequivocally. We feel that patients with MEN2A and FMTC should be 6 years of age to undergo surgery. Patients with MEN2B should undergo thyroidectomy during infancy because of the aggressiveness and earlier age of onset of MTC in these patients.[77] The likelihood of MTC recurrence in these patients is low, but patient follow-up over the next decades will need to be done. At present, it is advisable to follow these patients by evaluating stimulated plasma calcitonin levels every

1 to 2 years. These patients must also continue to be followed for the development of pheochromocytomas and hyperparathyroidism.

PERSISTENT OR RECURRENT MEDULLARY THYROID CANCER

Nonsurgical Management

Patients who present with palpable MTC often have elevated calcitonin levels following primary surgery, indicating residual or recurrent MTC. In the study by Block et al.[7] of patients who presented with palpable tumors, 15 (83%) of 18 patients with hereditary disease and 11 (55%) of 20 patients with sporadic tumors had persistent disease, as indicated by elevated calcitonin levels postoperatively.[7] Many patients with persistently high levels of calcitonin following thyroidectomy and node dissection continue to do well without other evidence of disease for many years.[78] By contrast, in a Norwegian study of 84 cases of MTC,[79] it was noted that more than 50% of patients who presented with cervical node metastases eventually died of the disease. Variations in outcome among patients with MTC may be explained by differences in the biologic virulence of the tumor, the extent of spread at the time of treatment, and the adequacy of surgical treatment.

Unlike differentiated thyroid cancer, radioactive iodine has not been found to be helpful in the treatment of patients with metastatic MTC, because C cells are not derived from thyroid follicles and do not concentrate iodine.[80] Several authors have advocated the use of external-beam radiation therapy for metastatic or recurrent MTC in the neck.[81-85] These studies, however, were retrospective and were done on small numbers of patients. Other studies have not supported the use of radiation therapy in MTC.[86-88] In the report by Samaan et al,[87] 202 patients were studied retrospectively. Despite the fact that the authors felt that the characteristics of the two groups were comparable, it was found that the patients who received external-beam radiation therapy had a worse outcome than patients who did not. The role of radiation therapy has not been well defined in MTC, and further studies are needed to define its role. Reoperation on a patient who has had external-beam radiation therapy is especially treacherous, and since surgery has been shown to be effective in treating these patients, we do not recommend radiation therapy unless all surgical options had been exhausted.

Chemotherapeutic agents have not been found to be consistently effective in patients with MTC.[89-95] Adriamycin alone, and in combination with other agents, has resulted in several partial responses and has been used in individuals without a surgical option.

Reoperation

Several groups have reported their experience with reoperation for persistent or recurrent MTC in the neck.[18,71,96-101] These groups reported a significant reduction in stimulated calcitonin levels following reoperation in most patients. In our two series of patients, from 1990 through 1992,[96] and from 1992 through 1996,[101] all patients had persistent or recurrent elevation of stimulated calcitonin levels following primary surgery for MTC.

SERIES 1 (1990 THROUGH 1992)

We reported our experience with 32 patients treated between 1990 and 1993.[96] These patients had previously undergone total thyroidectomy and most of the patients also had previously undergone lymph node dissections. All patients had elevated levels of calcitonin. Localization studies, including selected venous catheterization, computed tomographic scanning, and physical examination, were successful in localizing tumor in half the cases.

In all patients, the central zone of the neck, where the previous thyroidectomy had been performed, was explored and all residual soft tissue and lymph nodes were removed. Our technique of cervical exploration is as follows: The patient is placed in the reflex position with padding under the arms and torso. The head is placed in mild hyperextension. The previous thyroidectomy incision is excised and extended to the posterior borders of the sternocleidomastoid muscles. Superior and inferior subplatysmal flaps are developed and retracted. The recurrent laryngeal nerves are identified by a "back door" approach after medial reflection of the sternothyroid muscle. Once the nerves are identified, the strap muscles may safely be mobilized off of the central compartment. The strap muscles are divided on one side and occasionally on both sides, to enhance exposure. Central node dissection is done first. This is often tedious because of scarring. All residual thyroid tissue and nodal tissue within the central compartment is removed (level VI and VII nodes). This is carried out from the level of the hyoid bone, along the larynx, and along the recurrent nerves to a level below the innominate artery on the right side, and to a comparable level approaching the aortic arch behind the clavicle on the left side. All tissue on the anterior surface of the trachea, including any visible thymic tissue, is removed. The lateral boundaries of this part of the dissection are the carotid sheaths. In patients with functioning parathyroid tissue that has not been autotransplanted, a thorough search for parathyroid glands is carried out. This may take 1 hour or more, because no nodes are removed until parathyroid tissue is identified and confirmed by biopsy and frozen section. When normal parathyroid tissue is identified, it is either resected and preserved on ice for autotransplantation and viable freezing, or, in the case of viable superior glands with no evidence of nearby metastatic tumor, left in situ. Afterward, central node or unilateral or bilateral functional neck dissections (with removal of jugular nodes, levels II, III, IV, and V) are then carried out (Fig. 12-4). In this 1993 series, one patient had simultaneous median sternotomy and mediastinal node dissection. Three patients underwent subsequent median sternotomy with mediastinal node dissection as an additional procedure. Operative morbidity was low, and there were no deaths. In 28 of the 35 operations, the patient was discharged from the hospital 2 to 5 days after surgery. In nine patients (group 1), calcitonin was reduced to undetectable levels following reoperation. In 13 patients (group 2), postoperative calcitonin levels were decreased by 40% or more. In 10 patients (group 3), postoperative calcitonin levels were not improved.

To identify factors that could be used preoperatively to select patients likely to benefit from reoperation, results of surgery were correlated with patient age, sex, disease (hereditary vs. sporadic), number of nodes previously resected, characteristics of the primary tumor, calcitonin levels, and results of preoperative localization studies. Patient sex, disease, number of nodes previously resected, preoperative calcitonin levels, and preoperative localization study results were not significantly different among the three groups. Previously resected tumors from patients in group 3, however, were more likely to have demonstrated invasive features (invasion of adjacent structures, extranodal or extracapsular spread) than tumors from patients in groups 1 and 2 ($p < 0.05$, Fisher's exact test).

We concluded that reoperation with meticulous removal of residual nodal and tumor tissue in patients with persistent postoperative hypercalcitoninemia, resulted in normalization of calcitonin levels in 28% of patients, and a decrease in calcitonin levels by 40% or more in another 42% of patients.[96] The results also suggested that determination of the degree of invasiveness of the primary tumor may help in selecting patients likely to benefit from reoperative surgery for recurrent MTC.

We sought to improve our results through better selection of patients who would be likely to benefit from reoperation.[101] We achieved this by applying systematic metastatic workup, including routine computed tomography (CT) or magnetic resonance imaging (MRI) of the neck, chest, and abdomen; selective venous catheterization in selected patients; and by instituting routine liver laparoscopy and biopsy in all patients.

We found that diagnostic laparoscopy is extremely useful in detecting distant metastases in these patients.[102] In our series of 41 patients with hypercalcitoninemia following initial surgical treatment for MTC, all underwent

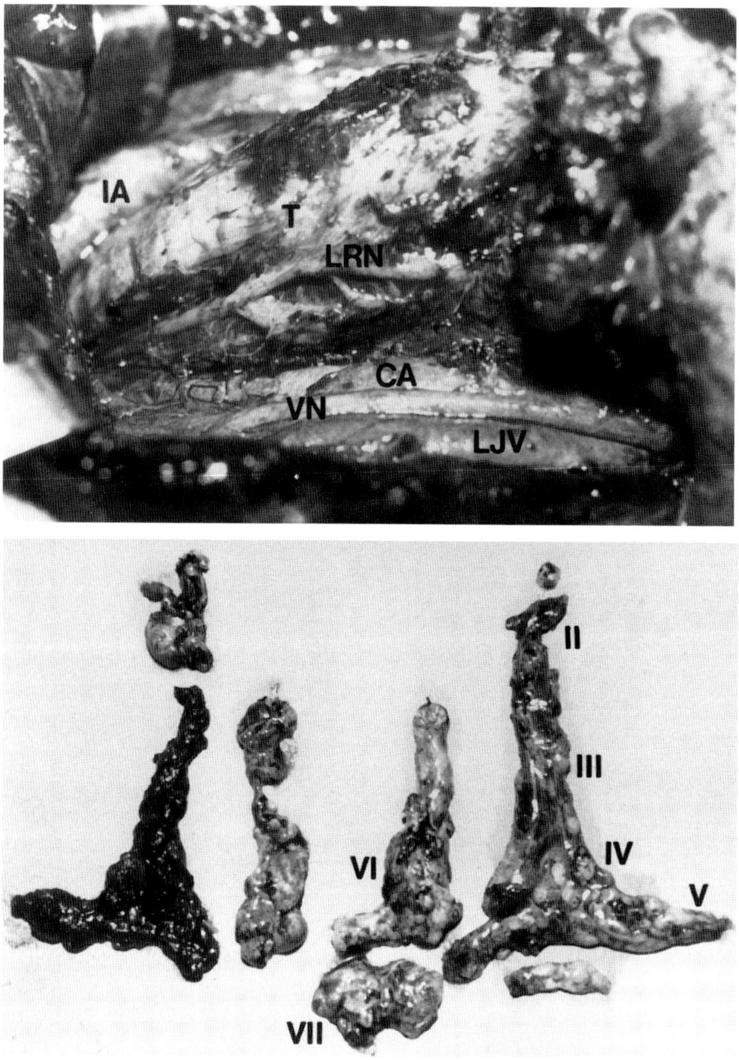

• **FIGURE 12-4** This patient with MEN2B had recurrent elevation of calcitonin levels 20 years after total thyroidectomy for MTC. Redo central neck dissection and bilateral functional neck dissections (microdissection) were performed. **A,** View of trachea and dissected central and left paratracheal compartment. Taken from the patient's left side; patient's head is to the right and chest is to the left. (*IA,* Innominate vein; *T,* trachea; *LRN,* left recurrent laryngeal nerve; *CA,* left carotid artery; *VN,* left vagus nerve; and *LJV,* left jugular vein.) Note markedly enlarged nerves characteristic of MEN2B. **B,** Surgical specimen from the same patient showing central and upper mediastinal nodes (level VII), bilateral paratracheal nodes (level VI), and bilateral jugular chain and posterior triangle nodes (levels II, III, IV, and V nodes). Microscopic foci of MTC were found in paratrachal dissection specimens. (From Moley JF. Medullary thyroid cancer. In Clark OH, Duh Q-Y, eds. Textbook of Endocrine Surgery. Philadelphia: WB Saunders, 1997.)

laparoscopic (n = 36) or open (n = 5) examination and biopsy of the liver. Thirty-seven of the 41 patients underwent imaging by CT and/or MRI of the liver, and 17 underwent selective venous catheterization with measurement of hepatic and peripheral vein–stimulated calcitonin levels. Liver metastases were found in eight patients, seven by laparoscopy and one by open examination. Seven of these patients had *normal* CT and/or MRI scans of the liver. Laparoscopy or open liver examination revealed metastases in two of 11 patients with elevated hepatic vein/peripheral vein–stimulated calcitonin ratios (above 1.3). Metastases appeared as small (less than 5 mm) bright white nodules on the surface of the liver (Fig. 12-5).

From this experience we concluded that direct examination and biopsy of the liver by laparoscopy may demonstrate small deposits of metastatic MTC in patients with an otherwise normal metastatic workup, and we apply this diagnostic modality in all patients who are considered for reoperation for MTC.

SERIES 2 (1992 THROUGH 1996)

Between August 1992 and November 1996, 115 patients with recurrently or persistently elevated calcitonin levels following primary surgery for MTC were evaluated.[101] In all patients, previous operative notes and pathology reports were reviewed. Fifty-three patients did not undergo reoperation. Of these, 10 were found to have distant metastases following radiologic evaluation. Three patients who had undergone extensive prior surgery and radiation therapy to the neck were not considered appropriate candidates for reoperation. Two patients were not thought to be candidates for reoperation because of severe underlying medical problems. Twenty-four patients declined further evaluation and consideration for reoperation, after discussion of treatment options with this surgeon and with the referring physician. Fourteen patients were undergoing evaluation and had not been operated on yet.

Sixty-two patients underwent surgery. In all of these patients except one, pathology slides from the patient's initial operation were obtained and reviewed. In 10 patients, laparoscopic or open examination of the liver revealed liver metastases (see Fig. 12-5). In seven patients, palliative debulking of cervical tumor was carried out. All but one of the patients who underwent a palliative operation are alive and well, with no evidence of airway compromise, or of bulky cervical recurrence. One patient died with massive liver involvement after a prolonged period characterized by weight loss, diarrhea, and inanition.

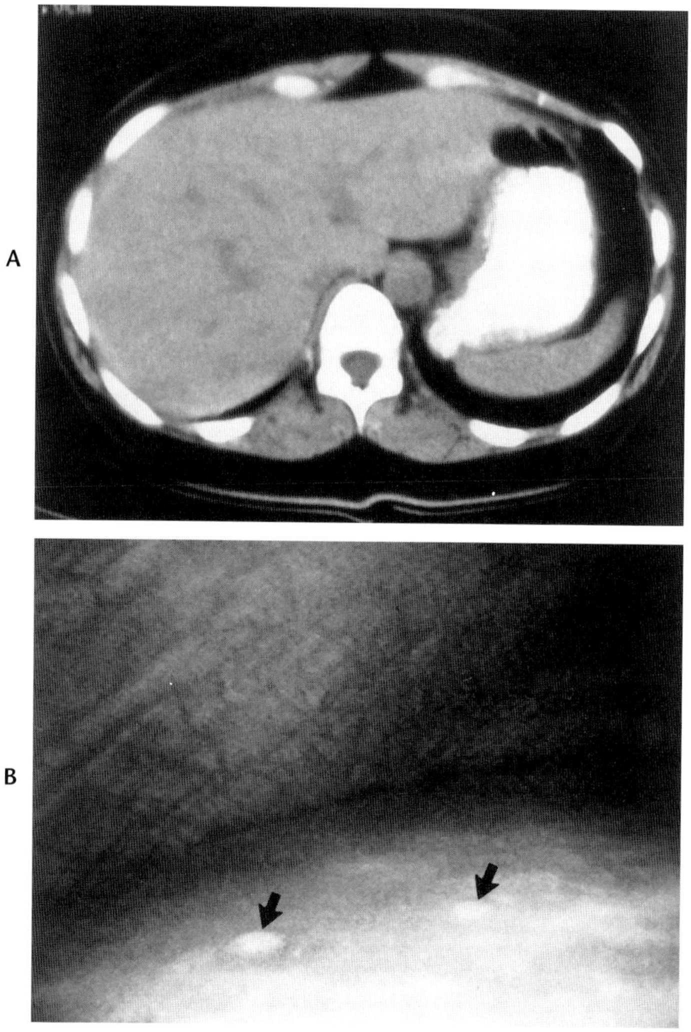

• **FIGURE 12-5** **A,** Computed tomographic scan of the liver from a patient with MEN2A, recurrent MTC, and elevated calcitonin levels; there is no evidence of liver metastases on the scan. **B,** Laparoscopic view of the liver from the same patient showing multiple small raised whitish lesions on and just beneath the surface of the liver, confirmed to be metastatic MTC by biopsy. These small, multiple metastases are usually not seen on routine CT scanning or nuclear scanning. (From Tung WS, Vesely, TM, and Moley JF. Laparoscopic detection of hepatic metastases in patients with residual or recurrent medullary thyroid cancer. Surgery, 118:1024, 1995.)

In 45 patients, 51 operations were carried out with curative intent. The mean age of these patients was 38.8 years (range, 10 to 60 years). Twenty-four patients had sporadic disease, 17 had MEN2A, and four had MEN2B. Direct examination of the liver was accomplished by laparoscopy in 44 patients and as an open procedure in three. Laparoscopy was carried out as previously described (see Fig. 12-5). If hepatic metastases were identified, cervical exploration was not done, unless there was evidence of central recurrence threatening the trachea or major arteries. If the liver was clear of apparent metastatic disease, cervical exploration was carried out. Our technique of cervical exploration was similar to that described in our first series. Central dissection (levels VI an VII nodes) was performed in all patients. Bilateral (30 patients) or unilateral (15 patients) functional neck dissections (levels II, III, IV, and V nodes) were also carried out (see Fig. 12-4).

Of the seven patients who had palliative cervical operations, one patient had persistent postoperative hypocalcemia. There were no other complications in that group. In the 45 patients who underwent reoperation with curative intent, there were no postoperative deaths and no transfusions were required. Thoracic duct leak occurred in four patients (8.9%). This required operative repair in each case. In two patients the duct had been ligated at the time of surgery but had leaked from a point proximal to the ligation. Operative ligation of the duct, through a cervical approach (three patients), or a thoracic approach (one patient), was successful in each case. Two patients have persistent hypocalcemia (in a follow-up of 3 months and 2 years). There were no permanent nerve injuries. Two patients had hoarseness that persisted for several weeks after the surgery but cleared up after 1 month. Two patients had transient Horner's syndrome, and one patient had an axillary nerve praxis that lasted for 1 month. One patient had right hypoglossal nerve praxis with deviation of the tongue that lasted for 2 months. The mean hospital stay was 4.2 ± 0.4 days (range, 1 to 14 days). All patients have resumed regular activity and work.

A calcium-pentagastrin–stimulated calcitonin test was carried out at our institution immediately before and 72 hours after the operation. For 1- and 2-year follow-up testing, patients either returned to our institution, where a calcium-pentagastrin–stimulated test was performed, or they were tested by a physician in their geographic area.

Of the 45 patients who underwent reoperation with curative intent, the mean decrease in postoperative stimulated calcitonin level was 73.1% (Fig. 12-6). In 22 (48%) of 45 patients, the postoperative stimulated calcitonin level dropped more than 90% compared with the preoperative value. Of these 45 patients, 17 (38%) had postoperative stimulated calcitonin levels that were within the normal range (group 1), and six (13%) had no significant decrease

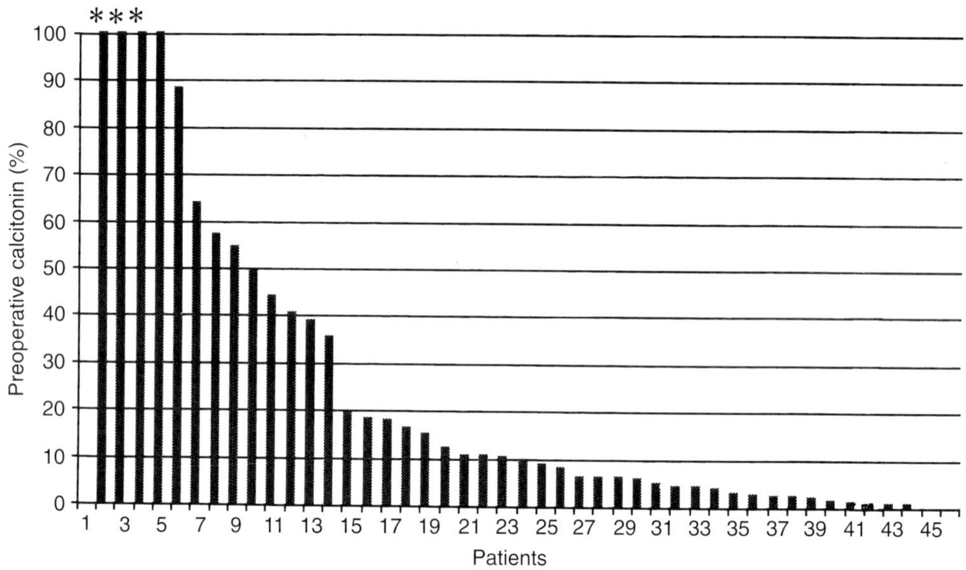

• **FIGURE 12-6** Postoperative change in peak stimulated calcitonin levels. The shaded bars indicate the postoperative stimulated calcitonin levels of the 45 patients who underwent curative cervical reexploration and dissection. The postoperative calcitonin level is expressed as a percentage of the preoperative calcitonin level (e.g., 100% indicates no change in calcitonin level; 10% indicates that the stimulated calcitonin level fell by 90%). (From Moley JF, Dilley WG, DeBenedetti MK. Improved results of cervical reoperation for medullary thyroid carcinoma. Ann Surg 225,734, 1997.)

in stimulated calcitonin levels (group 3). The remaining patients had a greater than 35% reduction in stimulated calcitonin levels (group 2). These three groups were compared with regard to age, sex, disease type (sporadic, MEN2A, or MEN2B), age at diagnosis, number of previous operations, tumor size, and tumor invasiveness (defined as whether or not the primary tumor or its nodal metastases demonstrated capsular invasion or invasion of adjacent structures). As in our earlier series, tumor invasiveness was the only parameter that correlated with failure to reduce postoperative calcitonin levels to the normal range ($p < 0.05$, Fisher's exact test). In group 1 patients, review of pathology from the primary operation did not reveal invasiveness in any case (0 of 17). In group 2 and 3 patients, invasiveness was identified in 8 of 28 cases.

Of the 17 patients who had normal postoperative stimulated calcitonin levels, 1-year follow-up levels are available for 12 patients. In 10 of the 12 patients the levels remained normal; two patients had recurrent elevation of calcitonin levels that have persisted after a 2-year follow-up. In five patients with normal calcitonin levels at 1 year, the stimulated calcitonin level remained normal at 2-year follow-up.

These results indicate an improvement in outcome following reoperation for persistent or recurrent MTC. In this series (1992 to 1996), 38% (17 of 45) of patients had normal postoperative stimulated calcitonin levels, compared with 28% (9 of 32) in the first series. In the most recent series, only 13% (6 of 45) of patients had no decrease in calcitonin levels following reoperation, compared with 31% (10 to 32) in the first series ($p = 0.07$, Fisher's exact test). This improvement has mainly occurred through better preoperative selection of patients, and the institution of routine laparoscopic liver examination preoperatively, which identified metastases in 10 patients, nine of whom had normal CT or MRI imaging of the liver and who would otherwise have undergone neck reoperation with curative intent.

In discussing reoperation with patients with elevated calcitonin levels following primary surgery, we describe the risks and options in detail. We always discuss the option of continuing observation and cite recent series that have demonstrated the frequently indolent nature of this tumor.[78] Many patients are comfortable with a nonoperative expectant approach. In this recent series of 115 patients, 24 decided not to undergo further evaluation or surgical intervention for this problem.[101] If a patient with elevated calcitonin levels has had an adequate previous operation and the results of imaging studies are normal, an expectant approach with routine yearly screening is appropriate in many cases. We do, however, feel that it is important to follow these patients closely with routine CT or MRI scanning of the neck and chest. This surveillance should be carried out because if patients develop a central recurrence, it can be resected. This will prevent death from invasion of the airway or great vessel in some patients.

Reoperation for recurrent or residual MTC in patients following primary procedures for MTC appears to be beneficial in the majority of patients who do not have distant metastatic disease and may result in improved local control rates, improved survival, and long-term cure in a significant number of patients. In this series, the designation "normal" for stimulated calcitonin levels is based on the normal range for patients who have not undergone thyroidectomy. The calcitonin levels after pentagastrin stimulation testing in patients who have undergone thyroidectomy for reasons other than MTC have not been well established. There is a great variation between laboratories and techniques of measurement. Close follow-up will be needed to elucidate the effect on calcitonin levels in the long run, and we cannot be sure that any of these patients have been cured until a follow-up of 5 to 10 years has been documented. A patient whose calcitonin levels remain elevated or become elevated again still benefits from operation, because disease is removed from the central neck. A patient who dies from MTC generally dies from central recurrence or distant metastases. Central recurrence with airway invasion and/or vascular invasion is a catastrophic but preventable complication. It is my feeling that even in the presence of distant MTC, local control by operative removal of tumor in the neck will result in improved survival and quality of life.

CONCLUSION

The identification of mutations in the RET proto-oncogene associated with MEN2A, MEN2B, and FMTC has led to a new paradigm in surgery—the performance of an operation based on the result of a genetic test. Prophylactic thyroidectomy based on direct mutation analysis appears to be curative in MEN2A and FMTC patients when they are screened at a young age. Since the introduction of microsurgical dissection for persistent hypercalcitoninemia in the 1980s, more accurate localization and staging studies have led to improved outcome and better patient selection for surgery.

REFERENCES

1. Grauer A, Raue F, Gagel RF. Changing concepts in the management of hereditary and sporadic medullary thyroid carcinoma. Endocrinol Metab Clin North Am 19:613, 1990.
2. Jaquet AJ. Ein Fall von metastasierenden Amyloidtumoren (Lymphosarcoma). Virchows Arch [Pathol Anat] 185:251, 1906.
3. Hazard JB, Hawk WA, Crile G. Medullar (solid) carcinoma of the thyroid—A clinicopathologic entity. J Clin Endocrinol Metab 19:152, 1959.
4. Saad MF et al. Medullary carcinoma of the thyroid. A study of clinical features and prognostic factors in 161 patients. Medicine 63:319, 1984.
5. Wolfe HJ et al. C-cell hyperplasia preceding medullary thyroid carcinoma. N Engl J Med 289:437, 1973.
6. Graze K et al. Natural history of familial medullary thyroid carcinoma. Effect of a program for early diagnosis. N Engl J Med 299:980, 1978.
7. Block MA, et al. Clinical characteristics distinguishing hereditary from sporadic medullary thyroid carcinoma: Treatment implications. Arch Surg 115:142, 1980.
8. Chong GC et al. Medullary carcinoma of the thyroid gland. Cancer 35:695, 1975.
9. Rossi RL et al. Nonfamilial medullary thyroid carcinoma. Am J Surg 139:554, 1980.
10. Rougier P et al. Medullary thyroid carcinoma: Prognostic factors and treatment. Int J Radiat Oncol Biol Phys 9:161, 1983.
11. Williams ED, Brown CL, Doniach I. Pathological and clinical findings in a series of 67 cases of medullary carcinoma of the thyroid. J Clin Pathol 19:103, 1966.
12. Shah JP. Cervical lymph node metastases—Diagnostic, therapeutic, and prognostic implications. Oncology 4:61, 1990.

13. Kallinowski F et al. Medullary carcinoma of the thyroid: Therapeutic strategy derived from fifteen years of experience. Surgery 114:491, 1993.
14. Musholt TJ, Moley JF. Management of recurrent medullary thyroid carcinoma after total thyroidectomy. Probl Gen Surg 14:89, 1997.
15. Buhr HJ et al. Microsurgical neck dissection for occultly metastasizing medullary thyroid carcinoma. Three-year results. Cancer 72:3685, 1993.
16. Gautvik KM et al. Early liver metastases in patients with medullary carcinoma of the thyroid gland. Cancer 63:175, 1989.
17. Bergholm U et al. Clinical characteristics in sporadic and familial medullary thyroid carcinoma. A nationwide study of 249 patients in Sweden from 1959 through 1981. Cancer 63:1196, 1989.
18. Tisell LE et al. Reoperation in the treatment of asymptomatic metastasizing medullary thyroid carcinoma. Surgery 99:60, 1986.
19. Howe JR, Norton JA, Wells SA, Jr. Prevalence of pheochromocytoma and hyperparathyroidism in multiple endocrine neoplasia type 2A: Results of long-term follow-up. Surgery 114:1070, 1993.
20. Farndon JR et al. Familial medullary thyroid carcinoma without associated endocrinopathies: A distinct clinical entity. Br J Surg 73:278, 1986.
21. Baylin SB et al. Inherited medullary thyroid carcinoma: A final monoclonal mutation in one of multiple clones of susceptible cells. Science 199:429-31, 1978.
22. Mathew CGP et al. A linked genetic marker for multiple endocrine neoplasia type 2A on chromosome 10. Nature 328:527, 1987.
23. Simpson NE et al. Assignment of multiple endocrine neoplasia type 2A to chromosome 10 by linkage. Nature 328:528, 1987.
24. Lairmore TC et al. Familial medullary thyroid carcinoma and multiple endocrine neoplasia type 2B map to the same region of chromosome 10 as multiple endocrine neoplasia type 2A. Genomics 9:181, 1991.
25. Norum RA et al. Linkage of the multiple endocrine neoplasia type 2B gene (MEN2B) to chromosome 10 markers linked to MEN2A. Genomics 8:313, 1990.
26. Gardner E. et al. Genetic linkage studies map the multiple endocrine neoplasia type 2 to a small interval on chromosome 10. Hum Mol Genet 2:241, 1993.
27. Mole SE et al. Localization of the gene from multiple endocrine neoplasia to a 480 kb region in the chromosome band 10q11.2. Hum Mol Genet 2:247, 1993.
28. Takahashi M, Ritz, J, Cooper GM. Activation of a novel human transforming gene ret by DNA arrangement. Cell 42:581, 1985.
29. Kwok JB et al. Structural analysis of the human ret protooncogene using exon trapping. Oncogene 8:2575, 1993.
30. Tahira T et al. Characterization of ret proto-oncogene mRNAs encoding two isoforms of the protein product in a human neuroblastoma cell line. Oncogene 5:97, 1990.
31. Tahira T et al. Expression of *proto-ret* mRNA in embryonic and adult rat tissues. Biochem Biophys Res Commun 153:1290, 1988.
32. Donis-Keller H et al. Mutations in the RET protooncogene associated with MEN2A and FMTC. Hum Mol Genet 2:851, 1993.
33. Mulligan LM et al. Germ-line mutations of the RET protooncogene in multiple endocrine neoplasia type 2A. Nature 363:458, 1993.
34. Eng C et al. A novel point mutation in the tyrosine kinase domain of the RET protooncogene in sporadic medullary thyroid carcinoma and in a family with FMTC. Oncogene 10:509, 1995.

35. Bolino A et al. RET mutations in exons 13 and 14 of FMTC patients. Oncogene 10:2415, 1995.
36. Santoro M et al. Activation of *RET* as a dominant transforming gene by germline mutations of MEN2A and MEN2B. Science 267:381, 1995.
37. Carlson KM et al. Single missense mutation in the tyrosine kinase catalytic domain of the RET protooncogene is associated with multiple endocrine neoplasia type 2B. Proc Natl Acad Sci USA 91:1579, 1994.
38. Hofstra RMW et al. A mutation in the RET protooncogene associated with multiple endocrine neoplasia type 2B and sporadic medullary thyroid carcinoma. Nature 367:375, 1994.
39. Smith, DP. Houghton, C, Ponder, BAJ. Germline mutation of RET codon 883 in two cases of de novo MEN2B. Oncogene 15:1213, 1997.
40. Musholt PB et al. "Cold" single-strand conformational variants for mutation analysis of the RET protooncogene. Surgery 122:363, 1997.
41. Schuchardt A et al. Defects in the kidney and enteric nervous system of mice lacking the tyrosine kinase receptor RET. Nature 367:377, 1994.
42. Sanchez MP et al. Renal agenesis and the absence of enteric neurons in mice lacking GDNF. Nature 382:70, 1996.
43. Pichel JG et al. Defects in enteric innervation and kidney development in mice lacking GDNF. Nature 386:73, 1996.
44. Moore MW et al. Renal and neuron abnormalities in mice lacking GDNF. Nature 382:76, 1996.
45. Trupp M et al. Functional receptor for GDNF encoded by the c-ret proto-oncogene. Nature 381:785, 1996.
46. Durbec P et al. GDNF signalling through the RET receptor tyrosine kinase. Nature 381:789, 1996.
47. Jing S et al. GDNF-induced activation of the Ret protein tyrosine kinase is mediated by GDNFR-a, a novel receptor for GDNF. Cell 85:1113, 1996.
48. Treanor JJS et al. Characterization of a multi-component receptor for GDNF. Nature 382:80, 1996.
49. Moley J et al. Oncogene and growth factor expression in MEN related tumors. Henry Ford Hosp Med J 40:284, 1992.
50. Roncalli M et al. Prognostic value of N-myc immunoreactivity in medullary thyroid carcinoma. Cancer 74:134, 1994.
51. Moley JF et al. Low frequency of ras gene mutations in neuroblastomas, pheochromocytomas, and medullary thyroid cancers. Cancer Res 51:1596, 1991.
52. Khosla S et al. Loss of heterozygosity suggests multiple genetic alterations in pheochromocytomas and medullary thyroid carcinomas. J Clin Invest 87:1691, 1991.
53. Moley J et al. Consistent association of 1p loss of heterozygosity with pheochromocytomas from patients with multiple endocrine neoplasia type 2 syndromes. Cancer Res 52:770, 1992.
54. Yang KP et al. Deletion mapping on the distal third region of chromosome 1p in multiple endocrine neoplasia type IIA. Anticancer Res 10:527, 1990.
55. Shin E et al. Deletion mapping of chromosome 1p and 22q in pheochromocytoma. Jpn J Cancer Res 84:402, 1993.
56. Mulligan LM et al. Genetic events in tumour initiation and progression in multiple endocrine neoplasia type 2. Genes Chromosom Cancer 6:166, 1993.

57. Dou S et al. Identification of chromosomal loci for tumor suppressor loci implicated in progression of pheochromocytoma and medullary thyroid carcinoma. Am J Hum Genet 55:A20, 1994.
58. Herfarth K et al. Abscence of p53 alterations in pheochromocytomas and medullary thyroid carcinomas. Genes Chromosom Cancer 20:24, 1997.
59. Telander RL et al. Medullary carcinoma in children. Results of early detection and surgery. Arch Surg 124:841, 1989.
60. Norton JA et al. Multiple endocrine neoplasia type IIb. The most aggressive form of medullary thyroid carcinoma. Surg Clin North Am 59:109, 1979.
61. Wells SA, Jr et al. Early diagnosis and treatment of medullary thyroid carcinoma. Arch Intern Med 145:1248, 1985.
62. Wells SA, Jr et al. The importance of early diagnosis in patients with hereditary medullary thyroid carcinoma. Ann Surg 195:595, 1982.
63. Wells SA, Jr et al. The early diagnosis of medullary thyroid carcinoma of the thyroid gland in patients with multiple endocrine neoplasia type II. Ann Surg 182:362, 1975.
64. Russell CF et al. The surgical management of medullary thyroid carcinoma. Ann Surg 197:42, 1983.
65. Telander RL et al. Results of early thyroidectomy for medullary thyroid carcinoma in children with multiple endocrine neoplasia type 2. J Pediatr Surg 21:1190, 1986.
66. Leape LL et al. Total thyroidectomy for occult familial medullary carcinoma of the thyroid in children. J Pediatr Surg 11:831, 1976.
67. Carney JA et al. Alimentary tract ganglioneuromatosis: A major component of the syndrome of multiple endocrine neoplasia type IIb. N Engl J Med 295:1287, 1976.
68. Khairi MR et al. Mucosal neuroma, pheochromocytoma and medullary thyroid carcinoma: Multiple endocrine neoplasia type 3. Medicine 54:89, 1975.
69. Wells S et al. Provocative agents and the diagnosis of medullary carcinoma of the thyroid gland. Ann Surg 188:139, 1978.
70. Wells SA Jr et al. Medullary thyroid carcinoma: Relationship of method of diagnosis to pathologic staging. Ann Surg 188:377, 1978.
71. Dralle H et al. Compartment-oriented microdissection of regional lymph nodes in medullary thyroid carcinoma. Surg Today 24:112, 1994.
72. Wells SA Jr et al. Transplantation of the parathyroid glands: Current status. Surg Clin North Am 59:167, 1979.
73. Wells SA Jr et al. Predictive DNA testing and prophylactic thyroidectomy in patients at risk for multiple endocrine neoplasia type 2A. Ann Surg 220:237, 1994.
74. Olson JA, Jr et al. Parathyroid autotransplantation during thyroidectomy. Results of long-term follow-up. Ann Surg 223:472, 1996.
75. Lips C et al. Clinical screening as compared with DNA analysis in families with multiple endocrine neoplasia type 2A. N Engl J Med 331:828, 1994.
76. Skinner MA et al. Medullary thyroid carcinoma in children with multiple endocrine neoplasia types 2A and 2B. J Pediatr Surg 31:177, 1996.
77. O'Riordain DS et al. Medullary thyroid carcinoma in multiple endocrine neoplasia types 2A and 2B. Surgery 116:1017, 1994.
78. van Heerden JA et al. Long-term course of patients with persistent hypercalcitoninemia after apparent curative primary surgery for medullary thyroid carcinoma. Ann Surg 212:395, 1990.
79. Normann T et al. Medullary carcinoma of the thyroid in Norway. Acta Endocrinol 83:71, 1976.

80. Saad MF, Guido JJ, Samaan NA. Radioactive iodine in the treatment of medullary carcinoma of the thyroid. J Clin Endocrinol Metab 57:124, 1983.
81. Rougier P et al. The values of calcitonin and carcinoembryonic antigen in the treatment and management of nonfamilial medullary thyroid carcinomas. Cancer 51:855, 1983.
82. Halnan KE. The non-surgical treatment of thyroid cancer. Br J Surg 62:769, 1975.
83. Simpson WJ. Radiotherapy in thyroid cancer. Can Med Assoc J 113:115, 1975.
84. Steinfeld AD. The role of radiation therapy in medullary carcinoma of the thyroid. Radiology 123:745, 1977.
85. Nguyen TD et al. Results of postoperative radiation therapy in medullary carcinoma of the thyroid: A retrospective study by the French Federation of Cancer Institutes—the Radiotherapy Cooperative Group. Radiother Oncol 23:1, 1992.
86. Chong GC et al. Medullary carcinoma of the thyroid gland. Cancer 35:695, 1975.
87. Samaan NA, Schultz PN, Hickey RC. Medullary thyroid carcinoma: Prognosis of familial versus nonfamilial disease and the role of radiotherapy. Horm Metab Res 21:20, 1989.
88. Williams ED, Brown CL, Doniach I. Pathological and clinical findings in a series of 67 cases of medullary carcinoma of the thyroid. J Clin Pathol 19:103, 1966.
89. Husain M et al. Failure of medullary carcinoma of the thyroid to respond to doxorubicin therapy. Horm Res 9:22, 1978.
90. Gottlieb JA, Hill DS Jr. Chemotherapy of thyroid cancer with adriamycin. Experience with 30 patients. N Engl J Med 290:193, 1974.
91. Scherubl H, Raue F, Ziegler R. Combination chemotherapy of advanced medullary and differentiated thyroid cancer. Phase II study. J Cancer Res Clin Oncol 116:21, 1990.
92. Petursson SR. Metastatic medullary thyroid carcinoma. Complete response to combination chemotherapy with dacarazine and 5-fluorouracil. Cancer 62:1899, 1988.
93. Orlandi F et al. Chemotherapy with dacarbazine and 5-fluorouracil in advanced medullary thyroid cancer. Ann Oncol 5:763, 1994.
94. Schlumberger M et al. Treatment of advanced medullary thyroid cancer with an alternating combination of 5 FU-streptozocin and 5 FU-dacarbazine. The Groupe D'Etudedes Tumeurs a Calcitonine (GETC). Br J Cancer 71:363, 1995.
95. Wu LT et al. Treatment of advanced medullary thyroid carcinoma with a combination of cyclophosphamide, vincristine, and dacarbazine. Cancer 73:432, 1994.
96. Moley JF et al. Reoperation for recurrent or persistent medullary thryoid cancer. Surgery 114:1090, 1993.
97. Norton JA, Doppman JL, Brennan MF. Localization and resection of clinically inapparent medullary carcinoma of the thyroid. Surgery 87:616, 1980.
98. Buhr HJ, et al. Microsurgical lymph node dissection for metastatic asymptomatic C-cell carcinoma. Henry Ford Hosp Med J 40:268, 1992.
99. Brumsen et al. Should patients with medullary thyroid carcinoma undergo extensive lymph node (re)operation to improve long-term survival? Henry Ford Hosp Med J 40:271, 1992.
100. Ellenhorn JD, Shah JP, Brennan MF. Impact of therapeutic regional lymph node dissection for medullary carcinoma of the thyroid gland. Surgery 114:1078, 1993.
101. Moley JF, Dilley WG, DeBenedetti MK. Improved results of cervical reoperation for medullary thyroid carcinoma. Ann Surg 225:734, 1997.
102. Tung WS, Vesely TM, Moley JF. Laparoscopic detection of hepatic metastases in patients with residual or recurrent medullary thyroid cancer. Surgery 118:1024, 1995.

CHAPTER

13

Locally Recurrent Thyroid Carcinoma

HIROYUKI YAMASHITA, M.D., Ph.D.

Differentiated thyroid cancer shows a wide range of biologic behavior, although it is commonly associated with low morbidity and mortality. The disease-specific survival rates at 10 years are about 90%.[1-5] Despite excellent prognosis, some patients have a recurrence of thyroid cancer locally, in the regional lymph nodes, and/or at distant sites; approximately half of the patients who develop recurrent thyroid cancer eventually die of the disease. The likelihood of a recurrence of disease varies with several prognostic factors based on clinical, surgical, and pathologic findings. Several scoring systems and risk-group definitions were proposed to identify prognostic factors for recurrence and survival.[1,3-10]

Approximately two thirds of initial recurrences are in the neck area, and local recurrence leads to a decreased life expectancy. Control of local cancer is important, because it avoids invasion and compression of surrounding tissues. The persistence of cancer increases the risk of distant metastasis.[11-13] Prevention and early detection of regional and/or local recurrence and adequate treatment of recurrent disease appear to improve the quality of life and survival of patients with differentiated thyroid cancer. The treatment of recurrent thyroid cancer of follicular cell origin consists of surgery, radioiodine therapy, and external-beam radiation, alone or in combination. At our institution, intraoperative irradiation therapy and/or percutaneous ethanol injection therapy have also been employed for locally advanced nonresectable tumors.

In this chapter I will describe the management of locally recurring differentiated thyroid cancer. Analyses of our data with respect to local recurrence, its predisposing factors, and prognosis were based on 2176 patients with differentiated thyroid cancer who underwent curative surgery between 1970 and 1989 at the Noguchi Thyroid Clinic.

INITIAL TREATMENT OF DIFFERENTIATED THYROID CANCER

Careful ultrasonographic examination enhances the clinical evaluation of cervical lymph nodes and identifies other nodules within the thyroid gland, helping the surgeon to plan the extent of thyroidectomy and lymph node dissection. Careful examination by palpation or combined with ultrasonography during surgery is also important for the appropriate initial treatment.

Initial surgical and medical therapy for thyroid cancer influences the outcome, in terms of prognosis and quality of life. The extent of thyroid surgery for differentiated thyroid cancer remains controversial, with methods ranging from lobectomy to total thyroidectomy with or without modified radical neck dissection. Because differentiated thyroid cancer is uncommon and generally indolent, long follow-up studies of large numbers of patients are necessary to evaluate various treatment strategies. Furthermore, the fact that a considerable number of patients with recurrent thyroid carcinoma can be cured by surgery alone and/or with ^{131}I therapy makes it more difficult to determine the appropriate treatment. Although no prospective randomized studies have compared the risks and benefits among the different operative procedures, those who favor thyroid-conserving procedures cite the low incidence of recurrence and fewer complications,[4,14-17] whereas those advocating total thyroidectomy note the advantages in postoperative monitoring with thyroglobulin, radioactive iodine treatment, and removal of undetected malignancy in the contralateral lobe.[2,5,18-21] Our standard practice for papillary carcinoma has been total lobectomy on the side of the tumor and subtotal thyroidectomy of the contralateral lobe with modified radical neck dissection of the affected side. This treatment is followed by external radiotherapy, if necessary, for persistent or recurrent disease. For patients with follicular carcinoma, who are diagnosed by pathologic examination in approximately one fifth of cases, the usual treatment has been total lobectomy. Radioiodine therapy, with or without completion thyroidectomy, has usually been performed only in patients with distant metastases. The extent of thyroidectomy and lymph node dissection, which is a main point of controversy among endocrine surgeons, was previously well described by analyzing a large number of patients treated at our clinic.[4,22]

Some basic considerations should be addressed for analyzing outcome after the treatment of differentiated thyroid cancer. As mentioned, our standard practice for differentiated thyroid cancer is lobectomy, or lobectomy plus subtotal thyroidectomy of the contralateral lobe. In some other institutions, total thyroidectomy followed by ^{131}I is the standard therapy for differentiated thyroid cancer. In the latter cases, there may be some patients with ^{131}I-proved metastases without other clinical evidence of disease after the initial surgery. Therefore the percentage of curative surgery is less than the former and the outcome must be different if it is compared with that of patients who underwent a curative operation. Similarly, the recurrence rate depends on the extent and duration of follow-up programs and modalities used to detect recurrent disease. We recently noted that recurrent disease was detected at an earlier stage at our institution by using sensitive ultrasonography, thallium scintigraphic scanning, and serum thyroglobulin measurement.[4]

RESULTS

The characteristics and results of our patients are shown in Table 13-1. These 2176 patients, who underwent potentially curative thyroid operations from 1970 to 1989, were followed until August 1997. The mean and median follow-up period for the patients known to be alive at the last follow-up visit was 14.7 years and 14.2 years, respectively. Although some authors advocate routine radioiodine ablation after total or near-total thyroidectomy, claiming a decreased incidence of recurrence and improved prognosis,[5,19] others disagree with this approach.[4,9,23,24] Our results (see Table 13-1) do not support using total thyroidectomy for all patients with differentiated thyroid carcinoma because we have obtained equally good or perhaps even better results with the use of subtotal thyroidectomy. Although it has been reported that total thyroidectomy can be carried out without significant morbidity,[19,20] we believe that any possible benefits of total thyroidectomy must balance out the increased risk of morbidity with benefits such as hypoparathyroidism and laryngeal nerve palsy. In this study we excluded patients with small thyroid cancers (tumor size less than 10 mm), because these tumors are usually found incidentally in surgical specimens, and ordinarily the patient has an excellent prognosis.[25] If we were to include 1106 patients with small

TABLE 13-1 Characteristics and Results of 2176 Patients With Differentiated Thyroid Cancer

Characteristic	Group (histologic type)		
	Papillary Cancer	Follicular Cancer	Papillary and Follicular Cancer
Patients	1903	273	2176
Sex (female:male ratio)	10:3	5:7	9:4
Mean age (yr)	45 (6-90)	46 (12-77)	45 (6-90)
Tumor size (mm)	26 (11-115)	32 (11-88)	28 (11-115)
Extracapsular adhesion or invasion (%)	35	19	38
Gross lymph node metastasis (%)	38	4	34
Histologic lymph node metastasis (%)	75	9	66
Disease-specific survival			
10-year (%)	97	95	97
20-year (%)	93	86	92
Recurrence-free survival			
10-year (%)	90	86	90
20-year (%)	83	83	82

differentiated thyroid cancers treated during the same period, the 10- and 20-year disease-specific survival rates for the entire group would be 98% and 94%, respectively.

RECURRENT THYROID CANCER

Diagnosis

Most recurrences develop within several years after thyroidectomy, and approximately half of our patients who developed recurrences did so within 5 years. Thallium-201 scintigraphy, CT scanning, and MRI are useful for follow-up of patients who have undergone less than total or near-total thyroidectomy. Radioiodine scanning is not useful in these patients because of the presence of the remnant thyroid. Our studies[26] and those of Aufferman et al.[27] document that recurrent thyroid cancer can be distinguished from fibrous tissue.

Serum thyroglobulin determination is also a useful tumor marker after total ablation of the thyroid gland, either surgically or after thyroidectomy, followed by ^{131}I ablation. The presence of thyroglobulin after total thyroidectomy suggests persistent disease. Monitoring of serum thyroglobulin levels is also helpful in patients who have been treated by less-than-total

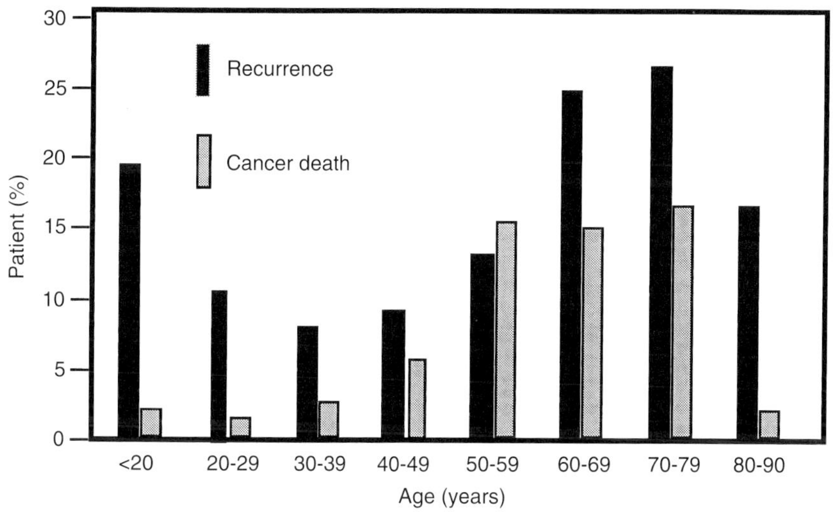

• **FIGURE 13-1** Recurrence and cancer death in patients with differentiated thyroid cancer in each age group.

thyroidectomy, especially when preoperative thyroglobulin values are available and sequential measurements are used during follow-up.[28-30] An increment or increasing thyroglobulin value suggests recurrent or persistent disease. Thyroglobulin levels may be inaccurate in 8% to 20% of patients because of antithyroglobulin antibodies.

Risk Factors

The concept of risk group definitions is extremely important for the understanding and management of differentiated thyroid cancers. Several studies of risk group analysis are available; these are described in Chapters 9 and 11.

Risk group definitions were based on disease-specific death after treatment. Few studies are available regarding prognostic factors for recurrent thyroid cancer,[9,15,30-32] because the time of recurrence often depends on the modality used for detection, and cancer death generally represents the risk group category more accurately than recurrence. Since most patients present with a recurrence before they die of thyroid cancer, a similar risk factor should be expected for both recurrence and death.

The exception is younger patients; even when nodal and lung cancer recurs, these patients appear to have a favorable prognosis. Fig. 13-1 shows that patients at the extremes of age have more recurrent thyroid cancer, although the cancer death rate was very low in the younger patient group, which is in agreement with many other reports.[5,32,33]

Papillary vs. Follicular Cancer

Several authors reported that papillary and follicular carcinomas behave differently.[8,34-36] Patients with papillary thyroid carcinomas tend to have frequent regional lymph node recurrences. In contrast, patients with follicular thyroid carcinomas are prone to metastases to the bone and the lungs with a regional recurrence rate of about 10%. Because papillary thyroid carcinoma comprises about 80% of differentiated thyroid cancer, the results obtained by analysis of differentiated thyroid cancer may reflect the nature of patients with papillary cancer but may not represent those with follicular cancer. Comparisons between patients with papillary and follicular cancer treated at our hospital are shown in Tables 13-1 and 13-2. Figs. 13-2 through 13-4 show the survival curves of patients with recurrent thyroid cancer (249 patients with papillary and 38 patients with follicular carcinomas). Approximately half of the patients with recurrent papillary cancer and two thirds of those with recurrent follicular cancer died of the disease during the study period.

Local Recurrence of Papillary Cancer

The following analyses were based on 1903 patients with papillary thyroid cancer. In Table 13-2, the sites of first recurrence in patients with differentiated thyroid cancer are shown. The incidence of local and/or regional recurrence (10.2%) in our studies is comparable to those of other reported series that ranged from 4% to 26%.[2,5,8,16,19] Fig. 13-5 illustrates the survival

TABLE 13-2 First Recurrence Sites of Patients With Differentiated Thyroid Cancer

	Group (histologic type)		
Site	Papillary Cancer Number (%)	Follicular Cancer Number (%)	Papillary and Follicular Cancer Number (%)
Patients	1903	273	2176
Neck area	194 (10.2)	15 (5.5)	209 (9.6)
Local	43 (2.3)	4 (1.5)	47 (2.2)
Regional	106 (5.6)	6 (2.2)	112 (5.1)
Locoregional	45 (2.4)	5 (1.8)	50 (2.3)
Distant	55 (2.9)	23 (8.4)	78 (3.6)
Total	249 (13.1)	38 (14.0)	287 (13.2)

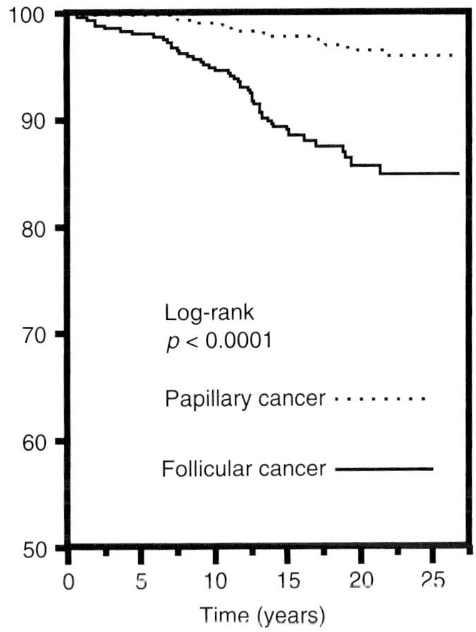

• **FIGURE 13-2** Disease-specific survival curves in patients with papillary thyroid cancer and follicular thyroid cancer.

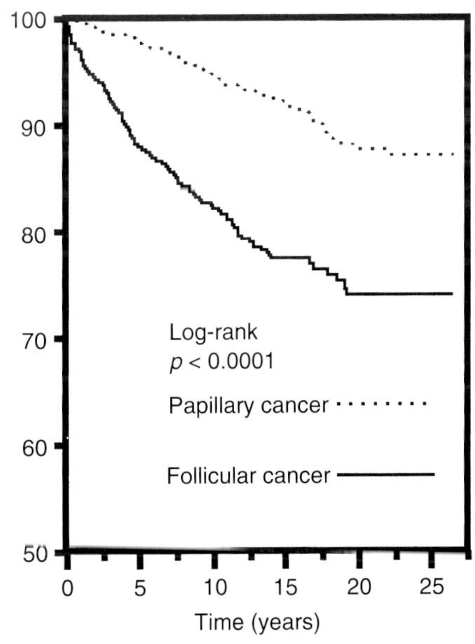

• **FIGURE 13-3** Disease-free survival curves in patients with papillary thyroid cancer and follicular thyroid cancer. There are significant differences in both disease-specific and disease-free survival rates between the two groups ($p < 0.0001$).

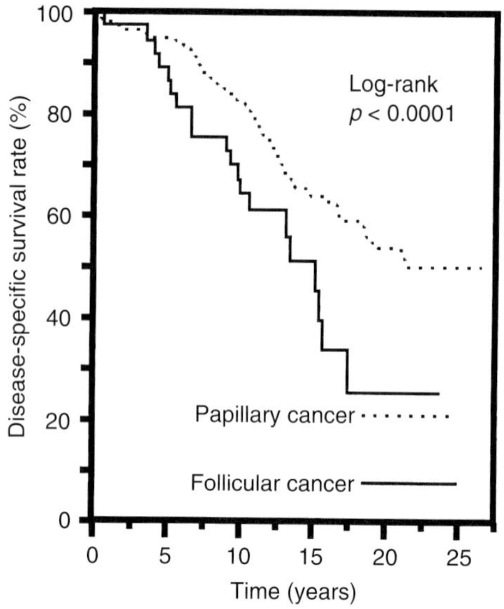

• **FIGURE 13-4** Disease-specific survival curves in patients with papillary and follicular thyroid cancer who developed metastasis.

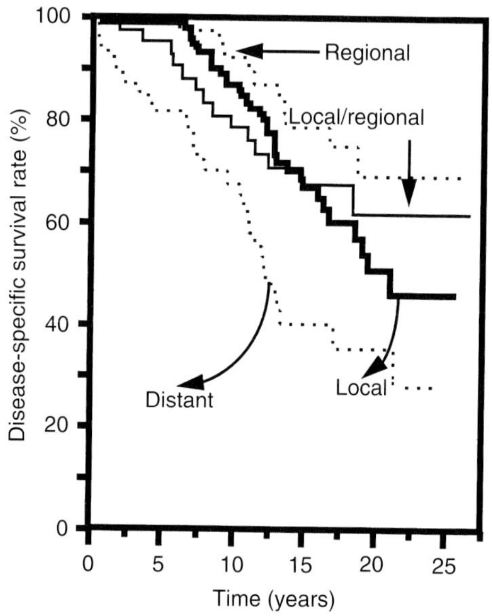

• **FIGURE 13-5** Disease-specific survival curves in patients with papillary thyroid cancer related to the first recurrent site.

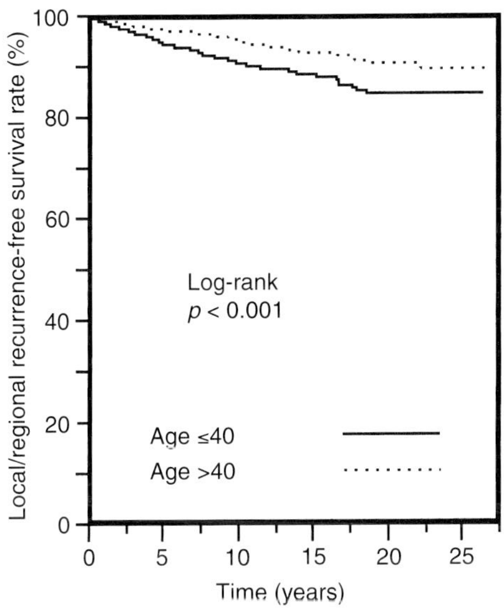

• **FIGURE 13-6** Local/regional recurrence-free survival curves in patients with papillary thyroid cancer related to age.

curves for 249 patients with recurrent papillary thyroid cancer after grouping them by the site of first recurrence. Figs. 13-6 through 13-8 show locoregional recurrence-free survival curves in patients with papillary thyroid cancer related to clinical factors and outcome of patients with recurrent thyroid cancer according to the site of first recurrence. Although some authors mentioned that postoperative recurrence limited to lymph nodes did not have an adverse affect on survival, a considerable number of patients with regional metastases as the first recurrence eventually presented with other recurrence sites (see Fig. 13-8, *A*). The results of univariate and multivariate analysis of risk factors for recurrence in the neck (locoregional) as the site of first recurrence are shown in Table 13-3. When univariate analysis was used, age, sex, tumor size, extracapsular adhesion/invasion, and gross nodal metastases were risk factors. When multivariate analysis was used, age, extracapsular adhesion/invasion, tumor size, and gross nodal metastasis remained significant predictors of survival, whereas sex no longer had a significant impact.

There is controversy about the influence of lymph node metastases on recurrence and survival in patients with papillary thyroid cancer. Our results suggest that lymph node involvement detected at initial surgery places patients in the high-risk group for locoregional recurrence.[4] Other authors have reported that the presence of clinical nodal metastases was associated

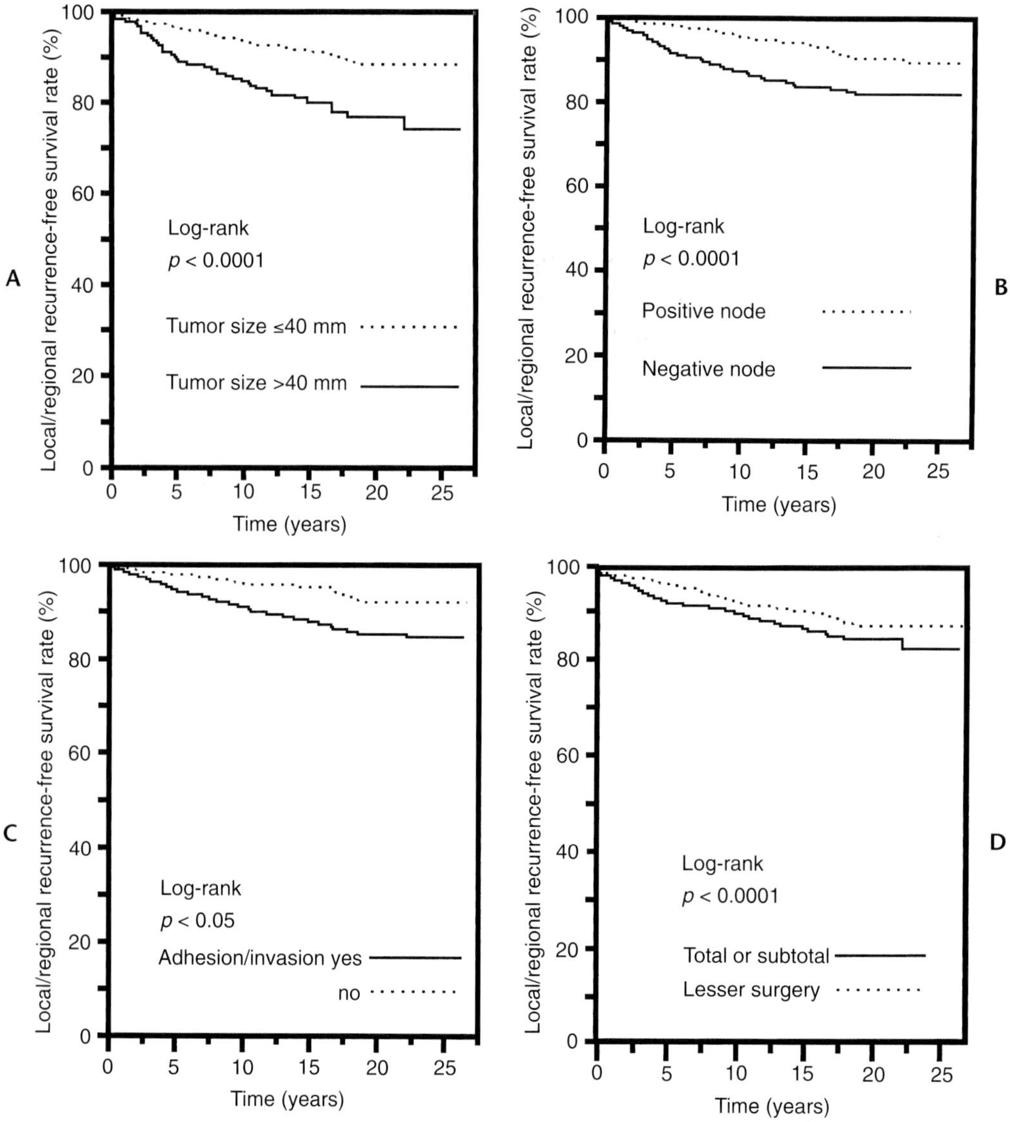

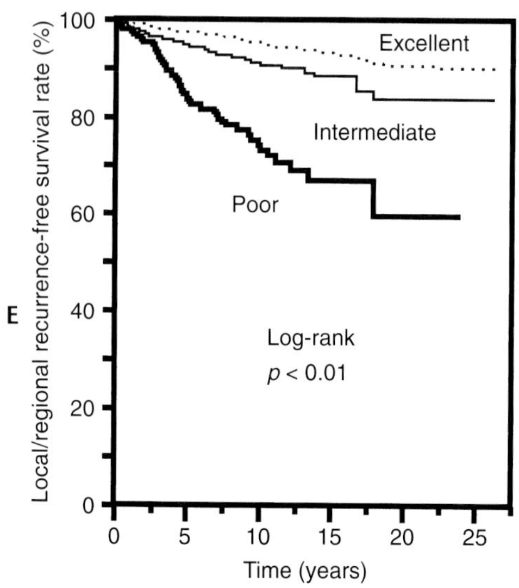

• **FIGURE 13-7** Local/regional recurrence-free survival curves in patients with papillary thyroid cancer according to the following groupings. **A,** By tumor size; **B,** by nodal involvement; **C,** By adhesion/ invasion; **D,** By extent of procedure; and **E,** By log-rank.

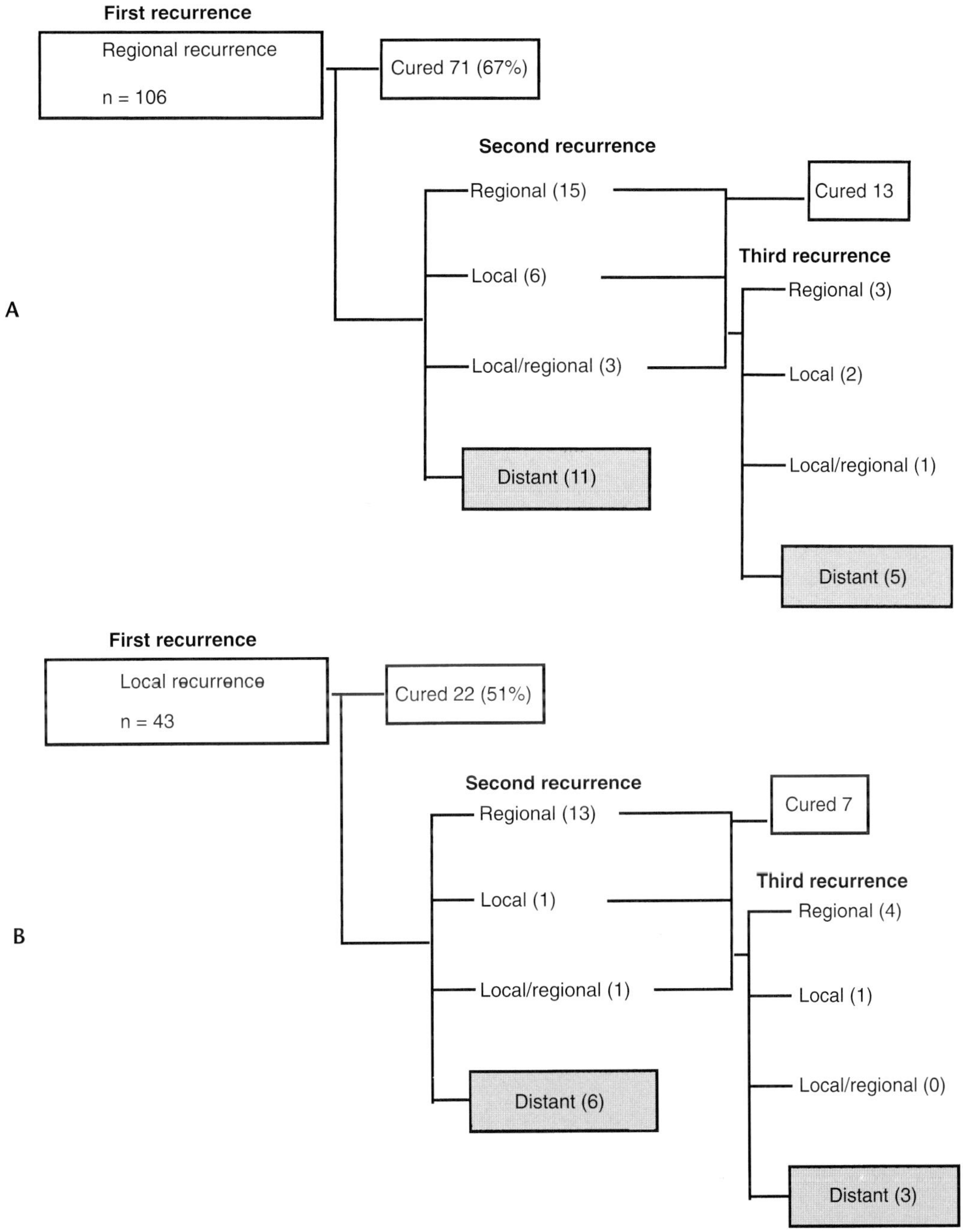

• **FIGURE 13-8** Outcome of patients with recurrent thyroid cancer according to site of first recurrence. **A,** Nineteen of 106 patients developed distant metastases during the study period. **B,** Twelve of 43 patients developed distant metastases during the study period.

Continued on p. 320.

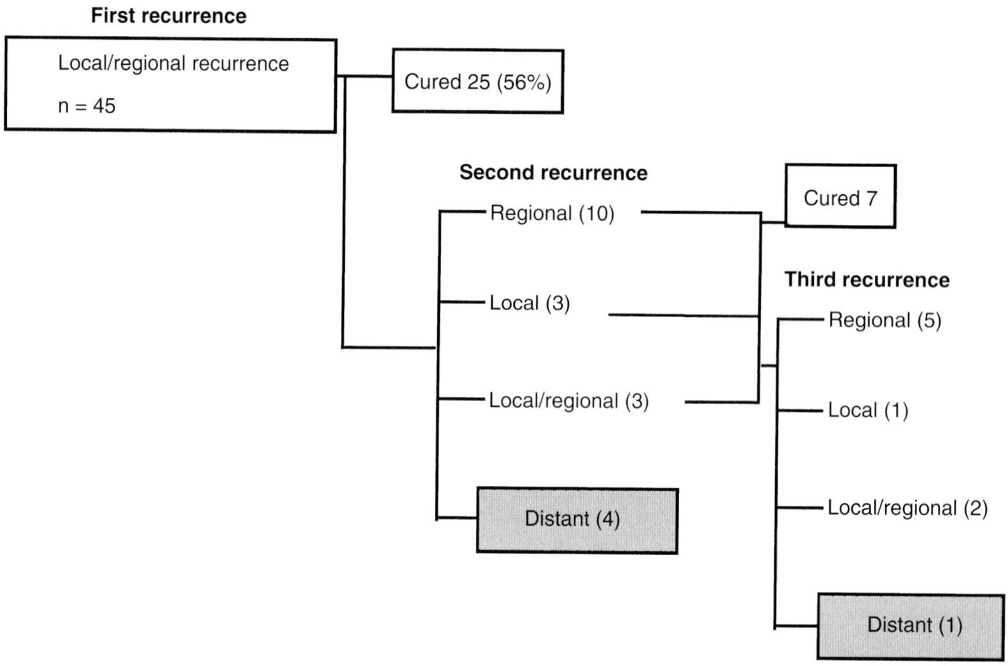

• **FIGURE 13-8 cont'd** C, Eight of 45 patients developed distant metastases during the study period.

with decreased survival rates[37,38] and with increased recurrence rates as well.[1,2,39-41] However, some studies have shown that the presence of nodal metastases has no adverse effect on survival[8,15,24] or may even be associated with an improved prognosis.[41-43]

One explanation would be that patients with clinically palpable metastases underwent more extensive surgical procedures, resulting in a prognosis comparable to that for patients without noticeable metastases. Alternatively, the results possibly depend on the percentage of younger patients included in the studied population, because more young patients present with clinically palpable nodal metastases despite having a better prognosis.

Extrathyroidal invasion/adhesion at the time of initial surgery predicts a worse prognosis. Our finding is in agreement with other studies that showed that the extrathyroidal spread of the tumor was associated with the highest risk of both recurrence and related death. Age was found to be the most important prognostic factor for local recurrence; this finding is in agreement

TABLE 13-3 Factors Affecting Local/Regional Recurrence-Free Survival in Univariate and Multivariate Analysis

Factor	No. of Patients	Univariate Analysis (*p* value)	Multivariate Analysis (*p* value)
Sex			
Males	169	0.017	0.105
Females	1734		
Age (yr)			
≤40	725	0.001	0.003
>40	1178		
Tumor size (mm)			
≤40	1664	0.0001	0.0001
>40	239		
Surgical procedure			
Total or subtotal	845	0.019	*
Lesser thyroidectomy	1055		
Multifocal			
No	1566	0.953	
Yes	337		
Adhesion/invasion			
No	1367	0.0001	0.005
Yes	536		
Gross nodal metastasis			
No	1207	0.0001	0.0001
Yes	696		

* Surgical procedure was not included in the multivariate analysis, because lesser thyroidectomies were employed for patients with an earlier tumor stage and had a significantly low rate of local recurrence.

with virtually all studies.[1,2,4-8,24,37,38,43-46] Some have stressed the importance of sex as one of the major determinants of outcome in patients with papillary thyroid cancer,[15,36,37] whereas others have reported that there are no significant differences between the sexes.[5,8] In our series, sex was found to be a significant risk factor for locoregional recurrence in univariate analysis, but not in multivariate analysis. As noted in Chapter 4, there was no significant difference in either recurrence or survival between the sexes in patients treated since 1970, contrary to our previous report based on patients treated between 1946 and 1971.[22] Therefore the discrepancy could be attributed to the difference in patient cohorts from one institution to another as well as the period for analysis.

TREATMENT OF LOCAL RECURRENT CANCER

Surgery

Patients with regional and/or local recurrent thyroid cancer should be treated surgically when this is technically possible. With regard to recurrence in the remnant thyroid gland, our results are described in Chapter 11. When patients present with distant metastasis in addition to the local/regional disease, completion thyroidectomy should be undertaken to use radioiodine to ablate metastatic deposits. Several studies have reported a higher complication rate in patients undergoing reoperation. When recurrent thyroid cancer is not resectable, other therapies should be considered and used, including radioiodine, external or intraoperative irradiation, and percutaneous ethanol injection therapy, based on the patient's quality of life and prognosis.

Postoperative Suppressive Therapy

Although no randomized trials are available for suppressive therapy using thyroxin as an adjunctive to surgical therapy, several studies have shown the beneficial effects of thyroid-stimulating hormone (TSH) suppression therapy.[5,46,47] We recommended thyroid hormone supplements for all patients, but suppressive doses were given only to patients with recurrent disease. Because there are adverse effects from TSH suppressive therapy,[48-52] we use this treatment only in patients who are likely to benefit from it. Because patients in low-risk groups do so well, it is difficult to demonstrate the benefit of TSH suppression therapy in this group. When TSH suppression therapy with thyroid hormones is indicated, bone mineral density and cardiac function should be carefully followed; bone metabolism and cardiac function are the main targets of subclinical hyperthyroidism.[48-52]

^{131}I Therapy

Radioiodine has been used as an adjunct to surgical therapy for ablation of remnant thyroid and to treat metastatic diseases. Some endocrinologists believe that the best method for minimizing recurrence and improving survival is total thyroidectomy with a postoperative ^{131}I whole-body scan to detect and treat metastatic diseases, and TSH suppressive therapy.[19] Although this approach theoretically seems appropriate, it has not been convincingly shown to decrease the recurrence rate or to improve overall survival. One reason is that the efficacy of radioiodine therapy depends on tumor uptake, and not all thyroid cancers concentrate radioiodine (up to 70% reported rate of uptake).[21] Older patients who are generally considered to be at higher risk also have tumors that tend to lose radioiodine avidity. Another issue is related to the occult recurrent diseases detected by the ^{131}I whole-body scan; these occult lesions would not appear as clinically recurrent cancer without any treatment.

At our institution, radioiodine therapy is used to treat patients with distant metastases and/or local recurrent tumors that are not surgically resectable. A disease diagnosed scintigraphically before it becomes palpable or symptomatic is more amenable to radioiodine therapy and some groups of patients can benefit from this aggressive therapy.[52,53] Approximately half the patients who present with a recurrence eventually die of thyroid cancer. Therefore another option to improve the outcome may be to adopt radioiodine therapy after completion thyroidectomy in addition to removing local recurrent tumors.

External-Beam Irradiation Therapy

External irradiation therapy has been used to treat patients with locally invasive, unresectable, or recurrent thyroid carcinomas that do not take up radioiodine. Tubiana et al.[54] reviewed 97 patients with differentiated thyroid carcinomas who received external radiotherapy after incomplete resection. Of the 97 patients, total survival rates were 78% and 57% at 5 and 15 years and disease-free survival rates were 58% and 39%, respectively. The incidence of local recurrence in those treated with adequate doses of radiation (50 Gy or more) was low with the probability of local recurrence being 11% at 15 years vs. 23% for patients treated with surgery alone, although the irradiated patients had larger and more extensive tumors. Simpson et al.[55] reported that local recurrence was highest among patients with papillary cancer treated by surgery alone (8.3%), compared with 5.6% for radioiodine, 6% for radiotherapy, and 3% for both therapies. However, Mazzaferri and Jhiang[5] reported that recurrence rates were highest following external radiation and lowest after ^{131}I. Thirty years after treatment, recurrence rates were 63% of 56 patients following external radiation, 40% of 151 patients following no medical therapy, 30% of 760 patients treated with thyroid hormone alone, and 15% of 388 patients treated with ^{131}I. An interpretation of this result is difficult, because these patients were treated according to the judgment of the attending physician without special protocols and external irradiation might have been used for patients with locally advanced tumors. In our series, most patients with local recurrence of cancer were treated with external irradiation (45 Gy for 5 weeks) following surgery.

CONCLUSION

Despite the excellent prognosis of most patients with papillary thyroid cancer, some of them have a recurrence, and approximately half of the patients who develop recurrence eventually die of the disease. Every effort should be made to improve survival of patients with recurrent disease, including early detection and complete resection of recurrent tumors, TSH suppression therapy, and adjuvant use of ^{131}I therapy, and external irradiation in high-risk patients. When patients present with distant metastasis in addition to the local/regional disease, completion thyroidectomy should be undertaken for the subsequent use of ^{131}I therapy. When the recurrent cancer is not resectable, other therapies, including radioiodine, external or intraoperative irradiation, and percutaneous ethanol injection therapy, should be used either singly or in combination.

REFERENCES

1. McCormick M et al. Natural history, treatment, and course of papillary thyroid carcinoma. J Clin Endocrinol Metab 71:414, 1990.
2. Samaan NA et al. The results of various modalities of treatment of well-differentiated thyroid carcinomas: A retrospective review of 1599 patients. J Clin Endocrinol Metab 75:714, 1992.
3. Hay ID et al. Predicting outcome in papillary thyroid carcinoma: Development of a reliable prognostic scoring system in a cohort of 1779 patients surgically treated at one institution during 1940 through 1989. Surgery 114:1050, 1993.
4. Noguchi S, Murakami N, Kawamoto H. Classification of papillary cancer of the thyroid based on prognosis. World J Surg 18:552, 1994.
5. Mazzaferri EL, Jhiang SM. Long-term impact of initial surgical and medical therapy on papillary and follicular thyroid cancer. Am J Med 97:418, 1994.
6. Cady B et al. Risk factor analysis in differentiated thyroid cancer. Cancer 43:810, 1979.
7. Tennvall J et al. Is the EORTC prognostic index of thyroid cancer valid in differentiated thyroid carcinoma? Retrospective multivariate analysis of differentiated thyroid carcinoma with long follow-up. Cancer 57:1405, 1986.
8. Simpson WJ et al. Papillary and follicular thyroid cancer. Prognostic factors in 1,578 patients. Am J Med 83:479, 1987.
9. Cady B, Rossi R. An expanded view of risk-group definition in differentiated thyroid carcinoma. Surgery 104:947, 1988.
10. Shaha AR, Loree TR, Shah JP. Intermediate-risk group for differentiated carcinoma of thyroid. Surgery 116:1036, 1994.
11. Anderson P, Dische S. Local tumor control and the subsequent incidence of distant metastatic disease. Int J Radiat Oncol Biol Phys 7:1645, 1981.
12. Suit H. Potential for improving survival rates for the cancer patient by increasing the efficacy of treatment of the primary lesion. Cancer 50:1227, 1982.
13. Asakawa H et al. Prognostic factors in patients with recurrent differentiated thyroid carcinoma. J Surg Oncol 64:202, 1997.
14. Wanebo HJ, Andrews W, Kaiser DL. Thyroid cancer: Some basic considerations. Cancer J Clin 33:87, 1983.

15. McConahey WM et al. Papillary thyroid cancer treated at the Mayo Clinic, 1946 through 1970: Initial manifestations, pathologic findings, therapy, and outcome. Mayo Clin Proc 61:978, 1986.
16. Grant CS et al. Local recurrence in papillary thyroid carcinoma: is extent of surgical resection important? Surgery 104:954, 1988.
17. Cady B. Papillary carcinoma of the thyroid. Semin Surg Oncol 7:81, 1991.
18. Perzik S. The place of total thyroidectomy in the management of 909 patients with thyroid disease. Am J Surg 132:480, 1976.
19. Clark OH. Total thyroidectomy: The treatment of choice for patients with differentiated thyroid cancer. Ann Surg 196:361, 1982.
20. Thompson NW. Total thyroidectomy in the treatment of thyroid carcinoma. In Thompson NW, Vinik AI, eds. Endocrine Surgery Update. New York: Grune & Stratton, 1983, pp 71-84.
21. Pacini F et al. Outcome of 309 patients with metastatic differentiated thyroid carcinoma treated with radioiodine. World J Surg 18:600, 1994.
22. Noguchi S, Murakami N. The value of lymph-node dissection in patients with differentiated thyroid cancer. Surg Clin North Am 67:251, 1987.
23. Cady B et al. Further evidence of the validity of risk group definition in differentiated thyroid carcinoma. Surgery 98:1171, 1985.
24. Hay ID et al. Ipsilateral lobectomy versus bilateral lobar resection in papillary thyroid carcinoma: A retrospective analysis of surgical outcome using a novel prognostic scoring system. Surgery 102:1088, 1987.
25. Noguchi S et al. Small carcinomas of the thyroid. A long-term follow-up of 867 patients. Arch Surg 131:187, 1996.
26. Ohnishi T et al. Detection of recurrent thyroid cancer: MR versus thallium-201 scintigraphy. Am J Neuroradiol 14:1051, 1993.
27. Auffermann W, Clark OH, Thurnher S, et al. Recurrent thyroid carcinoma: characteristics on MR images. Radiology 168:753-757, 1988.
28. Harvey RD et al. Measurement of serum thyroglobulin is of value in detecting tumour recurrence following treatment of differentiated thyroid carcinoma by lobectomy. Br J Surg 77:324, 1990.
29. Ruiz GJ et al. Thyroglobulin level as a predictive factor of tumoral recurrence in differentiated thyroid cancer. J Nucl Med 32:395, 1991.
30. Wyngaarden KV, McDougall IR. Is serum thyroglobulin a useful marker for thyroid cancer in patients who have not had ablation of residual thyroid tissue? Thyroid 7:343, 1997.
31. Ladurner D et al. Tumor recurrence at the neck in papillary thyroid gland cancer. A statistical analysis of the recurrence probability after radical surgery. Langenbecks Arch Chir 376:203, 1991.
32. Herrera MF et al. Papillary thyroid carcinoma in Mexican patients: Clinical aspects and prognostic factors. World J Surg 20:94, 1996.
33. Zimmerman D et al. Papillary thyroid carcinoma in children and adults: Long-term follow-up of 1039 patients conservatively treated at one institution during three decades. Surgery 104:1157, 1988.
34. Franssila KO. Is the differentiation between papillary and follicular thyroid carcinoma valid? Cancer 32:853, 1973.
35. Harness JK et al. Deaths due to differentiated thyroid cancer: A 46-year perspective. World J Surg 12:623, 1988.

36. Shaha AR, Shah JP, Loree TR. Patterns of nodal and distant metastasis based on histologic varieties in differentiated carcinoma of the thyroid. Am J Surg 172:692, 1996.
37. Tubiana M et al. Long-term results and prognostic factors in patients with differentiated thyroid carcinoma. Cancer 55:794, 1985.
38. Scheumann GF et al. Prognostic significance and surgical management of locoregional lymph node metastases in papillary thyroid cancer. World J Surg 18:559, 1994.
39. Kerr DJ et al. Prognostic factors in thyroid tumours. Br J Cancer 54:475, 1986.
40. McHenry CR, Rosen IB, Walfish PG. Prospective management of nodal metastases in differentiated thyroid cancer. Am J Surg 162:353, 1991.
41. Vickery AJ, Wang CA, Walker AM. Treatment of intrathyroidal papillary carcinoma of the thyroid. Cancer 60:2587, 1987.
42. Franssila KO. Prognosis in thyroid carcinoma. Cancer 36:1138, 1975.
43. Cady B et al. Changing clinical, pathologic, therapeutic, and survival patterns in differentiated thyroid carcinoma. Ann Surg 184:541, 1976.
44. Cady B et al. The effect of thyroid hormone administration upon survival in patients with differentiated thyroid carcinoma. Surgery 94:978, 1983.
45. Brooks JR et al. Surgical therapy for thyroid carcinoma: A review of 1249 solitary thyroid nodules. Surgery 104:940, 1988.
46. Dinneen SF et al. Distant metastases in papillary thyroid carcinoma: 100 cases observed at one institution during 5 decades. J Clin Endocrinol Metab 80:2041, 1995.
47. Clark OH. TSH suppression in the management of thyroid nodules and thyroid cancer. World J Surg 5:39, 1981.
48. Taelman P et al. Reduced forearm bone mineral content and biochemical evidence of increased bone turnover in women with euthyroid goitre treated with thyroid hormone. Clin Endocrinol 33:107, 1990.
49. Woeber KA. Thyrotoxicosis and the heart. N Engl J Med 327:94, 1992.
50. Biondi B et al. Cardiac effects of long term thyrotropin-suppressive therapy with levothyroxine. J Clin Endocrinol Metab 77:334, 1993.
51. Biondi B et al. Impaired cardiac reserve and exercise capacity in patients receiving long-term thyrotropin suppressive therapy with levothyroxine. J Clin Endocrinol Metab 81:4224, 1996.
52. Uzzan B et al. Effects on bone mass of long term treatment with thyroid hormones: A meta-analysis. J Clin Endocrinol Metab 81:4278, 1996.
53. Schlumberger M et al. Long-term results of treatment of 283 patients with lung and bone metastases from differentiated thyroid carcinoma. J Clin Endocrin Metab 63:960, 1986.
54. Tubiana M et al. External radiotherapy in thyroid cancers. Cancer 55:2061, 1985.
55. Simpson WJ et al. Papillary and follicular thyroid cancer: Impact of treatment in 1578 patients. Int J Radiat Oncol Biol Phys 14:1063, 1988.

CHAPTER

14

Multidisciplinary Treatment of Nonresectable Differentiated Thyroid Carcinoma

SHIN WATANABE, M.D.
SHIRO NOGUCHI, M.D., Ph.D.

The percentage of noncurative operations for differentiated thyroid carcinoma tends to increase with patient age. In our series of 5110 patients with papillary carcinoma treated between 1946 and 1996, the rate was 2.4% in patients aged 60 years or younger, 6.3% in patients from 61 to 70 years of age, and 18.6% in those older than 70 years of age. The higher rate of recurrence in older patients could be partially explained by the more extensive disease at presentation. For older patients, more extensive surgical resection was generally used, because the recurrence often involved local or distant metastases. Unfortunately, when patients were treated more aggressively because of more advanced disease, there was more postoperative morbidity.

During the past five decades we have observed a changing presentation of differentiated thyroid carcinoma in our patients, including age, tumor size, and extent of disease. The mean age of patients at first visit increased from 38 years in the 1940s to 53 years in the 1990s. It is anticipated that this trend will continue; therefore a therapeutic approach needs to be established for patients with nonresectable differentiated thyroid carcinoma, particularly in older patients (over 45 years of age) who are known to have a worse prognosis.

We generally use radioactive iodine (radioiodine) and external radiation therapy for patients who undergo noncurative surgery; these therapies can be used separately or in combination. We use intraoperative radiation therapy (IORT) and/or percutaneous ethanol injection therapy (PEIT) for patients with locally advanced unresectable tumors. In this chapter, we will describe our experience using these therapies combined with radioiodine treatment and/or arterial infusion chemotherapy for the management of unresectable invasive thyroid carcinoma and will report on our results with this treatment.

PATIENT CHARACTERISTICS

Patients undergoing noncurative surgery are classified into the following three groups based on the spread of thyroid carcinoma at the initial treatment: group 1, patients presenting with distant metastases; group 2, patients presenting with unresectable tumor in the neck without distant metastases; and group 3, patients presenting with both locally advanced nonresectable carcinoma and distant metastases. Patients suspected of having microscopic residual tumor after surgery were excluded.

Patients whose tumors take up radioiodine after total thyroidectomy and appropriate lymph node dissection should be treated with ^{131}I. Almost 42% to 63% of metastatic thyroid cancer in patients in Japan and up to 80% in the United States take up enough radioiodine for this treatment to be effective.[1-4] Radioiodine therapy is less effective for patients in groups 2 and 3, because radioiodine does not accumulate in the tumor until the normal thyroid tissue has been removed, and radioiodine treatment rarely eradicates large masses. External irradiation therapy is limited to patients with gross thyroid carcinoma.

Since 1987 and 1990, we have used PEIT with IORT, respectively. Multidisciplinary treatment using these therapies combined with radioiodine therapy and/or arterial infusion chemotherapy has been used since 1992. The goal of multidisciplinary treatment is to eradicate locally advanced tumor to improve the prognosis of patients and their quality of life.

THERAPIES

Percutaneous Ethanol Injection Therapy

PEIT has been used effectively for treating patients with hepatocellular carcinoma.[5-9] The injection of absolute ethanol directly into the tumor denatures cellular proteins with embolization of coagulated serum protein.[5] Porter in

1908 was the first to use PEIT for a patient with Graves' disease.[10] Results were inconsistent, and the procedure was basically abandoned.

Since the advent of ultrasound imaging, PEIT has again received attention as an alternative to surgery or radioiodine ablation for the treatment of patients with autonomous thyroid nodules.[11-15] It has also been used as sclerotherapy for thyroid cysts.[16-18] However, there have only been a few reports on the use of PEIT for patients with thyroid carcinoma.[19-22] The initial reports suggest that this therapy is effective in patients with unresectable thyroid carcinoma. PEIT appears to be applicable for most patients with unresectable thyroid carcinoma and for patients with superficial metastatic tumors identified by either palpation or ultrasonography, regardless of the number of tumors.

We perform PEIT under ultrasonographic guidance using a 7.5 MHz probe. Our PEIT procedure is as follows:

1. The patient is premedicated with antipyretic analgesic or pentazocine and then given lidocaine (0.5%).
2. A 5 or 10 ml syringe equipped with an extension tube and a 22-gauge needle is used.
3. After the needle is inserted into the tumor, 0.5 to about 10 ml of 99% ethanol is injected slowly, depending on the size of the tumor and the resistance pressure in injecting the site. The site of ethanol infusion is recognized as a hyperechoic area (Fig. 14-1). In patients with large tumors, ethanol is injected at several different sites of the tumor in one session.
4. The most important points are to stop the injection as soon as the patient complains of pain and to diminish the inside pressure of the tumor by leaving the needle alone in the tumor for several minutes after the injection. This procedure enables some ethanol to leak out from the needle and decreases the risk of skin necrosis resulting from this leakage of ethanol into the subcutaneous tissue along the needle tract.
5. PEIT is usually done two or three times per week until a satisfactory result is obtained.

Occasionally a patient may suffer from severe pain during the injection, as a result of leakage of injected ethanol into the surrounding normal tissue. In such a patient, a local anesthetic is usually insufficient for pain control, and further therapy is not used during the same session. We have recently tried PEIT or intraoperative ethanol injection therapy with the patient under general anesthesia, injecting a large amount of ethanol from multiple needle insertions in one treatment session.

PEIT may cause some sensorimotor or autonomic nerve paralysis if the ethanol comes in contact with nerves. One of our 18 patients treated by PEIT developed transient Horner's syndrome and another had recurrent

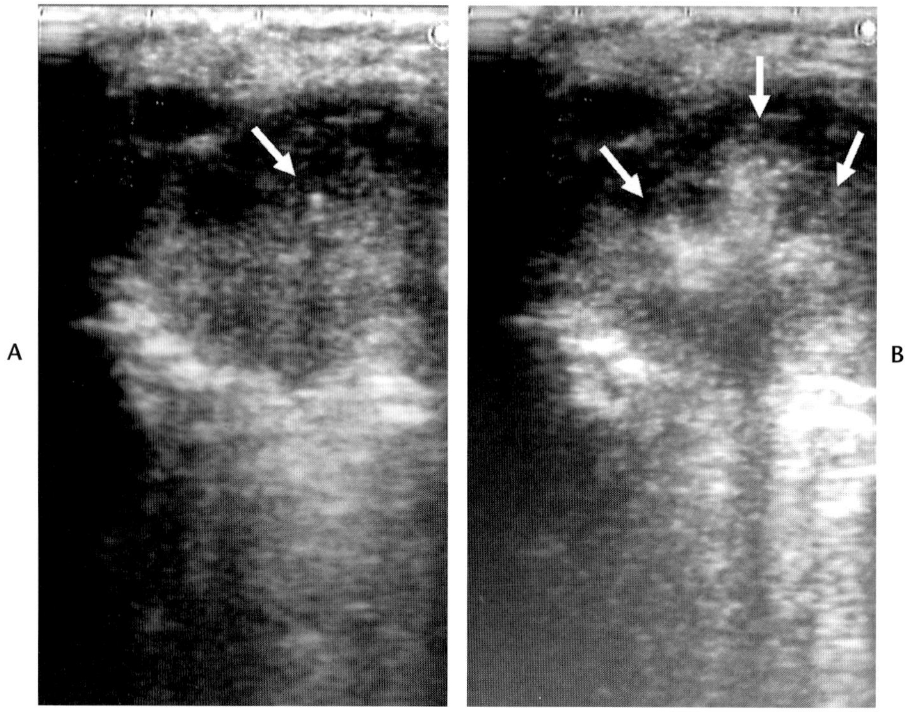

• **FIGURE 14-1** Ultrasonography of injecting ethanol. **A,** A needle is inserted into the tumor; a small, high echoic point can be seen *(arrow);* **B,** 1 ml of ethanol is injected. A penetrated part was recognized as a high echoic area *(arrows).*

nerve paralysis. Such complications would probably increase if patients were treated by larger amounts of ethanol under general anesthesia. For this reason, careful observation under ultrasonographic guidance in patients who are under general anesthesia is recommended during ethanol injections.

Edema and hemorrhage around tumors can occur after PEIT. Patients with a large tumor adjacent to the trachea can develop airway obstruction; therefore, after PEIT, administration of a prophylactic corticosteroid or a tracheotomy is recommended. Skin necrosis may also be induced by ethanol leakage into the subcutaneous tissues along the needle tract.

Case 1

The patient was a 78-year-old Japanese man who had undergone a subtotal thyroidectomy with modified radical neck dissection in 1990 and surgical resection for recurrent lymph node disease in 1992. He received radioiodine therapy (100 mCi) after the discovery of lung metastases in 1995. In 1996, he presented with a large tumor extending from the submandibular region

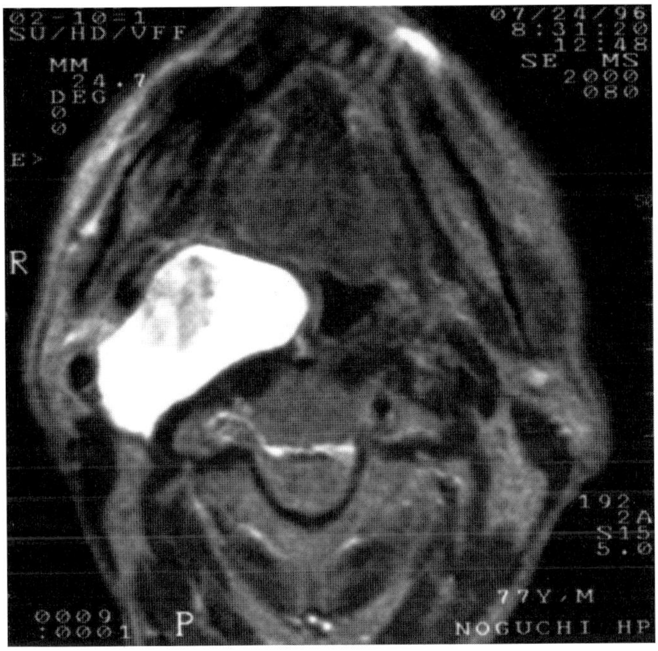

• **FIGURE 14-2** T2-weighted image on MRI of the tumor before PEIT.

to the pharynx, which resulted in severe airway compression (Fig. 14-2). The patient was successfully treated with PEIT twice (total dose, 17 ml) in August 1996 and radioiodine therapy (100 mCi). The airway compression was improved after a transient deterioration by local edema of surrounding tissue induced by PEIT (Fig. 14-3). His serum thyroglobulin level decreased from 1340 to 212 ng/ml.

Case 2

The patient was a 60-year-old Japanese woman who had locally advanced thyroid carcinoma (maximum diameter of the tumor, 110 mm) at presentation (Fig. 14-4). She was treated with IORT (20 Gy) in November 1993 (Fig. 14-5) and PEIT (total dose, 183 ml) from June to October 1994 (Fig. 14-6). A large skin defect (50 × 50 mm) developed during PEIT as a result of leakage of ethanol into the subcutaneous tissue after most of the tumor changed to necrotic tissue. However, her wound recovered completely on February 1995 (Fig. 14-7). Her serum thyroglobulin level decreased from 10,200 ng/ml to normal range (less than 55 ng/ml) and thereafter increased to 217 ng/ml. Radioiodine therapy and PEIT were given for her residual neck cancer and developing lung metastases during her course of treatment.

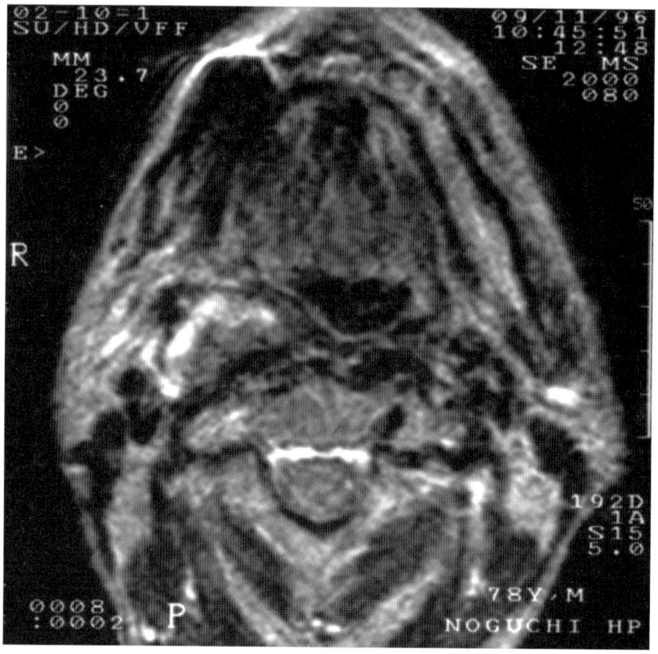

• **FIGURE 14-3** T2-weighted image on MRI after PEIT.

A

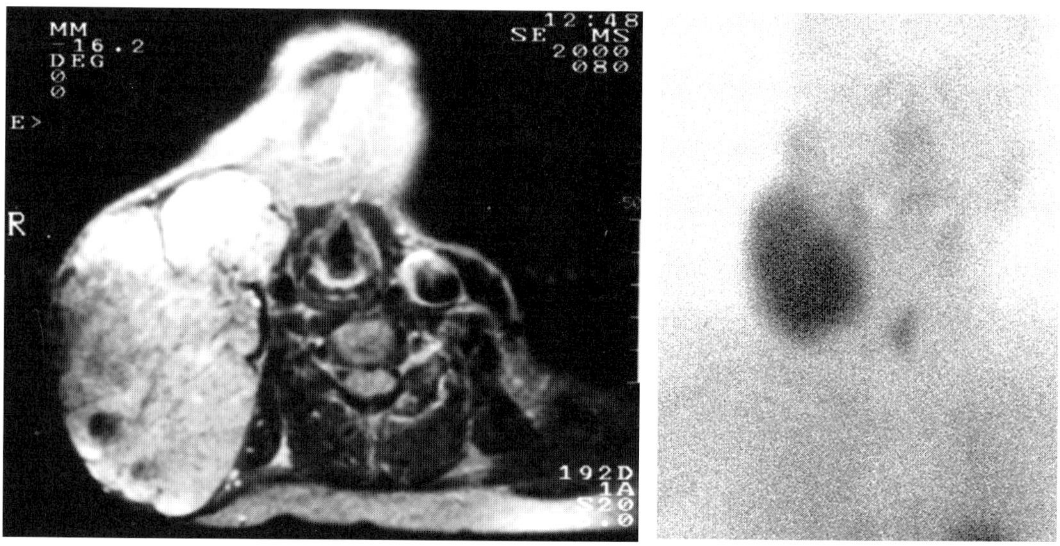

B

• **FIGURE 14-4** **A,** T2-weighted image on MRI at presentation; **B,** ^{201}T1 scintigraphy (early image) at presentation.

A

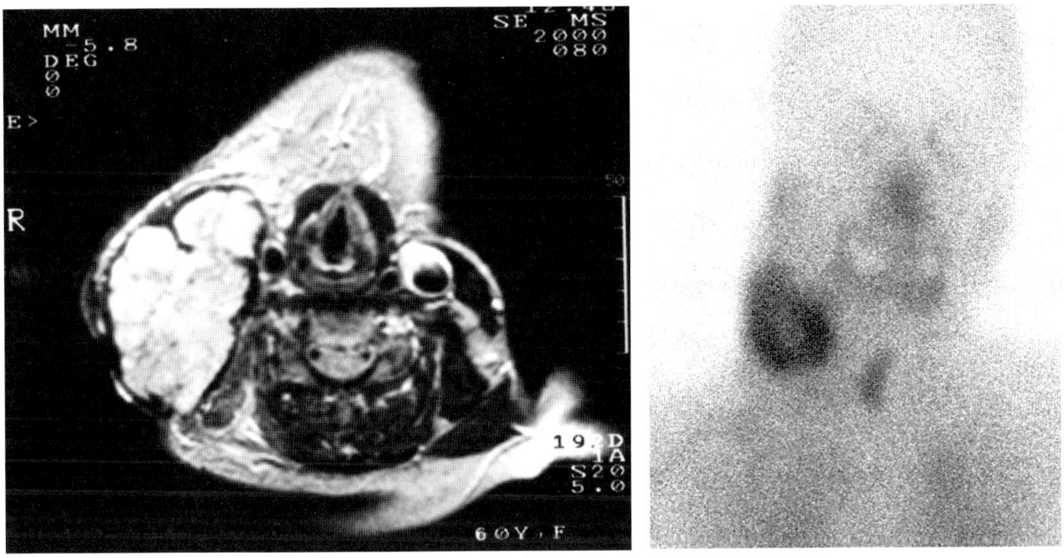

B

• **FIGURE 14-5** **A,** T2-weighted image on MRI after IORT; **B,** ^{201}T1 scintigraphy (early image) after IORT.

A

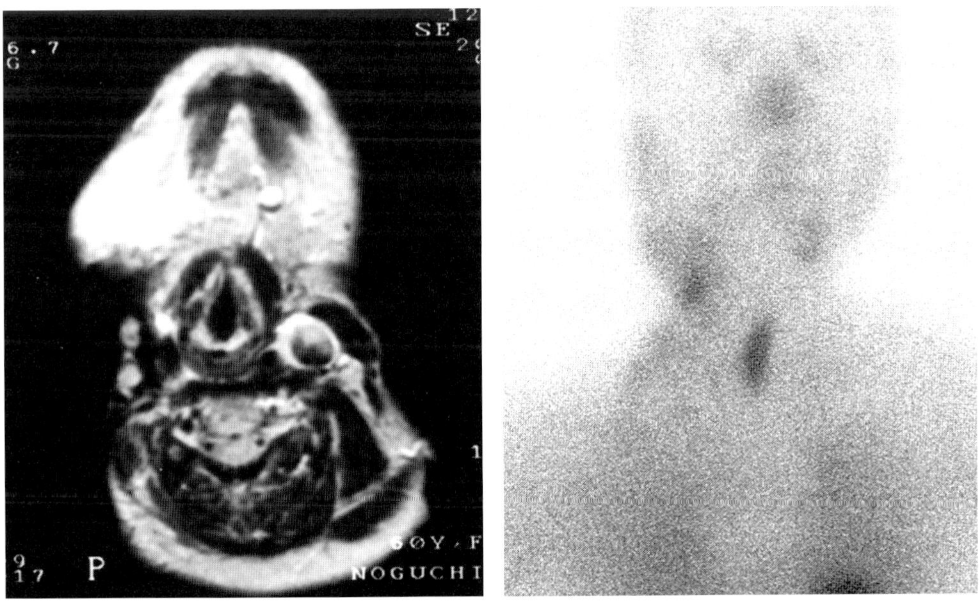

B

• **FIGURE 14-6** **A,** T2-weighted image on MRI after IORT and PEIT; **B,** ^{201}T1 scintigraphy (early image) after IORT and PEIT.

A

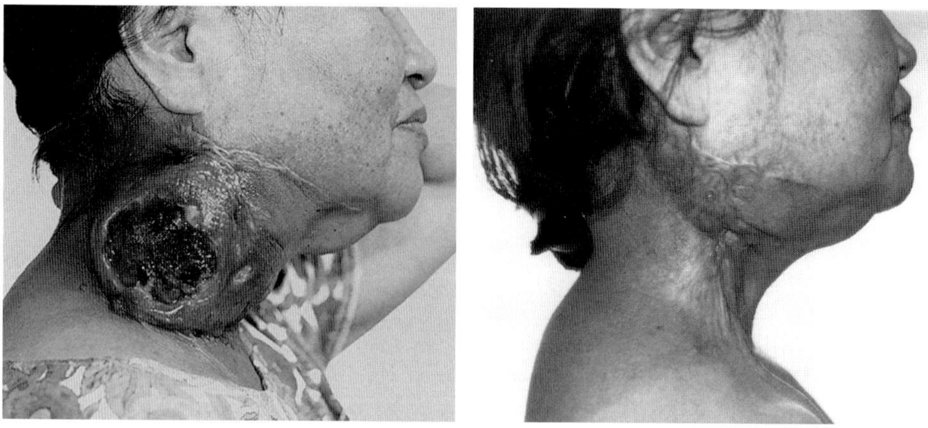

B

• **FIGURE 14-7** **A,** Large skin defect during PEIT; **B,** about 4 months after PEIT.

Intraoperative Radiotherapy

IORT is occasionally used in patients with carcinoma of the pancreas, digestive tract, urinary system, and other organs.[23-27] Tumoricidal radiation can be delivered by IORT to eradicate tumors completely. There are a few reports of IORT applied for differentiated thyroid carcinoma, in which 4 to 10 Gy of radiation was delivered after surgery and combined with postoperative external radiation or other therapies.[28,29] The target of IORT was mainly control of the local diseases after surgery for patients with microscopic residual disease at the resection margins. We have mainly used IORT for patients with unresectable bulky thyroid tumors.[3] We usually treat patients who have microscopic residual disease after thyroidectomy with external radiation therapy. Simpson et al.[30] reported that 90% of patients treated with postoperative radiation for microscopic residual papillary carcinoma became disease free.

An electron beam is commonly used for IORT to the superficial tumor after resection. However, we used x-ray from a 4 MeV linear accelerator because we considered x-ray therapy to be more suitable for our patient with a large tumor.

Our IORT procedure is as follows:

1. The area and angle of radiation are determined by the size of tumor and its anatomic relation to the vertebrae by routine x-ray examination and magnetic resonance imaging (MRI).
2. We make a skin flap at the site of the tumor to avoid the radiation dermatitis; a single dose of 15 to 25 Gy is delivered to the tumor.

We do not recommend using IORT for tumors in the central part of the neck because of the risk of radiation injury to the trachea, esophagus, and/or spinal cord, which is the organ most sensitive to radiation. Doses higher than 40 Gy may lead to radiation myelitis and paraplegia. In cases in which IORT is used for treatment of thyroid carcinoma in a submandibular lesion, great care should be taken to avoid radiation injury to the cerebellum and the mucous membranes of the oral cavity.

Tochner et al.[31] reported that an IORT dose of 25 Gy or more resulted in severe, prolonged, life-threatening esophagitis. Peripheral neuropathy has been reported after IORT using more than 20 Gy.[32] Powers et al.[33] irradiated the para-aortic region of beagle dogs with between 15 and 55 Gy intraoperatively using an electron beam; they observed a 50% decrease in the percentage of muscle fibers in cases of radiation over 20 Gy. We have not experienced these adverse effects of IORT, although our follow-up period is relatively short (mean follow-up, 20.5 months; range 1 to 57 months).

Case 3

The patient was a 68-year-old man who had previously undergone surgery for a papillary thyroid carcinoma at another hospital in 1991 and in 1995. He had large invasive tumors (maximum diameter, 70 mm) on the right side of the neck with mediastinum metastases (Fig. 14-8). The upper tumor was treated by PEIT alone (total dose, 21.5 ml) and the lower tumor was treated by both IORT (20 Gy) and intraoperative ethanol injection therapy (dose, 16.5 ml). Two months later he received radioiodine therapy (100 mCi). After these therapies, the tumor clearly decreased in size and ^{201}T1 scanning revealed uptake in a small part near the trachea (Fig. 14-9). His serum thyroglobulin level decreased from 2700 to 123 ng/ml. Repeat PEIT and radioiodine therapy are planned for the residual tumor.

Arterial Infusion Chemotherapy

There have been very few controlled studies using chemotherapy for the treatment of differentiated thyroid carcinoma. Several single agents such as doxorubicin, bleomycin, and cisplatin, as well as multiple combination regimens, have been evaluated for efficacy, but interpretation of the results is limited by the small number of treated patients. We have treated two patients with arterial infusion chemotherapy. These patients were evaluated by arteriography to determine whether the thyroid carcinoma could be removed because involvement of the common carotid artery was suggested by ultrasonography and MRI. Arterial infusion chemotherapy was performed for this unresectable tumor because of the presence of major feeding arterial vessels. Because of our use of IORT and PEIT, we have only limited experience with arterial infusion chemotherapy. Most tumors in our patients have several minor feeding arteries rather than a single major one, making arterial infusion chemotherapy less effective.

A B C

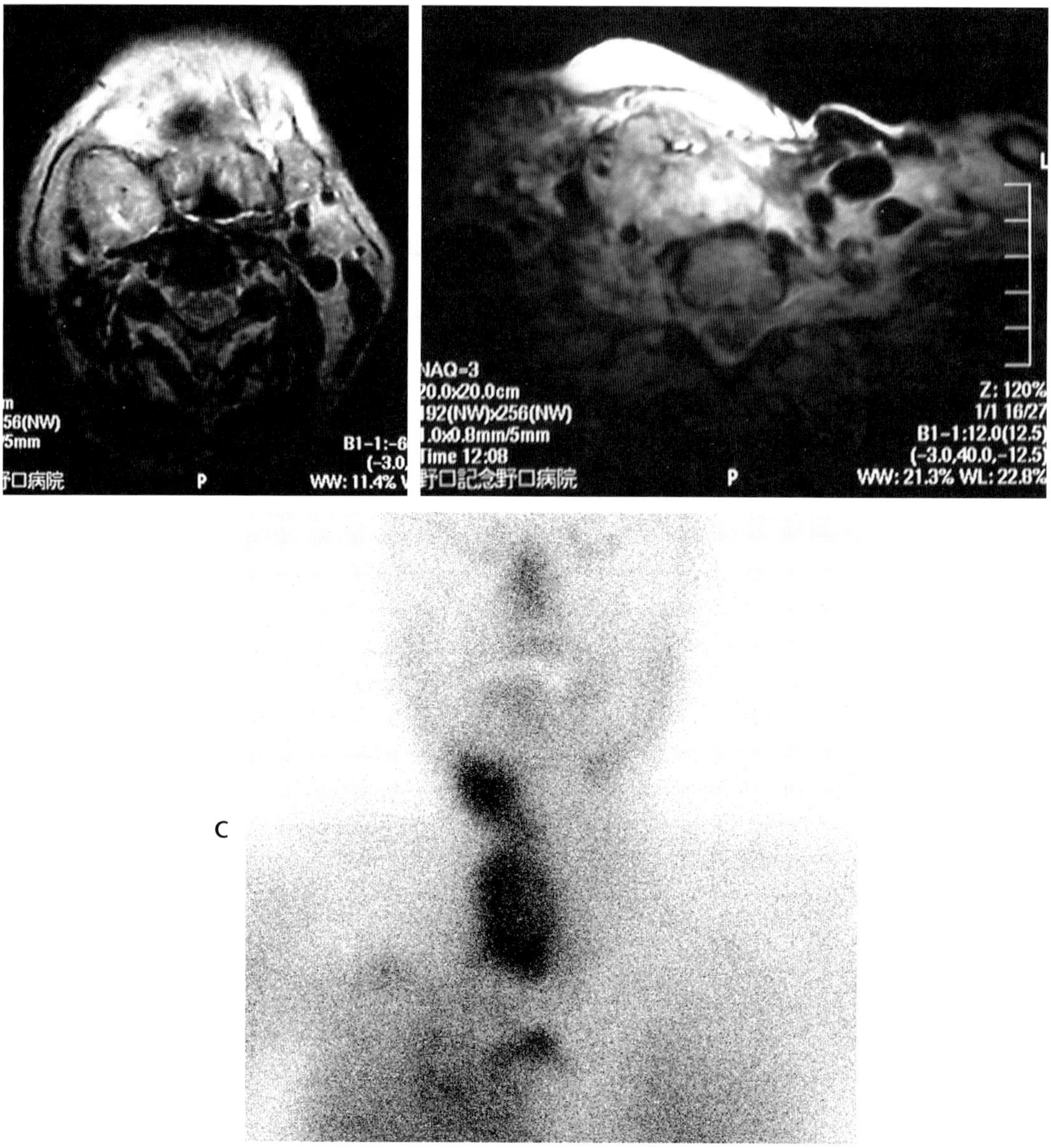

• **FIGURE 14-8** **A,** T2-weighted image on MRI of upper tumor before PEIT. **B,** T2-weighted image on MRI of lower tumor before IORT and PEIT; **C,** ^{201}T1 scintigraphy (early image) before multidisciplinary treatment.

Case 4

The patient was a 60-year-old woman who had unresectable invasive 70 mm thyroid carcinoma without distant metastasis when first seen (Fig. 14-10). During a period of 10 months, five sessions of arterial infusion chemotherapy were performed, and cystic degeneration of the tumor was observed. She was subsequently treated with IORT (20 Gy) and PEIT (total dose,

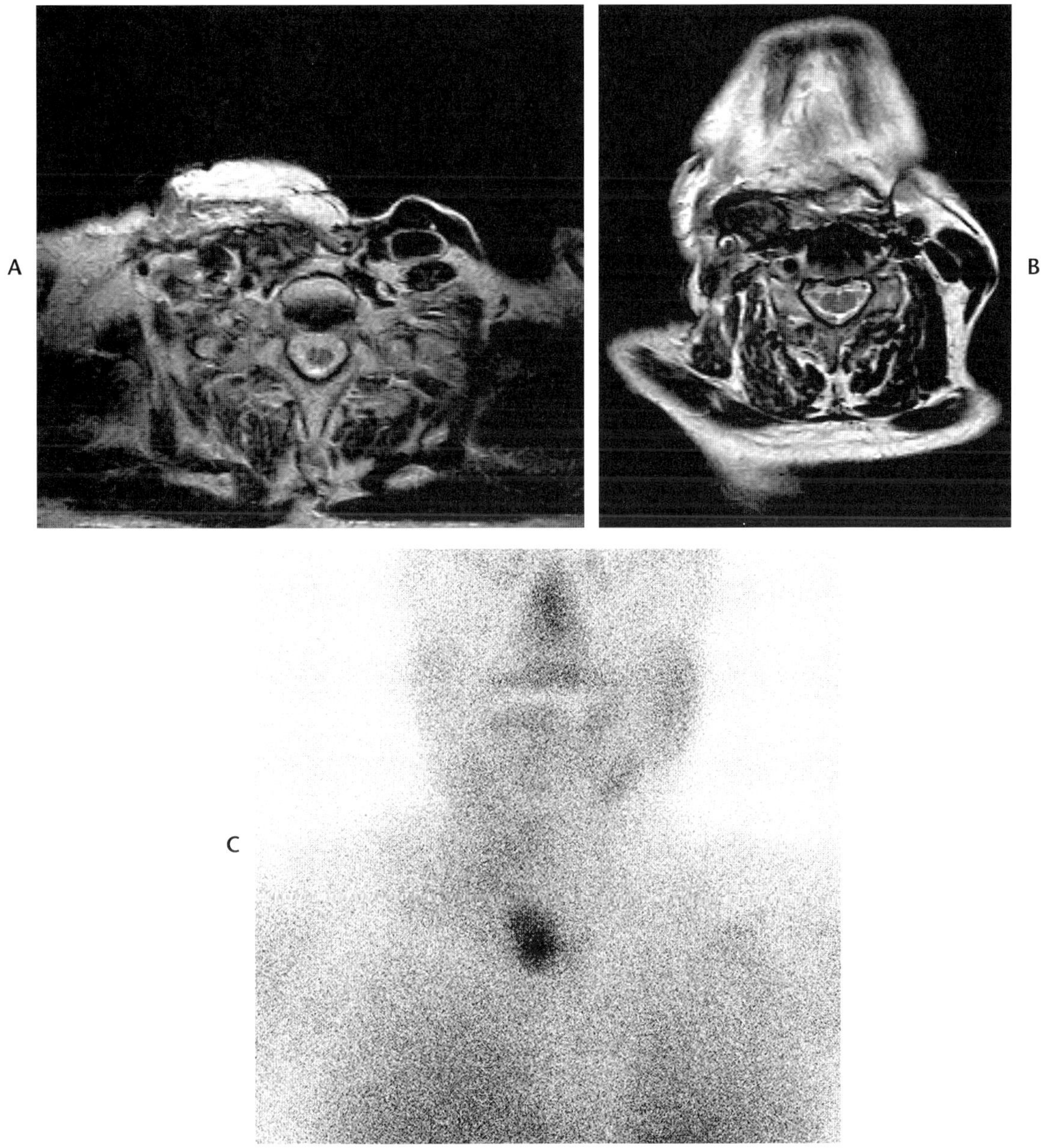

• **FIGURE 14-9** **A,** T2-weighted image on MRI of upper tumor after PEIT; **B,** T2-weighted image on MRI of lower tumor after IORT and PEIT; **C,** ^{201}T1 scintigraphy (early image) after multidisciplinary treatment.

160.5 ml). Although the size of the tumor did not change on MRI, there was no longer accumulation of ^{201}T1 and aspiration cytology failed to demonstrate any carcinoma cells (Fig. 14-11). During the 15-month period of treatment, her serum thyroglobulin level decreased from 25,400 to 212 ng/ml and she is considered to have achieved a complete remission.

A

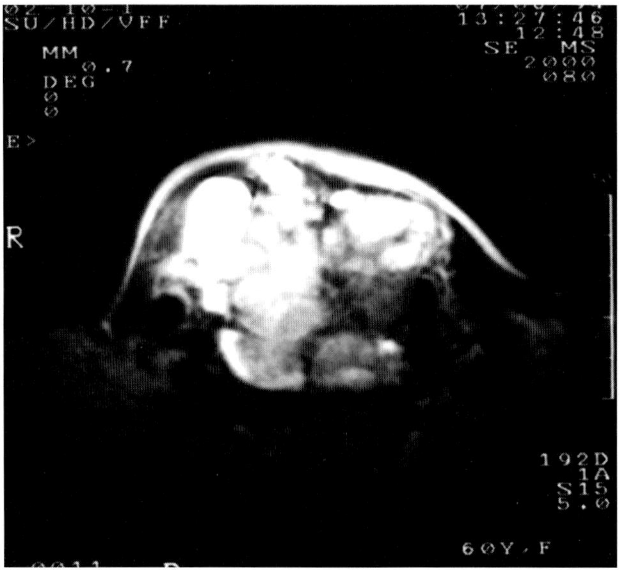

B

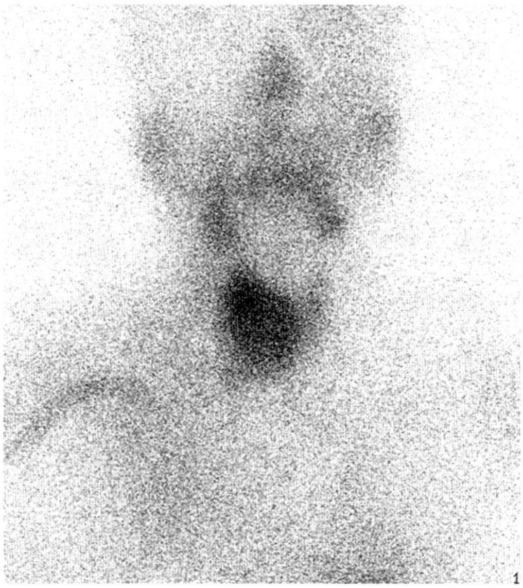

• **FIGURE 14-10** **A,** T2-weighted image on MRI at presentation; **B,** ^{201}T1 scintigraphy (early image) at presentation.

A

B

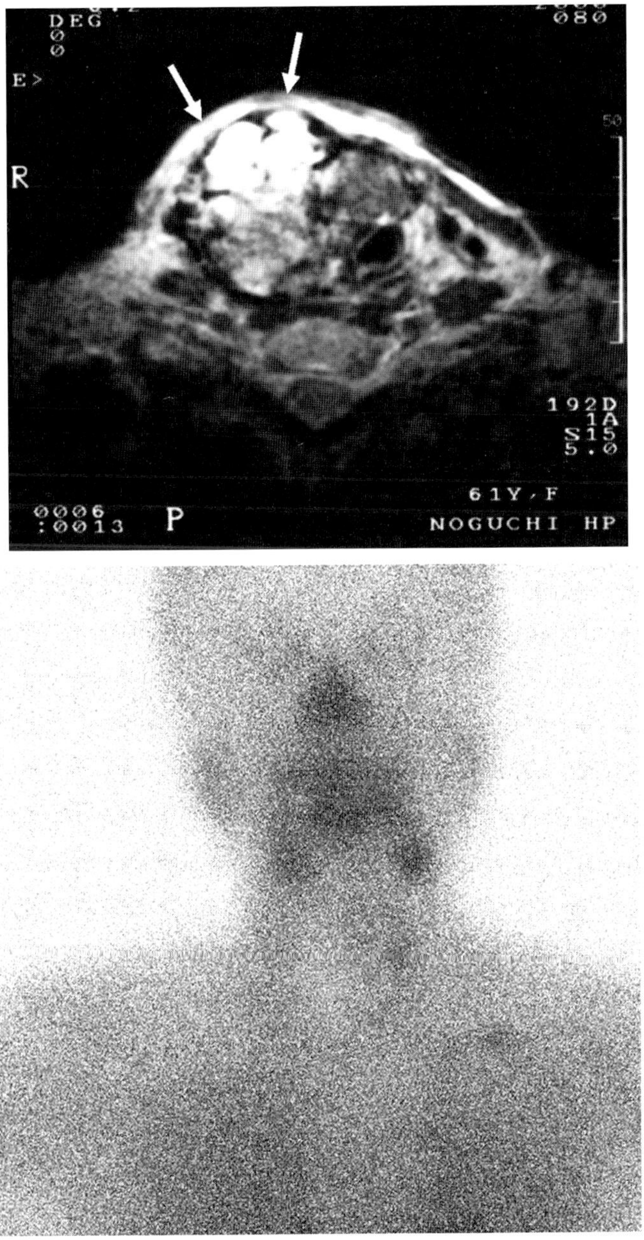

• **FIGURE 14-11** A, T2-weighted image on MRI after multidisciplinary treatment. The high signal area is the cystic part *(arrows)*, B, ^{201}T1 scintigraphy (early image) after multidisciplinary treatment.

EFFICACY OF MULTIDISCIPLINARY TREATMENT

Since 1990 we have evaluated the size and the viability of the carcinoma cells using ^{201}T1 scintigraphy and MRI as well as serum thyroglobulin measurements. Thyroid carcinoma generally has an extremely high signal on T2-weighted images and contrast enhancement on T1-weighted images using gadolinium on MRI. During treatment with IORT and PEIT, thyroid carcinoma sometimes became necrotic. We can therefore recognize what we believe is the viable part of the tumor using MRI. Accurate evaluation of the size of tumors after multidisciplinary treatment is sometimes difficult because of their various shapes. Successful effects of multidisciplinary treatment on the size of tumors were observed in all patients within a few months in our series. The time lag for the treatment and the effect can be explained by the time taken for the tumors to change to necrotic tissue after treatment and then to be gradually absorbed. Therefore there were some patients whose tumors had no accumulation of ^{201}T1 by scintigraphy despite the remaining tumor mass.

MULTIDISCIPLINARY TREATMENT SERIES

Twenty-six patients with unresectable differentiated thyroid carcinoma were treated using multiple therapies from 1992 to March 1997. Twenty-four were women and two were men. Their average age was 69 years (range, 39 to 86 years). Eight patients had known distant metastases at the beginning of treatment and three patients developed distant metastases during treatment. Distant metastases were present in the lungs (six patients), in the mediastinum (four patients), and in the bone (one patient). Four patients were diagnosed as having unresectable tumors on first examination, 10 more were judged to be unresectable at the time of surgery and 12 patients became unresectable when they developed recurrent tumor. Of the 10 patients diagnosed at operation, five received either IORT or PEIT at the same time in their operation. The average follow-up was 20.5 months. We generally use IORT first, and PEIT is the second choice for most patients who require multiple therapies.

Nine patients were treated by PEIT, eight patients by IORT, and nine patients by both PEIT and IORT. Of the nine patients who received both PEIT and IORT, one patient had previously been treated with arterial infusion chemotherapy. Radioiodine treatment was employed in six patients

TABLE 14-1 MRI Evaluation (N = 24)

	Decrease of Size (%)	Degeneration (%)
Slight	15(62.5)	6 (25)
Moderate	5 (20.8)	12 (50)
Considerable	4 (16.7)	6 (25)

with distant metastases. Among patients receiving PEIT or intraoperative ethanol injection, 14 patients were treated once and four patients twice. The total dose ranged from 2 to 183 ml, and the frequency ranged from 1 to 44. The cancers ranged from 1.5 to 9 cm, and 15 patients had tumors larger than 5 cm. Fourteen patients underwent IORT once (the dose was 15 Gy in nine, 20 Gy in four, and 25 Gy in one), and the remaining three patients received IORT twice (the total dose was 30 in two and 40 in one). The size of the field of IORT ranged from 3 × 3 to 9 × 8.5 cm. One patient received arterial infusion chemotherapy; pirarubicin hydrochloride 30 mg plus mitomycin C 20 mg were infused into the superior thyroid artery five times during a 10-month period.

During and after multidisciplinary treatment, 24 patients were evaluated by MRI and/or ^{201}T1 scintigraphy; one patient was evaluated by ultrasonography only. One patient was not evaluated because of her apparent progressive disease during the course of treatment.

Tumor size was diminished in nine patients, and the degeneration in most of the tumor was observed in 18 of 24 patients by MRI assessment (Table 14-1). The accumulation of ^{201}T1 disappeared or distinctly decreased in 13 of 16 patients.

The serum thyroglobulin level was regarded as a tumor marker in 17 of 26 patients. In 17 patients, their preoperative thyroglobulin level ranged from 103 to 25,400 ng/ml, it was more than 1000 ng/ml in 10 of 17 patients. After multiple treatments, the thyroglobin level was normal in four patients and decreased to less than half of the pretreatment values in eight of 17 patients. Of the remaining nine patients, five had interfering antithyroglobulin antibodies, and four patients had exhibited normal serum thyroglobulin levels before treatment, so thyroglobulin levels were not helpful.

Of six patients with distant metastases who received radioiodine therapy, radioiodine uptake was observed in distant metastases and neck tumors in four patients and was observed only in the neck tumor in two patients. In one patient, radioiodine uptake in the distant metastases became more evident when the tumor in the neck was reduced by multidisciplinary treatment.

TABLE 14-2 Total Evaluation (N = 26)

	Number (%)
Complete remission	4 (15.4)
Partial response	11 (42.3)
No change	4 (15.4)
Partial response/progressive disease	4 (15.4)
Progressive disease	3 (11.5)

From these findings, complete remission or partial response was seen in 15 patients (57.7%), whereas 11 patients had either no change or progressive disease (Table 14-2). Four patients who had a partial response sequentially developed progressive disease. Of seven patients with progressive disease, three were diagnosed by aspiration cytology as having anaplastic carcinoma during the therapy, and two had lymph node metastases in the mediastinum that could not be treated by multidisciplinary treatment. The remaining two had massive involvement of the esophagus or the brachial plexus. Five patients died of thyroid carcinoma; their survival time ranged from 10 to 55 months. The remaining 14 patients continue to receive multiple therapies.

COMPLICATIONS AND RESULTS

Because the survival rate for patients with thyroid carcinoma who are categorized as low risk is greater than 95% at 20 years, these tumors behave almost like benign tumors. By contrast, in high-risk and elderly patients, thyroid carcinoma is much more aggressive.

Some patients present with unresectable thyroid carcinoma when diagnosed and others develop recurrences. Many patients with unresectable tumors must suffer pain, discomfort, and mental distress for a prolonged period. The recurrent or persistent masses are usually clearly visible to the patients and others, which is emotionally difficult for patients and their families and friends.

Total thyroidectomy with or without lymph node dissection followed by radioiodine treatment has been a management of choice for patients with distant metastases at presentation. Management of patients with unresectable locally invasive thyroid carcinoma who also have distant metastases is extremely difficult. Repeat surgery, chemotherapy, radioiodine therapy, and external radiation can be palliative but are often not curative.

The 10-year survival rate at our medical center was 66.3% in 71 patients who had or developed distant metastases among 2035 patients with papillary carcinoma treated between 1970 and 1989. However, the survival time of patients with differentiated thyroid carcinoma is considerably longer than that of patients with other types of malignancies. Because of this fact, they warrant multiple therapies if they are effective. A complete remission rate of up to 30% has been reported in patients with distant metastases whose primary tumor could be resected by total thyroidectomy.[2] Some experts believe that for patients with distant metastases, aggressive surgery combined with total laryngectomy and/or esophagectomy for patients who also have locally advanced tumors, was not indicated, considering the quality of life after surgery. We have used IORT and PEIT for treatment of such patients to improve the duration of survival and the patient's quality of life. It is possible that the result of radioiodine may be more effective for distant metastases if the locally recurring or persisting cancer is removed.

Sixteen of our 26 patients with advanced local tumor did not have clinical evidence of distant metastases. Four of the 16 patients underwent noncurative surgery because thyroid cancer invaded the common carotid artery, prevertebral fascia, trachea, or larynx, and the remaining 12 patients were diagnosed as having nonresectable tumors as demonstrated on preoperative MRI, arteriography, or esophagography and physical examination. A partial or complete response was obtained in 11 (69%) of 16 patients by using IORT, PEIT, ^{131}I, and some other therapies.

For most patients, fine-needle aspiration cytology was used to determine the type and differentiation of the carcinoma. We had some difficulty, however, in judging the extent of local invasion and size of the unresectable thyroid carcinoma. In three of our patients, cytologic examination revealed undifferentiated or squamous thyroid carcinoma. All of them died of these cancers within 9 months of initial diagnosis despite multiple therapies. Three other patients with undifferentiated thyroid carcinoma also died within 21 months despite the use of thyroidectomy, IORT, PEIT, and other therapies. These patients were considered to have very aggressive thyroid cancer because of the rapid growth of these tumors before treatment. Our remaining 21 patients with differentiated thyroid cancer appeared to benefit from multiple treatments as described above. Unfortunately, the precise indications for IORT, PEIT, external radiation, ^{131}I, and chemotherapy are not clearly defined. We judged the effectiveness of this treatment by the clinical response.

The diagnosis made by fine-needle aspiration cytology in many of our patients may not have revealed the most aggressive cancer, since differentiated and undifferentiated thyroid cancers can occur within the same tumor.

Despite this fact, as mentioned, most patients with unresectable thyroid cancer received excellent palliation.

Unfortunately IORT and PEIT could not be used in some patients because of the location of the primary tumor. Patients whose tumors are located around the submandibular gland are difficult: these patients usually complain of severe pain during PEIT and IORT, and there is increased risk of irradiating the central nervous system.

We have used MRI, and ^{201}Tl scintigraphy with serum thyroglobulin measurement for assessment of tumors and evaluation of responses to multidisciplinary treatment. These two imaging modalities help to distinguish the portion of the tumor that is composed of viable thyroid carcinoma cells from necrotic tissue. Complete remission has been observed in four of our patients; two were treated with IORT alone, one with PEIT alone, and two with both IORT and PEIT. The tumor size in the two patients treated with IORT alone was relatively small (2 cm). Although our numbers are small, we believe that complete remission can be achieved in patients who have tumors smaller than 2 cm. We recommend using PEIT for patients with larger tumors. Our data suggest that in some patients who appear to have unresectable thyroid cancer, treatment with surgery, IORT, PEIT, ^{131}I, and other therapies can be curative. Therefore, surgical resection of metastatic tumors should be considered when possible.

CONCLUSION

When we initially used IORT and PEIT, there were some patients who died of airway obstruction. We have subsequently avoided this situation by better staging of our patients with MRI, ^{201}Tl, and other means. We currently arrange for either IORT or PEIT for patients who are thought to have unresectable thyroid cancer. Although our results with IORT and PEIT in patients who have unresectable thyroid carcinoma are encouraging, further studies are needed to establish a more efficient approach in terms of dosage and frequency of IORT and PEIT. Considering the rarity of this condition, a multidisciplinary study should be established to determine the overall effectiveness of this treatment.

REFERENCES

1. Zohar Y, Strauss M. Occult distant metastases of well-differentiated thyroid carcinoma. Head Neck 16:438, 1994.

2. Schlumberger M et al. Radioactive iodine treatment and external radiotherapy for lung and bone metastases from thyroid carcinoma. J Nucl Med 37:598, 1996.
3. Nakahara H et al. Intraoperative radiotherapy for unresected differentiated thyroid carcinoma. Endocr Surg 12:141, 1995.
4. Miyamoto S et al. [Results of radioiodine therapy in 47 patients with distant metastases of differentiated thyroid carcinoma]. [Japanese]. Nippon Igaku Hoshasen Gakkai Zasshi. Nippon Acta Radiol 51:810, 1991.
5. Shiina S et al. Percutaneous ethanol injection therapy for hepatocellular carcinoma. A histopathologic study. Cancer 68:1524, 1991.
6. Shiina S et al. Multiple-needle insertion method in percutaneous ethanol injection therapy for liver neoplasms. Gastroenterology 26:47, 1991.
7. Shimada M et al. Needle track seeding after percutaneous ethanol injection therapy for small hepatocellular carcinoma. J Surg Oncol 58:278, 1995.
8. Tapani E et al. Complications following high-dose percutaneous ethanol injection into hepatic tumors. Acta Radiol 37:655, 1996.
9. Livraghi T, et al. Percutaneous ethanol injection in the treatment of hepatocellular carcinoma in cirrhosis: A study on 207 patients. Cancer 69:925, 1992.
10. Dralle H. Histologische und aktuelle Aspekte alternativer Operationsverfahren bei der immunogenen Hyperthyreose. Endocr Surg 11:363, 1994.
11. Lippi F et al. Treatment of solitary autonomous thyroid nodules by percutaneous ethanol injection: Results of an Italian multicenter study. The Multicenter Study Group. J Clin Endocrinol Metab 81:3261, 1996.
12. Papini E, Pacella CM, Verde G. Percutaneous ethanol injection (PEI): What is its role in the treatment of benign thyroid nodules. Thyroid 5:147, 1995.
13. Paracchi A et al. Percutaneous intranodular ethanol injection: A new treatment for autonomous thyroid adenoma. J Endocrinol Invest 15:353, 1992.
14. Monzani F et al. Percutaneous ethanol injection treatment of autonomous thyroid adenoma: Hormonal and clinical evaluation. Clin Endocrinol 36:491, 1992.
15. Di Lelio A et al. Treatment of autonomous thyroid nodules: Value of percutaneous ethanol injection. Am J Radiol 164:207, 1995.
16. Monzani F et al. Percutaneous aspiration and ethanol sclerotherapy for thyroid cysts. J Clin Endocrinol Metab 78:800, 1994.
17. Yasuda K et al. Treatment of cystic lesion of the thyroid by ethanol instillation. World J Surg 16:958, 1992.
18. Verde G et al. Ultrasound guided percutaneous ethanol injection in the treatment of cystic thyroid nodules. Clin Endocrinol 41:719, 1994.
19. Goletti O et al. Percutaneous ethanol injection treatment of the postsurgical recurrence of a 'cold' thyroid nodule. J Endocrinol Invest 14:13, 1991.
20. Goletti O et al. Inoperable thyroid carcinoma: palliation with percutaneous injection of ethanol. Eur J Surg 159:639, 1993.
21. Nakada K et al. Treatment of radioiodine-negative bone metastasis from papillary thyroid carcinoma with percutaneous ethanol injection therapy. Ann Nucl Med 10:441, 1996.
22. Yamauchi T et al. An ethanol injection therapy for tumors of inoperable patients with a differentiated thyroid carcinoma. Jpn J Cancer Clin 37:1035, 1991.
23. Di Carlo V et al. Intraoperative and postoperative radiotherapy in pancreatic cancer. Int J Pancreatol 21:53, 1997.

24. Nishimura A et al. Intraoperative radiotherapy for advanced carcinoma of the pancreas. Cancer 54:2375, 1984.
25. Takahashi M et al. Intraoperative radiotherapy in the definitive treatment of localized carcinoma of the prostate. Int J Radiat Oncol Biol Phys 11:147, 1985.
26. Matsutani M et al. Intra-operative radiation therapy for malignant brain tumours: Rationale, method, and treatment results of cerebral glioblastomas. Acta Neurochir 131:80, 1994.
27. Spaeth J et al. Intra-operative radiotherapy—5 years of experience in the palliative treatment of recurrent and advanced head and neck cancers. Oncology 54:208, 1997.
28. Wolf G et al. Intraoperative radiation therapy in advanced thyroid cancer. Eur J Surg Oncol 21:357, 1995.
29. Wolf G et al. Intraoperative radiation therapy, endotracheal hyperthermia and IR-192-brachytherapy in patients with advanced thyroid cancer. Acta Med Austriaca 23:76, 1996.
30. Simpson WJ et al. Papillary and follicular thyroid cancer: Impact of treatment in 1578 patients. Int J Radiat Oncol Biol Phys 14:1063, 1988.
31. Tochner ZA et al. Long-term tolerance of thoracic organs to intraoperative radiotherapy. Int J Radiat Oncol Biol Phys 22:65, 1992.
32. Kinsella TJ et al. Threshold dose for peripheral neuropathy following intraoperative radiotherapy (IORT) in a large animal model. Int J Radiat Oncol Biol Phys 20:697, 1991.
33. Powers BE et al. Muscle injury following experimental intraoperative irradiation. Int J Radiat Oncol Biol Phys 20:463, 1991.

PART

V

ADVANCES IN MOLECULAR BIOLOGY

CHAPTER

15

The Role of Basic Science Research

ORLO H. CLARK, M.D.

Two questions are addressed in this chapter: Has basic science research had any impact on the treatment of patients with differentiated thyroid cancer? Should surgeons be educated and trained in basic science? Historically, improved care of patients with surgical thyroid disorders, as well as patients with other surgical conditions, occurred because of better anesthesia, antisepsis, and improved instrumentation. Also, surgeons and their colleagues who treated numerous patients with various thyroid disorders accurately recorded the results of these operations.[1] These exciting medical and surgical advances influenced many intelligent students to seek careers in surgery.

HISTORICAL BACKGROUND

Experiments by physiologist Morris Schiff of Switzerland in the 1850s suggested that transplanting thyroid tissue in dogs prevented hypothyroidism.[2] This information was quickly forgotten because of the high incidence of infection that occurred during these experiments and because few thyroid operations were done on patients because of an excessive mortality rate. Subsequent experiments in thyroid transplantation by surgeon Victor Horsley of England in monkeys, and by surgeons Sir Felix Semon, Jacques-Louis Reverdin, and Theodore Kocher in humans, suggested that the clinical manifestations of hypothyroidism that develop after total thyroidectomy, including weakness, pallor, anemia, and facial edema, were associated with an absence or dysfunction of the thyroid.[1,3-5] A committee was established to investigate the cause of myxedema.[6] The members reviewed 109 reports of myxedematous patients and also studied the effects of thyroidectomy in animals. In 1888, the committee stated that cretinism, myxedema, and cachexia strumipriva were caused either by the absence or degeneration of the thyroid.[6] In 1891, a student of Horsley, George Murray[7] of Newcastle, injected sheep's thyroid in glycerine into a myxedematous woman. Her condition improved. Fox,[8] MacKenzie,[9] and Vermeluen[10] in 1892 and 1893 reported that giving thyroid by mouth was beneficial for hypothyroid patients. Once diagnosed, hypothyroidism was no longer a problem. This observation now enabled surgeons to remove all of the thyroid gland.

Theodore Kocher[11] from Berne, Switzerland contributed much to the development of safe thyroidectomy. His clinical observations in numerous patients on the development of myxedema after total thyroidectomy also helped elucidate the hormone-producing function of the thyroid gland; without it patients developed myxedema (Fig. 15-1). Numerous other surgeons, often in collaboration with pathologists, endocrinologists, and other clinicians, made important contributions to the improvement of patient care. One such surgeon was Dunhill[12] in Australia, who made advances in the treatment of patients with Graves' disease (Fig. 15-2).

To make these important contributions, these surgeons and their colleagues needed to treat numerous patients with similar problems. They had to be careful observers and to record their failures as well as their successes. They often worked closely with other specialists in medicine who evaluated the same clinical problems from a different perspective.

Accurate and reproducible measurement of responses to therapy also added greatly to patient care. For example, there was considerable controversy about whether preoperative treatment of patients with hyperthyroidism with iodine was therapeutically effective. Henry Stanley Plummer and Walter Meredith Boothby[13] at the Mayo Clinic measured the basic metabolic rate of hyperthyroid patients who were treated preoperatively with iodide solution. Documentation of the return of the basal metabolic rate to normal eliminated any further debate about whether iodine should be used preoperatively in hyperthyroid patients (Fig. 15-3).

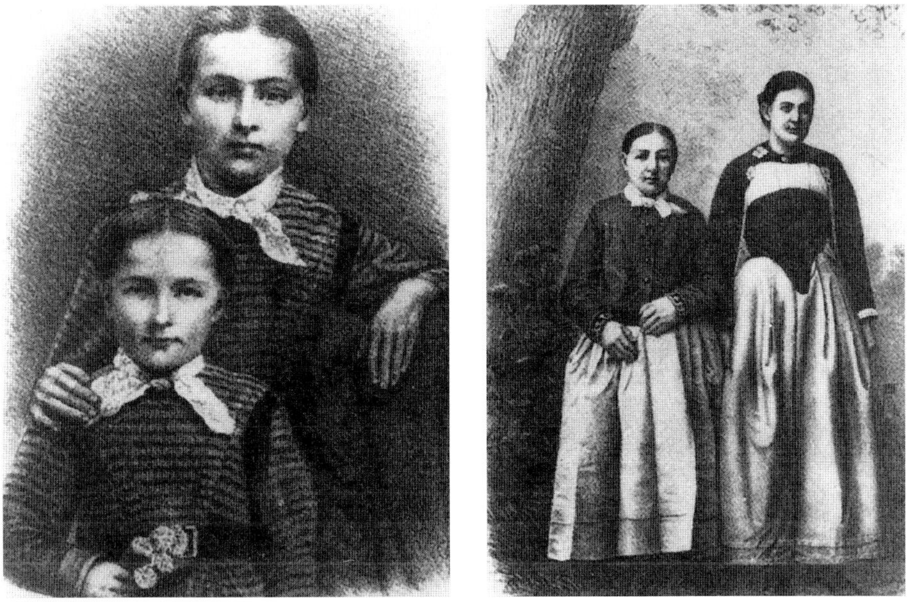

A B

• **FIGURE 15-1** Kocher's patients—the Bischsel sisters. **A,** Before operation (Marie on right). **B,** After operation (Marie on left). (From Kocher, TL. Über Kropf-exstripation und ihre Folgen. Arch klin Chir 29:254, 1883.)

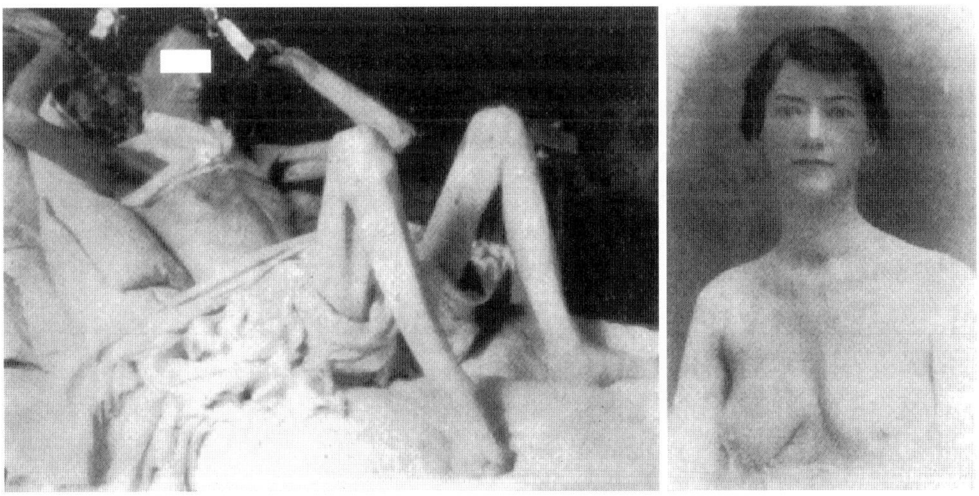

A B

• **FIGURE 15-2** Woman with gross wasting and cardiac involvement. **A,** 10 days after operation, **B,** 90 days after operation.

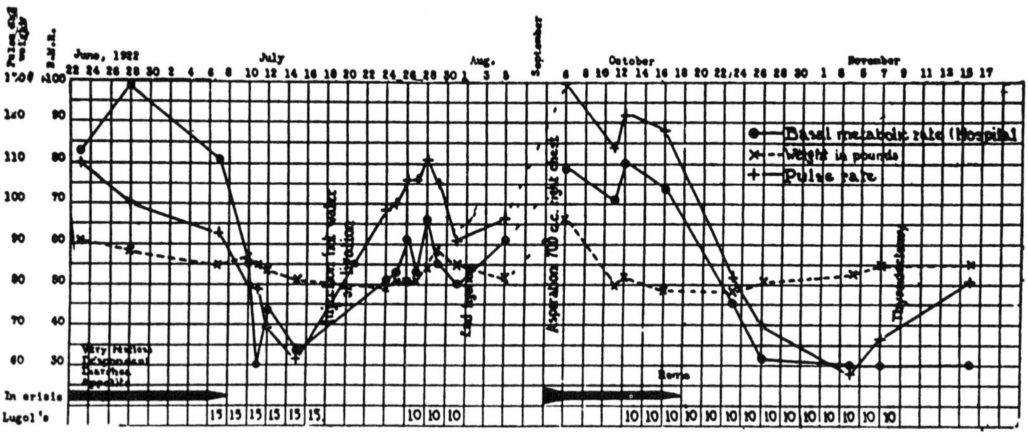

• **FIGURE 15-3** Basal metabolic rate (BMR) in 2 patients with Graves' disease documenting decrease in BMR in response to Lugol's iodine solution in two patients.

IMPACT ON SURGICAL TRAINING

I want to briefly discuss why being a good technician is not the same thing as being a good surgeon. One of my professors when I was a student at Cornell Medical College, the late Professor Walsh McDermott, stated: "One would not want to be operated upon by a surgeon who was only educated and not trained, or by a surgeon who was trained but not educated." A surgeon must know not only how to operate, but also when to operate, what tests need to be done preoperatively, what the preferred operation is, and when the operation is completed.

When operating with residents and students on patients with thyroid cancer, I frequently remark that surgeons must think like Winston Churchill. By this I mean one must consider "the battle," or the objective of the specific operation being done, and "the war," or what is best for the patient in the long run. For example, performing a thyroid lumpectomy and exposing the recurrent laryngeal nerve and parathyroid glands might initially save time. However, if this nodule turned out to be a thyroid carcinoma on permanent histologic examination, the patient would be at a disadvantage at subsequent resection because of the high risk of complications such as hypoparathyroidism and permanent hoarseness from operating in a previously operated field.[14] By contrast, if a total thyroid lobectomy was performed as the initial operation, there should be little increased risk at reoperation, because the parathyroid glands and recurrent laryngeal nerve on the other side are in unviolated territory.

Another example of the importance of a good surgical education is illustrated in the following case. A 28-year-old woman presents with a thyroid nodule. Should she have a fine-needle biopsy for cytologic examination? If the cytologic examination reveals medullary thyroid cancer, does she require any further testing before thyroidectomy? Would it be correct to operate on her without further tests, such as a serum calcitonin level, to confirm the diagnosis, a RET oncogene test to determine whether she has familial disease, a serum calcium level to see if she has hyperparathyroidism (MEN2), and, most important, a 24-hour urine test to rule out a coexisting pheochromocytoma? A thyroidectomy in such a patient who has MEN2A or MEN2B with a coexistent pheochromocytoma without preoperative preparation might precipitate a hypertensive crisis and sudden death.

It is essential today that all patients with medullary thyroid carcinoma be screened for familial disease.[15] About 25% of patients with medullary thyroid carcinoma have familial disease, and as many as 9% of patients with MEN2A and more with MEN2B have a de novo mutation.[16,17] It should be evident from this example that to be a good surgeon, one must be not only a good technician but must also understand both the pathophysiology of the disorder and the rapidly developing field of molecular medicine.

Technology is changing rapidly, and it is to be hoped that in the future we will treat patients with thyroid cancer with even better techniques than we are using today. This is yet another reason to support the need for education beyond technical training. Many businesses today are hiring students with a broad education rather than those with a focused technical training, because they know that even the best technical training will be rendered obsolete within a few years.

For surgical residents to become future leaders in surgery, it is essential that they conduct research in basic science. The knowledge they gain will not only enable them to understand the exciting new world of molecular biology and molecular medicine, but it will also help them carefully evaluate the research of others. It will also help them to create healthy collaborative investigations with colleagues in other disciplines of medicine or basic science. Such collaborations should lead to important new findings that will benefit patients with thyroid cancer and other problems. Developing special expertise in a particular field also makes colleagues aware of the authorities in that field; it will also result in local, national, and international recognition, since surgeons are interested in new information. Most important is that it will benefit our patients.

Despite my opinions, there are few data documenting the benefits of basic science for a surgeon in training. Most previous surgical leaders, at least in the United States, have done some basic science research during their training. It is difficult to know whether these surgeons became surgical leaders because they had done this research or whether they would have become leaders anyway because of their intellectual capability and energy. The answer is probably unimportant, because the results of this experience seem to speak for themselves.

IMPACT ON CLINICAL MANAGEMENT

To return to the basic question of whether basic science research has any impact on the treatment of patients with differentiated thyroid cancer, one has to look no farther than to the changing management of patients with medullary thyroid cancer (MTC). As mentioned, 25% of patients with MTC have familial disease. These patients can now be diagnosed by a blood test for documenting a specific missense mutation, a RET point mutation on chromosome 10 (Fig. 15-4).[18] It is thus no longer necessary to screen first-degree relatives with yearly calcitonin tests after provocative testing with pentagastrin and/or calcium. The specific mutations responsible for familial MTC and MEN2A were first identified in 1987 by linkage analysis.[19,20] Subsequent mapping located the gene for MEN2A and later for familial MTC, and MEN2B adjacent to the centromere on chromosome 10.[21] Patients with familial disease have a specific germline (DNA) mutation, and more than 95% can be precisely diagnosed by gene (RET) testing.[15,16,18] Some sporadic medullary thyroid cancers have somatic, tumor-specific mutations that are the same mutations that are found in patients with MEN2B. Such somatic mutations may or may not predict a worse prognosis. Clinical observation and molecular science have also documented that familial MTC and MEN2A are associated with Hirschsprung's disease, and MEN2A is associated with lichen planus amyloidosis.[22,23]

Studies of papillary thyroid cancer (PTC) have also documented that there are somatic chromosomal rearrangements on chromosome 10 (RET/PTC 1,2,3) that to date have only been found in the tumors, but not as germline mutations in the blood (Fig. 15-5).[24-27] Familial nonmedullary thyroid cancers, most of which are papillary thyroid cancers, account for about 6% of all papillary thyroid cancers.[28-32] In most articles,[29,30] these familial cancers are reported to be slightly more aggressive than sporadic thyroid cancers. Some studies disagree.[31] The germline mutation responsible

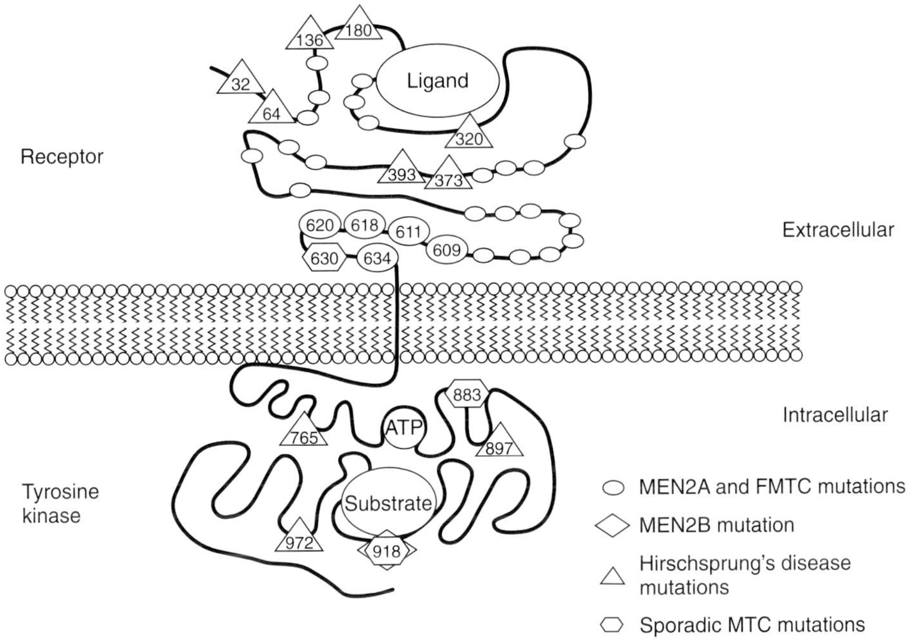

• **FIGURE 15-4** Graphic representation of the RET proto-oncogene protein domains and mutations associated with disease: MEN2A, MEN2B, FMTC, sporadic MTC, and Hirschsprung's mutations in the RET proto-oncogene. The RET proto-oncogene encodes a transmembrane tyrosine kinase receptor *(upper panel).* The receptor has five components, a cadherin-like region, extracellular region, a cysteine-rich extracellular domain, a transmembrane (TM) domain, and two intracellular tyrosine kinase domains (TK1 and TK2). In approximately 30% of papillary thyroid carcinomas, a chromosome 10 rearrangement places one of three promoters (RET-PTC1, RET-PTC2, and RET-PTC3) upstream of the intracellular TK1 and TK2 sequences. This rearrangement results in continuous activation of the tyrosine kinase domains shown in the upper panel. (From Doris-Keller H et al. Mutations in the ret proto-oncogene are associated with MEN2A and FMTC. Hum Mol Genet 2:851, 1993.)

for these mutations has not, as yet, been identified but it appears to be inherited as an autosomal dominate trait.[33] Other chromosomal mutations have also been identified in papillary and other nonmedullary differentiated thyroid cancers, including trk on chromosome 1,[34] met or hepatocyte growth factor,[35] and MTS-1 on chromosome 9.[36,37] In general, current investigations suggest that specific oncogenes are related to specific thyroid cancers and that various oncogenes or combinations of oncogenes may correlate with tumor behavior.[38,39] For example, thyroid-stimulating hormone receptor (TSH-R) and gsp mutations are generally associated with "hot" or

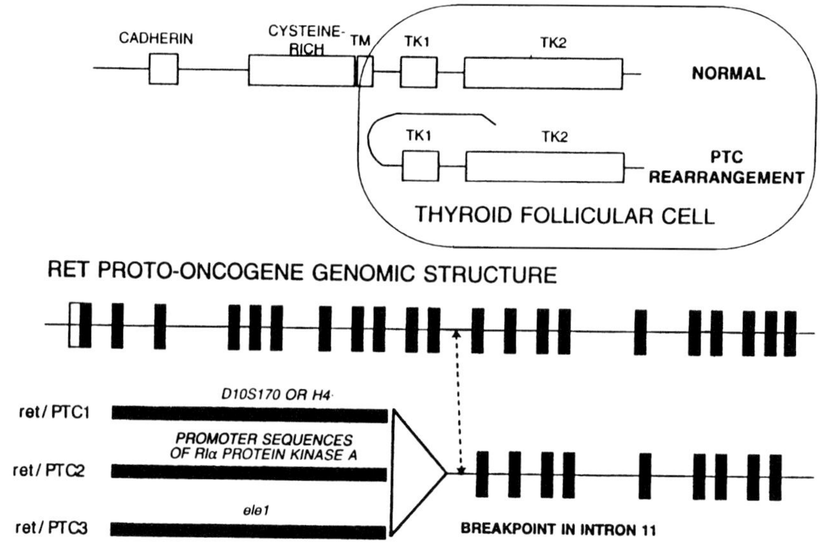

• **FIGURE 15-5** RET proto-oncogene rearrangements found in papillary thyroid cancer (see caption). (From Santoro M et al. Molecular characterization RET/PTC3; a novel rearranged of the RET proto-oncogene in a human thyroid papillary carcinoma. Oncogene 9:509, 1994.)

"autonomous" follicular thyroid adenomas.[40-42] One might expect that more TSH-R or gsp mutations would be present in thyroid tumors in patients from endemic goiter areas, since these patients' thyroid glands must use iodine more efficiently to maintain the euthyroid state. Goretzki et al.[38] documented that patients from iodine-poor Marburg and Dusseldorf, Germany are more likely to have gsp mutations in papillary thyroid cancers than are papillary thyroid cancers in comparable patients from iodine-rich San Francisco. In this study, the frequency of ras mutations was similar within both groups.

However, Shi et al.[43] reported more ras mutations in patients with thyroid tumors from iodine-poor Hungary than those from iodine-rich Newfoundland. Other studies suggest that ras mutations are more common in follicular thyroid neoplasms and possibly more common in follicular thyroid cancers.[44] The combination of both ras and gsp mutations has been reported to be more common in papillary thyroid cancers that are more aggressive.[38] K ras mutations have also been reported to occur more frequently in thyroid tumors from patients and animals who have been exposed to low-dose therapeutic radiation in most[45,46] but not all studies.[47] RET rearrangements have been documented to occur in 3% to 33% of papillary

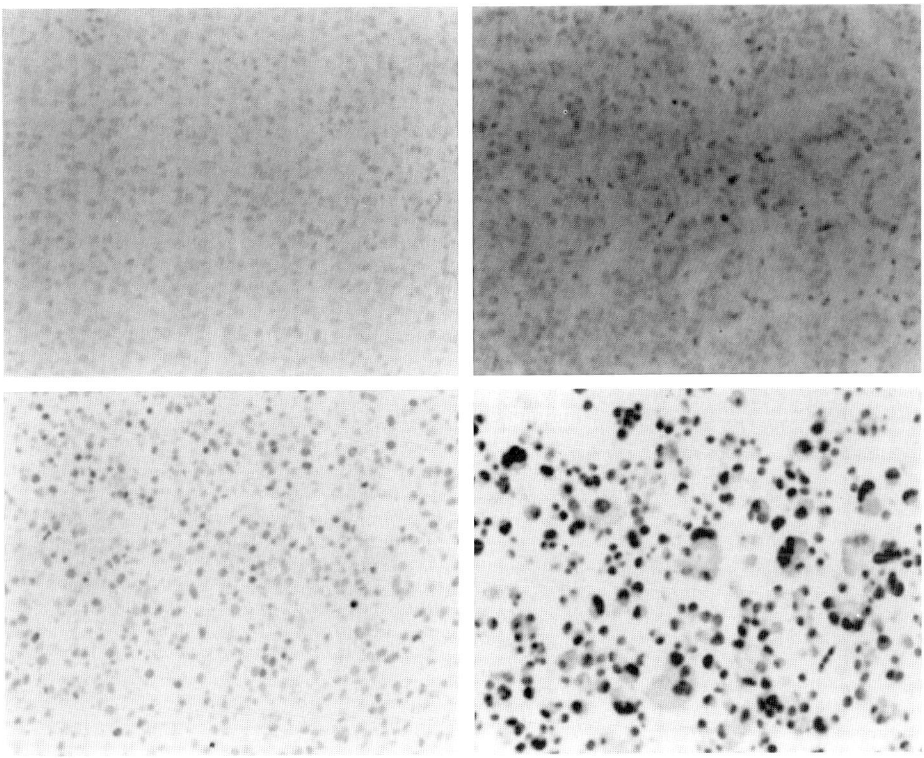

• **FIGURE 15-6** p53 immunocytochemistry (ICC) in a patient with metastatic Hürthle cell carcinoma. Note absence of positive nuclei in the right thyroid lobe Hürthle cell adenoma *(upper left)*, few positive nuclei in the left thyroid lobe Hürthle cell carcinoma *(upper right)*, and intense homogenous nuclear reactivity in the breast metastasis from which the cell line was derived *(lower left)* and in the cell line HTC-UC 1.3 *(lower right)*. (From Jossert GH et al., Immunocytochemical detection of p53 in human thyroid carcinomas is associated with mutation and immortalization of cell lines. J Clin Endocrinol Metab 81;3498, 1996, © The Endocrine Society.)

thyroid carcinomas not associated with irradiation[24-26,48] and in about 60% to 80% of children with thyroid cancer after exposure to irradiation in Belarus or after low-dose external radiation treatment.[49] Interestingly, most of the RET changes in children from Chernobyl have been mostly RET/PTC3 rearrangements, whereas in papillary thyroid cancers that occur after external radiation, most tumors contain a RET/PTC1 rearrangement.[50,51] p53 and MTS-1 tumor suppressor gene mutations have been almost exclusively confined to anaplastic thyroid cancers or in thyroid cancer cell lines (Fig. 15-6).[36,52-54] Additional studies are obviously needed to further clarify the relationship of specific oncogenes or tumor suppressor genes with the propensity to develop specific tumors and with tumor behavior.

The specific oncogenes or tumor suppressor genes found in various thyroid tumors function by altering signal transduction pathways within these tumors. To understand, one might compare these systems to a car being driven down a high hill. The car will go faster when the driver steps on the gas pedal or releases the brake. Thus RET mutations increase protein kinase activity in papillary thyroid cancers; gsp mutations block gtp-ase activity, which results in constitutive activation of the adenylate cyclase transduction system in thyroid neoplasms of follicular cell origin.[24,25,40,55] Constitutive activation means that the system is "turned on" almost maximally, so that further hormonal activation does not result in further activation. Tumor suppressor genes such as p53 or MTS-1 function by releasing the brake and allowing more cells to divide and grow. Anaplastic thyroid cancers often have p53 or MTS-1 mutations.[36,37,52-54]

In our studies of the adenylate cyclase system in differentiated thyroid cancers of follicular thyroid origin, we noted that locally invasive tumors and primary tumors associated with distant metastases often appeared to be constitutively activated; that is, these tumors had a higher basal activity and lower adenylate cyclase response to TSH.[55,56] By contrast, benign follicular neoplasms generally had a high adenylate cyclase response to TSH whether they were "autonomous" or "nonfunctioning" (see Chapter 6). We therefore studied 24 thyroid neoplasms for the presence of gsp oncogenes.[40] We initially anticipated that the thyroid cancers that were constitutively activated and were more aggressive would have gsp mutations because of their higher basal activity and lower adenylate cyclase response to TSH. Most of the tumors that we initially studied were therefore aggressive papillary thyroid cancers that had a constitutively activated adenylate cyclase system. One "autonomous" follicular adenoma with a high adenylate cyclase response to TSH was included as a control, and this tumor was the only tumor among these 24 tumors that contained a gsp oncogene.[40] Subsequent studies documented that gsp oncogenes occur most frequently in "autonomous" follicular neoplasms and most hot nodules have TSH-R or gsp mutations.[41,42] Suarez et al.[57] were successful in documenting that two of three follicular thyroid cancers and one of three papillary thyroid cancers that they studied that had constitutively activated cAMP levels also had gsp mutations. Although we had done numerous previous studies, we could not identify any specific correlation between constitutively activated adenylase activity and gsp mutations. We and others have recently identified TSH-R mutations in "hot" follicular, Hürthle, and insular thyroid cancers.[58-62] Thus, TSH-R

TABLE 15-1 Thyroid Growth Factor

Stimulation	Inhibition
Insulin life growth factor	Transforming growth factor-beta (TGFβ)
Epidermal growth factor	
Human chorionic gonadotropin	Somatostatin
Fibroblast growth factor	Retenoic acid

mutations, although apparently only found in "autonomously" functioning thyroid nodules, can occur in these rare tumors when malignant.[62]

Numerous factors other than TSH and thyroid-stimulating immunoglobulins appear to stimulate thyroid growth (Table 15-1). In some in vitro systems, TSH has no effect on thyroid cell growth unless epidermal growth factor or serum is present.[63] Insulin-like growth factor also has been reported to be important for thyroid tumor growth.[64] Vasoactive intestinal polypeptide (VIP) binds to specific receptors in normal and neoplastic thyroid tissue and stimulates adenylate cyclase activity.[65] Perhaps more important clinically is the fact that transforming growth factor-beta (TGF-β), vitamin A and retinoic acid, somatostatin, adenosine, lithium, and alpha-adrenergic agents inhibit thyroid cell growth.[66-68] We and others have documented that somatostatin dramatically inhibited basal and stimulated adenylate cyclase response to TSH as well as neoplastic cell growth and invasion,[67,69,70] but this unfortunately does not occur in patients with progressive thyroid cancer of differentiated cell origin or in nude mice with malignant human thyroid tumors.[69,71] Promising studies have recently documented that treatment of patients with retinoic acid causes some thyroid cancers to trap more iodine and regress after treatment with ^{131}I.[68]

CONCLUSION

As surgical scientists we know the critical questions that need to be answered concerning the best management of patients with thyroid cancer. The widely varying behavior of these tumors, their usual responsiveness to TSH stimulation and treatment with radioiodine, as well as their association with specific oncogenes or tumor suppressor genes, makes further studies essential, both for correlating specific oncogenes and tumor suppressor genes with tumor behavior and for developing potential targets for gene therapy and better methods of treatment. Surgical scientists in collaboration with basic scientists must remain involved with this and other basic research. Studies correlating genotype-phenotype relationships will help to improve the medical and surgical treatment of our patients.

REFERENCES

1. Welbourn RB. The History of Endocrine Surgery. New York: Praeger, 1990.
2. Merke F. History and Iconography of Endemic Goitre and Cretinism. Boston: MTP Press, 1984.
3. Semon F. The Autobiography of Sir Felix Semon. London: Jarrolds, 1926.
4. Horsley V. On the function of the thyroid gland. Prog R Soc Lond 389:5, 1884.
5. Horsley V, Foster M. Further research into the function of the thyroid gland and into the pathological state produced by removal of the same. Prog R Soc Lond 40:6, 1986.
6. Ord WM et al. Myxedema report. Trans Clin Soc 21 (Suppl): 1888.
7. Murray GR. Treatment of myxedema by injections of extract of thyroid of sheep. Br Med J 2:796, 1891.
8. Fox EL. Myxedema treated by extract of thyroid by mouth. Br Med J 2:941, 1892.
9. MacKenzie HWG. Myxedema treated with great benefit by feeding thyroid glands. Br Med J 2:940, 1892.
10. Vermeluen F. Treatment of myxedema by feeding thyroid glands. Br Med J 1:266, 1893.
11. Kocher TL. Uber Kropf Exstirpatioen und ihre Folgen. Arfch Klin Chir 29:254, 1883.
12. Dunhill TP. Surgical treatment of Graves' disease. Med J Aust 15:625, 1910.
13. Plummer HS, Boothby WM. Value of iodine in exophthalmic goiter. Collect Paper Mayo Clin 15:565, 1923.
14. Levin KE et al. Reoperative thyroid surgery. Surgery 111:604, 1992.
15. Marsh DJ, Learoyd DL, Robinson BG. Medullary thyroid carcinoma: Recent advances and management update. Thyroid 5:407, 1995.
16. Wells SA Jr et al. Predictive DNA testing and prophylactic thyroidectomy in patients at risk for multiple endocrine neoplasia type 2A. Ann Surg 220:237, 1994.
17. Schuffenecker I et al. Prevalence and parental origin of de novo RET mutations in multiple endocrine neoplasia type 2A and familial medullary thyroid carcinoma. Le Groupe d'Etude des Tumeurs a Calcitonine [letter]. Am J Hum Genet 60:233, 1997.
18. Doris-Keller H et al. Mutations in the RET proto-oncogene are associated with MEN 2A and FMTC. Hum Mol Genet 2:851, 1993.
19. Mulligan LM et al. Germ-line mutations of the RET proto-oncogene in multiple endocrine neoplasia type 2A. Nature 353:458, 1993.
20. Hofstra RMW et al. A mutation in the RET proto-oncogene associated with multiple endocrine neoplasia type 2B and sporadic medullary thyroid cancer. Nature 367:375, 1994.
21. Carlson KM et al. Single missense mutation in the tyrosine kinase catalytic domain of the RET proto-oncogene is associated with multiple endocrine neoplasia type 2B. Proc Natl Acad Sci 91:1579, 1994.
22. Mulligan LM et al. Diverse phenotypes associated with exon 10 mutations of the RET proto-oncogene. Hum Mol Genet 3:2163, 1994.
23. Gagel RF et al. Multiple endocrine neoplasia type 2A associated with cutaneous lichen amyloidosis. Ann Intern Med 111:802, 1989.

24. Fusco A et al. A new oncogene in human thyroid papillary carcinomas and then lymph node metastases. Nature 328:170, 1987.
25. Bongarzone I et al. Molecular characterization of a thyroid tumor-specific transforming sequence formed by the fusion of ret tyrosine kinase and the regulatory subunit RI alpha of cyclic AMP-dependent protein kinase. Mol Cell Biol 13:358, 1993.
26. Santoro M et al. Molecular characterization of RET/PTC3; a novel rearranged version of the RET proto-oncogene in a human thyroid papillary carcinoma. Oncogene 9:509, 1994.
27. Wohllk N et al. Application of genetic screening information to the management of medullary thyroid carcinoma and multiple endocrine neoplasia type 2. Endocrinol Metab Clin North Am 25:1, 1996.
28. Ozaki O et al. Familial occurrence of differentiated, nonmedullary thyroid carcinoma. World J Surg 12:565, 1988.
29. Grossman R et al. Familial non-medullary thyroid cancer: An emerging entity that warrants aggressive treatment. Arch Surg 130:892, 1995.
30. Takami H, Ozaki D, Ito K. Familial non-medullary thyroid cancer: An emerging entity that warrants aggressive treatment [letter]. Arch Surg 131:676, 1991.
31. Loh KC. Familial nonmedullary thyroid carcinomas: A meta-review of case series. Thyroid 7:107, 1997.
32. Kraimps JL et al. Familial papillary carcinoma of the thyroid. Surgery 121:715, 1997.
33. Burgess JR et al. Two families with an autosomal dominant inheritance pattern for papillary carcinoma of the thyroid. J Clin Endocrinol 82:345, 1997.
34. Pierotti MA et al. Rearrangements of TRK proto-oncogene in papillary thyroid carcinomas. J Clin Endocrinol Invest 18:130, 1995.
35. DiRenzo MF et al. Overexpression of the c-MET/HGF receptor in human thyroid carcinoma derived from the follicular epithelium. J Endocrinol Invest 18:134, 1995.
36. Jones CJ et al. High-frequency deletion of the tumor suppressor gene P161NK4a (MTS1) in human thyroid cancer cell lines. Mol Cell Endocrinol 116:115, 1996.
37. Tung WS et al. Infrequent CDKN2 mutation in human differentiated thyroid cancers. Mol Carcinog 15:5, 1996.
38. Goretzki PE et al. Mutational activation of RAS and GSP oncogenes in differentiated thyroid cancer and their biological implications. World J Surg 116:576, 1992.
39. Hara H, et al. N-ras mutation: An independent prognosis factor for aggressiveness of papillary thyroid carcinoma. Surgery 116:1010, 1994.
40. Lyons J et al. Two G protein oncogenes in human endocrine tumors. Science 249:655, 1990.
41. O'Sullivan C et al. Activating point mutations of the gsp oncogene in human thyroid adenomas. Mol Carcinog 4:345, 1991.
42. Parma J et al. Somatic mutations causing constitutive activity of the thyrotropin receptor are the major cause of hyperfunctioning thyroid adenomas: Identification of additional mutations activating both the cyclic adenosine 3′ × 5′-monophosphate and inositol phosphate–Ca2+ cascades. Mol Endocrinol 9:725, 1995.
43. Shi YF et al. High rates of ras codon 61 mutation in thyroid tumors in an iodide-deficient area. Cancer Res 51:2690, 1991.
44. Lemoine NR et al. High frequency of ras oncogenes activation in all stages of human thyroid tumor genesis. Oncogene 4:159, 1989.
45. Wright PA et al. Radiation-associated and 'spontaneous' human thyroid carcinomas show a different pattern of ras-oncogene mutation. Oncogene 6:471, 1991.

46. Sarne D, Schneider AB. External radiation and thyroid neoplasia. Endocrinol Metab Clin North Am 25:181, 1996.
47. Challeton C et al. Pattern of ras and gsp oncogene mutations in radiation-associated human thyroid tumors. Oncogene 11:601, 1995.
48. Sugg SL et al. Ret/PTC-1, -2, and -3 oncogene rearrangements in human thyroid carcinomas: Implications for metasatic potential? J Clin Endocrinol Metab 81:3360, 1996.
49. Nikiforov Y, Gnepp DR, Fagin JA. Thyroid lesions in children and adolescents after the Chernobyl disaster: Implications for the study of radiation tumorigenesis. J Clin Endocrinol Metab 81:9, 1996.
50. Fugazzola L et al. Oncogenic rearrangements of the RET proto-oncogene in papillary thyroid carcinomas from children exposed to the Chernobyl nuclear accident. Cancer Res 55:5617, 1995.
51. Bounacer A et al. High prevalence of activating ret proto-oncogene rearrangements in thyroid tumors from patients who had received external radiation. Oncogene 15:1263, 1997.
52. Ito T et al. Unique association of p53 mutations with undifferentiated but no differentiated carcinomas of the thyroid gland. Cancer Res 52:1369, 1992.
53. Fagin JA et al. High prevalence of mutations of the p53 gene in poorly differentiated human thyroid carcinomas. J Clin Invest 91:179, 1993.
54. Jossert GH et al. Immunocytochemical detection of p53 in human thyroid carcinomas is associated with mutation and immortalization of cell lines. J Clin Endocrinol Metab 81:3498, 1996.
55. Siperstein AE et al. Adenylate cyclase activity as a predictor of thyroid tumor aggressiveness. World J Surg 12:528, 1988.
56. Siperstein AE et al. Adenylate cyclase activity as a predictor of thyroid tumor aggressiveness. World J Surg 12:528, 1988.
57. Suarez HG et al. gsp mutations in human thyroid tumors. Oncogene 6:677, 1991.
58. Baloch Z, Livolsi VA. Detection of an activating mutation of the thyrotropin receptor in a case of an autonomously hyperfunctioning thyroid insular carcinoma [letter]. J Clin Endocrinol Metab 82:3906, 1997.
59. Schroeder S, Marthaler B. Autonomous function and malignancy in thyroid tumors: A critical analysis of data in the literature on the existence of hyperfunctioning follicular and papillary thyroid carcinomas. Pathologe 17:349, 1996.
60. Russo D, Arturi F, Filetti S. Thryoid stimulating hormone receptor gene mutations and polymorphisms in thyroid disease. Curr Opin Endocrinol Diabetes 5:428, 1996.
61. Russo D et al. Detection of an activating mutation of the TSH receptor in a case of an autonomously functioning thyroid insular carcinoma. J Clin Endocrinol Metab 82:735, 1997.
62. Russo D et al. A Val 677 activating mutation of the thyrotropin receptor in a Hürthle cell thyroid carcinoma associated with thyrotoxicosis. Thyroid 9:13-17, 1999.
63. Westermark K et al. EGF-receptors in human normal and pathological thyroid tissue. Histopathology 28:221, 1996.
64. Williams DW, Williams ED, Wynford-Thomas D. Loss of dependence on IGF-1 for proliferation of human thyroid adenoma cells. Br J Cancer 57:535, 1988.
65. Siperstein AE, Miller RA, Clark OH. Stimulatory effect of vasoactive intestinal polypeptide on human normal and neoplastic thyroid tissue. Surgery 104:985, 1988.
66. Duh QY, Clark OH. Growth factor for thyroid neoplasms. Prog Surg 19:205, 1988.

67. Siperstein AE et al. Effect of somatostatin on adenylate cyclase activity in normal and neoplastic thyroid tissue. World J Surg 16:791, 1992.
68. Simon D et al. Redifferentiation therapy with retinoids: Therapeutic option for advanced follicular and papillary thyroid carcinoma. World J Surg 22:569, 1998.
69. Hoelting T et al. Somatostatin analog octreotide inhibits the growth of differentiated thyroid cancer cells in vitro, but not in vivo. J Clin Endocrinol Metab 81:2638, 1996.
70. Weber C et al. Effects of tamoxifen and somatostatin analogue on growth of human medullary, follicular, papillary thyroid carcinoma cell lines: Tissue culture and nude mouse xenograft studies. Surgery 109:1065, 1990.
71. Zlock DW et al. Octreotide therapy in advanced thyroid cancer. Thyroid 4:427, 1994.

CHAPTER

16

Oncogenes and Tumor Suppressor Genes in Differentiated Thyroid Cancer

PETER E. GORETZKI, M.D.
CORNELIA DOTZENRATH, M.D.
KLAUS M. SCHULTE, M.D.
DIETMAR SIMON, M.D.
HANS D. RÖHER, M.D.

Differentiated thyroid cancer (DTC) is currently the cause of death in less than 1% of all patient deaths from malignant diseases. Therefore, to some people, DTC seems to be more important as a scientific issue than as a national health hazard. Much is known about thyroid cell physiology as well as about external and internal growth-stimulating and growth-inhibiting factors in normal, hyperplastic, and neoplastic thyroid tissue. Today the genes of many growth factor receptors have been cloned so that they can be investigated in normal and mutated thyroid cells. Environmental factors such as exposure to low-dose therapeutic radiation or to radiation fallout after the accidental release of radiation at the nuclear power plant in Chernobyl, in 1986, cause mutations in thyroid cells and dramatically increase the risk that exposed individuals will develop thyroid cancer. Correlating altered growth-regulating genes with the development and progression of thyroid neoplasms should serve as a useful example for the investigation of thyroid and other neoplasms.

CYTOGENETIC SCREENING

Genetic investigations in DTC initially focused primarily on DNA analysis of cell ploidy; malignant thyroid tumors that had an aneuploid cellular DNA pattern appeared to be more aggressive.[1-9] One could not determine whether a thyroid tumor was benign or malignant, however, based on tumor ploidy.[1] Subsequently, studies of loss of heterozygosity (LOH) in marker regions of the total cellular DNA in differentiated thyroid tumors were performed.[4-9] In 1998, Ward et al.[9] demonstrated that there were major differences in chromosomal instability between follicular and papillary thyroid cancers; that is, follicular cancers had more genetic instability (more LOH-positive findings in almost all tested chromosomes) than papillary thyroid cancer did. The increased chromosomal instability in these follicular cancers increases the risk of acquiring additional mutations to the already present mutations; such changes can lead to further cell dedifferentiation and more aggressive tumor behavior. Differences in chromosomal instability, at least in part, may thus account for the general observation that patients with follicular thyroid cancer present in a more advanced stage and have a worse prognosis than do patients with papillary thyroid cancer (PTC). The data on chromosomal instability also remind us of the fact that follicular and papillary cancers have different oncogenes and are biologically different tumors despite the fact that they originate from the same thyroid cell. Therefore these tumors should be clearly defined histologically and investigated and discussed separately. Ward et al.,[9] in their studies of chromosomal instability, did not identify significant differences in LOH patterns between benign and malignant thyroid neoplasms. This is of interest because earlier studies of cell ploidy, as mentioned, also documented that one could not differentiate follicular thyroid carcinomas from follicular thyroid adenomas using this technique. To date, LOH investigations, like ploidy studies, do not appear to be useful in differentiating between benign and malignant thyroid tumors. Whether investigations of specific chromosomal changes will provide more information about behavior of DTC is of interest. Most investigators today using molecular-genetic studies are studying the sites of known oncogenes and tumor suppressor genes or specific LOH findings situated on the chromosomal arms 2p, 2q, 3p, 10q, 11q, and 17q that harbor specific tumor suppressor genes.[4-8] Such investigations should identify specific alterations or mutations that are responsible or related to the induction and/or progession of thyroid tumors in humans.

MUTATIONS IN PHYSIOLOGIC PATHWAYS

Primary molecular genetic research concerning the physiologic pathway of thyroid-stimulating hormone TSH[10] focused on activating mutations in the TSH receptor (TSH-R) and in the alpha subunit of the guanonucleotide-stimulating protein (gsp) that stimulate adenylate cyclase. Previous biochemical studies demonstrated an enhanced adenylate cyclase response to TSH and an increased cyclic adenosine monophosphate (cAMP) production after TSH in well-differentiated benign tumors and in some malignant thyroid tumors when compared with normal tissue from the same patient.[11,12] Therefore it was hypothesized that this phenomenon could be explained by constitutive activation of the TSH-R or gsp protein because of specific mutations. It was further hypothesized that constitutive activation of adenylate cyclase activity should not only enhance thyrocyte function but should also stimulate thyrocyte growth.[10-15] cAMP has been shown to stimulate the growth in vitro of normal and neoplastic human thyrocytes.[10,12-14]

Mutations of the TSH-R and the Gs-protein causing constitutively overactive adenylate cyclase were subsequently identified in differentiated human thyroid tumors.[15-22] gsp and TSH-R mutations, however, were primarily found in autonomous functioning thyroid follicular adenomas but were uncommon in DTC.[15,17-19,23-25] The clinical relevance of TSH-R and gsp mutations in autonomously functioning adenomas is well accepted, whereas the importance of these mutations in DTC is questioned. Some of the reported differences in the prevalence of these mutations in DTC could partially be explained by technical problems. Many of the former investigations used the technique of "dot blot hybridization," which is associated with a high incidence of false positive and false negative results.[21,22,26,27] These problems have subsequently been overcome by sequencing all amplified DNA. The process of sequencing at least positive dot blot results is now warranted, since neither microdissection of tissue fractions before DNA extraction nor polymerase chain reaction (PCR) amplification of undigested DNA after "wild-type specific digestion" nor asymmetric PCR amplification of extracted DNA is able to eliminate false positive findings.[26,28] This is especially important in PCR reactions when amplified DNA is obtained from formalin-fixed paraffin-embedded tissue, since formalin induces DNA breakages that may lead to additional technical problems in mutation analysis.[27]

There is little information available documenting that transfection of mutated TSH-R or mutated gsp into human thyrocytes increases cell replication or reduces cell apoptosis. These data are generally required before these mutations can be accepted as oncogenes responsible for the development of thyroid cancer.

MUTATIONS IN ras GENES

ras genes were among the first oncogenes to be investigated in human malignancies. The three different ras genes, Kirsten-ras (Ki-ras), Harvey-ras (H-ras), and N-ras, encode for three different proteins with amino acid similarity. The oncogenes demonstrate tissue specificity and result from mutations of codons 12, 13, and 61. All three mutations increase the ras-GTP state rather than the ras-GDP state, the former increasing adenylate cyclase activity. The Ki-ras mutation is found mainly in epithelial cancers, such as in the pancreas. N-ras mutations are found predominantly in hematologic malignancies. Human thyroid neoplasms have been reported to have all three ras mutations. Only minor differences in the number and distribution of this ras mutations have been found in benign and malignant tumors and in papillary and follicular thyroid cancers (Table 16-1).[21,29-34] The differences in frequency of ras gene mutations in benign and malignant thyroid neoplasms probably relate to the techniques used (dot blot hybridization of PCR-amplified archival tissue DNA) and also possibly the result of geographic differences in the distribution of ras gene mutations.[30,32,35,36] Despite this confusing picture of ras gene mutations in human thyroid cancer, further

TABLE 16-1 Prevalence of Mutations in ras Genes Ki-ras, Ha-ras, or N-ras in Thyroid Tumors

Reference	Year	Goiter (n/N)	Adenoma (n/N)	Follicular Cancer (n/N)	Papillary Cancer (n/N)
Suarez et al.[29]	1988	—	8/24	4/5	2/10
Lemoine et al.[30]	1989	—	0/4	1/2	2/3
Wright et al.[31]	1989	—	—	8/15	3/17
Namba et al.[32]	1990	4/19	6/25	0/3	3/14
Schark et al.[33]	1990	—	1/24	7/46	—
Karga et al.[34]	1991	—	0/9	2/14	11/15
Goretzki et al.[21]	1992	6/15	—	4/8	5/25
TOTAL		10/34	15/86	26/93	16/84
Percentage		29	17	28	19

n, Number of mutation positive samples; N, number of all investigated samples.

studies would be of interest comparing ras-positive tumors in different research laboratories. The transfection of H-ras genes in rodents interestingly resulted in the development of follicular thyroid tumors.[37]

Fogelfeld et al.[36] demonstrated an increased incidence of Ki-ras mutations in radiation-associated human thyroid cancers, suggesting that environmental factors may result in specific oncogenes and tumors. The studies of TSH-R, gsp, and ras activating mutations in the initiation and promotion of DTC are still inconclusive. The observation that Ki-ras mutations are more common after external radiation and gsp and TSH-R mutations occur after exposure to nitrosamines supports the association of environmental factors and thyroid neoplasms.[38]

Other growth-stimulating mutations in human thyrocytes such as epidermal growth factor may be of more importance in the growth and behavior of thyroid neoplasms.[39] Epidermal growth factor and other locally active growth factors bind to specific tyrosine kinase receptors that activate second messengers other than cAMP, such as the phosphoinositol pathway.

MUTATION AND EXPRESSION OF TYROSINE KINASE RECEPTORS

Mutations of the epidermal growth factor receptor (EGF-R) have not been demonstrated in thyroid tumors,[40-44] but Haugen et al.[42] found overexpression of the EGF-R in PTC. This overexpression in DTC correlated with high tumor burden and with tumor dedifferentiation. Overexpression of EGF-R was also associated with a higher probability of clinical recurrence after thyroidectomy and postoperative radioiodine therapy.[43]

Overexpression of tyrosine kinase receptors other than the EGF-R was also found for the hepatocyte growth factor receptor (HGF-R/c-met).[45] DiRenzo et al.[45,46] and Belfiori et al.[47] reported that overexpression of this receptor correlated with a poor prognosis in DTC. Our own experiments using human thyrocytes in culture failed to show any enhanced effect of HGF in DTC cells when compared with cells from benign thyroid tumors, which brings into question the effect of HGF in DTC.[48] More information is necessary before a definitive statement can be made regarding the overexpression of HGF-R and its impact on the behavior of DTC. The molecular basis for EGF-R and HGF-R overexpression in thyroid tissues is unknown. Further investigations are needed before drawing conclusions concerning the overexpression of EGF-R and HGF-R and the secondary effects of receptor overexpression in DTC. In contrast to the current data regarding the tyrosine kinase receptors EGF-R and HGF-R and their clinical importance, the

TABLE 16-2 Prevalence of RET/PTC Rearrangement in Papillary Thyroid Cancer

Reference	Country	Year	PTC Rearrangement n/N	(RET/PTC) %
Ishizaka et al.[51]	Japan	1991	1/38	3
Wajjwalku et al.[52]	Japan	1992	1/11	9
Santoro et al.[53]	France	1992	8/70	11
Zou et al.[54]	Emirate	1993	1/40	3
Bongarzone et al.[55]	Italy	1994	18/52	34
Jhiang and Mazzaferri[56]	United States	1994	4/36	11
Sugg et al.[57]	Canada	1996	3/57	5
Bounacer et al.[58]	France	1997	3/20	15
Mayr et al.[59]	Germany	1997	8/99	8
Klugbauer[60]	Belarus	1998	rad$^+$ 33/38	87
			rad$^-$ 12/16	71

RET/PTC Rearrangement in papillary thyroid cancer from different regions; n, Number of PTC-positive tumors; N, number of all investigated tumors.
rad = radiation positive (+) or negative (–)

clinical importance of RET/PTC kinase receptor in papillary thyroid cancer has been proved.

In NIH 3T3 cells transfected with RET/PTC oncogenes, Donghi et al.[49] and Grieco et al.[50] demonstrated malignant transformation. They also reported that the RET/PTC oncogene is specific for papillary thyroid cancer. PTC is a rearranged RET proto-oncogene. About 20% to 30% of Italian and American patients with PTC have RET/PTC rearrangements (Table 16-2).[51-60] In other European countries, only about 4% to 8% of patients with papillary thyroid cancers have been found to be RET/PTC positive.[61-62]

Three different RET/PTC rearrangements (H4, RI alpha, and ele 1) have been identified,[57-59,60,63-65] resulting in different expression of RET and different phosphorylation of RET (Fig. 16-1). The RET/PTC3 rearrangement has been found in at least 60% of the PTC in children from Belarus near Chernobyl.[58,60] The incidence of RET rearrangement overall in these tumors was as high as 87%.[60] Even in patients with non–radiation-induced PTC from the Belarus region, RET rearrangements exceeded the 4% to 8% normally found in most other European patients. Thus Klugbauer et al.[60] found 71% PTC positivity in PTC patients with no known history of radiation exposure; two thirds of these rearrangements were RET/PTC1.

Interestingly, the behavior of the radiation-induced PTC in children from Belarus correlated with their histologic structure. In only 18% was a typical PTC histologic picture found, whereas an increased number of follicular and

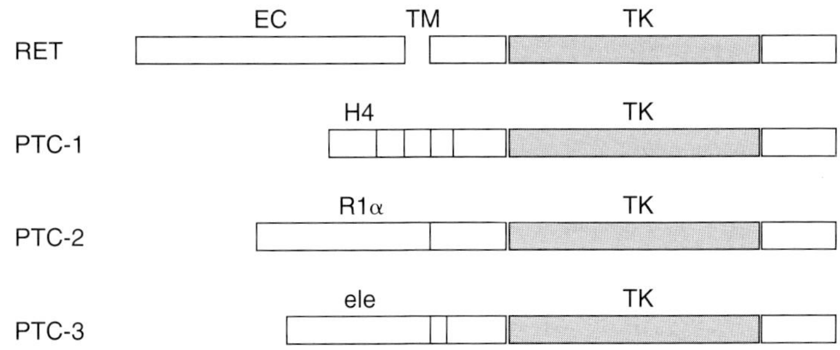

• **FIGURE 16-1** Rearrangement of ret oncogene tyrosine kinase with genes H4, R1-alpha, and ele results in three new oncogenes specific for papillary thyroid cancer (PTC-1 to PTC-3)

solid PTC variants were identified; RET/PTC3 mutations were more common in follicular and solid variants of PTC than thyroid cancer with a typical histologic picture. Therefore it is evident that radiation exposure (at least the radiation released from the Chernobyl nuclear plant accident) induced RET/PTC3 rearrangements in vivo that appear to cause PTC of a more aggressive "solid and follicular" variant type.

In contrast to the marked increase in RET/PTC3 rearrangements in PTC in children from the Chernobyl area, RET/PTC rearrangements in other regions do not appear to correlate with tumor behavior.[54] Therefore RET/PTC1 is thought to represent an early event in the development of PTC and may cause follicular thyroid cells to develop papillary structures that behave similarly to PTC without RET/PTC mutations. Further mutations may be required for these tumors to develop a more aggressive clinical behavior.[57,59,62,64-66] Of interest, mice transfected with PTC1 develop PTC or at least thyroid tumors with a papillary structure.[67]

The clinical detection of PTC as a tumor-specific oncogene with three different subtypes—of which one is activated by radiation exposure and then causes a histologically specific solid variant of PTC with a poorer prognosis—demonstrates a very important genotype-phenotype relationship. The correlation between these animal studies and in vitro experiments, with regard to PTC and the PTC oncogenes, makes this system an excellent cancer oncogene model for the investigation of other human cancers.[57-60,63-67]

TUMOR SUPPRESSOR GENES

Investigations regarding the tumor suppressor gene p53 were the first studies in differentiated human thyroid cancer.[68,69] Numerous authors studied

TABLE 16-3 Overexpression of p53 and Genetically Proved p53 Mutations Give Different Results in the Prevalence of p53 Mutations in Thyroid Cancer

	Benign*		Differentiated Thyroid Cancer*		Poorly Differentiated Cancer*	
p53 Detection	n/N	%	n/N	%	n/N	%
IHC	0/141	—	56/527	11	69/170	41
Sequencing	0/68	—	17/257	7	43/70	61
Rad + Sequencing			4/22	18		

p53 overexpression (IHC) and p53 mutations sequencing in thyroid tumors
p53 mutations are more common in radiation-induced thyroid carcinomas.
*Cumulative data from eight (IHC) and six (sequencing) references.
IHC, Immunohistochemistry-measured overexpression of p53; sequencing, sequencing of 53 gene; Rad + Sequencing, sequencing of p53 gene in tumor from patient with history of radiation exposure.

p53 point mutations in anaplastic thyroid cancers. The incidence of p53 overexpression was never higher than approximately 10%, and the incidence of genetically proved mutations in DTC was even smaller and can be assumed to be less than 6%.[54,68-72] Selected patients with DTC and a history of external radiation (Table 16-3) were reported by Fogelfeld et al.[73] to harbor p53 mutations in 10% to 25% of cases. p53 mutations are late mutations and appear to be of minor importance in the development of DTC. However, they appear to have a more important role in anaplastic thyroid cancers, where p53 mutations are found in more than 75% of tumors.[69,70,72] Other tumor suppressor genes including the cell cycle–specific kinase inhibitors p15 (INK4B) and p16 (INK4A)[74-78] have been studied in DTC. p53 or p16 tumor suppressor genes have been found in established thyrocyte cell lines.[76] p16 and p15 failed to be of any clinical importance in DTC or in metastatic thyroid cancers.[77] A similar finding was observed in squamous cell tumors of the head and neck and their cell lines.[78] It is possible, however, that a small number of normal (wild-type) cells such as occur in circulating cells and vessels may mask the presence of mutant genes. Although as mentioned there is a high incidence of LOH in many chromosomes and general chromosomal instability, especially in follicular thyroid cancers, proof is lacking for a tumor suppressor gene that is important for the development of DTC. More studies are obviously necessary.

The sodium/iodide symporter (SIS) is a possible candidate gene with possible tumor-suppressing abilities.[79-81] SIS is necessary to accumulate iodide in thyrocytes for thyroid hormone production. Since most thyroid cancers accumulate less iodide than the surrounding normal thyroid tissue ("cold nodule") and since the cell growth of primary cultures of normal human thyrocytes is inhibited by iodide, numerous groups have investigated the expression and possible mutation of the recently cloned SIS in normal and pathologic thyroid tissues.[79-85] To date, only decreased expression of SIS mRNA has been demonstrated in thyroid cancer. No specific SIS mutations have been found in either benign or malignant thyroid tumors. The importance of SIS in the development of DTC, and possible mutations in the SIS gene, await further investigation.

INTRANUCLEAR ONCOGENES

There is limited information regarding the functional integrity of nuclear oncogenes c-fos, c-myc, and c-jun in DTC. It is known, however, that c-fos and c-jun inhibit the thyroid hormone receptor T3-R;[78,85] this receptor may act as a tissue-specific tumor suppressor gene, possibly like SIS. Redifferentiation of thyroid cell lines from a follicular thyroid cancer and in tumors from these cell lines growing in nude mice have been demonstrated after the administration of retinoic acid.[85] Since retinoic acid receptor and T3-R are part of a common receptor family, further investigations focused on the subtype of retinoic acid receptor and T3-R are of interest. However, morphogenetic and functional studies of T3-R, failed to show any T3-R mutations in DTC.

CONCLUSION

DTC develops more frequently in humans and animals after exposure to low-dose therapeutic radiation and can be related to specific ras and RET/PTC oncogenes and p53 tumor suppressor genes.[38] Epidemiologic studies demonstrate a greater prevalence of DTC in women than in men. There is also an increased prevalence of cancer with advancing age and a higher proportion of follicular to papillary thyroid cancer in patients from iodine-deficient areas. Molecular-genetic studies will have to relate these observations to specific candidate genes (oncogenes as well as tumor suppressor genes) that may be related to sex, aging, and the histologic structure of the tumor. In the future, the identification of specific mutations and genotype-phenotype relationships may help us direct more selective or specific preventive or clinical treatment (Fig. 16-2).[86-90]

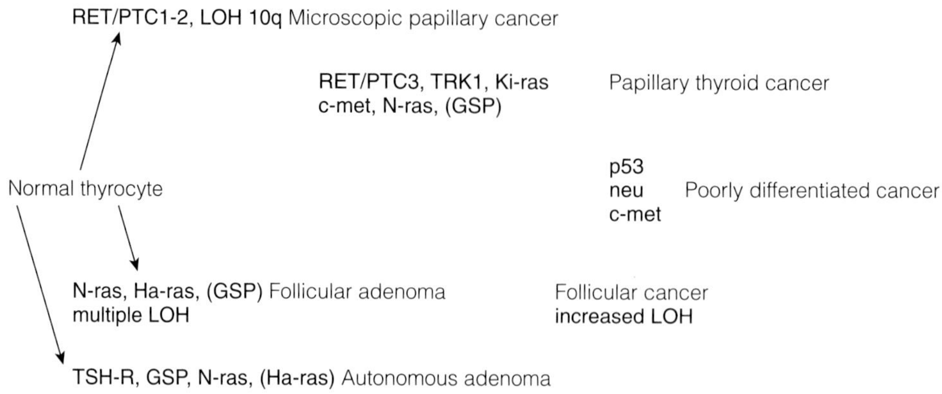

• **FIGURE 16-2** Mutations in proto-oncogenes and tumor suppressor genes that have been described in thyroid adenoma, papillary and follicular thyroid cancer, and poorly differentiated thyroid cancer.

Molecular-genetic studies of DTC have demonstrated activating TSH mutations in autonomous functioning "hot" thyroid adenomas. Locally active growth factors such as epidermal growth factor, insulin-like growth factor, and hepatocyte growth factor, are also present in some thyroid neoplasms RET/PTC mutations that are specific for PTC. Environmental factors such as radiation have been documented to induce specific mutations in Ki-ras, PTC, and p53 genes. Further investigations regarding oncogenes and tumor suppressor genes in thyroid cancer may help us understand why and how these tumors develop, how they can be prevented, and which mutations are associated with a good or bad outcome.

REFERENCES

1. Zedenius J et al. Follicular tumors of the thyroid gland: Diagnosis, clinical aspects and nuclear DNA analysis. World J Surg 16:589, 1992.
2. Grant CS et al. Diagnostic and prognostic utility of flow cytometric DNA measurements in follicular thyroid tumors. World J Surg 14:283, 1990.
3. Schelfbout LJDM et al. Frequency and degree of aneuploidy in benign and malignant thyroid neoplasms. Int J Cancer 45:16, 1990.
4. Jenkins RB et al. Frequent occurrence of cytogenetic abnormalities in sporadic non-medullary thyroid carcinoma. Cancer 66:1213, 1990.
5. Bondeson L et al. Chromosome studies in thyroid neoplasia. Cancer 64:680, 1989.
6. Herrmann ME et al. Genetic markers in thyroid tumors. Surgery 110:941, 1991.
7. Marsh DJ et al. Differential loss of heterozygosity in the region of the cowden locus within 10q22-23 in follicular thyroid adenomas and carcinomas. Cancer 57:500, 1997.
8. Herrmann ME et al. Cytogenetic study of a papillary thyroid carcinoma with a rearranged chromosome 10. Cancer Genet Cytogenet 57:209, 1991.

9. Ward LS et al. Studies of allelic loss in thyroid tumors reveal major differences in chromosomal instability between papillary and follicular carcinomas. J Clin Endocrinol Metab 83:525, 1998.
10. Roger P et al. Mitogenic effect of thyrotropin and adenosine 3′5″-monophosphate in differentiated normal human thyroid cells in vitro. J Clin Endocrinol Metab 66:1158, 1988.
11. Clark OH et al. Characterization of the thyrotropin receptor-adenylate cyclase system in neoplastic human thyroid tissue. J Clin Endocrinol Metab 57:140, 1983.
12. Goretzki PE et al. Growth regulation of normal thyroids and thyroid tumors in man. Recent Results Cancer Res 118:48, 1990.
13. Ledent C et al. The TSH cyclic AMP cascade in the control of thyroid cell proliferation: The story of a concept. Thyroidology 3:97, 1991.
14. Maenhaut C et al. Activation of the cyclic AMP cascade as an oncogenic mechanism: The thyroid example. Biochemie 73:29, 1991.
15. Bourne HR, Sanders DA, McCormick F. The GTPase superfamily: A conserved switch for diverse cell functions. Nature 348:125, 1990
16. Parmentier M et al. Molecular cloning of the thyrotropin receptor. Science 246:1620, 1989.
17. Parma J et al. Somatic mutations in the thyrotropin receptor gene cause hyperfunctioning thyroid adenomas. Nature 365:649, 1993.
18. Kopp P et al. Congenital hyperthyroidism caused by a mutation in the thyrotropin receptor area. N Engl J Med 222:150, 1995.
19. Paschke R et al. Identification and functional characterization of two new somatic mutations causing constitutive activation of the thyrotropin receptor in hyperfunctioning autonomous adenomas of the thyroid. J Clin Endocrinol Metab 79:1785, 1994.
20. Lyons J et al. Two G protein oncogenes in human endocrine tumors. Science 249:655, 1990.
21. Goretzki PE et al. Mutational activation of ras and gsp oncogenes in differentiated thyroid cancer and their biological implications. World J Surg 16:576, 1992.
22. Suarez HG et al. gsp mutations in human thyroid tumours. Oncogene 6:667, 1991.
23. Ringel MD et al. Absence of activating mutations of the genes encoding the alpha subunits of GI I and Gq in thyroid neoplasia. J Clin Endocrinol Metab 83:554, 1998.
24. Spambalg D et al. Structural studies of the thyrotropin receptor and Gs-alpha in human thyroid cancers: Low prevalence of mutations predicts infrequent involvement in malignant transformation. J Clin Endocrinol Metab 81:3898, 1996.
25. Waldmann V et al. Absence of Gs-alpha gene mutations in childhood thyroid tumors after Chernobyl in contrast to sporadic adult thyroid neoplasia. Cancer 57:2358, 1997.
26. Gorelov VN et al. Distribution of Gs-alpha activating mutations in human thyroid tumors measured by subcloning. J Cancer Res Clin Oncol 122:453, 1996.
27. Goretzki PE et al. Mutation and expression of alpha Gs in differentiated thyroid carcinoma (DTC) and medullary thyroid carcinoma (MTC). Exp Clin Endocrinol 101:54, 1993
28. Gorelov VN, Röher HD, Goretzki PE. A method to increase the sensitivity of mutation-specific oligonucleotide hybridization using asymmetric polymerase-chain reaction (PCR). Biochem Biophys Res Commun 200:365, 1994.
29. Suarez HG et al. Detection of activated ras oncogenes in human thyroid carcinomas. Oncogene 2:403, 1988.

30. Lemoine NR et al. High frequency of ras oncogene activation in all stages of human thyroid tumorigenesis. Oncogene 4:159, 1989.
31. Wright PA et al. Papillary and follicular thyroid carcinomas show a different pattern of ras oncogene mutation. Br J Cancer 60:576-577, 1989.
32. Namba H, Rubin SA, Fagin JA. Point mutations of ras oncogenes are an early event in thyroid tumorigenesis. Mol Endocrinol 4:1474, 1990.
33. Schark C, Fulton N, Jacoby RF. N-ras 61 oncogene mutations in Hürthle cell tumors. Surgery 108:994, 1990.
34. Karga H et al. Ras oncogene mutations in benign and malignant thyroid neoplasms. J Clin Endocrinol Metab 73:832-836, 1991.
35. Wright PA et al. Radiation-associated and 'spontaneous' human thyroid carcinomas show a different pattern of ras oncogene mutation. Oncogene 6:471, 1991.
36. Fogelfeld L et al. Prevalence of K-ras point mutations in radiation-induced thyroid cancer. 67 American Thyroid Association meeting, Tampa, Fla, 1993; abstract 66.
37. Burns JS et al. Stepwise transformation of primary thyroid epithelial cells by a mutant Ha-ras oncogene. An in vitro model of tumor progression. Mol Carcinog 6:129, 1992.
38. Kitahori Y et al. Genetic alterations in N-bis (2-hydroxypropyl) nitrosamine induced rat transplantable thyroid carcinoma lines: Analysis of the TSH-R, G-alpha-s, ras and p53 genes. Carcinogenesis 18:265, 1997.
39. Duh QY, Gum ET, Gerend PL. Epidermal growth factor receptors in normal and neoplastic thyroid tissue. Surgery 98:1000, 1985.
40. DePotter CR et al. The neu-oncogene protein as a predictive factor for haematogenous metastases in breast cancer patients. Int J Cancer 45:55, 1990.
41. Lemoine NR et al. Abnormalities of the EGF receptor system in human thyroid neoplasia. Int J Cancer 49:558, 1991.
42. Haugen DRF et al. Expression of c-erbB-2 protein in papillary thyroid carcinoma. Br J Cancer 65:832, 1992.
43. Simon D, Goretzki PE, Röher HD. The significance of c-neu and p53 in endocrine tumors. Langenbecks Arch Chir (Suppl 69), 1993.
44. Auguste U et al. Oncogene expression in follicular neoplasms of the thyroid. Am J Surg 164:592, 1992.
45. DiRenzo MF et al. Overexpression of the c-MET/HGF-receptor in human thyroid carcinomas derived from the follicular epithelium. J Endocrinol Invest 18:134, 1995.
46. DiRenzo MF et al. Expression of the met/HGF receptor in normal and neoplastic human tissues. Oncogene 6:1997, 1991.
47. Belfiori A et al. Low/absent Met/HGF-R expression in papillary thyroid carcinoma: A prognostic factor for distant metastasis. J Endocrinol Invest 19:57, 1996.
48. Schulte KM et al. Differential regulation of the HGF-receptor (c-met) mRNA in human thyroid cells. J Endocrinol Invest 20(Suppl):5, 1997.
49. Donghi R et al. The oncogene associated with human papillary thyroid carcinoma (PTC) is assigned to chromosome 10q11-q12 in the same region as the multiple endocrine neoplasia type 2A (MEN2A). Oncogene 4:321, 1989.
50. Grieco M et al. PTC is novel rearranged from the ret proto-oncogene and is frequently detected in vivo in human thyroid papillary carcinomas. Cell 60:557, 1990.
51. Ishizaka Y et al. Detection of retTPC/PTC transcripts in thyroid adenomas and adenomatous goiter by an RT-PCR method. Oncogene 6:1667, 1991.
52. Wajjwalku W et al. Low frequency of rearrangements of the ret and trk proto-oncogenes in Japanese thyroid papillary carcinomas. Jpn J Cancer Res 83:671, 1992.

53. Santoro M et al. Ret oncogene activation in human thyroid neoplasms is restricted to the papillary cancer subtype. J Clin Invest 89:1517, 1992.
54. Zou M, Shi Y, Farid NR. p53 mutations in all stages of thyroid carcinomas. J Clin Endocrinol Metab 77:1054, 1993.
55. Bongarzone I et al. Frequent activation of ret protooncogene by fusion with a new activating gene in papillary thyroid carcinomas. Cancer Res 54:2979-2985, 1994.
56. Jhiang SM, Mazzaferri EL. The ret/PTC oncogene in papillary thyroid carcinoma. J Lab Clin Med 123:331-337, 1994.
57. Sugg SL et al. RET/PTC-1, -2, and -3 oncogene rearrangements in human thyroid carcinoma: Implications of metastatic potential? J Clin Endocrinol Metab 81:3360, 1996.
58. Bounacer A et al. High prevalence of activating ret proto-oncogene rearrangements in thyroid tumors from patients who had received external radiation. Oncogene 15:1263, 1997.
59. Mayr B et al. Ret/PTC-1, -2, and -3 oncogene rearrangements in human thyroid carcinomas: Implications for metastatic potential? J Clin Endocrinol Metab 82:1306, 1997.
60. Klugbauer S et al. Molecular analysis of new subtypes of ELE/RET rearrangements, their reciprocal transcripts and breakpoints in papillary carcinoma of children after Chernobyl. Oncogene 16:671, 1998.
61. Zou M, Shi Y, Farid NR. Low rate of ret proto-oncogene activation (PTC/ret-TPC) in papillary thyroid carcinomas from Saudi Arabia. Cancer 73:176, 1994.
62. Mayr B et al. Expression of Ret/PTC, 1, -2, -delta3, and -4 in German papillary thyroid carcinoma. Br J Cancer 77:903, 1998.
63. Ito T et al. In vitro irradiation is able to cause RET oncogene rearrangement. Cancer Res 53:2940, 1993.
64. Tallini G et al. Ret/PTC oncogene activation defines a subset of papillary thyroid carcinoma lacking evidence of progression to poorly differentiated or undifferentiated tumor phenotypes. Clin Cancer Res 4:287, 1998.
65. Nikiforov YE et al. Distinct pattern of ret oncogene rearrangement in morphological variants of radiation-induced and sporadic thyroid papillary carcinomas in children. Cancer Res 57:1690, 1997.
66. Bongarzone I et al. RET/NTRK1 rearrangements in thyroid gland tumors of the papillary carcinoma family: Correlation with clinicopathological features. Clin Cancer Res 4:232, 1998.
67. Santoro M et al. Development of thyroid papillary carcinomas secondary to tissue-specific expression of the RET/PTC1 oncogene in transgenic mice. Oncogene 12:1821, 1996.
68. Wright PA et al. Mutations of the p53 gene in a differentiated human thyroid carcinoma cell line, but not in primary thyroid tumours. Oncogene 6:1693, 1991.
69. Nakamura T et al. p53 gene mutations associated with anaplastic transformation of human thyroid carcinomas. Jpn J Cancer Res 83:1293, 1992.
70. Ito T et al. Unique association of p53 mutations with undifferentiated but not with differentiated carcinomas of the thyroid gland. Cancer Res 52:1369, 1992.
71. Fagin JA et al. High prevalence of mutations of the p53 gene in poorly differentiated human thyroid carcinomas. J Clin Invest 91:179, 1993.
72. Hermann M et al. p53 gene alterations in differentiated thyroid cancers. Oncol Rep 2:741, 1995.
73. Fogelfeld L et al. p53 gene mutations in radiation-induced thyroid cancer. J Clin Endocrinol Metab 81:3039, 1996.

74. Goretzki PE et al. A frequent mutation/polymorphism in tumor suppressor gene INK4B (MTS-2) in papillary and medullary thyroid cancer. Surgery 120:1081, 1996.
75. Schulte KM et al. INT-2 gene amplification in differentiated human thyroid cancer. Exp Clin Endocrinol Diabetes 104:101, 1996.
76. Jones CJ et al. High frequency deletion of the tumor suppressor gene p16 INK4a (MTS1) in human thyroid cancer cell lines. Mol Cell Endocrinol 116:115, 1996.
77. Schulte KM et al. Loss of heterozygozity for MTS2 (p15) is rare in human thyroid malignancy cancer. Thyroid 7:682, 1997.
78. Zhang SY et al. Higher frequency of alterations in the p16/CDNKN2 gene in squamous cell carcinoma cell lines than in primary tumors of the head and neck. Cancer Res 54:5050, 1994.
79. Zhang XK et al. Novel pathway for thyroid hormone receptor action through interaction with jun and fos oncogene activities. Mol Cell Biol 11:6016, 1991.
80. Levy O et al. Characterization of the thyroid Na+/I-symporter with an anti-COOH terminus antibody. Proc Natl Acad Sci USA 94:5568, 1997.
81. Smanik P et al. Expression, exon-intron organization, and chromosome mapping of the human sodium iodide symporter. Endocrinology 138:3555, 1997.
82. Smanik PA, et al. Cloning of human sodium/iodide transporter and mechanism of the loss of radioiodine uptake activity in thyroid tumors. Thyroid 7:312, 1997.
83. Kim HK et al. Sodium-iodide symporter mRNA measurements by RT-PCR in thyroid tumors. Thyroid 7:47, 1997.
84. Yoshida A et al. Different electrophysiological character of I-, CI04-, and SCN-in the transport by Na+/I-symporter. Biochem Biophys Commun 231:731, 1997.
85. Schmutzler C et al. Functional retinoid and thyroid hormone receptors in human thyroid carcinoma cell lines and tissues. Int J Cancer 76:368-376, 1998.
86. Wynford-Thomas D. In vitro models of thyroid cancer. Cancer 16:115, 1993.
87. Fagin JA. Molecular human thyroid neoplasms. Annu Rev Med 45:45, 1994.
88. Farid NR, Shi Y, Zou M. Molecular basis of thyroid cancer. Endocr Rev 15:202, 1994.
89. Said S, Schlumberger M, Suarez H. Oncogenes and anti-oncogenes in human epithelial tumors. J Endocrinol Invest 17:371, 1994.
90. Nikifarov YE, Fazin JA. Risk factors for thyroid cancer. Trends Endocrinol Metab 8:20-25, 1997.

CHAPTER

17

Angiogenesis and Thyroid Neoplasms

QUAN-YANG DUH, M.D.
EU YOUNG SOH, M.D.

Thyroid cancer is characterized by uncontrolled growth, local invasion, and distant metastasis. Various genetic changes, such as oncogene activation and tumor suppressor gene inactivation, have been implicated in the development of thyroid cancer.[1] In addition, various growth factors have also been found to modulate the development of thyroid cancer via autocrine, juxtacrine, paracrine, or endocrine action, through various cellular signaling pathways.[2] Some of these growth factors promote tumor growth by stimulating angiogenesis. Angiogenesis is a prerequisite for the growth of both primary cancer and metastases. In this chapter we will review the concept of tumor angiogenesis and angiogenesis factors, especially vascular endothelial growth factor (VEGF). We will emphasize the important role of angiogenesis in thyroid cancer and speculate on the potential treatments for thyroid cancer that target tumor angiogenesis using some of the newly developed angiogenesis inhibitors.

TUMOR ANGIOGENESIS

Angiogenesis is the development of new blood vessels from surrounding tissues. Angiogenesis creates new blood vessels out of existing blood vessels. This is in contrast to vasculogenesis, when new blood vessels are developed de novo in embryogenesis. Angiogenesis involves proliferation and migration of normal endothelial cells, usually in response to local conditions or paracrine factors secreted by other cells. Angiogenesis occurs in many normal processes, such as endometrial growth, follicular development, organ regeneration, and wound healing. It also occurs in some pathologic processes, such as diabetic retinopathy, hemangiomas, psoriasis, and rheumatoid arthritis.[3-8]

Angiogenesis is a prerequisite for tumor growth, because new blood vessels are needed to provide nutrients and oxygen to the growing tumor mass. Diffusion alone is only sufficient for a few millimeters. Without angiogenesis all solid tumors would be necrotic at the center and have a thin shell of viable tissue only a few millimeters thick.

Tumor angiogenesis has certain interesting aspects that challenge our usual perspectives on tumor growth. Angiogenesis is regulated by paracrine action. For example, tumor cells secrete angiogenesis factors, and the endothelial cells in the normal surrounding tissue then respond to these growth factors by proliferation and migration. Angiogenesis requires the normal endothelial cells to proliferate, then "invade" abnormal tumor tissue—the opposite of how we think of cancer, in which cancer cells proliferate and invade the normal surrounding tissue.

ANGIOGENESIS AND THE THYROID

Angiogenesis plays an important role in the growth of benign thyroid tissue, as in multinodular goiter[9] and Graves' disease,[10] and thyroid cancer. Thyroid cancers are vascular tumors. Angiogenesis allows the primary tumor and the metastases to grow in size. The size of the tumor is a prognostic factor for patients with thyroid cancer—that is, the larger the tumor, the worse the prognosis.[11] In fact, papillary thyroid cancers smaller than 0.5 cm are clinically insignificant and rarely invade or metastasize.[12] This benign course has been postulated to be caused by the lack of angiogenesis in these "occult cancers."

Microvasculature and Thyroid Cancer

The extent of tumor angiogenesis can be estimated by counting the number of microvessels in the histologic sections of the cancer tissue. The endothelial cells are identified by immunohistochemical staining using antibodies against factor VIII, CD31, or CD34, which are expressed in the endothelial cells. Tumor microvessel count has been found to correlate with tumor metastasis and patient prognosis for many cancers including breast cancer,[13] lung cancer,[14] colon cancer,[15] prostate cancer,[16] bladder cancer,[17] astroglial brain tumors,[18] and squamous cell cancer of the head and neck.[19,20]

Tumor microvasculature may also have prognostic significance in endocrine tumors. Tumor microvessel count was found to correlate with the invasive behavior of pheochromocytoma.[21] On the other hand, adrenocortical carcinomas have increased endothelial cell proliferation but do not have a higher microvessel count in comparison to adrenocortical adenomas or normal adrenocortical tissue.[22] The microvessel count in thyroid cancers is increased when compared with normal thyroid tissue. Microvessel count was found to correlate with the prognosis for patients with medullary thyroid cancer (MTC).[23] That is, tumors from patients who died of MTC contained significantly more microvessels than those from patients who did not die of MTC. In these patients, the microvessel count was the only clinically significant prognostic indicator besides TNM stage. Interestingly, however, in the same study, microvessel count did not correlate with prognosis in patients who had papillary, follicular, or undifferentiated thyroid cancer. These findings may reflect type II errors due to low or high mortality rates for the differentiated and undifferentiated thyroid cancers, respectively.

Although both benign (hyperplastic or neoplastic) and malignant thyroid tissues can have increased angiogenesis,[9,10] malignant and invading tissues may stimulate more angiogenesis. In microinvasive follicular thyroid carcinomas, Segal et al.[24] found that pleomorphic areas and areas adjacent to capsular penetration by the tumor had increased microvasculature, whereas there are no areas of increased microvasculature in follicular adenomas.

Angiogenesis Factors in Thyroid Tissue

Angiogenesis can be induced by various physiologic and pathologic conditions. For example, hypoxia is one of the most potent stimulators of angiogenesis.[25] Various growth factors produced by the cancer cells also stimulate tumor angiogenesis via paracrine action.[4] The best studied angiogenesis growth factor is VEGF, which will be discussed in detail in the next section. Other angiogenesis growth factors that are found in thyroid tissue or cancer are discussed below.

Basic fibroblast growth factor (bFGF, FGF-2) is a potent mitogenic factor for endothelial cells. Although it was initially identified in fibroblasts, basic FGF is present in many tissues in the body. The effect of bFGF and acidic FGF (aFGF, FGF-1) are mediated through the FGF receptor-1 (FGFR-1). Because bFGF does not have a secretory peptide, its action via the paracrine mechanism has been questioned. Basic FGF, however, is probably secreted by cancer cells, since it is found in the condition media of cell culture and is measurable in the plasma and urine of cancer patients.

Thyroid cells produce both bFGF and its receptor FGFR-1. Since bFGF has a mitogenic effect on both thyroid cells and endothelial cells, it has both an autocrine (stimulates thyroid cells themselves) and paracrine (stimulates endothelial cells) effect.

Rats treated with methimazole and placed on a low-iodine diet develop goiters. Immunohistochemical staining of these experimental goiters shows that the increased angiogenesis is accompanied by increased immunohistochemical staining of angiogenesis stimulators, bFGF, and transforming growth factor-beta 1 TGF-β1), and decreased immunohistochemical staining for an angiogenesis inhibitor, thrombospondin-1 (TSP-1).[9] Normal porcine thyroid cells produce bFGF, and bFGF is a growth factor for the FRTL-5 thyroid cells in culture.[26]

Development of human goiter is accompanied by increased angiogenesis. Thyroid follicular cells from multinodular goiter has an increased expression of bFGF, aFGF, and FGFR-1 compared with normal thyroid tissue.[27,28] Interestingly, in adenomatous goiter, FGFR-1 is more frequently expressed than bFGF; that is, some goiters may respond more to the paracrine stimulation of bFGF from neighboring tissue than from autocrine stimulation.[29]

In human differentiated thyroid cancers, both bFGF and FGFR-1 are highly expressed.[29,30] Immunohistochemical staining of bFGF in the thyroid cells is most intense for thyroid cancers, followed by adenomas, followed by normal thyroid tissue.[30] Expression of bFGF may correlate with the degree of malignancy in differentiated thyroid cancer—the more intensely the cells stain for bFGF, the more extensive the lymphnode metastasis.[31,32]

The stimulation of bFGF on endothelial cells involves both a direct paracrine and an indirect autocrine mechanism. Basic FGF stimulates the endothelial cell directly via the FGF receptor. It also induces VEGF expression by the endothelial cells. VEGF then stimulates the endothelial cells in an autocrine fashion. Neutralizing anti-VEGF antibody can dramatically reduce the angiogenesis induced by bFGF.[33]

Placental-derived growth factor (PIGF) mRNA is expressed in the normal thyroid gland and goiter. PIGF is a dimeric glycoprotein similar to VEGF. PIGF-1 and PIGF-2 are splice variants that differ only in the carboxyl terminal. PIGF-1 induces angiogenesis in the rabbit cornea and chick chorioallantoic membrane assays, and it stimulates the migration and proliferation of endothelial cells in the bovine coronary postcapillary venules and human umbilical vein assays. PIGF-1 induced angiogenesis in a dose-dependent manner, and it had an effect comparable with that of VEGF and bFGF under similar conditions and concentrations.[34]

Other growth factors, such as epidermal growth factor (EGF), transforming growth factor-alpha and beta (TGF-α and TGF-β), angiogenin and tumor necrosis factor-alpha (TNF-α) have also been implicated in tumor angiogenesis. These factors do not directly stimulate proliferation of endothelial cells, and probably induce angiogenesis indirectly.

Nonthyroid cells within the thyroid cancer tissue, such as the tumor-infiltrating lymphocytes, also secrete angiogenesis factors and may contribute to tumor angiogenesis.[35]

VASCULAR ENDOTHELIAL GROWTH FACTOR

VEGF is a unique angiogenesis factor because it is a true paracrine growth factor.[36-39] Cancer cells secrete VEGF. VEGF then stimulates neighboring noncancer endothelial cells to grow, to produce proteases, to migrate, and to make new capillaries. VEGF, however, has no significant direct mitogenic effect on the cancer cells themselves.

VEGF is a 34 to 42 kDa, heat- and acid-stable, dimeric, heparin-binding glycoprotein.[40,41] The different splice variants of VEGF account for the different molecular weights. VEGF binds to membrane VEGF receptors 1 and 2 (flt1 and flk1/KDR) that are receptor tyrosine kinases, and activates the phospholipase C signaling system.[42] Embryologically VEGF promotes vasculogenesis by stimulating the cells via VEGF receptors 1 and 2. In existing blood vessels, such as those at the edge of a cancer, VEGF promotes angiogenesis in cooperation with angiopoietin 2, which inhibits the Tie 2 receptor. Tie 1 and Tie 2 receptors are also receptor tyrosine kinases that are structurally similar to VEGF receptors.[43] Tie 2 binds to angiopoietins. These receptor tyrosine kinases are crucial for embryologic development; transgenic mice overexpressing angiopoietin 2 or knockout mice without functioning VEGF receptors or Tie receptors do not survive.[44]

VEGF may be the final common pathway for other growth factors that have been found to stimulate angiogenesis, for example, hypoxia-inducible factor-1alpha (HIF-1α)[25] and bFGF.[33]

VEGF not only stimulates proliferation of endothelial cells but also increases vascular permeability, and was also named vascular permeability factor (VPF). This increase in vascular permeability also facilitates angiogenesis. Extravasation of plasma proteins and deposition of fibrin create an extravascular fibrin gel matrix that supports the in-growth of new blood vessels.[40,45]

The Role of VEGF in Thyroid Tissue

VEGF expression in thyroid cell lines can be analyzed by Northern blot for VEGF mRNA and Western blot for VEGF protein synthesis. Secretion of VEGF can be measured in the culture media by enzyme-linked immunosorbent assay. VEGF expression in thyroid cells can also be localized in histologic sections by immunohistochemical staining with anti-VEGF antibody. For example, human cell lines from fibrosarcoma (HT1080), histiocytic lymphoma (U937), and rhabdomyosarcoma (A673) have been found to express VEGF mRNA and secrete VEGF in vitro.

Sato et al.[10] were the first to show that normal and Graves' thyroid tissue expressed VEGF mRNA. Viglietto et al.[46] showed that thyroid cancer cell lines expressed VEGF and that VEGF expression paralleled the tumorigenic potential of the cell lines. They also found that VEGF was most highly expressed in the anaplastic thyroid cancer cell line.

In our own studies, we found higher VEGF mRNA expressions and VEGF production and secretion in the thyroid cancer cell lines (papillary, follicular, Hürthle, and medullary cancer cell lines) than in the primary cultures of normal thyroid cells.[47] We found that thyroid cancer cell lines of follicular cell origin expressed more VEGF than those of parafollicular cell origin. Primary and metastatic thyroid cancers, however, appeared not to differ in their VEGF expression. Immunohistochemical staining of papillary, follicular, and Hürthle cell cancers for VEGF was also stronger than that of medullary thyroid cancers, benign tissue, or hyperplastic (Graves' disease) thyroid tissue.[47]

Although most of the experimental data support the paracrine action of VEGF (from the thyroid cells to the endothelial cells) and have identified VEGF receptors only in the endothelial cells, some studies showed VEGF receptors in thyroid cells. Wang et al.[48] identified VEGF receptors on FRTL-5 rat thyroid cells and postulated a negative autocrine effect of VEGF on the thyroid cell. In the FRTL-5 cells, VEGF inhibited the TSH-stimulated uptake of thymidine.

Regulation of Vascular Endothelial Growth Factor Expression in Thyroid Tissue

Growth factors (e.g., TSH, EGF), inhibitors (e.g., tamoxifen), and activating oncogenes (e.g., ras) that are known to modulate thyroid cancer cell growth may also have an indirect effect on thyroid cancer tumor growth and metastasis by regulating the expression of VEGF and tumor angiogenesis. TSH stimulates the production and secretion of VEGF by the thyroid cell via both the adenylate cyclase and the protein kinase C signal transduction pathways.[10] When rats were made hypothyroid by propylthiouracil (PTU), and have an elevated serum level of TSH, the thyroid cells expressed more VEGF mRNA, whereas the endothelial cells from the thyroid gland expressed more VEGF receptors.[48]

Thyroid cancers, in general, secrete more VEGF than normal thyroid cells. In our studies of human thyroid cancer cell lines, we found some to have a constitutively elevated VEGF secretion and others to have an exaggerated increase in VEGF secretion in response to TSH stimulation.[49] XTC-1 Hürthle cell cancer cell line[50] has a threefold higher basal VEGF secretion than normal thyroid cells. TPC-1 (papillary), FTC-133 (follicular), and MTC 1.1 (medullary) thyroid cancer cell lines secreted significantly more (twofold to fivefold) VEGF than normal thyroid cells when stimulated with TSH. Therefore TSH may promote growth in some thyroid cancers by stimulating VEGF secretion and angiogenesis.[49] In these cell lines, we also found that VEGF secretion is stimulated by epidermal growth factor and inhibited by tamoxifen.

The ras oncogene, which is activated in some thyroid cancers and follicular adenomas,[1] may also have an effect on angiogenesis via VEGF. H-ras transformed rat intestinal epithelial cells have an increased expression of VEGF. When the mutant ras protein was disrupted by treatment with L-739, 749 (a protein farnesyltransferase inhibitor), the expression of VEGF was suppressed.[51]

ANGIOGENESIS INHIBITORS

Since angiogenesis is essential for the growth of localized and metastatic cancers, inhibiting angiogenesis may prevent cancer growth, and it potentially can be used to treat patients with cancer. There are theoretical advantages that make antiangiogenesis therapy appealing for cancer treatment. The target of antiangiogenesis is the normal endothelial cells that are homogeneous, genetically stable, and have a low mutation rate. It is therefore less likely to develop resistance to treatment. By contrast, standard chemotherapy that targets tumor cells usually become less effective with repetitive use, because the cancer cells are more heterogeneous, genetically unstable, and have a higher mutational rate.[52] Another interesting aspect is that anti-invasive agents not only can block invasion by the tumor cells but also can block the invasion by the newly formed vessels into the tumor (tumor angiogenesis).

Inhibitors of invasion can therefore indirectly block the growth of primary tumor and metastasis by blocking angiogenesis.[53]

Any potential antiangiogenesis drug for cancer treatment requires multistep testing before clinical trials in humans are begun. First, it must be tested to determine whether it inhibits proliferation of endothelial cells in culture. Second, it must be determined whether the drug inhibits angiogenesis in bioassays, for example, in rabbit cornea or chick embryo chorioallantoic membrane. Third, it must be determined whether the drug has an antitumor effect in xenotransplanted human cancers in nude mice, such as preventing primary tumor growth, formation of metastases, or shrinking or obliterating the tumor mass. Before a drug is used in human trials, it must demonstrate a significant anticancer effect. In addition, since angiogenesis is required for normal physiologic processes, such as endometrial growth and wound repair, potential toxicity should be monitored.

Next we will review some of the antiangiogenesis drugs that have an anticancer effect. Some of them are already involved in clinical trials and may potentially be useful for treating advanced or aggressive thyroid cancers.

TNP-470 (AGM-1470)

TNP-470, 6-O-(N-chloroacetyl-carbamoyl)-fumagillol, is a semisynthetic analog of fumagillin that inhibits in vivo tumor growth. The exact mechanism of action for TNP-470 is unknown, although it inhibits the methionine aminopeptidase activity of type 2 methionine aminopeptidase (MetAP2).[54] TNP-470 has been found to prevent the development of liver metastases from xenotransplanted human colon cancer[55,56] and stomach cancer[57] in nude mice and bone metastases from xenotransplanted breast cancer.[58] Clinical trials are ongoing for the treatment of a variety of cancers with TNP-470. Complete remission of metastatic cervical cancer after treatment with TNP-470 has also been reported.[59]

Hama et al.,[60] in an experimental model of thyroid cancer, treated xenotransplanted human anaplastic thyroid carcinoma in nude mice with injection of TNP-470. Intratumoral injection of TNP-470 completely inhibited tumor growth. Peritumoral injection also significantly inhibited tumor growth, whereas subcutaneous and intraperitoneal injections were less effective.

Protease inhibitors may inhibit angiogenesis, since proteolysis is an important aspect of invasion and angiogenesis. Degradation of the extracellular matrix facilitates cell migration. Rats injected with Dunning MAT-LyLu prostate cancer cells develop lung metastases.[61] Serine protease urokinase (u-PA) stimulates tumor angiogenesis. To determine the role of u-PA in cancer, gene coding for a mutant u-PA, which binds to the receptor but has no proteolytic activity, was used to transfect these prostate cancer cells. Rats injected with the transfected cells had smaller tumors and fewer metastases.[61] Matrix metalloproteinase (MMP) may also stimulate tumor angiogenesis. The activity of MMP is inhibited by tissue inhibitor of metalloproteinases-1 (TIMP-1). TIMP-1 has been found to have antiangiogenesis effects.[62]

Tyrosine Kinase Inhibitors

Antiangiogenesis drugs may also target downstream in the signaling pathway of the angiogenesis factor. PD 166866, 6-aryl-pyrido[2,3-d] pyrimidine, is a specific inhibitor of the human fibroblast growth factor-1 receptor (FGFR-1) tyrosine kinase.[63] Similarly, wortmannin is a fungal metabolite that selectively inhibits phosphatidylinositol 3-kinase, and it has been found to inhibit angiogenesis in bioassays of chick embryo chorioallantoic membranes.[64]

Anti-VEGF Antibody

Kim et al.[65] and Warren et al.[66] showed that murine monoclonal anti-VEGF antibody inhibited the growth of xenotransplanted human cancer cells in nude mice and prevented liver metastases. In our own study,[47,49] we injected nude mice subcutaneously with human thyroid cancer cells (papillary TPC-1, follicular FTC-133, and Hürthle XTC-1). These mice developed large subcutaneous tumors, and some developed systemic metastases. For the treatment group, we began intraperitoneal injection with anti-VEGF antibody when the tumor became apparent (2 mm). Treatment with anti-VEGF antibody dramatically inhibited tumor angiogenesis and prevented the growth of subcutaneous tumors and development of metastases. The humanized form of anti-VEGF antibody is currently being used in clinical trials for treatment of various cancers.

Angiostatin and Endostatin

Some interesting new angiogenesis inhibitors are those produced by the cancer cells themselves. The clinical observation that distant metastases frequently remain dormant until the primary cancer is removed led to the hypothesis of tumor-produced antiangiogenesis factors that suppress the growth of distant metastases via an endocrine mechanism. This hypothesis was proved true when O'Reilly et al.[67] isolated angiostatin from a primary Lewis lung carcinoma and found it to be a potent angiogenesis inhibitor that suppressed the growth of its own lung metastases. Angiostatin is produced by cancer-mediated proteolysis by urokinase (u-PA) that converts plasminogen to angiostatin.[68,69] In addition to systemic administration, gene therapy using angiostatin is another potential treatment. Gene transfer of a cDNA coding for mouse angiostatin into murine T241 fibrosarcoma cells suppressed primary and metastatic tumor growth in vivo.[70]

A potential disadvantage of antiangiogenesis therapy is that it may only be tumoristatic and not tumoricidal. Endostatin is a 20 kDa C-terminal fragment of collagen XVIII that specifically inhibits endothelial proliferation, tumor angiogenesis, and tumor growth. It was identified from a hemangioendothelioma using a strategy similar to that used for identifying angiostatin.[71] When mice bearing Lewis lung carcinoma, T241 fibrosarcoma, or B16F10 melanoma were treated with endostatin, the tumors regressed. When the tumors regrew, the mice were retreated with endostatin. After two to six treatment cycles, the tumors no longer recurred. This ability to treat repeatedly without developing drug resistance and to induce prolonged tumor dormancy after repeated treatment showed that antiangiogenesis therapy might have advantages over conventional chemotherapy.[52]

Other Angiogenesis Inhibitors

There are numerous other angiogenesis inhibitors. FR-118487 suppressed liver metastasis by inhibiting angiogenesis in a rabbit colon cancer model.[72] Clarithromycin is a macrolide antibiotic. It suppressed tumor-induced angiogenesis by inhibiting endothelial cell tube formation.[73] Eriochrome Black T (EBT) is an analog of suramin, a cancer chemotherapeutic agent. EBT inhibited angiogenesis in the chick chorioallantoic membrane assay with more potency and less toxicity than suramin.[74] Irsogladine is used clinically as an anti-gastric ulcer agent. It inhibited tumor growth and angiogenesis in xenotransplants of human glioma and hepatoma cells.[75] The endogenous estrogen metabolite 2-methoxyoestradiol inhibited endothelial cell proliferation and migration in vitro and angiogenesis and growth of solid tumors in mice.[76] SR 25989 is a member of the thienopyridine family. It inhibits angiogenesis by upregulating thrombospondin-1, probably mediated by p53.[77] Thrombospondin-1 is a 430 kDa glycoprotein that is a component of the extracellular matrix and a potent inhibitor of angiogenesis both in vitro and in vivo.[78]

CONCLUSION

As in most other solid tumors, growth and metastasis of thyroid cancer depend on tumor angiogenesis. Various paracrine factors, such as VEGF and bFGF, are produced by the cancer cells and stimulate the normal endothelial cells to proliferate and migrate and to develop new vessels that provide nutrients to the growing tumor. Microvasculature count is a prognostic factor in many solid tumors and may have prognostic importance in some thyroid cancers. Production and secretion of angiogenesis factors by thyroid cancer cells are likely to be regulated by thyroid-stimulating hormone and its associated signaling pathways that also regulate thyroid cell function and growth. Antiangiogenesis therapy, such as TNP-470, anti-VEGF antibody, angiostatin, and endostatin, may in the future be an option for treatment of advanced or aggressive thyroid cancers.

REFERENCES

1. Fagin JA. Molecular genetics of human thyroid neoplasms. Annu Rev Med 45:45, 1994.
2. Hoelting T, Duh QY. Thyroid tumor growth, invasion and metastasis in vivo and in vitro. In Clark OH, Duh QY, eds. Textbook of Endocrine Surgery. Philadelphia: WB Saunders, 1997.
3. Folkman J. What is the evidence that tumors are angiogenesis dependent? J Natl Cancer Inst 82:4, 1990.
4. Risau W. Angiogenic growth factors. Prog Growth Factor Res 2:71, 1990.
5. Bouck N. Tumor angiogenesis: The role of oncogenesis and tumor suppressor genes. Cancer Cells 2:179, 1990.
6. Folkman J et al. Induction of angiogenesis during the transition from hyperplasia to neoplasia. Nature 339:58, 1989.
7. Folkman J, Shing Y. Angiogenesis. J Biol Chem 267:10931, 1992.
8. Shifren JL et al. In the human fetus, vascular endothelial growth factor is expressed in epithelial cells and monocytes, but not vascular endothelium: Implications for mode of action. J Clin Endocrinol Metab 79:316, 1994.
9. Patel VA et al. Changes in the immunohistochemical localisation of fibroblast growth factor-2, transforming growth factor-beta 1 and thrombospondin-1 are associated with early angiogenic events in the hyperplastic rat thyroid. J Endocrinol 148:485, 1996.
10. Sato K et al. Stimulation by thyroid-stimulating hormone and Graves' immunoglobulin G of vascular endothelial growth factor mRNA expression in human thyroid follicles in vitro and flt mRNA expression in the rat thyroid in vivo. J Clin Invest 96:1295, 1995.
11. Hay ID et al. Predicting outcome in papillary thyroid carcinoma: Development of a reliable prognostic scoring system in a cohort of 1779 patients surgically treated at one institution during 1940 through 1989. Surgery 114:1050, 1993.
12. Cady B, Rossi R. Surgery of the thyroid and parathyroid gland. In Silverman ML, ed. Pathology of the thyroid and parathyroid gland, 3rd ed. Philadelphia: WB Saunders, 1991.
13. Weidner N et al. Tumor angiogenesis and metastasis—Correlation in invasive breast carcinoma. N Engl J Med 324:1, 1991.
14. Harpole DH Jr et al. Angiogenesis and molecular biologic substaging in patients with stage I non-small cell lung cancer. Ann Thorac Surg 61:1470, 1996.
15. Frank RE et al. Tumor angiogenesis as a predictor of recurrence and survival in patients with node-negative colon cancer. Ann Surg 222:695, 1995.

16. Weidner N et al. Tumor angiogenesis correlates with metastasis in invasive prostate carcinoma. Am J Pathol 143:401, 1993.
17. Jaeger TM et al. Tumor angiogenesis correlates with lymph node metastases in invasive bladder cancer. J Urol 154:69, 1995.
18. Leon SP, Folkerth RD, Black PM. Microvessel density is a prognostic indicator for patients with astroglial brain tumors. Cancer 77:362, 1996.
19. Williams JK et al. Tumor angiogenesis as a prognostic factor in oral cavity tumors. Am J Surg 168:373, 1994.
20. Eisma RJ, Spiro JD, Kreutzer DL. Vascular endothelial growth factor expression in head and neck squamous cell carcinoma. Am J Surg 174:513, 1997.
21. Liu Q et al. Tumor angiogenesis in pheochromocytomas and paragangliomas. Surgery 120:938, 1996.
22. Sasano H et al. Vascularity in human adrenal cortex. Mod Pathol 11:329, 1998.
23. Fontanini G et al. Microvessel count: An indicator of poor outcome in medullary thyroid carcinoma but not in other types of thyroid carcinoma. Mod Pathol 9:636, 1996.
24. Segal K et al. Angiogenesis in follicular tumors of the thyroid. J Surg Oncol 63:95, 1996.
25. Carmeliet P et al. Role of HIF-1 alpha in hypoxia-mediated apoptosis, cell proliferation and tumour angiogenesis. Nature 394:485, 1998.
26. Emoto N et al. Identification and characterization of basic fibroblast growth factor in porcine thyroids. Endocrinology 128:58, 1991.
27. Becks GP et al. Increase of basic fibroblast growth factor (FGF) and FGF receptor messenger RNA during rat thyroid hyperplasia: Temporal changes and cellular distribution. J Endocrinol 142:325, 1994.
28. Thompson SD et al. Fibroblast growth factors 1 and 2 and fibroblast growth factor receptor 1 are elevated in thyroid hyperplasia. J Clin Endocrinol Metab 83:1336, 1998.
29. Shingu K et al. Expression of fibroblast growth factor-2 and fibroblast growth factor receptor-1 in thyroid diseases: Difference between neoplasms and hyperplastic lesions. Endocr J 45:35, 1998.
30. Eggo MC et al. Expression of fibroblast growth factors in thyroid cancer. J Clin Endocrinol Metab 80:1006, 1995.
31. Kodama M et al. Immunohistochemical localization of acidic and basic fibroblast growth factors in human benign and malignant thyroid lesions. Jpn J Clin Oncol 24:66, 1994.
32. Shingu K et al. Expression of basic fibroblast growth factor in thyroid disorders. World J Surg 18:500, 1994.
33. Seghezzi G et al. Fibroblast growth factor-2 (FGF-2) induces vascular endothelial growth factor (VEGF) expression in the endothelial cells of forming capillaries: An autocrine mechanism contributing to angiogenesis. J Cell Biol 141:1659, 1998.
34. Ziche M et al. Placenta growth factor-1 is chemotactic, mitogenic, and angiogenic. Lab Invest 76:517, 1997.
35. Herrmann G et al. T lymphocytes, CD68-positive cells and vascularisation in thyroid carcinomas. J Cancer Res Clin Oncol 120:651, 1994.
36. Conn G et al. Purification of a glycoprotein vascular endothelial cell mitogen from a rat glioma-derived cell line. Proc Natl Acad Sci USA 87:1323, 1990.
37. Leung DW et al. Vascular endothelial factor is a secreted angiogenic mitogen. Science 246:1306, 1989.
38. Jakeman LB et al. Binding sites for vascular endothelial growth factor are localized on endothelial cells in adult rat tissues. J Clin Invest 89:244, 1992.

39. Weinder K, Marme D, Weich H. AIDS-associated Kaposi's sarcoma cells in culture express vascular endothelial growth factor. Biochem Biophys Res Commun 183:1167, 1992.
40. Senger DR et al. Purification and NH_2-terminal amino acid sequence of guinea pig tumor-secreted vascular permeability factor. Cancer Res 50:1774, 1990.
41. Yeo T-K et al. Glycosylation is essential for efficient secretion but not for permeability enhancing activity of vascular permeability factor (vascular endothelial growth factor). Biochem Biophys Res Commun 179:1568, 1991.
42. Brock TA, Dvorak HF, Senger DK. Tumor-secreted vascular permeability factor increases cytosolic Ca^{2+} and von Willebrand factor release in human endothelial cells. Am J Pathol 138:213, 1991.
43. Lin P et al. Inhibition of tumor angiogenesis using a soluble receptor establishes a role for Tie2 in pathologic vascular growth. J Clin Invest 100:2072, 1997.
44. Maisonpierre PC et al. Angiopoietin-2, a natural antagonist for Tie2 that disrupts in vivo angiogenesis. Science 277:55, 1997.
45. Nagy JA et al. Pathogenesis of tumor stroma generation: A critical role for leaky blood vessels and fibrin deposition. Biochem Biophys Acta 948:305, 1988.
46. Viglietto G et al. Upregulation of vascular endothelial growth factor (VEGF) and down regulation of placental growth factor (PLGF) associated with malignancy in human thyroid tumors and cell lines. Oncogene 11:1569, 1995.
47. Soh EY et al. Vascular endothelial growth factor expression is higher in differentiated thyroid cancer than in normal or benign thyroid. J Clin Endocrinol Metab 82:3741, 1997.
48. Wang JF et al. Presence and possible role of vascular endothelial growth factor in thyroid cell growth and function. J Endocrinol 157:5, 1998.
49. Soh EY et al. Thyroid-stimulating hormone promotes the secretion of vascular endothelial growth factor in thyroid cancer cell lines. Surgery 120:944, 1996.
50. Zielke A et al. Establishment of a highly differentiated thyroid cancer cell line of Hürthle cell origin. Thyroid 8:475, 1998.
51. Rak J et al. Mutant ras oncogenes upregulate VEGF/VPF expression: Implications for induction and inhibition of tumor angiogenesis. Cancer Res 55:4575, 1995.
52. Boehm T et al. Antiangiogenic therapy of experimental cancer does not induce acquired drug resistance. Nature 390:404, 1997.
53. Kohn EC, Liotta LA. Molecular insights into cancer invasion: Strategies for prevention and intervention. Cancer Res 55:1856, 1995.
54. Griffith EC et al. Methionine aminopeptidase (type 2) is the common target for angiogenesis inhibitors AGM-1470 and ovalicin. Chem Biol 4:461, 1997.
55. Tanaka T et al. Prevention of hepatic metastasis of human colon cancer by angiogenesis inhibitor TNP-470. Cancer Res 55:836, 1995.
56. Konno H et al. Efficacy of an angiogenesis inhibitor, TNP-470, in xenotransplanted human colorectal cancer with high metastatic potential. Cancer 77(Suppl):1736, 1996.
57. Kanai T et al. Effect of angiogenesis inhibitor TNP-470 on the progression of human gastric cancer xenotransplanted into nude mice. Int J Cancer 71:838, 1997.
58. Sasaki A et al. Angiogenesis inhibitor TNP-470 inhibits human breast cancer osteolytic bone metastasis in nude mice through the reduction of bone resorption. Cancer Res 58:462, 1998.
59. Kudelka AP, Verschraegen CF, Loyer E. Complete remission of metastatic cervical cancer with the angiogenesis inhibitor TNP-470. N Engl J Med 338:991, 1998.

60. Hama Y et al. Therapeutic efficacy of the angiogenesis inhibitor O-(chloroacetyl-carbamoyl) fumagillol (TNP-470; AGM-1470) for human anaplastic thyroid carcinoma in nude mice. Exp Toxicolo Pathol 49:239, 1997.
61. Evans CP et al. Inhibition of prostate cancer neovascularization and growth by urokinase-plasminogen activator receptor blockade. Cancer Res 57:3594, 1997.
62. Thorgeirsson UP et al. Breast cancer: Tumor neovasculature and the effect of tissue inhibitor of metalloproteinases-1 (TIMP-1) on angiogenesis. In Vivo 10:137, 1996.
63. Panek RL et al. In vitro biological characterization and antiangiogenic effects of PD 166866, a selective inhibitor of the FGF-1 receptor tyrosine kinase. J Pharmacol Exp Ther 286:569, 1998.
64. Oikawa T, Shimamura M. Potent inhibition of angiogenesis by wortmannin, a fungal metabolite. Eur J Pharmacol 318:93, 1996.
65. Kim KJ et al. Inhibition of vascular endothelial growth factor-induced angiogenesis suppresses tumor growth in vivo. Nature 362:841, 1993.
66. Warren RS et al. Regulation by vascular endothelial growth factor of human colon cancer tumorigenesis in a mouse model of experimental liver metastasis. J Clin Invest 95:1789, 1995.
67. O'Reilly MS et al. Angiostatin: A novel angiogenesis inhibitor that mediates the suppression of metastases by a Lewis lung carcinoma. Cell 79:315, 1994.
68. Gately S et al. Human prostate carcinoma cells express enzymatic activity that converts human plasminogen to the angiogenesis inhibitor, angiostatin. Cancer Res 56:4887, 1996.
69. Gately S et al. The mechanism of cancer-mediated conversion of plasminogen to the angiogenesis inhibitor angiostatin. Proc Natl Acad Sci USA 94:10868, 1997.
70. Cao Y et al. Expression of angiostatin cDNA in a murine fibrosarcoma suppresses primary tumor growth and produces long-term dormancy of metastases. J Clin Invest 101:1055, 1998.
71. O'Reilly MS et al. Endostatin: An endogenous inhibitor of angiogenesis and tumor growth. Cell 88:277, 1997.
72. Eda I et al. The suppression of postoperative liver metastasis caused by the continuous intraportal infusion of angiogenesis inhibitor FR-118487 in a rabbit colon cancer model. Surg Today 28:273, 1998.
73. Yatsunami J et al. Clarithromycin is a potent inhibitor of tumor-induced angiogenesis. Res Exp Med 197:189, 1997.
74. Morris AD et al. Eriochrome Black T, structurally related to suramin, inhibits angiogenesis and tumor growth in vivo. Anticancer Drugs 8:746, 1997.
75. Ono M et al. Inhibition of tumor growth and neovascularization by an antigastric ulcer agent, irsogladine. Cancer Res 56:1512, 1996.
76. Fotsis T et al. The endogenous oestrogen metabolite 2-methoxyoestradiol inhibits angiogenesis and suppresses tumour growth. Nature 368:237, 1994.
77. Klein-Soyer C et al. Angiogenesis inhibitor SR 25989 upregulates thrombospondin-1 expression in human vascular endothelial cells and foreskin fibroblasts. Biol Cell 89:295, 1997.
78. Grossfeld GD et al. Thrombospondin-1 expression in bladder cancer: Association with p53 alterations, tumor angiogenesis, and tumor progression. J Natl Cancer Inst 89:219, 1997.

CHAPTER

18

Genetic Basis of Medullary Thyroid Carcinoma

SHINYA UCHINO, M.D., Ph.D.

Medullary thyroid carcinoma (MTC) is a relatively rare malignant thyroid disease that accounts for approximately 1% to 5% of all thyroid carcinomas.[1,2] Approximately 75% of MTCs develop as sporadic tumors and 25% are familial. MTC was first reported as a distinct clinicopathologic entity of thyroid cancer by Hazard et al.[3] in 1959. In 1961, Sipple[4] reported a high incidence of thyroid cancer in patients with pheochromocytomas. The association of MTC with pheochromocytoma and hyperparathyroidism was found to be a characteristic combination of hereditary disease of MEN2.[5,6]

Patients with familial MTC (FMTC) are classically divided into three types according to the phenotype of the disease. The first is multiple endocrine neoplasia type 2A (MEN2A), characterized by three endocrine tumors in different combinations: MTC, pheochromocytoma, and hyperparathyroidism. Approximately 50% of MTCs occur in combination with pheochromocytoma and 15% to 30% with hyperparathyroidism.[7] In most MEN2A patients, MTC is the initial presentation and the major cause of morbidity and mortality. The second form is MEN2B, characterized by MTC, pheochromocytoma, multiple mucosal neuromas of the lips and tongue, intestinal ganglioneuromatosis, and eye and skeletal (marfanoid habitus) abnormalities. MEN2B is the most lethal form among the three types and presents earlier in childhood. The third form is FMTC with no other endocrine disease in a minimum of four members. FMTC develops later in life and is more indolent than MEN2A and MEN2B. These familial forms are inherited as an autosomal dominant mutation with nearly complete penetrance. A child of an affected parent has a 50% chance of inheriting the causative gene and developing MTC.

Clinically, sporadic MTC is characterized by a negative family history in a patient whose MTC is usually diagnosed when in his or her fifties or sixties.[8] Some patients with MTC are diagnosed with MTC postoperatively. The major histologic differences between familial and sporadic MTC are that hereditary MTC develops bilaterally in the superior portion of the thyroid lobes and is multicentric, whereas sporadic MTC usually presents as a single nodule.

C-CELL STIMULATION TEST

The former method for the identifying asymptomatic individuals at risk for MEN2A, MEN2B, and FMTC was by performing provocative tests with infusion of pentagastrin or calcium to measure a patient's serum calcitonin levels. An abnormal increase in the calcitonin level suggests the presence of C-cell hyperplasia or MTC. Careful assessment of the results of C-cell stimulation test is necessary, because there are physiologic and neoplastic C-cell hyperplasias as well as varied numbers of C cells, so an individual's response to C-cell stimulation may differ in the normal population. An increased number of C cells in normal subjects is not uncommon and may represent a physiologic form of C-cell hyperplasia rather than a neoplastic hyperplasia. Neoplastic C-cell hyperplasia is the precursor of MTC associated with MEN2A, MEN2B, and FMTC.[9] In gene carriers of MEN2A, MEN2B, or FMTC, neoplastic C-cell hyperplasia often occurs early in life. Physiologic forms cannot be recognized with conventional hematoxylin and eosin staining and require calcitonin immunostaining for diagnosis. Neoplastic forms consist of mildly to moderately atypical C cells that can usually be identified with hematoxylin & eosin-stained sections.

Provocative testing that uses pentagastrin and/or calcium to diagnose patients with C-cell hyperplasia or early MTC was helpful. However, subsequent studies have documented that total thyroidectomy was performed in 5% to 10% of individuals at risk for MEN2A who had abnormal results of C-cell stimulation tests, but that were subsequently documented to be RET gene negative.[10-13] It seems that slightly high calcitonin levels after stimulation could not accurately discriminate between a false positive response or the presence of MTC or neoplastic C-cell hyperplasia.[14-19]

RET GENE

The gene responsible for MEN2A has been localized on chromosome 10q11.2 by linkage analysis.[20-24] In 1993, germline point mutations of RET proto-oncogene were identified and have subsequently been found in family members affected with MEN2A, MEN2B, and FMTC.[25-27]

The RET proto-oncogene encodes a protein structurally related to transmembrane receptors with a cytoplasmic tyrosine-kinase domain. This gene contains two cadherin-like repeats in the extracellular region, a cysteine-rich domain upstream of the transmembrane domain, and a tyrosine-kinase domain in the cytoplasmic region (Fig. 18-1). Its overall architecture is similar to that of epidermal growth factor, platelet-derived growth factor, and nerve growth factor receptors.[28,29] The RET gene is located on chromosome 10q11.2[30,31] and is composed of at least 20 exons distributed along 30 kb of genomic DNA.[30-34] It was first isolated by transfection of NIH3T3 cells with a human T-cell lymphoma DNA, and was activated by the fusion of the tyrosine-kinase domain of this gene to the 5′-terminal portion of one of the other genes.[35] RET rearrangements are also found in papillary thyroid carcinomas.[36,37] To date, three genes capable of rearrangement with RET gene have been found: H4 gene (RET/PTC1),[38] the regulatory subunit RIα of cAMP-dependent protein kinase A (RET/PTC2),[39] and ELE1 gene (RET/PTC3)[40,41]

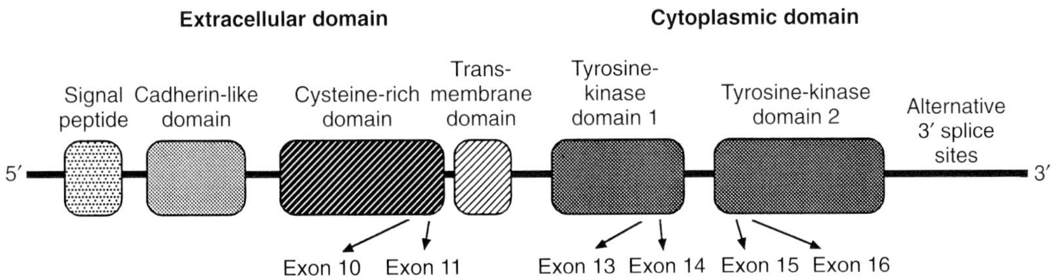

• **FIGURE 18-1** Schematic representation of the RET receptor tyrosine kinase. There is a signal peptide, cadherin-like domain, and cysteine-rich domain in the extracellular domain and two tyrosine-kinase domains in the cytoplasmic domain. Exons of RET proto-oncogene in which germline or somatic mutations have been reported are indicated by arrows.

Recent investigations have revealed that glial cell line–derived neurotrophic factor (GDNF), a member of the transforming growth factor-β superfamily, is the natural ligand for the RET receptor tyrosine kinase. It acts through a multimeric receptor complex, which also includes a novel glycosyl phosphoinositol–linked protein GDNF receptor-α.[42,43] It has been postulated that GDNF is the ligand for a heterotetrameric complex of RET and GDNFR-α in which GDNFR-α provides the ligand-binding capacity for GDNF, and RET provides the signaling function. No GDNF mutation was found in MEN2 families and sporadic endocrine tumors without a RET mutation.[44,45]

GERMLINE MUTATIONS IN MEN2A, MEN2B, AND FMTC FAMILIES

Actually, more than 95% MEN2A families have a germline RET point mutation. Mutations are concentrated on five cysteine codons: 609, 611, 618, and 620 in exon 10, and 634 in exon 11, mapping in a cysteine-rich domain of the extracellular domain of the RET protein (Table 18-1 and Fig. 18-2).[25,26] In the study of the International RET Mutation Consortium, germline mutations in the above five cysteine codons were found in 199 (98%) of 203 MEN2A families.[46] Among the five cysteine residues, codon 634 is most commonly mutated (in 85% of MEN2A families). The most frequent mutation at codon 634 in MEN2A families is TGC → CGC (52%) resulting in the amino acid substitution of arginine for cysteine.

Approximately 95% of families with MEN2B had a germline mutation at codon 918; ATG → ACG resulting in the substitution of methionine for threonine in exon 16 of the RET gene (see Table 18-1 and Fig. 18-2).[27,47] A germline two-base substitution GCT (Ala) → TTT (Phe) at condon 883 was also found in a few MEN2B families.[48] In more than 50% of MEN2B patients, the mutation is de novo (new germinal mutation), whereas only about 10% of MEN2A are de novo mutations. In studies of parent-of-origin effects in MEN2B, it was demonstrated that almost all patients had a paternally derived de novo codon 918 mutation.[49,50] A RET allele may be more susceptible to mutation when inherited from the father.

Germline RET mutations have been found in 88% of FMTC families (see Table 18-1 and Fig. 18-2). The majority of mutations in FMTC families occur in the same five cysteine codons as for MEN2A mutations.[25,46] Mutations in FMTC families show a relatively equal distribution compared with that of MEN2A families. Codon 630 is another cysteine codon and was reported to be mutated in one FMTC case.[51] Mutations have also been

TABLE 18-1 Germline RET Mutations in MEN2A, MEN2B, and FMTC

Exon	Codon	Nucleotide Change	Amino Acid Change	Restriction Enzyme
MEN2A and FMTC				
10	609	TGC → CGC	Cys → Arg	BspMI, AciI
		TGC → TAC	Cys → Tyr	BspMI
	611	TGC → TAC	Cys → Tyr	(–)
		TGC → TGG	Cys → Trp	NlaIV
	618	TGC → AGC	Cys → Ser	AluI, EarI
		TGC → GGC	Cys → Gly	(–)
		TGC → CGC	Cys → Arg	CfoI, HaeII, HhaI, HinPI
		TGC → TAC	Cys → Tyr	RsaI
		TGC → TCC	Cys → Ser	(–)
		TGC → TTC	Cys → Phe	MboII
	620	TGC → GGC	Cys → Gly	(–)
		TGC → CGC	Cys → Arg	AciI, BstUI
		TGC → TAC	Cys → Tyr	(–)
		TGC → TCC	Cys → Ser	(–)
		TGC → TTC	Cys → Phe	TaqI, MboII
11	630	TGC → TTC	Cys → Phe	TaqI
	634	TGC → AGC	Cys → Ser	DdeI, EspI, Bpu11021
		TGC → GGC	Cys → Gly	HaeIII
		TGC → CGC	Cys → Arg	CfoI, HhaI, HinPI
		TGC → TAC	Cys → Tyr	RsaI, AciI
		TGC → TCC	Cys → Ser	Fnu4HI, Eam11051
		TGC → TTC	Cys → Phe	Fnu4HI, AciI
		TGC → TGG	Cys → Trp	CfoI + Fnu4HI, HhaI, HinPI
FMTC				
13	768	GAG → GAC	Glu → Asp	MaeIII
14	804	GTG → TTG	Val → Leu	(–)
		GTG → ATG	Val → Met	NlaIII
15	891	TCG → GCG	Ser → Ala	(–)
MEN2B				
15	883	GCT → TTT	Ala → Phe	AluI, DdeI
16	918	ATG → ACG	Met → Thr	FokI

found in noncysteine codons in the intracellular tyrosine-kinase domain. Missense mutations at codon 768 of exon 13, GAG → GAC replacing glutamic acid with asparatic acid, have been found in some FMTC families,[52-55] as have mutations at codon 804 in exon 14, GTG (Val) → TTG (Leu) and GTG (Val) → ATG (Met).[53,56] Although the effects of these mutations have not been clearly documented, it is suggested that codon 768 mutation

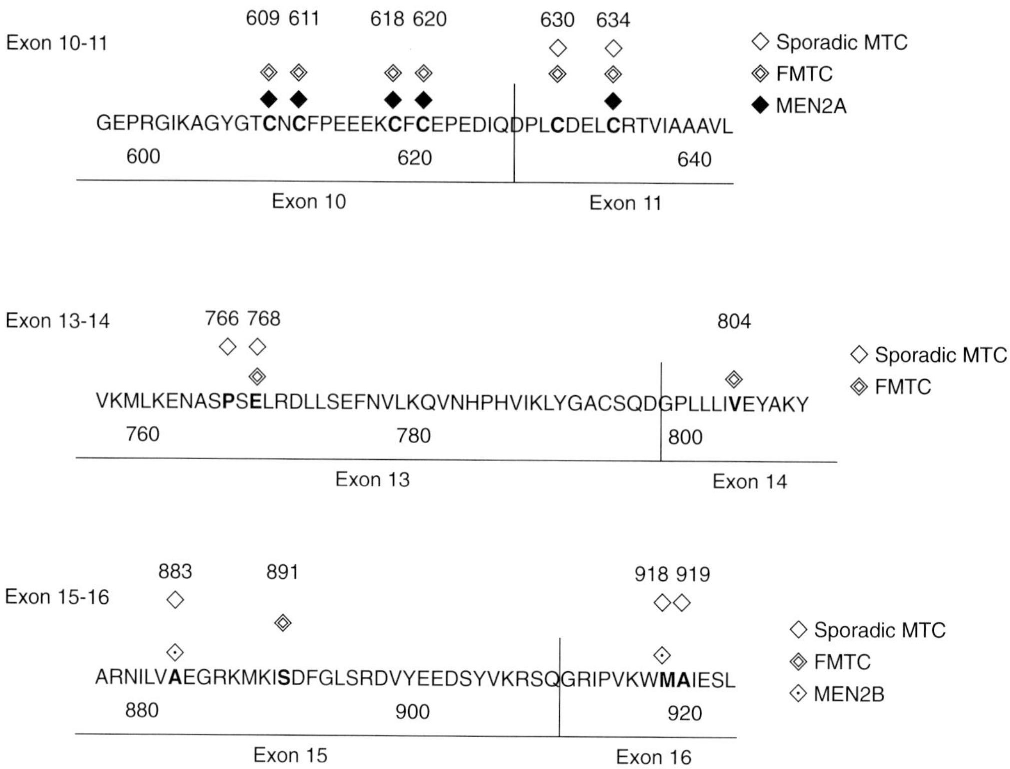

• **FIGURE 18-2** Distribution of RET mutation in MEN2A, MEN2B, FMTC, and sporadic MTC. Each of the missense mutations described in Tables 13-1 and 13-2 is indicated as follows: ◆(MEN2A), ◇(MEN2B), ◈(FMTC), and ◇(sporadic MTC). Abbreviations for the amino acid residues are as follows: A (Ala), C (Cys), D (Asp), E (Glu), F (Phe), G (Gly), H (His), I (Ile), K (Lys), L (Leu), M (Met), N (Asn), P (Pro), Q (Gln), R (Arg), S (Ser), T (Thr), V (Val), W (Trp), and Y (Tyr).

modifies tyrosine-kinase activity by changing the substrate specificity or the ATP-binding capacity of the receptor, and codon 804 mutation activates the receptor by altering the kinetics of interactions between RET and substrates or modifying the range of substrates phosphorylated.[7,52] Furthermore, germline mutation at codon 891 in exon 15, TCG (Ser) → GCG (Ala), was recently reported in an FMTC family.[57] In a small number of MEN2A, MEN2B, and FMTC families, the germline RET mutation could not be identified.

Patients with hereditary MTC may occasionally be treated as sporadic MTC. RET germline mutations have recently been found in apparently sporadic MTCs; this frequency ranges from 1.5% to 24.0%.[51,58-61] In our series, 6 (15%) of 40 cases had germline RET point mutations.[62] Genetic testing for RET mutations in peripheral blood leukocytes and tumor DNA is indispensable for preoperative or postoperative MTC patients and has replaced provocative testing for calcitonin increase.

BIOLOGIC ASPECTS OF RET

Expression of RET gene plays an important role in normal development. The function of RET locus has been conserved throughout higher and lower vertebrates.[63] RET is considered to be closely associated with renal organogenesis and enteric neurogenesis.[64] The increased expression of this gene is associated with nervous system cells, hematopoietic cell proliferation, and differentiation.[28,65] RET transcripts have been detected in normal thyroid tissue and the adrenal medulla as well as tumors of neuroectodermal origin, including MTC, pheochromocytomas, and neuroblastomas.[66-69] Both normal and mutant alleles are expressed in normal lymphocytes and tumor tissues of MEN2A patients.[70] However, RET expression was not found in gliomas or in Ewing's sarcomas, which also are believed to be of neuroectodermal origin.[67]

Two types of RET isoforms, 1072 and 1114 amino acids, are well known.[71] The C-terminal nine amino acids of the smaller protein were changed to 51 unrelated amino acids in the larger protein as a result of change in the coding sequence due to alternative splicing.[28] A third RET isoform that differs in the C terminus by 43 amino acids has also been found.[34] Each RET isoform is thought to have different biologic activities. The transforming activity of the longer isoform (1114 amino acids) of MEN2B-type mutation was much higher than that of its shorter isoform (1072 amino acids) and lower than that of both isoforms of MEN2A-type mutation.[72,73] It is expected that the two additional tyrosine residues present in the larger protein may have been implicated in RET autophosphorylation.[74,75]

Wild-type RET exists normally in an undimerized form. RET protein with MEN2A mutation, mutated in the cysteine residues, forms aberrant disulfide bonds with other mutant RET molecules and thus creates a homodimerization of RET with constitutive activation of its kinase and transforming activities.[76,77] MEN2B mutation occurs in the tyrosine-kinase domain and the catalytic core region of the RET protein. No RET dimerization is detectable in RET protein with MEN2B mutation and altered RET catalytic properties have been shown.[77] The mutation of both MEN2A and MEN2B exerts dominant transforming activities in NIH3T3 cells as a consequence of constitutive activation of the RET kinase. NIH3T3 stable transfectants expressing RET with a mutation of MEN2A or MEN2B gained a transformed morphology, formed colonies in soft agar, and gained tumorigenicity in nude mice.[77,78] Transgenic mouse expressing a MEN2A mutation develops bilateral C-cell hyperplasia and subsequently bilateral MTCs.[79] Both the amount of RET homodimers and RET kinase activity are higher in cysteine codon 634 mutation than mutations in cysteine codons 609, 618, or 620.[64,80]

GENOTYPE-PHENOTYPE CORRELATION

The correlation between the nature of RET oncogene mutation and the prevalence of pheochromocytoma or hyperparathyroidism in MEN2A has been investigated by several groups. In the study by the International RET Mutation Consortium, a significant association between the presence of a mutation at codon 634 and the presence of either pheochromocytoma or hyperparathyroidism has been shown.[46] Patients with codon 634 mutations, a specific TGC (Cys) → CGC (Arg) mutation, were most likely to develop parathyroid disease.[46,81,82] In studies of French and German MEN2A and FMTC families, the prevalence of pheochromocytoma and hyperparathyroidism was also significantly higher in families with a mutation of cysteine 634, but a specific codon 634 mutation has not been identified.[83,84]

Patients with MEN2A or FMTC patients with RET mutations of codons 618 and 620 in exon 10 generally have less aggressive MTC than patients with mutations of cysteine codon 634 in exon 11. Moers et al.[85] claimed that MEN2A should not be subclassified into MEN2A and FMTC, but rather according to the specific RET mutation, because the diagnosis of MTC-only applies to small families with cysteine codon mutations, and other endocrine tumors may be found in large FMTC families. Recently a duplication of 12 base pairs between codon 634 and 635, resulting in the insertion of four amino acids and creating an additional cysteine codon, has been found in a MEN2A family without pheochromocytoma but with a high incidence of parathyroid disease.[86] Tumor development and progression of MTC differ among individuals from the same families with MEN2A, MEN2B, and FMTC; thus other genetic factors as well as RET mutation may have a role in the development of these endocrine tumors.

PREDICTIVE DNA TESTING AND TREATMENT

Rapid, accurate genetic information about RET mutations from peripheral blood leukocytes is helpful for discriminating gene carriers from non-gene carriers in families with a history of MEN2A, MEN2B, or FMTC. Many gene carriers for MEN2A do not manifest the disease, even in old age. More than 90% of MTCs for MEN2A gene carriers can be detected by 30 years of age by use of biochemical screening tests, whereas only about two thirds of all MEN2A gene carriers will present clinically by the age of 70.[87]

Total thyroidectomy with central neck lymph node dissection is the recommended surgical procedure for asymptomatic gene carriers with MTC. Early thyroidectomy performed before biochemical or clinical evidence of MTC is usually curative. Thyroid specimens from gene carriers with elevated serum calcitonin levels contain either neoplastic C-cell hyperplasia or microscopic or macroscopic MTC, supporting prophylactic total thyroidectomy for gene carriers.[88-91] However, an indicator for immediate total thyroidectomy for gene carriers with normal basal and stimulated calcitonin levels remains to be established.[10,92]

Skinner et al.[91] reported that 1 of 17 children with MEN2A, having undergone total thyroidectomy for MTC based on an elevated stimulated plasma calcitonin level, had metastases to the cervical lymph nodes when the tumor was discovered. Wells et al.[88] found that 21 of 58 MEN2A members had RET mutations. Total thyroidectomy was performed in 13 patients, ranging in age from 6 to 20 years. There was no metastatic MTC in regional lymph nodes, and postoperative stimulated plasma calcitonin values were normal. They recommended total thyroidectomy for children as young as 5 years of age, with repeat C-cell stimulation testing at 2 and 5 years after thyroidectomy. When plasma calcitonin levels remain normal, continued provocative testing would appear unnecessary.

Lips et al.[12] reported their experience of total thyroidectomy in eight gene carriers of MEN2A, 4 to 18 years of age, who had negative or equivocal stimulation test results. Sections of thyroid tissue from these patients revealed small foci of MTCs. They documented that it is justified to postpone surgery until after the plasma calcitonin stimulation test results become positive or until the patient is 12 to 13 years of age, because the majority of their patients who were operated on after test results became positive have not had a recurrence of the disease.

We have observed three patients, 70, 33, and 15-years of age, with MEN2A and RET germline mutations who had no clinical manifestations but did have positive calcitonin stimulation tests. At total thyroidectomy, no lymph node metastases were identified. Three additional patients treated in our hospital for suspected sporadic MTC, subsequently discovered to have germline RET mutation and MEN2A, did not undergo total thyroidectomy and to date have had no recurrence of MTC.

Although MTC is the major cause of death in patients with MEN2A, MTC in Japanese patients with MEN2A generally shows the milder course.

In our experience the prognosis of Japanese MEN2A patients is favorable compared with that of their counterparts in Europe and the United States.[93] We must more carefully consider the timing of the operation in MEN2A or FMTC gene carriers with no evident thyroid tumor or elevated calcitonin levels.

The MTC associated with MEN2B is more virulent than that related to MEN2A or FMTC. MTC generally develops earlier in patients with MTC, and thyroidectomy for MTC has been suggested in infancy for these patients. Approximately half of the patients with MEN2B had metastatic MTC at the time of diagnosis.[88] Moreover, the incidence of recurrent MTC and death from MTC, even after thyroidectomy, is high among patients with MEN2B. Therefore treatment of patients with MEN2B is recommended as soon as the diagnosis is confirmed. However, patients with MEN2B must continue to be screened for the development of pheochromocytomas and patients with MEN2A for pheochromocytomas and hyperparathyroidism.

The most common surgical complication of total thyroidectomy is injury to the parathyroid glands, with permanent hypoparathyroidism and recurrent nerve paralysis. Concomitant surgical hypoparathyroidism would reduce or abolish the increased rate of bone loss. Calcitonin has an uncertain physiologic role in the preservation of bone mass. Surgical thyroidectomy abolishes the calcitonin secretion in response to calcium, and several authors have found a reduced bone mineral density compared with age-matched controls.[94,95] Other investigators have not found increased osteoporosis after total thyroidectomy.[96] Almost all patients who undergo total thyroidectomy for thyroid cancer receive exogenous thyroid hormone to suppress TSH secretion and thyroid stimulation. Thyroid replacement diminishes the bone mineral density of hypothyroid patients, but its effect on euthyroid subjects is controversial. These observations suggest that patients undergoing total thyroidectomy must be followed carefully for bone disorders.

SOMATIC RET MUTATION IN SPORADIC MTC

In approximately one third of sporadic MTCs, somatic ATG → ACG mutation at codon 918 resulting in the substitution of methionine for threonine, which is also found in most MEN2B families, has been reported (Table 18-2 and Fig. 18-2).[27,47,51,56,97-99] This somatic mutation has been documented to correlate with tumor recurrence or poor prognosis.[100,105,106] In contrast, we have detected somatic mutations at codon 918 in only 2(6%) of 34 sporadic MTCs. The correlation of codon 918 mutation with poor prognosis could

TABLE 18-2 Summary of Somatic RET Gene Mutations in Sporadic MTCs

Exon	Codon	Nucleotide Change	Amino Acid Change	References
11	630	TGC → CGC	Cys → Arg	100
	634	TGC → TGG	Cys → Trp	100
	634	TGC → CGC	Cys → Arg	101
	592-607	48 bp deletion		102
	630	6 bp deletion		26
	632-633	3 bp deletion		103
	632-633	6 bp deletion		102
	633-635	9 bp deletion		104
13	766	CCG → TCG	Pro → Ser	62
	768	GAG → GAC	Glu → Asp	52
15	883	GCT → TTT	Ala → Phe	99
16	918	ATG → ACG	Met → Thr	27,47
	919	GCA → GTA	Ala → Val	62

not be confirmed in our series. Differences in the incidence of RET somatic mutations at codon 918 and in association with tumor recurrence or prognosis suggest that other unknown factors are associated with development or progression of sporadic MTC.

Various somatic mutations in both the cysteine-rich domain and tyrosine-kinase domain of the RET gene have been identified in sporadic MTCs (see Table 18-2 and Fig. 18-2). Missense mutations in the cysteine-rich domain were reported in a small number of sporadic MTCs: TGC (Cys) → CGC (Arg) at codons 630 and 634, and TGC (Cys) → TGG (Trp) at codon 634.[100,101] Interestingly, deletion of some of the nucleotide sequence in the cysteine-rich domain is also found in certain sporadic MTCs: a 6 bp deletion at codon 630, a 3 bp deletion occurring from the second letter of codon 632 to the first letter of codon 633, and a 27 bp deletion in exon 10.[26,103,107] Recently Ceccherini et al.[102] found a case of sporadic MTC with a 6 bp deletion removing codon 632 and 633 and a case with a 48 bp deletion removing 16 amino acids from codons 592 to 607. They also showed that expression of a RET carrying one of two deletions resulted in strong transforming activity in NIH3T3 cells. Alemi et al.[104] reported that 14 of 15 sporadic MTCs had a deletion of 9 bp at positions 1825 and 1830-7 within the cysteine-rich domain resulting in the loss of codons 633 to 635 (Leu-Cys-Arg) with amino acid substitutions in codons 632 (Glu to Ser) and 636 (Thr to Ser). All of these alterations are in frame mutations with or without amino acid substitutions. It is estimated that the deletion event around the cysteine-rich region results in the constitutive activation of the tyrosine-kinase of RET.

In the intracellular tyrosine-kinase domain, GAG (Glu) → GAC (Asp) mutation at codon 768 of exon 13, which is also found in some FMTC families and GCT (Ala) → TTT (Phe) mutation at codon 883 of exon 15 were reported as somatic mutations.[52,99] We found novel point mutations in two cases of sporadic MTC. One showed two simultaneous point mutations, ATG (Met) → ACG (Thr) at codon 918 and GCA (Ala) → GTA (Val) at codon 919. The other showed a mutation in exon 13, a CCG (Pro) → TCG (Ser) mutation at codon 766.[62]

Second Somatic Event in MTC

In MTC as in other tumors, accumulation of genetic alterations, activation of oncogenes, and functional loss of tumor suppressor genes contribute to tumor development. Tumor suppressor genes are thought to play an important role in tumor development by means of inactivation mechanisms consisting of loss of one chromosomal allele containing a tumor suppressor gene and mutation of the gene in the remaining allele.[108] Loss of heterozygosity has been examined to explore chromosomal numeric and structural abnormalities of MTCs. Allelic loss on chromosome 10q in which RET gene is located is found rarely both in hereditary and sporadic MTCs.[109-113] Frequent loss of heterozygosity on chromosomes 1p and 22q in hereditary and sporadic MTCs was reported by several researchers.[112-116] Alterations in other genes may also contribute to progression of hereditary and sporadic MTCs or phenotypic variation among families with MEN2A. One case of sporadic MTC in our series had two simultaneous point mutations at codons 918 and 919 with loss of the wild-type allele, and these results also suggest that both alleles at the RET locus were altered.

In the study by Landsvater et al.,[117] no somatic RET mutations were identified on examination of the entire coding region of the RET gene in four tumors of MTC or pheochromocytoma from MEN2A and MEN2B patients examined. However, several groups have documented the somatic RET mutation besides the germline mutation in MTC of MEN2A and FMTC patients. Both simultaneous germline mutations in exon 10 or 11 and somatic mutations at codon 918 of RET have been reported in some MTCs from patients with MEN2A.[118,119] Miyauchi et al.[55] reported sporadic GCA (Ala) → CCA (Pro) mutation at codon 919 in addition to the germline GAG (Glu) → GAC (Asp) mutation at codon 768 in an FMTC patient. Eng et al.[119] found an intratumor heterogeneity of codon 918 mutation and heterogeneity among subsets of multiple metastases. It appears that a germline RET mutation is necessary for C-cell hyperplasia, but it is probable that the second genetic event in RET gene in tumor tissue is related to MTC development or progression.

NEUROENDOCRINE AND PARATHYROID TUMORS

Somatic mutations of RET gene in sporadic pheochromocytomas were detected at codon 918, an ATG (Met) → ACG (Thr) substitution, and the frequency of this mutation ranges from 8% to 15%.[103,120,121] Loss of heterozygosity was reported on chromosomes 1p, 3p, 11p, 11q, 17p, and 22q in pheochromocytomas.[112,115,122,123] In small cell lung carcinomas, RET mutation from GCC (Ala) to GAC (Asp) at codon 664 in exon 11 was reported.[124] No RET point mutations were found in the other neuroendocrine tumors, such as pituitary adenomas, pancreatic neuroendocrine tumors, pulmonary carcinoids, gastrointestinal carcinoids, neuroblastomas, malignant melanomas, and schwanomas.[121]

In sporadically occurring benign or malignant parathyroid lesions, RET mutations at hot spots of exons 10, 11, and 16 are not involved in tumor development.[125-127] It appears that either mechanisms of RET activation are involved, or RET plays a more minor role in growth control in parathyroid cells than in pheochromocytes or C-cells.

HIRSCHSPRUNG'S DISEASE

RET is also involved in the pathogenesis of Hirschsprung's disease (HSCR), a developmental disorder of the automatic innervation of the gut. Point mutations scattered along the RET sequence were found in several cases of familial and sporadic HSCR.[128-131] In the study by Attié et al.[131] germline mutations of the RET gene were found in 50% of familial HSCR and somatic mutations in 35% of sporadic HSCR. Several lines of evidence support a gain of function mechanism for tumorigenesis in the MEN2 syndromes but a loss of function mechanism for aganglionosis in Hirschsprung's disease. There is no obvious relationship between the nature of RET gene mutations and the HSCR phenotype.[130,131] Germline mutations at cordon 618 or 620 were found in a kindred with MEN2A and Hirschsprung's disease.[90,130,132-134] Considering the low penetrance of the mutant RET gene and the lack of a genotype-phenotype correlation, other genetic and/or epigenetic factors may contribute to HSCR development.

CONCLUSION

Germline mutations in the RET gene have been shown to be the underlying cause of MEN2A, MEN2B, and FMTC. These mutations cause constitutive kinase activation of the RET. Gene carriers of these families can be detected by genetic testing for RET gene point mutations. In MEN2B, immediate total thyroidectomy is necessary as soon as the diagnosis is confirmed. In MEN2A and FMTC, detection of gene carriers at the presymptomatic stage with elevated serum calcitonin levels facilitates a complete cure by total thyroidectomy and/or central neck dissection. We believe, however, that careful consideration must be given to the indications of immediate total thyroidectomy among gene carriers of MEN2A and FMTC without thyroid tumors as demonstrated by ultrasonograpy and without elevated calcitonin levels in response to pentagastrin or calcium stimulation.[135]

Somatic RET mutations of this gene are found in about one third of sporadic MTCs. Other alterations in RET gene or alterations in other genes may also contribute to the development or progression of MTC. Furthermore, phenotypic variation and different aggressiveness of MTC among families with MEN2 and the same RET germline mutation have not been explained fully. More information must therefore be obtained about alterations in coding or intronic regions throughout the entire RET gene, loss of heterozygosity at the site of candidate tumor suppressor genes, and activation of other oncogenes in MTCs.

REFERENCES

1. Hill CS Jr. et al. Medullary (solid) carcinoma of the thyroid gland: An analysis of the M.D. Anderson Hospital experience with patients with the tumor, its special features and its histogenesis. Medicine 52:141, 1973.
2. Ezaki H et al. Analysis of thyroid carcinoma based on material registered in Japan during 1977-1986 with special reference to predominance of papillary type. Cancer 70:808, 1992.
3. Hazard JB, Hawk WA, Crile G Jr. Medullary (solid) carcinoma of the thyroid—A clinicopathologic entity. J Clin Endocrinol Metab 19:152, 1959.
4. Sipple JH. The association of pheochromocytoma with carcinoma of the thyroid gland. Am J Med 31:163, 1961.
5. Williams ED. A review of 17 cases of carcinoma of the thyroid and pheochromocytoma. J Clin Pathol 18:288, 1965.
6. Schimke RN, Hartmann WH. Familial amyloid-producing medullary thyroid carcinoma and pheochromocytoma: A distinct genetic entity. Ann Intern Med 63: 1027, 1965.
7. Eng C. The RET proto-oncogene in multiple endocrine neoplasia type 2 and Hirschsprung's disease. N Engl J Med 335:943, 1996.

8. Ledger GA et al. Genetic testing in the diagnosis and management of multiple endocrine neoplasia type II. Ann Intern Med 122:118, 1995.
9. Perry A, Molberg K, Albores-Saavedra J. Physiologic versus neoplastic C-cell hyperplasia of the thyroid: Separation of distinct histologic and biologic entities. Cancer 77:750, 1996.
10. Gagel RF et al. Clinical use of molecular information in the management of multiple endocrine neoplasia type 2A. J Intern Med 238:333, 1995.
11. Lichter JB et al. Presymptomatic testing using DNA markers for individuals at risk for familial multiple endocrine neoplasia 2A. J Clin Endocrinol Metab 74:368, 1992.
12. Lips CJM et al. Clinical screening as compared with DNA analysis in families with multiple endocrine neoplasia type 2A. N Engl J Med 331:828, 1994.
13. Gagel RF. The abnormal pentagastrin test. Clin Endocrinol (Oxf) 44:221, 1996.
14. Lips CJM et al. Thyroid C-cell hyperplasia and micronodules in close relatives of MEN-2A patients: Pitfalls in early diagnosis and reevaluation of criteria for surgery. Henry Ford Hosp Med J 35:133, 1987.
15. Gagel RF et al. The clinical outcome of prospective screening for multiple endocrine neoplasia type 2A. An 18-year experience. N Engl J Med 318:478, 1988.
16. Landsvater RM et al. The clinical implications of a positive calcitonin test for C-cell hyperplasia in genetically unaffected members of an MEN2A kindred. Am J Hum Genet 52:335, 1993.
17. Barbot N et al. Pentagastrin stimulation test and early diagnosis of medullary thyroid carcinoma using an immunoradiometric assay of calcitonin: Comparison with genetic screening in hereditary medullary thyroid carcinoma. J Clin Endocrinol Metab 78:114, 1994.
18. Marsh DJ et al. The identification of false positive responses to the pentagastrin stimulation test in RET mutation negative members of MEN 2A families. Clin Endocrinol (Oxf) 44:213, 1996.
19. Hernández G et al. False-positive results of basal and pentagastrin-stimulated calcitonin in non-gene carriers of multiple endocrine neoplasia type 2A. Thyroid 7:51, 1997.
20. Simpson NE et al. Assignment of multiple endocrine neoplasia type 2A to chromosome 10 by linkage. Nature 328:528, 1987.
21. Mathew CG et al. A linked genetic marker for multiple endocrine neoplasia type 2A on chromosome 10. Nature 328:527, 1987.
22. Gardner E et al. Genetic linkage studies map the multiple endocrine neoplasia type 2 loci to a small interval on chromosome 10q11.2. Hum Mol Genet 2:241, 1993.
23. Mole SE et al. Localisation of the gene for multiple endocrine neoplasia type 2A to a 480 kb region in chromosome band 10q11.2. Hum Mol Genet 2:247, 1993.
24. Yamamoto M et al. Tight linkage of the ret proto-oncogene with the multiple endocrine neoplasia type 2A locus. Jpn J Clin Oncol 21:149, 1991.
25. Mulligan LM et al. Germline mutations of the RET proto-oncogene in multiple endocrine neoplasia type 2A. Nature 363:458, 1993.
26. Donis-Keller H et al. Mutations in the RET proto-oncogene are associated with MEN 2A and FMTC. Hum Mol Genet 2:851, 1993.
27. Hofstra RMW et al. A mutation in the RET proto-oncogene associated with multiple endocrine neoplasia type 2B and sporadic medullary thyroid carcinoma. Nature 367:375, 1994.
28. Takahashi M et al. Cloning and expression of the RET proto-oncogene encoding a tyrosine kinase with two potential transmembrane domains. Oncogene 3:571, 1988.

29. Takahashi M, Buma Y, Hiai H. Isolation of RET proto-oncogene cDNA with an amino-terminal signal sequence. Oncogene 4:805, 1989.
30. Donghi R et al. The oncogene associated with human papillary thyroid carcinoma (PTC) is assigned to chromosome 10q11-q12 in the same region as multiple endocrine neoplasia type 2A (MEN 2A). Oncogene 4:521, 1989.
31. Ishizaka Y et al. Human ret proto-oncogene mapped to chromosome 10q11.2. Oncogene 4:1519, 1989.
32. Kwok JBJ et al. Structural analysis of the human RET proto-oncogene using exon trapping. Oncogene 8:2575, 1993.
33. Ceccherini I et al. DNA polymorphisms and conditions for SSCP analysis of the 20 exons of the RET proto-oncogene. Oncogene 9:3025, 1994.
34. Myers SM et al. Characterization of RET proto-oncogene 3′ splicing variants and polyadenylation sites: A novel C-terminus for RET. Oncogene 11:2039, 1995.
35. Takahashi M, Ritz J, Cooper GM. Activation of a novel human transforming gene, RET, by DNA rearrangement. Cell 42:581, 1985.
36. Grieco M et al. PTC is a novel rearranged form of the RET proto-oncogene and is frequently detected in vivo in human thyroid papillary carcinomas. Cell 60:557, 1990.
37. Sugg SL, Zheng L, Rosen IB, et al. RET/PTC-1, -2, and -3 oncogene rearrangements in human thyroid carcinomas: Implications for metastatic potential? J Clin Endocrinol Metab 81:3360, 1996.
38. Pierotti MA et al. Characterization of an inversion on the long arm of chromosome 10 juxtaposing D10S170 and RET and creating the oncogenic sequence RET/PTC. Proc Natl Acad Sci USA 89:1616, 1992.
39. Bongarzone I et al. Molecular characterization of a thyroid tumor-specific transforming sequence formed by the fusion of RET tyrosine kinase and the regulatory subunit RIα of cyclic AMP-dependent protein kinase A. Mol Cell Biol 13:358, 1993.
40. Bongarzone I et al. Frequent activation of ret protooncogene by fusion with a new activating gene in papillary thyroid carcinomas. Cancer Res 54:2979, 1994.
41. Jhiang SM, Smanik PA, Mazzaferri EL. Development of a single-step duplex RT-PCR detecting different forms of RET activation, and identification of the third form of in vivo RET activation in human papillary thyroid carcinoma. Cancer Lett 78:69, 1994.
42. Trupp M et al. Functional receptor for GDNF encoded by the c-RET proto-oncogene. Nature 381:785, 1996.
43. Durbec P et al. GDNF signalling through the RET receptor tyrosine kinase. Nature 381:789, 1996.
44. Dahira PLM et al. Mutation analysis of glial cell line-derived neurotrophic factor (GDNF), a ligand for the RET/GDNF receptor α complex, in sporadic pheochromocytomas. Cancer Res 57:310, 1997.
45. Marsh DJ et al. Mutation analysis of glial cell line-derived neurotrophic factor, a ligand for an RET coreceptor complex, in multiple endocrine neoplasia type 2 and sporadic neuroendocrine tumors. J Clin Endocrinol Metab 82:3025, 1997.
46. Eng C et al. The relationship between specific RET proto-oncogene mutations and disease phenotype in multiple endocrine neoplasia type 2. International RET mutation consortium analysis. JAMA 276:1575, 1996.
47. Carlson KM et al. Single missense mutation in the tyrosine kinase catalytic domain of the RET protooncogene is associated with multiple endocrine neoplasia type 2B. Proc Natl Acad Sci USA 91:1579, 1994.

48. Smith DP, Houghton C, Ponder BAJ. Germline mutation of RET codon 883 in two cases of de novo MEN 2B. Oncogene 15:1213, 1997.
49. Carlson KM et al. Parent-of-origin effects in multiple endocrine neoplasia type 2B. Am J Hum Genet 55:1076, 1994.
50. Kitamura Y et al. Two maternally derived missense mutations in the tyrosine kinase domain of the RET protooncogene in a patient with de novo MEN 2B. Hum Mol Genet 4:1987, 1995.
51. Komminoth P et al. Analysis of RET protooncogene point mutations distinguishes heritable from nonheritable medullary thyroid carcinomas. Cancer 76:479, 1995.
52. Eng C et al. A novel point mutation in the tyrosine kinase domain of the RET proto-oncogene in sporadic medullary thyroid carcinoma and in a family with FMTC. Oncogene 10:509, 1995.
53. Bolino A et al. RET mutations in exons 13 and 14 of FMTC patients. Oncogene 10:2415, 1995.
54. Boccia LM et al. Mutation of RET codon 768 is associated with the FMTC phenotype. Clin Genet 51:81, 1997.
55. Miyauchi A et al. A novel somatic mutation in the RET proto-oncogene in familial medullary thyroid carcinoma with a germline codon 768 mutation. Jpn J Cancer Res 88:527, 1997.
56. Fink M et al. Distinction between sporadic and hereditary medullary thyroid carcinoma (MTC) by mutation analysis of the proto-oncogene. Int J Cancer 69:312, 1996.
57. Hofstra RMW et al. A novel point mutation in the intracellular domain of the ret protooncogene in a family with medullary thyroid carcinoma. J Clin Endocrinol Metab 82:4176, 1997.
58. Eng C et al. Low frequency of germline mutations in the RET proto-oncogene in patients with apparently sporadic medullary thyroid carcinoma. Clin Endocrinol (Oxf) 43:123, 1995.
59. Zedenius J et al. Somatic and MEN 2A de novo mutations identified in the RET proto-oncogene by screening of sporadic MTCs. Hum Mol Genet 3:1259, 1994.
60. Decker RA et al. Progress in genetic screening of multiple endocrine neoplasia type 2A: Is calcitonin testing obsolete? Surgery 118:257, 1995.
61. Wohllk N et al. Relevance of RET proto-oncogene mutations in sporadic medullary thyroid carcinoma. J Clin Endocrinol Metab 81:3740, 1996.
62. Uchino S et al. Novel point mutations and allele loss at the RET locus in sporadic medullary thyroid carcinomas. Jpn J Cancer Res 89:411, 1998.
63. Marcos-Guitiérrez CV et al. The zebrafish homologue of the RET receptor and its pattern of expression during embryogenesis. Oncogene 14:879, 1997.
64. Schuchardt A et al. Defects in the kidney and enteric nervous system of mice lacking the tyrosine kinase receptor RET. Nature 367:380, 1994.
65. Pachnis V, Mankoo B, Costantini F. Expression of the c-RET proto-oncogene during mouse embryogenesis. Development 119:1005, 1993.
66. Takahashi M, Cooper GM. RET transforming gene encodes a fusion protein homologous to tyrosine kinases. Mol Cell Biol 7:1378, 1987.
67. Santoro M et al. The RET proto-oncogene is consistently expressed in human pheochromocytomas and thyroid medullary carcinomas. Oncogene 5:1595, 1990.
68. Nagao M et al. Expression of RET protooncogene in human neuroblastomas. Jpn J Cancer Res 81:309, 1990.

69. Miya A et al. Expression of the RET proto-oncogene in human medullary thyroid carcinomas and pheochromocytomas of MEN 2A. Henry Ford Hosp Med J 40:215, 1992.
70. Quadro L et al. Frequent RET protooncogene mutations in multiple endocrine neoplasia type 2A. J Clin Endocrinol Metab 79:590, 1994.
71. Tahira T et al. Characterization of RET proto-oncogene mRNAs encoding two isoforms of the protein product in a human neuroblastoma cell line. Oncogene 5:97, 1990.
72. Asai N et al. A mutation at tyrosine 1062 in MEN2A-RET and MEN2B-RET impairs their transforming activity and association with shc adapter proteins. J Biol Chem 271:17644, 1996.
73. Rossel M et al. Distinct properties of two RET isoforms activated by MEN 2A and MEN 2B mutations. Oncogene 14:265, 1997.
74. Borello MG et al. The oncogenic versions of the Ret and Trk tyrosine kinases bind Shc and Grb2 adaptor proteins. Oncogene 9:1661, 1994.
75. Romano A et al. The high transforming potency of erbB-2 and RET is associated with phosphorylation of paxillin and a 23 kDa protein. Oncogene 9:2923, 1994.
76. Asai N et al. Mechanism of activation of the RET proto-oncogene by multiple endocrine neoplasia 2A mutations. Mol Cell Biol 15:1613, 1995.
77. Santoro M et al. Activation of RET as a dominant transforming gene by germline mutations of MEN 2A and MEN 2B. Science 267:381, 1995.
78. Xing S et al. Characterization of RET oncogenic activation in MEN2 inherited cancer syndromes. Endocrinology 137:1512, 1996.
79. Michiels FM et al. Development of medullary thyroid carcinoma in transgenic mice expressing the RET protooncogene altered by a multiple endocrine neoplasia type 2A. Proc Natl Acad Sci USA 94:3330, 1997.
80. Carlomagno F et al. The different RET-activating capability of mutations of cysteine 620 or cysteine 634 correlates with the multiple endocrine neoplasia type 2 disease phenotype. Cancer Res 57:391, 1997.
81. Mulligan LM et al. Specific mutations of the RET proto-oncogene are related to disease phenotype in MEN 2A and FMTC. Nat Genet 6:70, 1994.
82. Heshmati HM et al. Genetic testing in medullary thyroid carcinoma syndromes: Mutation types and clinical significance. Mayo Clin Proc 72:430, 1997.
83. Schuffenecker I et al. RET proto-oncogene mutations in French MEN 2A and FMTC families. Hum Mol Genet 3:1939, 1994.
84. Frank-Raue K et al. Mutations of the RET proto-oncogene in German multiple endocrine neoplasia families: Relation between genotype and phenotype. J Clin Endocrinol Metab 81:1780, 1996.
85. Moers AM et al. Familial medullary thyroid carcinoma: Not a distinct entity? Genotype-phenotype correlation in a large family. Am J Med 101:635, 1996.
86. Höppner W, Ritter MM. A duplication of 12 bp in the critical cysteine rich domain of the RET proto-oncogene results in a distinct phenotype of multiple endocrine neoplasia type 2A. Hum Mol Genet 6:587, 1997.
87. Ponder BAJ et al. Risk estimation and screening in families of patients with medullary thyroid carcinoma. Lancet 1:397, 1988.
88. Wells SA Jr et al. Predictive DNA testing and prophylactic thyroidectomy in patients at risk for multiple endocrine neoplasia type 2A. Ann Surg 220:237, 1994.
89. Pacini F et al. Early treatment of hereditary medullary thyroid carcinoma after attribution of multiple endocrine neoplasia type 2 gene carrier status by screening for RET gene mutations. Surgery 118:1031, 1995.

90. Borst MJ et al. Mutational analysis of multiple endocrine neoplasia type 2A associated with Hirschsprung's disease. Surgery 117:386, 1995.
91. Skinner MA et al. Medullary thyroid carcinoma in children with multiple endocrine neoplasia types 2A and 2B. J Pediatr Surg 31:177, 1996.
92. Frilling A et al. Presymptomatic DNA screening in families with multiple endocrine neoplasia type 2 and familial medullary thyroid carcinoma. Surgery 118:1099, 1995.
93. Iihara M et al. A nationwide clinical survey of patients with multiple endocrine neoplasia type 2 and familial medullary thyroid carcinoma in Japan. Jpn J Clin Oncol 27:128, 1997.
94. McDermott MT et al. Reduced bone mineral content in totally thyroidectomized patients: Possible effect of calcitonin deficiency. J Clin Endocrinol Metab 56:936, 1983.
95. Gonzalez DC et al. Bone mass in totally thyroidectomized patients. Role of calcitonin deficiency and exogenous thyroid treatment. Acta Endocrinol (Copenh) 124:521, 1991.
96. Hurley DL et al. Axial and appendicular bone mineral density in patients with long-term deficiency or excess of calcitonin. N Engl J Med 317:537, 1987.
97. Eng C et al. Mutation of the RET protooncogene in sporadic medullary thyroid carcinoma. Genes Chromosom Cancer 12:209, 1995.
98. Blaugrund JE et al. RET proto-oncogene mutations in inherited and sporadic medullary thyroid cancer. Hum Mol Genet 3:1895, 1994.
99. Marsh DJ et al. Somatic mutations in the RET proto-oncogene in sporadic medullary thyroid carcinoma. Clin Endocrinol (Oxf) 44:249, 1996.
100. Romei C et al. Somatic mutations of the RET protooncogene in sporadic medullary thyroid carcinoma are not restricted to exon 16 and are associated with tumor recurrence. J Clin Endocrinol Metab 81:1619, 1996.
101. Bugalho MJ et al. Molecular analysis of the RET proto-oncogene in patients with sporadic medullary thyroid carcinoma: A novel point mutation in the extracellular cysteine-rich domain. Eur J Endocrinol 136:423, 1997.
102. Ceccherini I et al. Somatic in frame deletions not involving juxtamembranous cysteine residues strongly activate the RET proto-oncogene. Oncogene 14:2609, 1997.
103. Hofstra RMW et al. Extensive mutation scanning of RET in sporadic medullary thyroid carcinoma and of RET and VHL in sporadic pheochromocytoma reveals involvement of these genes in only a minority of cases. J Clin Endocrinol Metab 81:2881, 1996.
104. Alemi M et al. A complex nine base pair deletion in RET exon 11 common in sporadic medullary thyroid carcinoma. Oncogene 14:2041, 1997.
105. Zedenius J et al. Mutations of codon 918 in the RET proto-oncogene correlate to poor prognosis in sporadic medullary thyroid carcinomas. J Clin Endocrinol Metab 80:3088, 1995.
106. Jhiang SM et al. RET mutation screening in MEN2 patients and discovery of a novel mutation in a sporadic medullary thyroid carcinoma. Thyroid 6:115, 1996.
107. Kalinin V, Frilling A. 27-bp deletion in the ret proto-oncogene as a somatic mutation associated with medullary thyroid carcinoma. J Mol Med 76:365, 1998.
108. Knudson AG. Antioncogenes and human cancer. Proc Natl Acad Sci USA 90:10914, 1993.
109. Landsvater RM et al. Development of multiple endocrine neoplasia type 2A does not involve substantial deletions of chromosome 10. Genomics 4:246, 1989.
110. Nelkin BD et al. Low incidence of loss of chromosome 10 in sporadic and hereditary human medullary thyroid carcinoma. Cancer Res 49:4114, 1989.

111. Okazaki M et al. Allele loss on chromosome 10 and point mutation of ras oncogenes are infrequent in tumors of MEN2A. Henry Ford Hosp Med J 37:112, 1989.
112. Khosla S et al. Loss of heterozygosity suggests multiple genetic alterations in pheochromocytomas and medullary thyroid carcinomas. J Clin Invest 87:1691, 1991.
113. Mulligan LM et al. Genetic events in tumour initiation and progression in multiple endocrine neoplasia type 2. Genes Chrom Cancer 6:166, 1993.
114. Mathew CGP et al. Deletion of genes on chromosome 1 in endocrine neoplasia. Nature 328:524, 1987.
115. Takai S et al. Loss of genes on chromosome 22 in medullary thyroid carcinoma and pheochromocytoma. Jpn J Cancer Res 78:894, 1987.
116. Yang K-P et al. Deletion mapping on the distal third region of chromosome 1p in multiple endocrine neoplasia type 2A. Anticancer Res 10:527, 1990.
117. Landsvater RM et al. Somatic mutations of the RET proto-oncogene are not required for tumor development in multiple endocrine neoplasia type 2 (MEN 2) gene carriers. Cancer Res 56:4853, 1996.
118. Marsh DJ et al. Germline and somatic mutations in an oncogene: RET mutations in inherited medullary thyroid carcinoma. Cancer Res 56:1241, 1996.
119. Eng C et al. Heterogeneous mutation of the RET proto-oncogene in subpopulations of medullary thyroid carcinoma. Cancer Res 56:2167, 1996.
120. Eng C et al. Point mutation within the tyrosine kinase domain of the RET proto-oncogene in multiple endocrine neoplasia type 2B and related sporadic tumours. Hum Mol Genet 3:237, 1994.
121. Komminoth P et al. RET proto-oncogene point mutations in sporadic neuroendocrine tumors. J Clin Endocrinol Metab 81:2041, 1996.
122. Yokogoshi Y, Yoshimoto K, Saito S. Loss of heterozygosity on chromosomes 1 and 11 in sporadic pheochromocytomas. Jpn J Cancer Res 81:632, 1990.
123. Moley JF et al. Consistent association of 1p loss of heterozygosity with pheochromocytomas from patients with multiple endocrine neoplasia type 2 syndromes. Cancer Res 52:770, 1992.
124. Futami H et al. A novel somatic point mutation of the RET proto-oncogene in tumor tissues of small cell lung cancer patients. Jpn J Cancer Res 86:1127, 1995.
125. Padberg B-C et al. Absence of RET proto-oncogene point mutations in sporadic hyperplastic and neoplastic lesions of the parathyroid gland. Am J Pathol 147:1600, 1995.
126. Pausova Z et al. Role of the RET proto-oncogene in sporadic hyperparathyroidism and in hyperparathyroidism of multiple endocrine neoplasia type 2. J Clin Endocrinol Metab 81:2711, 1996.
127. Williams GH et al. Analysis of the RET proto-oncogene in sporadic parathyroid adenomas. J Pathol 180:138, 1996.
128. Romeo G et al. Point mutations affecting the tyrosine kinase domain of the RET proto-oncogene in Hirschsprung's disease. Nature 367:377, 1994.
129. Edery P et al. Mutations of the RET proto-oncogene in Hirschsprung's disease. Nature 367:378, 1994.
130. Angrist M et al. Mutation analysis of the RET receptor tyrosine kinase in Hirschsprung disease. Hum Mol Genet 4:821, 1995.
131. Attié T et al. Diversity of RET proto-oncogene mutations in familial and sporadic Hirschsprung disease. Hum Mol Genet 4:1381, 1995.

132. Caron P et al. C618R mutation in exon 10 of the RET proto-oncogene in a kindred with multiple endocrine neoplasia type 2A and Hirschsprung's disease. J Clin Endocrinol Metab 81:2731, 1996.
133. Blank RD et al. Clinical presentations and RET protooncogene mutations in seven multiple endocrine neoplasia type 2 kindreds. Cancer 78:1996, 1996.
134. Mulligan LM et al. Diverse phenotypes associated with exon 10 mutations of the RET proto-oncogene. Hum Mol Genet 3:2163, 1994.
135. Uchino S et al. Presymptomatic detection and treatment of Japanese carriers of the multiple endocrine neoplasia type 2A gene. Surg Today 29:862, 1999.

CHAPTER

19

Thyroid-stimulating Hormone Suppression Therapy

ORLO H. CLARK, M.D.

There are differences of opinion about the therapeutic value of TSH (thyroid-stimulating hormone) suppression therapy for the treatment of patients with differentiated thyroid carcinoma of follicular cell origin.[1-4] There is also considerable controversy about the therapeutic benefits of TSH suppressive therapy for patients with benign thyroid nodules.[3-7]

The principal question I will address in this chapter is whether suppression of TSH causes some thyroid cancers to decrease in size and other thyroid cancers to stop growing or at least decrease their growth rate. I will specifically analyze the currently available clinical and basic science data regarding whether TSH suppressive therapy should be used in patients with differentiated thyroid cancer of follicular cell origin. I will only briefly discuss information regarding TSH suppressive therapy in benign thyroid neoplasms or in nodular goiter.[1,3,4] I will include historical data, animal and human data, and more recent information concerning basic science experiments relating to TSH and the metabolism, growth, and invasion of thyroid cancers as well as its effects on apoptosis.

CLINICAL BACKGROUND

In 1894, Von Eiselberg[8] reported that a 38-year-old woman with thyroid cancer developed myxedema following a total thyroidectomy; however, she became euthyroid when she developed recurrent metastatic thyroid cancer in her sternum. This situation made her physicians question whether her thyroid tumor and the thyroid gland were making a substance that was required to prevent myxedema. At that time the function of the thyroid gland was still being debated, although a committee chaired by William Miller Ord and including the surgeons Victor Horsley and Felix Semon in 1888 concluded that removal of the thyroid gland caused myxedema, cretinism, and cachexia strumipriva.[9-10]

In 1896, Paul Bruns from Tubingen, Germany reported that among the patients he treated with thyroid hormone, in about 67% of patients the nodules decreased in size, in approximately 8% the nodules disappeared, and in 25% the nodules failed to respond.[11] Diffuse goiters responded best, and when the thyroid hormone was discontinued, most of the nodules or goiters recurred.

In 1937, Sir Thomas Dunhill, in his Lettsomian lectures,[12] described two children 5 and 8 years of age who developed recurrent papillary thyroid cancer after thyroidectomy; one also received interstitial therapy. In both patients, the metastatic thyroid cancer disappeared when Dunhill treated the children with relatively large doses of thyroid hormone. In 1939, he reported the marked regression of a papillary thyroid cancer involving the lymph nodes and pulmonary parenchyma in another child following treatment with thyroid hormone. The patient was apparently without clinical evidence of recurrent thyroid cancer 17 years later.[2]

Subsequent publications by Balme,[13] Crile,[14] Thomas,[15] and others[16,17] also confirmed that some differentiated thyroid cancers of follicular cell origin regressed or disappeared in adults as well as in children when they were treated with thyroid hormone. Some of these patients, however, were probably hypothyroid after their thyroid operations, and their elevated TSH levels presumably stimulated these thyroid cancers more than normal levels of TSH would.[14,17]

Although most patients, especially young patients, with papillary and other well-differentiated thyroid cancers of follicular cell origin do well, this is not always the case. Some low- and high-risk patients, as identified by the TNM or AGES classifications, eventually die from these tumors.[18-21] Thyroid cancer, in fact, is responsible for more cancer deaths than any other endocrine tumor except the ovary.[19] It is also clear that some thyroid cancers respond only transiently to TSH suppressive therapy and others fail to respond. Thus the response of thyroid cancers to TSH suppressive therapy is similar to the response of patients with breast cancer when treated with tamoxifen.

Studies by Mazzaferri et al.,[21,22] Staunton and Greening,[23] and others[24-27] document that patients with differentiated thyroid cancer who are treated with thyroid hormone have fewer recurrences and improved survival. These retrospective studies probably underestimate the therapeutic value of TSH suppressive therapy, since patients with more aggressive tumors who received extensive surgical treatment were more likely to receive thyroid hormone and still had fewer recurrences and an improved survival.[1] A recent investigation by Pjol et al.[28] documented that among 141 patients treated with thyroid hormone after thyroidectomy for differentiated thyroid of follicular cell origin, the relapse-free survival was longer in the group with constantly suppressed TSH levels ($p < 0.05$ mU/L, n = 18) than in the group with nonsuppressed TSH levels (all TSH valued greater than or equal to $p < 0.01$, 1 mU/L, n = 15). Patients' ages, gender, and tumor stage were similar in these two groups. Using multivariate analysis including TSH suppression, age, gender, histology, and tumor stage, the degree of TSH suppression predicted relapse-free survival independent of other factors ($p = 0.02$). The authors concluded that a lesser degree of TSH suppression was associated with a higher relapse rate. These findings strongly support the use of TSH suppression in patients with thyroid cancer.[28]

Other clinical data supporting the concept that TSH stimulates the growth and function of thyroid cancers indicate that higher than normal levels of TSH are required for the uptake of radioiodine in metastatic thyroid cancers. TSH is also the best stimulator of the secretion of thyroglobulin by metastatic thyroid cancers.[29] Thyroglobulin is the most sensitive marker for diagnosing the presence of persistent thyroid cancer.[30,31] Clinicians make use of this information and render patients, after total or near-total thyroidectomy, hypothyroid in preparation for thyroid scanning and ablative treatment with radioiodine. For the most sensitive evaluation of whether the serum thyroglobulin concentration is truly normal, it should be less than 10 ng/ml when the patient is hypothyroid and less than 3 ng/ml while the patient is receiving thyroid hormone after a total thyroidectomy.[29]

Recombinant TSH is now available so that blood TSH levels can be increased without the necessity of making patients hypothyroid.[32,33] Unfortunately, some patients, when their thyroid hormone therapy is discontinued to make them transiently hypothyroid in preparation for scanning or treatment, rapidly develop bone pain or clinical evidence of new metastatic deposits or the growth of suspected metastases. Other relatively asymptomatic patients may develop symptoms from their metastases when they become hypothyroid. Overall, approximately 70% of patients with metastatic thyroid cancer of follicular cell origin will take up radioiodine in their metastatic deposits, and approximately 95% of these patients will have increased serum thyroglobulin concentrations in response to high serum TSH levels.[7,30,34-37]

Chronic stimulation of the thyroid gland with TSH probably leads to carcinogenesis in humans and animals as individuals with hyperplastic congenital goiters have developed carcinomas.[37] Numerous investigations have documented that treatment with thyroid hormone prevents or decreases the number of radiation-induced thyroid cancers in animals.[38-40] Animals that have previously been given carcinogens rapidly develop thyroid cancers when their TSH levels are increased.[41] Thyroid tumors induced in animals by ^{131}I are initially TSH dependent and can also only be transplanted successfully in thyroidectomized animals with high TSH levels.[37] Murphy et al.[42] reported that detectable thyroid abnormalities develop less frequently in patients given thyroid hormone. Fogelfeld et al.[43] reported that in a follow-up investigation of persons exposed to low-dose therapeutic radiation treatment with thyroid hormone decreased the number of benign thyroid nodules but did not decrease the number of thyroid cancers. Therefore any nodule that develops or is present in a patient who is receiving thyroid hormone and has been exposed to low-dose therapeutic radiation must be viewed with more suspicion of being cancerous. Approximately 40% of persons with thyroid nodules and a history of radiation exposure will have thyroid cancer.[44,45] DeGroot and Stanbury[37] also reported that treatment with thyroid hormone failed to prevent the formation of thyroid cancers in humans conflicting with the data found in animals.

Some studies,[46,47] but not all,[48] suggest that patients with Graves' disease and thyroid cancer have more aggressive thyroid cancers. Thyroid-stimulating immunoglobulins like TSH may stimulate the differentiation, growth, and invasion of some thyroid cancers. More recent articles suggest that patients with Hashimoto's thyroiditis and thyroid cancer have fewer recurrences and improved survival.[49-52] It therefore appears that there are stimulating and inhibiting antibodies that influence the behavior of at least some thyroid cancers.

TSH BINDING AND ADENYLATE CYCLASE

TSH stimulates thyroid function as well as the growth of thyroid cells primarily through activation of adenylate cyclase (AC) and phospholipase

C (PLC).[52] TSH also activates both the cyclic AMP (cAMP) and the PIP2 cascades in Chinese hamster ovary (CHO) cells transfected with human cDNA from the TSH receptor.[53] TSH activates AC via G proteins that link the receptor to AC.[54] The binding of TSH to the TSH receptor is specific in both normal and neoplastic thyroid tissue of follicular cell origin.[55] In contrast, most medullary thyroid cancers and anaplastic thyroid cancers lack TSH receptors and fail to increase AC in response to TSH.[56,57]

Normal and neoplastic thyroid tissue also have receptors for epidermal growth factor (EGF), insulin-like growth factor (IGF), vasoactive intestinal polypeptide (VIP), somatostatin, estrogen, androgen, and tamoxifen.[58-64] Most benign and malignant thyroid neoplasms maintain their ability to discriminate between various growth factors similar to normal thyroid tissues.[55]

Our experiments in normal and neoplastic human thyroid tissue documented that the AC response to TSH, above basal activity, is greater in follicular adenomas and in papillary and follicular thyroid cancers confined to the thyroid gland (class I tumors) than in normal thyroid tissue from the same patients.[65] As these differentiated thyroid cancers became more invasive or spread to the lymph nodes, lung, or bone, the AC response to TSH decreased (Fig. 19-1). Some of this decreased response in the more extensive tumors is because the basal AC activity in these tumors is already high and therefore cannot appreciably increase further; that is, these tumors appear to be constitutively activated.[65] Some thyroid neoplasms also have increased stimulatory G protein activity, which could explain why the basal AC activity was increased (Fig 19-2).[66]

We and other investigators previously reported that most normal and neoplastic thyroid tissues desensitize in response to repeated or continuous exposure to TSH.[67,68] This process of a decreased response to the same stimulus is called *homologous desensitization.* We questioned whether some thyroid cancers of follicular origin may continue to grow because they fail to desensitize or only partially desensitize in response to TSH stimulation. Our initial studies documented that most thyroid cancers desensitized similar to normal thyroid tissue from the same patients. Thus the AC response to TSH decreased appreciably on repeated exposure to TSH (Fig 19-3).[67] However, some metastatic thyroid cancers from lymph nodes, failed to desensitize.[67] Subsequent investigations by our group suggested that there are both quantitative and qualitative differences in the AC desensitization of neoplastic thyroid tissues in primary culture.[68] The decreased desensitization to TSH may account for the continued growth of some thyroid neoplasms in patients with relatively low or intermittently low serum TSH levels. Nagayama et al.[69] recently studied desensitization in rat thyroid FRTL5 cells

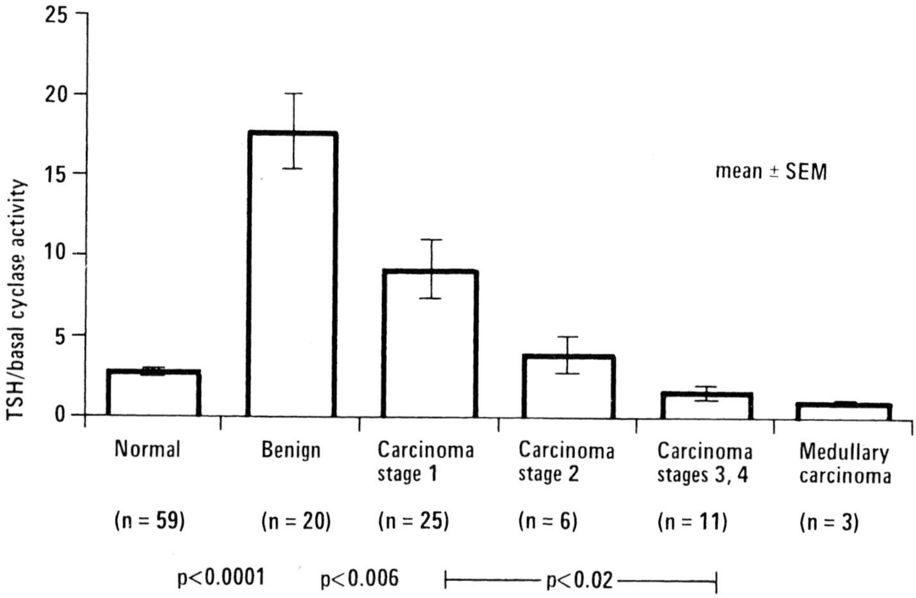

• **FIGURE 19-1** Effect of TSH on adenylate cyclase (AC) activity in thyroid cell membranes from a patient with poorly differentiated follicular carcinoma. Maximal AC response over basal AC activity in benign thyroid neoplasms, stages 1, 2, 3, and 4 thyroid carcinomas, and in medullary carcinoma. As the stage of the thyroid carcinoma increases, the maximal AC/basal activity decreases. (From Clark OH et al. Guanyl nucleotide regulatory proteins in neoplastic and normal human thyroid tissue. World J Surg 12:538, 1988. Reproduced with permission.)

and suggested that G protein–coupled receptor kinases (GRKs) and arrestins (beta-arrestin-1) are involved in TSH-receptor homologous desensitization. TSH in their experiments also caused down regulation of GRK5, but not beta-arrestin-1 expression. Whether there are alterations in GRK5 and in beta-arrestin-1 in malignant thyroid neoplasms is, to my knowledge, unknown at this time.

There appears to be "cross-talk" between various signal transduction pathways. For example, EGF has no appreciable effect on AC activity. EGF, however, causes desensitization of the TSH-AC signal transduction system in human neoplastic thyroid cells in culture.[67] Protein kinase C (PKC) activity appears to be involved, since inhibitors of PKC activity such as staurosporine block the effect of EGF on TSH-AC desensitization. Thus both homologous and heterologous (a decreased response to another growth factor) desensitization occurs in some thyroid neoplasms.

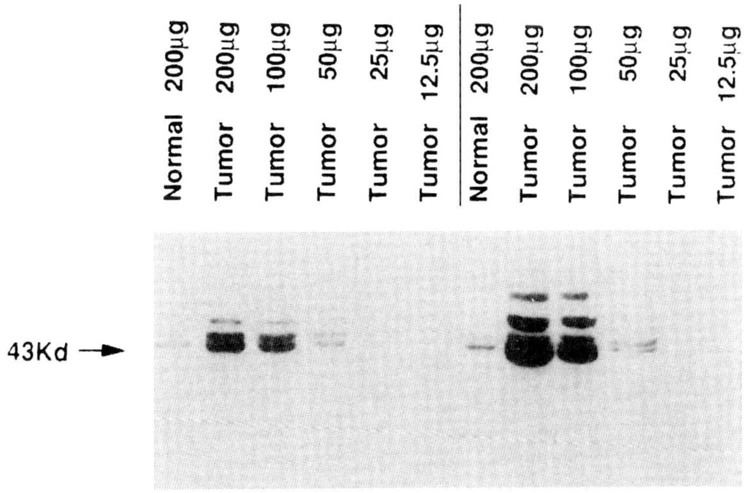

• **FIGURE 19-2** Western blots of normal and neoplastic thyroid tissue from two patients probed with antibody against the alpha subunit of Gs; 200 µg of normal membrane is compared with 200, 100, 50, 25, and 12.5 µg of tumor membrane. This semiquantitative method allows for an estimate of the fold increase in Gs seen in thyroid tumors.

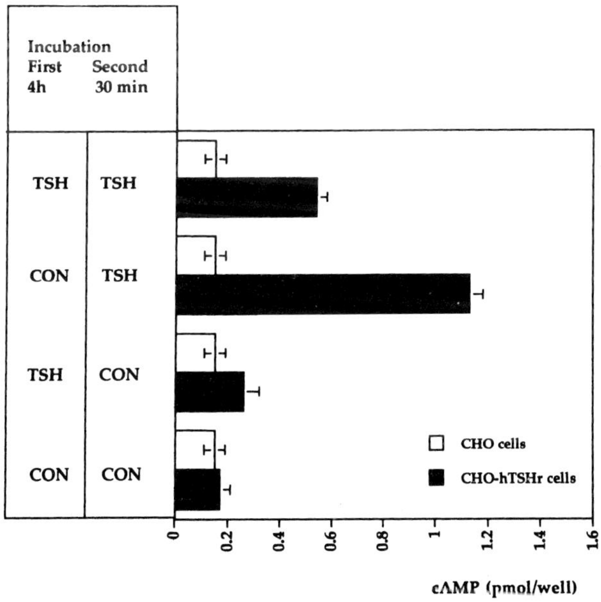

• **FIGURE 19-3** Homologous desensitization of cAMP response to thyrotropin stimulation. Each bar represents the mean ± SD of six experiments. CHO-hTSHr cells showed desensitization after pretreatment with thyrotropin *(TSH)* for 4 hours, whereas nontransfected CHO cells did not show thyrotropin stimulation. (*CON*, control medium; *CHO*, Chinese hamster ovary.)

TSH AND PROTEIN KINASE C ACTIVATION

Investigations have documented that TSH not only stimulates AC activity but also stimulates the generation of the phospholipid intermediate, inositol-1,4,5-triphosphate in human thyroid slices, independent of AC stimulation.[70] TSH also increases diacylglycerol levels in FRTL cells[71] and increases PLC levels in normal and neoplastic human thyroid membranes (Fig. 19-4).[72] TSH causes the translocation of PKC from its inactive cytostolic form to an active membrane-bound form.[73,74] In most thyroid systems, including human thyroid slices, TSH has a higher affinity for AC activation (from 0.1 to 1 mU/ml

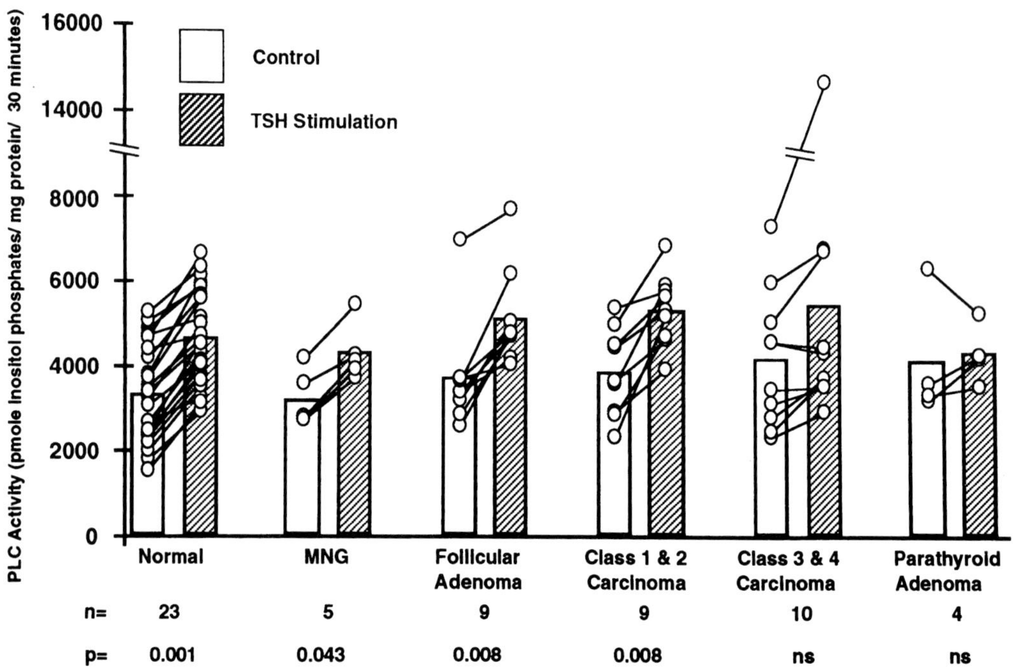

• **FIGURE 19-4** Phospholipase C *(PLC)* responsiveness to TSH in normal, hyperplastic, and neoplastic thyroid membranes. Control (basal) and TSH-stimulated PLC activity was assayed in 56 thyroid and four parathyroid adenoma specimens. Patients were stratified into histologic categories (normal thyroid, multinodular goiter *[MNG]*, follicular adenoma, carcinoma, and parathyroid adenoma). Carcinomas were stratified further by clinical stage (DeGroot classes 1 and 2 and classes 3 and 4). All carcinomas were either papillary, follicular, or Hürthle cell. Number of patients in each group is listed below each category.

TSH) than for PLC (from 1 to 10 mU/ml TSH). The same affinities of TSH for AC activation and PLC activation, as just mentioned, were documented in CHO cells transfected with cDNA from the human TSH receptor.[53] These findings strongly support the concept that a single signal transduction unit encodes receptor molecules coupled to both signaling cascades.

TSH also influences PKC activation by the tumor promoter phorbol ester, 12-0-tetradecanoylphorbol-13 acetate.[74] TPA also inhibits TSH-mediated iodine metabolism in rat FRTL thyroid cells.[75] Thus "cross-talk" between TSH-AC-PKA signaling and TSH-PLC-PKC signaling occurs in both directions.

Stimulation of the TSH-AC system is usually associated with cellular differentiation, whereas stimulation of the TSH-PKC system is associated with cellular dedifferentiation.[76] Tumor-promoting phorbol esters that stimulate the PKC system generally inhibit TSH-stimulated iodide organification in ovine and[77] porcine thyroid cells,[78] and thyroglobulin mRNA accumulation in canine thyroid cells.[79]

TSH, ONCOGENES, AND TUMOR SUPPRESSOR GENES

Numerous oncogenes including TSH-R, gsp, ras, RET/PTC, trk, met, and tumor suppressor genes, including p53 RB and MTS-1, are present in thyroid neoplasms.[80-98] These are discussed in more detail in Chapter 16. Of interest and probable importance is that RET/PTC has only been found in papillary thyroid cancers, and up to 50% of all papillary thyroid cancers, at least in Italy, have either a RET/PTC or trk mutation (rearrangement).[98] RET/PTC and trk mutations increase met expression.[99] RET/PTC mutations occur more frequently in papillary thyroid cancer in children and after radiation exposure.[100] Autonomous or "hot" follicular neoplasms causing hyperthyroidism usually have TSH receptor or gsp mutations.[84,101-104] Two patients with malignant "hot" thyroid cancers and hyperthyroidism have also recently been reported.[105,106]

TSH and other thyroid growth factors cause a rapid and transient increase of Fos. Fos gene expression is also increased in benign lesions and less so in malignant thyroid neoplasms.[103,104] Proliferating thyroid tumor cells have increased myc gene expression, and myc expression correlates positively with tumor dedifferentiation and more aggressive tumor behavior.[104]

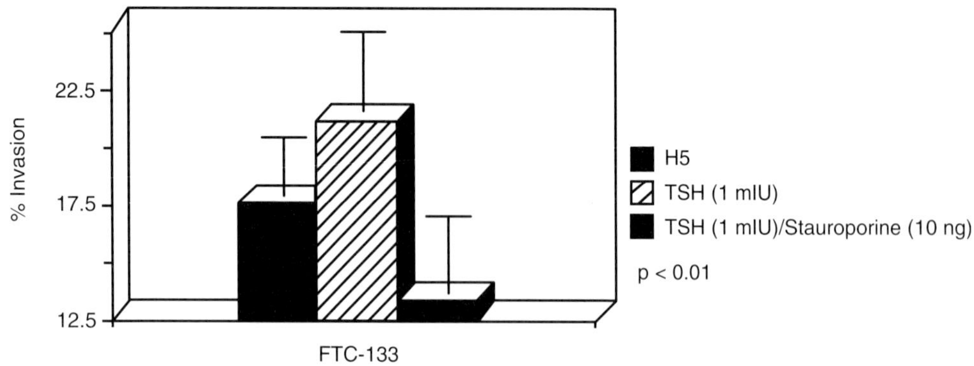

• **FIGURE 19-5** Stimulating effect of TSH on invasion of FTC-133 is reversed by staurosporine. Results are expressed as percentage of cancer cells that invaded through the polycarbonate membrane covered with reconstituted basement membrane (Matrigel).

TSH AND INVASION

We have studied the effects of TSH on invasion of papillary, follicular, and Hürthle cancer cell lines in vitro and in vivo.[106,107] Most of these studies were done using cell lines FTC-133, FTC-236, and FTC-238, provided by Peter Goretzki, M.D., Department of Surgery, Dusseldorf, Germany. All three of these cell lines were from one patient with a follicular thyroid cancer (FTC-133) with metastases to regional lymph nodes (FTC-236) and lung (FTC-238). The in vivo studies were done using these cell lines in nude mice.[106,107] As seen in Fig. 19-5, TSH (1 mIU/ml) significantly increased invasion in the FTC-133 cell line. Of interest, higher TSH concentrations (100 mIU/ml) inhibited invasion (data not shown). Stauroporine, a potent PKC antagonist, inhibited invasion indicating an important role for PKC and invasion in this cell line. As seen in Fig. 19-6, EGF and TSH (1 mIU/ml) increased invasion.[106] The tyrosine kinase antagonist genistein (1 μg/ml) dramatically inhibited EGF-stimulated invasion (column 3 in Fig. 19-6), whereas it failed to inhibit the increased invasion caused by TSH. These studies suggest that EGF stimulates tyrosine kinase activity and invasion via the phosphoinositol transduction pathways. These studies regarding invasion should offer useful models for developing new medications to treat patients with thyroid cancer by blocking invasion.

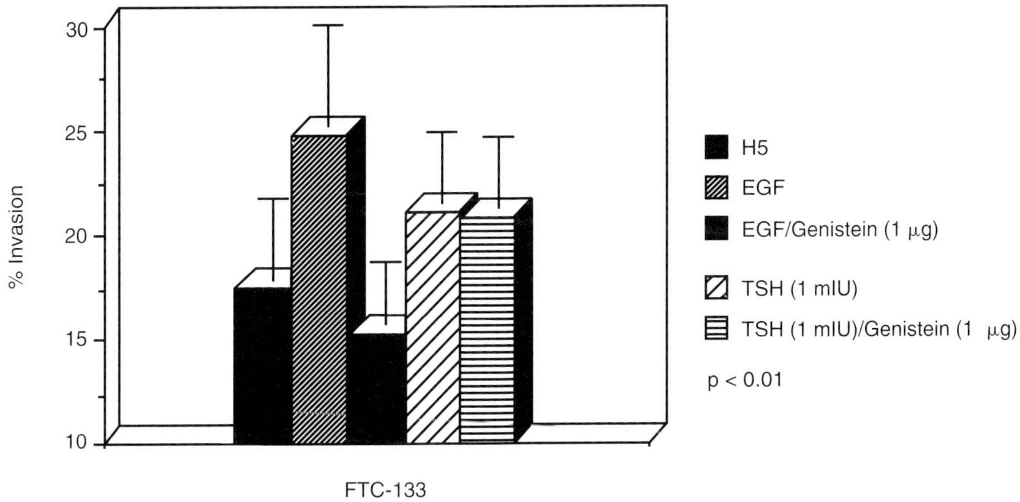

• **FIGURE 19-6** Tyrosine kinase antagonist genistein reverses the stimulating effect of EGF on invasion of FTC-133, but it has no effect on TSH stimulation.

TSH, ANGIOGENESIS, AND VASCULAR ENDOTHELIAL GROWTH FACTOR

For thyroid cancers or other tumors to grow to an appreciable size, or to invade and metastasize locally or to distant sites, they must develop a support system of new vessels from existing vasculature or angiogenesis.[107] This process is mediated either directly or indirectly by activation of growth factors produced by tumor cells.[108] Since some tumors such as hemangiomas have marked neovascularization and angiogenesis, yet are benign, angiogenesis by itself does not appear to cause cancer. Angiogenesis in breast cancer, however, correlates with metastases and prognosis. Anaplastic thyroid cancers also express more vascular endothelial growth factor (VEGF) than do papillary or follicular thyroid cancers.[109]

VEGF, also known as vascular permeability factor, is unique among angiogenic factors because it is both a vascular endothelial cell–specific mitogen and is secreted by cancer cells.[110,111] VEGF stimulates PLC by binding to a membrane receptor (flt-1, KDR) and causes proliferation of endothelial cells.[112] VEGF also increases vascular permeability, causing extravasation of plasma proteins and deposition of fibrin, which supports the ingrowth of new blood vessels.[113-117] (See Chapter 17.)

Hypoxia, phobol esters, basic fibroblast growth factor, and transforming growth factor (alpha and beta) all stimulate VEGF expression and angiogenesis. Transforming growth factor alpha and TGF-beta and basic fibroblast growth factor induce angiogenesis by both a direct effect on vascular endothelial cells and an indirect synergetic upregulation of VEGF messenger RNA expression during hypoxia.

Studies in our laboratory by Soh et al.[118,119] using human thyroid cell lines from a follicular thyroid cancer (FTC-133), provided by Dr. Goretzki, a papillary thyroid cancer provided by Dr. Nobno Sotah, Japan, and a metastatic Hürthle cell cancer (XTC) developed in our laboratory, as well as primary cultures from a medullary thyroid cancer (MTC 1.1) and normal thyroid tissue (NT 1.0), demonstrated that VEGF secretion is constitutively activated in some thyroid cancers and that VEGF secretion is stimulated by TSH. As seen in Fig. 19-7, TSH increased VEGF secretion in cell lines from both the follicular FTC-133 papillary (TPC-1) thyroid cancers, but there was no appreciable increase in the XTC-1 cell line. This cell line had very high basal VEGF activity, suggesting constitutive activation in this tumor; that is, VEGF secretion was already stimulated maximally, so secretion could not increase further. There was no appreciable increase in VEGF secretion in normal thyroid tissue in primary culture. Surprisingly, the medullary thyroid cancer in primary culture significantly increased VEGF secretion in response to TSH despite the absence of TSH receptors in medullary thyroid carcinomas.[118,119]

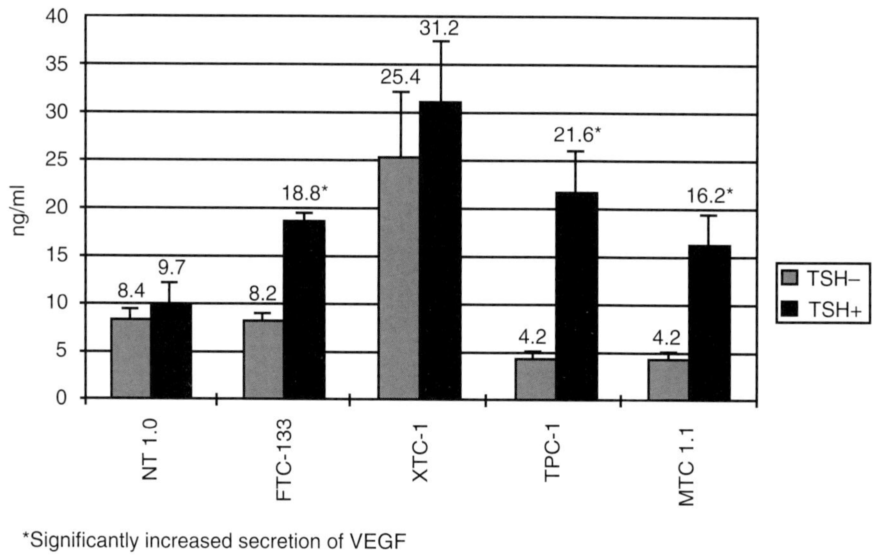

• **FIGURE 19-7** Studies by Soh et al.[118,119] and our group. Effects of TSH on VEGF secretion in thyroid cell lines are shown.

The mechanism of this increase is unknown. The response in FTC-133 and TPC-1 thyroid cancers is also of interest, because TSH receptors are markedly reduced or absent in thyroid cancer cell lines, including this one.

These studies demonstrate that TSH stimulates VEGF secretion and promotes angiogenesis in some thyroid cancers, and in some thyroid cancers VEGF expression is constitutively activated.

TSH AND APOPTOSIS

In both normal and pathologic situations, cells are programmed to die as a result of an orderly cascade of cellular events.[120] Programmed cell death is genetically regulated. Recently cell death in mice with acute liver necrosis was reversed by inhibition of apoptosis.[121,122] In the Nematode Caenorhabditis elegans molecules CED-3 and CED-4 are required for programmed cell death and CED-9 is an inhibitor of CED-4 and prevents death-inducing activity of CED-3.[123] In mammals, CED-9 corresponds to the Bc1-2 molecules and CED-3 to interleukin-1 beta–converting enzyme currently termed caspases.[124] During programmed cell death or apoptosis, cytoplasmic and chromatin condensation occur with DNA fragmentation. It seems that apoptosis requires at least four components: CED-3/caspases, CED-9/Bc1-2S, CED-4, and mitochondria. Of interest is that CED-4–induced mammalian cell death can be blocked by overexpression of Bc1-XL (a death-protective Bc1-2S) and by caspase inhibitors.[120]

Kawakami et al.[125] reported that Fas antigen was expressed in approximately 40% of unstimulated human thyrocytes, and the expression was significantly inhibited by the addition of TSH in a dose-dependent manner. The effect of TSH was mimicked by 8-bromo-cAMP, suggesting that the inhibitory effect of TSH on Fas antigen expression was mediated by protein kinase A. Treatment of thyrocytes with either interleukin-1 beta (IL-1 beta) or interferon gamma (IFN gamma), in contrast, dramatically increased Fas antigen expression and these effects were inhibited in the presence of TSH. The expression of Bc1-2 was not influenced by the addition of TSH, 8-bromo-cAMP, IL-1 beta, IFN gamma, or a combination of TSH and IL-1 beta or IFN gamma. Treatment of thyrocytes that had been stimulated by either IL-1 beta or IFN gamma with anti-Fas IgM antibody committed the cells to apoptosis, whereas the addition of TSH significantly inhibited apoptosis. Thus Fas antigen is functionally expressed on the surface of the thyrocytes, and TSH inhibits Fas antigen–mediated apoptosis of human thyrocytes apparently through the inhibitory effect of Fas antigen expression, resulting in the promotion of growth of the thyroid gland. Whether this process is involved in thyroid cancer is, to my knowledge, unknown. It appears, however, that TSH increases the growth of normal and neoplastic thyroid tissues and also inhibits programmed cell death. Increased apoptosis or programmed cell death has also been reported to occur in patients with Hashimoto's thyroiditis.[126]

TSH AND TRANSGENIC MICE

Coppee et al.,[127] created transgenic mice that expressed both the oncogenic Tg-A2aR and Tg-E7 transgenes. Previous experiments had documented that transgenic mice expressing the Tg-A2aR simulated G alpha S–coupled A2a adenosine receptor constitutively activated adequate cyclase and promoted a hyperfunctioning thyroid gland; after about 18 months, these animals developed malignant thyroid tumors.[128] Transgenic mice expressing an inhibitor of RB1 protein by the HPVG E-7 oncoprotein developed large differentiated thyroid goiters. Some of these animals by 18 months also developed thyroid cancers with metastases. Transgenic mice that expressed both Tg-A2aR and Tg-E7 developed larger goiters than those found in either parental line and severe hypothyroidism. The main feature of the Tg-A2aR/Tg-E7 mice was the rapid development of malignant thyroid neoplasms that metastasized to the lung. Tumors were obvious in mice at 2 months of age, and by 3 months 75% of the mice had malignant and metastatic tumors. Electron microscopic studies documented nuclear features similar to those found in papillary thyroid carcinomas in humans. This is the first transgenic model where the expression of two oncogenes resulted in the development of metastatic papillary thyroid carcinomas. Constitutive stimulation of the adenylate cyclase system in the Tg-A2aR mice certainly appears to be involved in thyroid tumor oncogenesis in this model. There is also an additive effect of these two transgenes on thyroid cell proliferation.

POTENTIAL COMPLICATIONS OF TSH SUPPRESSION

Although there is general agreement regarding the usefulness of employing thyroxine (L-T4) to suppress TSH stimulation of thyroid cancer growth and invasion, there is controversy regarding how such suppression is required for optimal results.[129] Hyperthyroidism associated with Graves' disease or toxic nodular goiter certainly results in bone loss and cardiac problems, but whether TSH suppression without elevated T3 and T4 levels or symptoms is detrimental to the bones or heart is controversial. A meta-analysis of cross-sectional studies found that bone mass on average was approximately 9% lower in postmenopausal women with biochemical evidence of thyroid excess.[130] A recent study of older women with hyperthyroidism also found a 70% increased risk of subsequent hip fractures compared to women without hyperthyroidism.[131] This report and others support the use of estrogen in postmenopausal women taking suppressive doses of thyroid hormone. Other studies suggest that if postmenopausal women with biochemical evidence of thyroid excess have more osteoporosis, it is minimal.[132-134] A recent prospective study of thyroid function and fracture risk found that there were no statistically significant differences in baseline bone mass of the calcaneus, spine, or femural neck or trochanteric hip regions in older women with persistently low TSH levels taking thyroid hormone than in persons with TSH levels in the normal range.[135]

Hyperthyroidism, as briefly mentioned above, can cause increased cardiac arrhythmias.[136] One must therefore balance the benefits of using thyroid hormone to suppress TSH with its possible risks. Based on the currently available evidence, we would recommend suppressing serum TSH levels to approximately 0.1 ml/L for patients with low-risk thyroid cancers (based on the TNM, AGES, or MACIS classifications) and to less than 0.1 mU/L and more than 0.03 mU/L for patients considered to be at higher risk.

CONCLUSION

There is considerable clinical and laboratory evidence supporting the use of L-thyroxine to suppress serum TSH levels in patients with thyroid cancer. This therapy appears to be similar to using tamoxifen for premenopausal women with breast cancer. It is effective and palliative for most but not all patients. Further studies are necessary to determine which tumors will respond and to what level TSH needs to be suppressed. Until such information is available, it seems advisable to give enough thyroid hormone to suppress TSH for virtually all patients who have had thyroid cancer.

REFERENCES

1. Clark OH. TSH suppression in the management of thyroid nodules and thyroid cancer. World J Surg 5:39, 1981.
2. Thomas CG Jr. Role of thyroid stimulating hormone suppression in the management of thyroid cancer. Semin Surg Oncol 7:115, 1991.

3. Zbar AP, O'Higgins NJ. Use and abuse of thyroid stimulating hormone suppressive therapy in patients with nodular goiter and benign or malignant thyroid neoplasms. In Clark OH, Duh QY, eds. Textbook of Endocrine Surgery. Philadephia: WB Saunders, 1997.
4. Burch HB. Evaluation and management of the solid thyroid nodule. Endocrinol Metab Clin North Am 24:663, 1995.
5. Gharib H. Management of thyroid nodules: Another look. Thyroid Today 20:1, 1997.
6. Gharib H et al. Suppressive therapy with levothyroxine for solitary thyroid nodules. A double-blind controlled clinical study. N Engl J Med 317:70-75, 1987.
7. Berghout A et al. Comparison of placebo with L-thyroxine alone or with carbinazole for treatment of sporadic non-toxic goiter. Lancet 336:193, 1990.
8. Von Eiselberg AF. Über physiologische Function einerim Sternum zur Entwicklung gekommen krebsigen Schilddrüsen-Metastase Arch Klin Chir 48:485, 1894.
9. Ord WM et al. Myxoedema report. Trans Med Soc Lond 21(Suppl), 1888.
10. Welbourn RB. The History of Endocrine Surgery. New York: Praeger, 1990.
11. Bruns P. Beobachtungen und Untersuchungen über die Schilddrüsen-behandlung des Kropfes. Beitr Klin Clir 16:521, 1896.
12. Dunhill T. Surgery of the thyroid gland: Lettsomian lectures. Trans Med Soc Lond 60:234, 1937.
13. Balme HW. Metastatic carcinoma of the thyroid successfully treated with thyroxine. Lancet 1:812, 1954.
14. Crile G Jr. Endocrine dependency of certain thyroid cancers. Cancer 10:1119, 1957.
15. Thomas CG Jr. Hormonal treatment of thyroid cancer. J Clin Enocrinol Metab 17:232, 1957.
16. Hill LD et al. Thyroid suppression. Arch Surg 108:403, 1974.
17. Crile G Jr. Changing end results in patients with papillary carcinoma of the thyroid. Surg Gynecol Obstet 132:450, 1971.
18. Hay ID. Papillary thyroid cancer in thyroid carcinoma. Endocrinol Metab Clin North Am 19:545, 1990.
19. Robbins J et al. Thyroid cancer: A lethal endocrine neoplasm. Ann Intern Med 115:133, 1991.
20. Ain KB. Papillary thyroid carcinoma: Etiology, assessment, and therapy. Endocrinol Metab Clin North Am 24:711, 1995.
21. Mazzaferri EL, Jhiang SM. Long term impact of initial surgical and medical therapy on papillary and follicular thyroid cancer. Am J Med 97:418, 1994.
22. Mazzaferri EL et al. Papillary thyroid carcinoma: The impact of therapy in 576 patients. Medicine (Baltimore) 56:171, 1977.
23. Staunton MD, Greening WP. Treatment of thyroid cancer in 293 patients. Br J Surg 63:253, 1976.
24. Staunton MD. Thyroid cancer: A multivariate analysis on influence of treatment on long-term survival. J Surg Oncol 20:613, 1994.
25. Cunningham MP et al. Survival discriminants for differentiated thyroid cancer. Am J Surg 160:344, 1990.
26. Szántó J et al. Follicular cancer of the thyroid gland. Oncology 48:483, 1991.
27. Simpson WJ et al. Papillary and follicular thyroid cancer: Impact of treatment in 1578 patients. Int J Radiat Oncol Biol Phys 14:1063, 1988.
28. Pjol P et al. Degrees of thyroid tropin suppression as a prognostic determinent in thyroid cancer. J Clin Endocrinol Metab 81:4318, 1996.

29. Clark OH, Hoelting T. Management of patients with differentiated thyroid cancer who have positive serum thyroglobulin levels and negative radioiodine scars. Thyroid 4:501, 1994.
30. DeVathaire F, Blanchon S, Schlumberger M. Thyroglobulin helps to predict recurrence after lobo-isthmusectomy in patients with differentiated thyroid carcinoma. Lancet 1:52, 1988.
31. Ross DS. Long-term management of differentiated thyroid cancer. Endocrinol Metab Clin North Am 19:719, 1990.
32. Ladenson PW et al. Comparison of thyroid hormone for radioactive iodine scanning in patients with thyroid carcinoma. N Engl J Med 337:928, 1997.
33. Utiger RD. Follow-up of patients with thyroid carcinoma [editorial comments]. N Engl J Med 337:888, 1997.
34. Clark OH. Thyroid nodules and thyroid cancer. In Clark OH, ed. Endocrine Surgery of the Thyroid and Parathyroid Glands. St. Louis: Mosby, 1985.
35. Mazzaferri EL, Young RL. Papillary thyroid carcinoma: A ten-year followup report of the impact of therapy in 576 patients. Am J Med 70:511, 1981.
36. Schlumberger M. Detection and treatment of lung metastases of differentiated thyroid carcinoma in patients with normal chest x-rays. J Nucl Med 29:1790, 1988.
37. DeGroot LJ, Stanbury JB. The Thyroid and Its Diseases. New York: Wiley & Sons, 1975.
38. Nichols CW Jr et al. Induction of neoplasms in rat thyroid glands by x-radiation of a single lobe. Arch Pathol Lab Med 80:177, 1965.
39. Doniach I, Williams ED. Development of thyroid and pituitary tumors in the rat two years after partial thyroidectomy. Br J Cancer 16:222, 1962.
40. Goldberg RC et al. Induction of neoplasms in the thyroid gland of the rat by subtotal thyroidectomy and by injection of one microcurie of I-131. Cancer Res 24:35, 1964.
41. Oshima M, Ward MJ. Dietary iodine deficiency as a tumor promotor and carcinogen in male F 334/N Cr rats. Cancer Res 46:877, 1986.
42. Murphy ED et al. Thyroid hormone administration in irradiated patients. J Surg Oncol 31:214, 1986.
43. Fogelfeld L et al. Recurrence of thyroid nodules after surgical removal in patients irradiated in childhood for benign conditions. N Engl J Med 320:835, 1989.
44. Witt TR et al. The approach to the irradiation thyroid. Surg Clin North Am 59:45, 1979.
45. Schneider AB et al. Radiation-induced tumors of the head and neck following childhood irradiation: Prospective studies. Medicine 64:1, 1985.
46. Belfiore A et al. Increased aggressiveness of thyroid cancer in patients with Graves' disease. J Clin Endocrinol Metab 70:830, 1990.
47. Ozaki O et al. Thyroid carcinoma in Graves' disease. World J Surg 14:437, 1990.
48. Hales IB et al. Does Graves' disease or thyrotoxicosis affect the prognosis of thyroid cancer. J Clin Endocrinol Metab 75:886, 1992.
49. Baker JR. The immune response to papillary thyroid cancer. J Clin Endocrinol Metab 80:3419, 1995.
50. Matsubayashi S et al. The correlation between papillary thyroid carcinoma and lymphocytic infiltration in the thyroid gland. J Clin Endocrinol Metab 80:3421, 1995.
51. Fiumara A et al. In situ evidence of neoplastic cell phagocytosis by macrophages in papillary thyroid cancer. J Clin Endocrinol Metab 82:1615, 1997.

52. Dumont JE et al. Physiological and pathological regulation of thyroid cell proliferation and differentiation by thyrotropin and other factors. Physiol Rev 72:667, 1992.
53. Van Sande J et al. Thyrotropin activates both the cyclic AMP and the PIP2 cascades in CHO cells expressing the human cDNA of TSH receptor. Mol Cell Endocrinol 74:R1, 1990.
54. Clark OH et al. Guanyl nucleotide regulatory proteins in neoplastic and normal human thyroid tissue. World J Surg 12:538, 1988.
55. Clark OH et al. Characterization of the TSH receptor adenylate cyclase system in neoplastic human thyroid tissue. J Clin Endocrinol Metab 57:140, 1983.
56. Ishikawa Y et al. Presence of TSH receptor in thyroid neoplasms. J Clin Endocrinol Metab 42:395, 1976.
57. Abe Y et al. Thyrotropin (TSH) receptor and adenlyate cyclase activity in human thyroid tumors. Absence of high affinity receptors and loss of TSH responsiveness in undifferentiated thyroid carcinoma. J Clin Endocrinol Metab 52:23, 1981.
58. Duh QY et al. Epidermal growth factor receptors in normal and neoplastic thyroid tissue. Surgery 98:1000, 1985.
59. Wynford-Thomas D, Williams ED, eds. Thyroid Tumors. Molecular Basis of Pathogenesis. Edinburgh: Churchill Livingstone, 1989.
60. Siperstein AE, Miller RA, Clark OH. Stimulatory effect of vasoactive intestinal polypeptide on human normal and neoplastic thyroid tissue. Surgery 104:985, 1988.
61. Siperstein AE. Effect of somatostatin on adenylate cyclase activity in normal and neoplastic thyroid tissue. World J Surg 16:791, 1992.
62. Clark OH et al. Estrogen and thyroid stimulating hormone (TSH) receptors in neoplastic and non-neoplastic human thyroid tissue. Surg Res 38:89-96, 1988.
63. Prinz RA, Sandberg L, Chandhuri PK. Androgen receptors in human thyroid tissue. Surgery 96:996, 1984.
64. Gross C et al. Presence of a specific antiestrogen binding site on human follicular thyroid carcinoma cell line (UCLA RO 82 W-1): Inhibition by an endogenous ligand present in human serum. J Clin Endocrinol Metab 77:1361, 1993
65. Siperstein AE et al. Adenylate cyclase activity as a predictor of thyroid tumor aggressiveness. World J Surg 12:528, 1988.
66. Siperstein AE et al. Increased stimulatory G protein in neoplastic thyroid tissues. Surgery 110:949, 1991.
67. Tezelman S et al. Desensitization of cyclic adenasine 3,5′-monophosphate response to thyrotropin in normal and primary or metastatic papillary thyroid cancer cells in vitro. Surgery 120:926, 1996.
68. Al-Sobhi S et al. Management of thyroid carcinosarcoma. World J Surg 122:548, 1997.
69. Nagayama Y et al. Expression and regulation of G protein-coupled receptor kinase 5 and beta-arrestinin-1 rat thyroid FRTL5 cells. Thyroid 6:627, 1996.
70. Laurent E et al. Dual activation by thyrotropin of the phospholinase C and cyclic AMP cascades in human thyroid. Mol Cell Endocrinol 52:273, 1987.
71. Brenner-Gati L, Berg KA, Gershengorn MC. Thyroid-stimulating hormone and insulin-like growth factor-1 synergize to elevate 1, 2-diacylglycerol in rat thyroid cells. Stimulation of DNA synthesis via interaction between lipid and adenylyl cyclase signal transduction systems. J Clin Invest 82:1144, 1988.
72. Shaver JK et al. Thyroid stimulating hormone activates phospholipase C in normal and neoplastic thyroid. Surgery 114:1064, 1993.

73. Tanabe A et al. Thyroid cell responses to thyrotropin and 12-0-tetradecanoyl-phorbol-13-acetate: Translocation of protein kinase C and phosphorylation of thyroid cell polypeptide substrates. Arch Biochem Biophys 243:92, 1985.
74. Ginsberg J, Murry PG. Effects of protein kinase C activators on the in vitro action of thyrotropin in pigs. Endocrinology 118:199, 1988.
75. Lombardi A et al. Independent and interactive effects of tetradecanoylphorbol acetate on growth and differentiated functions of FRTC cells. Endocrinology 123:1544, 1988.
76. Haraguchi K, Endo T, Duaya T. Effect of phorbol ester on protein phosphorylation and free T3 release by mouse thyroid lobes. Acta Endocrinol (Copenh) 112:217, 1986.
77. Bachrach LK et al. Phorbol esters stimulate growth and inhibit differentiation in cultured thyroid cells. Endocrinology 116:1603, 1985.
78. Ginsberg J, Murray PG. Protein kinase C activators modulate differentiated thyroid function in vitro. FEBS Lett 206:309, 1986.
79. Roger PP et al. Stimulation of cell proliferation and inhibition of differentation expression by tumor-promoting phorbol esters in dog thyroid cells in primary cultures. Cancer Res 46:898, 1986.
80. Gallo A et al. Ras and protein kinase C dedifferentiate thyroid cells by down-regulating nuclear cAMP-dependent protein kinase A. Genes Dev 6:1621-1630, 1992.
81. Weiss SJ et al. Thyroid-stimulated iodide transport mediated by adenosine 3′5′-monophosphate and dependent on protein synthesis. Endocrinology 114:1099, 1984.
82. Lombardi A et al. Independent and interactive effects of tetradecony l phorbol acetate on growth and differentiated functions of FRTL 5 cells. Endocrinology 1233:1544, 1988.
83. Parma J et al. Somatic mutations causing constitutive activity of the thyrotropin receptor are the major cause of hyperfunctioning thyroid adenomas. Identification of additional mutations activating both the cyclic adenosine 3′5′-monophosphate and inositol phosphage-Ca 2^{+} cascades. Mol Endocrinol 9:725, 1995.
84. Russo D et al. Genetic alterations in thyroid hyperfunctioning adenomas. J Clin Endocrinol Metab 80:1347, 1995.
85. Lyons J et al. Two G-protein oncogenes in human endocrine tumors. Science 249:655, 1990.
86. Goretzki PE et al. Mutational activation of ras and gsp oncogenes in differentiated thyroid cancer and their biological implications. World J Surg 116:576, 1992.
87. Suarez HG et al. gsp mutations in human thyroid tumors. Oncogene 6:677, 1991.
88. Lemoine NR et al. High frequency of ras oncogene activation in all stages of human thyroid tumor genesis. Oncogene 4:159, 1989.
89. Namba H et al. H ras proto-oncogene mutations in human thyroid neoplasms. J Clin Endocrinol Metab 71:223, 1990.
90. Fusco A et al. A new oncogene in human thyroid papillary carcinomas and their lymph node metastases. Nature 328:170, 1987.
91. Bongarzone I et al. High frequency of activation of tyrosine kinase oncogenes in human papillary thyroid carcinoma. Oncogene 4:1457, 1989.
92. Greco A et al. TRK T1 is a novel oncogene formed by the fusion of TPR and TRK genes in human papillary thyroid carcinomas. Oncogene 7:237, 1992.
93. Belfiore A et al. Negative low expression of the Met/hepatocyte growth factor receptor identifies papillary thyroid carcinomas with high risk of distant metastases. J Clin Endocrinol Metab 82:2322, 1997.

94. Jones CJ et al. High frequency deletion of the tumor suppressor gene P16-INK 4a (MTS1) in human thyroid cancer cell lines. Mol Cell Endocrinol 116:115, 1996.
95. Tung WS et al. In frequent CD KN2 mutations in human differentiated thyroid cancers. Mol Carcinog 15:5, 1996.
96. Jossart GH et al. Immunocytochemical detection of p53 in human thyroid carcinomas is associated with mutation and immortalization of cell lines. J Clin Endocrinol Metab 81:3498, 1996.
97. Ito T et al. Unique association of p53 mutations with undifferentiated but not with differentiated carcinomas of the thyroid gland. Cancer Res 52:1369, 1992.
98. Pierotti MA et al. Rearrangements of TRK proto-oncogene in papillary thyroid carcinomas. J Endocrinol Invest 18:130, 1995.
99. DiRenzo MF et al. Overexpression of the C-MET/HGF receptor gene in human thyroid carcinomas. Oncogene 7:2549, 1992.
100. Fugazzola L et al. Oncogenic rearrangements of the RET proto-oncogene in papillary thyroid cancers from children exposed to the Chernobyl nuclear accident. Cancer Res 55:5617, 1995.
101. Parma J et al. Somatic mutations in the thyrotropin receptor gene cause hyperfunctioning thyroid adenomas. Nature 365:649, 1993.
102. O'Sullivan C et al. Activating point mutations of the gsp oncogene in human thyroid adenoma. Mol Carcinog 4:345, 1991.
103. Farid NR, Zou M, Shi Y. Genetics of follicular thyroid cancer. Endocrinol Metab Clin North Am 24:865, 1995.
104. Farid NR, Sho Y, Zou M. Molecular bases of thyroid cancer. Endocrinol Rev 15:202, 1994.
105. Russo D et al. Detection of an activating mutation of the thyrotropin receptor in a case of an autonomously hyperfunctioning thyroid insular carcinoma. J Clin Endocrinol Metab 82:735, 1997.
106. Russo D et al. A VAL 677 activating mutation of the thyrotropin receptor in a Hürthle cell thyroid carcinoma associated with thyrotoxicosis Thyroid 1:13-17, 1999.
107. Hoelting T et al. Thyrotropin stimulates invasion and growth of follicular thyroid cancer cells via PKC rather than PKA activation. Biochem Biophy Res Commun 195:1230, 1993.
108. Hoelting T et al. Biphasic effects of thyrotropin on invasion and growth in papillary and follicular thyroid cancer in vitro. Thyroid 5:35, 1995.
109. Hoelting T et al. EGF and TGF alpha-stimulated invasion and growth of follicular thyroid cancer cells can be blocked by antagonism to the EGF receptor and the tyrosine kinase in vitro. Eur J Endocrinol 132:229, 1995.
110. Folkman J. Angiogenesis. J Biol Chem 267:10931, 1992.
111. Raj JW, St. Croix BO, Kerbel RS. Consequences of angiogenesis for tumor progression, metastases and cancer therapy. Anticancer Drugs 6:3, 1995.
112. Viglietto G et al. Upregulation of vascular endothelial growth factor (VEGF) and downregulation of placental growth factor (PIGF) associated with malignancy in human thyroid tumors and cell lines. Oncogene 11:1569, 1996.
113. Leung DW et al. Vascular endothelial growth factor is a secreted angiogenic mitogen. Science 246:1306, 1989.
114. Jakeman LB et al. Binding sites for vascular endothelial growth factor are localized on endothelial cells in rat tissues. J Clin Invest 89:244, 1992.

115. Brock TA, Dvorak HF, Senger DR. Tumor-secreted vascular permeability factor increases cytosolic $Ca2^+$ and von Willebrand factor release in human endothelial cells. Am J Pathol 138:213, 1991.
116. Senger DR et al. Purification and NH2-terminal amino acid sequence of guinea pig tumor secreted vascular permeability factor. Cancer Res 50:1774, 1990.
117. Nagy JA et al. Pathogenesis of tumor stroma generation: A critical role for leaky blood vessels and fibrin deposition. Biochem Biophys Acta 948:305, 1988.
118. Soh EY et al. Thyroid stimulating hormone promotes the secretion of vascular endothelial growth factor in thyroid cancer cell lines. Surgery 120:944, 1996.
119. Soh EY et al. Vascular endothelial growth factor expression is higher in differentiated thyroid cancer than in normal or benign thyroid. J Clin Endocrinol Metab 82:3741, 1997.
120. Goldstein P. Controlling cell death. Science 275:1081, 1997.
121. Rouquet N et al. ICE inhibitor YVADcmk is a potent therapeutic agent against in vivo liver apoptosis. Curr Biol 6:1192, 1996.
122. Shaham S, Horvitz HR. Developing Caenorhabditis elegans neurons may contain both cell-death protective and killer activities. Genes Dev 10:578, 1996.
123. Chinnaiyan AM et al. Interaction of CED-4 with CED-3 and CED-9: A molecular framework for cell death. Science 275:1122, 1997.
124. Alnemri ES et al. Human ICE/CEd-3 protease nomenclature [letter]. Cell 87:171, 1996.
125. Kawakami A et al. Thyroid stimulating hormone inhibits Fas antigen-mediated apoptosis of human thyrocytes in vitro. Endocrinology 137:3163, 1996.
126. Giordano C. Potential involvement of Fas and its ligand in the pathogenesis of Hashimoto thyroiditis. Science 275:960, 1997.
127. Coppee F et al. Early occurrence of metastatic differentiated thyroid carcinoma in transgenic mice expressing A2 adenoma receptor gene and the human papillamatous type 16E-7 oncogene. Oncogene 13:1471, 1996.
128. Ledent C et al. Differentiated carcinomas develop as a consequence of the thyroid specific expression of a thyroglobulin-human papillomavirus type 16 E7 transgene. Oncogene 10:1789, 1995.
129. Burmeister LA et al. Levothyroxine dose requirements for thyrotropin suppression with treatment of differentiated thyroid cancer. J Clin Endocrinol Metab 75:344, 1992.
130. Faber J, Galloe AM. Changes in bone mass during prolonged subclinical hyperthyroidism due to L-thyroxine treatment: A meta-analysis. J Endocrinol 130:350, 1994.
131. Cummings S et al. Risk factors for hip fractures in white women. N Engl J Med 332:767, 1995.
132. Greenspan SL et al. Skeletal integrity in premenopausal and postmenopausal women receiving long term L-thyroxine therapy. Am J Med 91:5, 1991.
133. Grant DJ et al. Suppressed TSH levels secondary to thyroxine replacement therapy are not associated with osteoporosis. Clin Endocrinol (Oxf) 39:529, 1993.
134. Hawkins F et al. Spinal bone mass after long term treatment with L-thyroxine in postmenopausal women with thyroid cancer and chronic lymphocytic thyroiditis. Calcif Tissue Int 54:16, 1994.
135. Bauer DC. Low thyrotropin levels are not associated with bone loss in older women: A prospective study. J Clin Endocrinol Metab 82:2931, 1997.
136. Sawin CT et al. Low serum thyrotropin concentrations as a risk factor for atrial fibrillation in older persons. N Engl J Med 331:1249, 1994.

Index

A

Ablative therapy
  imaging before, 167
  iodine-131 for, 178-180
Acidic fibroblast growth factor, 381, 382
Adenoma
  atypical, 236
  follicular, 112-113
    characteristics of, 24
    fine-needle aspiration cytology of, 54-57
    histology of, 133
    illustration of, 132
    surgery for, 28-29
  Hürthle cell, 72-73, 74
  magnetic resonance imaging of, 197
  minimally invasive cancer and, 236
  papillary, 63
Adenomatous goiter, 115
Adenomatous hyperplasia, 197
Adenylase cyclase system, 358
Adenylate cyclase, 418-419
Adhesion of primary tumor, 260
Adhesion/invasion of tumor, 320-321
Adriamycin, 295
Age, papillary cancer and, 67
AGES score, 231, 243
AGM-1470, 386-387
Algorithm for solitary nodule, 165
Amino acids in RET mutations, 399
Amyloid, 83
Anaplastic cancer
  classification of, 8
  fine-needle aspiration cytology of, 78-82, 148
  illustration of, 147
  invading through skin, 148
  thyroid thymoma *vs.*, 88-89
  total thyroidectomy and, 233
Anatomic landmarks in neck, 282
Angiogenesis, 379-389
  inhibitors of, 385-388
  thyroid and, 379-383
  thyroid-stimulating hormone and, 425-427
  vascular endothelial growth factor and, 383-385
Angiosarcoma, 91-92
Angiostatin, 387-388
Antibody, anti-VEGF, 387
Antiemetic with iodine-131 therapy, 186
Antigen, carcinoembryonic
  anaplastic carcinoma and, 79-80
  medullary cancer and, 151
  medullary carcinoma and, 85
Anti-VEGF antibody, 387
Apoptosis, thyroid-stimulating hormone and, 427-428
Architecture, papillary, 63
Arterial infusion chemotherapy, 335-338
Artifact of radionuclide scan, 172-173
Aspiration, fine-needle; *see* Cytology, fine-needle aspiration
Autonomously functioning nodule, 32-33
Autopsy, 4
Autotransplantation of parathyroid glands, 291-292

B

Basic fibroblast growth factor, 381-382
Basic science research, 349-360
  historical background of, 349-352
Basic science research—cont'd
  impact of
    on clinical management, 354-359
    on surgical training, 352-354
Benign neoplasm
  adenoma; *see* Adenoma
  adenylase cyclase system in, 358
  colloid nodule, 129
  ultrasonography of, 218
Bilateral lobectomy *vs.* thyroidectomy, 247
Binding, thyroid-stimulating hormone, 418-419
Biopsy, 292; *see also* Cytology, fine-needle aspiration
Bladder cancer, radionuclide therapy causing, 187
Bleomycin, 335
Blood vessel, angiogenesis and, 379-389; *see also* Angiogenesis
Bone, follicular cancer in, 143
Bone marrow, 186
Bone scan, 177
Branchial rest, 88
Breast, radionuclide concentrated in, 172-173

C

Calcitonin, in medullary cancer, 84, 279, 289, 290
  after thyroidectomy, 296, 297, 299
  testing for, 290, 301-303
Camera, scintillation, 163
  variables affecting scan sensitivity, 167-168
Capsular invasion of follicular carcinoma, 111
Carcinoembryonic antigen
  anaplastic carcinoma and, 79-80

Carcinoembryonic antigen—cont'd
medullary cancer and, 151
medullary carcinoma and, 85
Carcinoma; *see* Follicular cancer; Papillary cancer
CASTLE lesion, 88
C-cell lesion
fine-needle aspiration cytology of
hyperplasia and, 86-87
medullary carcinoma and, 82-86
hyperplastic, 86
medullary cancer and, 40, 279, 290
microcancer and, 114
mixed follicular, 87
C-cell stimulation test, 394-395
Cell
follicular epithelial, 39-40
Hürthle; *see* Hürthle cell *entries*
Central compartment, medullary cancer in, 280
Cervical exploration technique, 296-297
c-fos oncogene, 373
Chemotherapy
for nonresectable differentiated cancer, 335-338
for recurrent medullary cancer, 295
Chest x-ray for metastasis, 139
Child
cancer incidence in, 9-10
thyroidectomy in, 251
Chromatin in papillary cancer, 66
Chromosome in parathyroid tumor, 157
Cisplatin, arterial infusion with, 335
c-jun oncogene, 373
Clarithromycin, 388
Classification of thyroid cancer, 242
Clinical cancer, incidence of, 106-109
Clonality in medullary cancer, 284
c-myc oncogene, 373
Cold nodule
malignancy with, 166-167
radionuclide imaging of, 135, 164, 166
Collimeter, 163
Colloid nodule, benign, 129
Color Doppler ultrasonography, 220-222
Colorectal cancer, 187
Columnar cell variant papillary carcinoma, 70
Compartment, central, medullary cancer in, 280
Complications
of iodine-131 therapy, 184-187
of thyroid-stimulating hormone suppression therapy, 428-429
of total thyroidectomy, 230
Computed tomography
of nodule, 23-24
single-photon emission, uses of, 164
Congenital tumorlike lesion, cytology of, 44-46
Cyst, metastasis *vs.*, 173-174
Cystic nodule, risk of malignancy of, 23
Cystic papillary cancer, 68, 216, 217
Cytogenetic screening, 366
Cytokeratin
anaplastic carcinoma and, 79-80
immunostaining for, 69-70
Cytology, fine-needle aspiration, 39-93
of anaplastic cancer, 148
of anaplastic carcinoma, 78-82
of C-cell lesions
hyperplastic, 86-87
medullary, 82-86
of follicular cancer, 142
of Hürthle cell carcinoma, 72-76, 146
of lymphoma, 150
of medullary cancer, 153
of metastatic carcinoma, 90
of nodule, 165, 167
in euthyroid patient, 167
of nonepithelial neoplasms
lymphoma, 90-91
sarcoma, 91-92
nonresectable cancer and, 343-344
of papillary lesions, 62-72, 138
carcinoma, 63-68
Cytology, fine-needle aspiration—cont'd
of papillary lesions—cont'd
carcinoma variants and, 68-72
hyperplasia and, 62-63
of poorly differentiated carcinoma, 76-77
of primary mucoepidermoid carcinoma, 89
of primary thyroid thymoma, 88-89
significance of, 21-22
of squamous cell carcinoma, 88
thyroid follicular hyperplasia and neoplasia and, 51-61
follicular adenoma and, 54-57
follicular carcinoma and, 57-61
nodular goiter and, 51-54
of thyroid nodule, 22-23, 40-44
ultrasonography with, 210, 222

D

Dedifferentiation, 82
Desensitization, homologous, 419
Diet, low-iodine, 169
Differentiated cancer
adenylase cyclase system in, 358
conservative *vs.* comprehensive approach to, 252
cytogenetic screening for, 366
follicular; *see* Follicular cancer
intranuclear oncogenes in, 373
locally recurrent, 309-324; *see also* Recurrent cancer
mutations in
physiologic pathways, 367-368
ras genes, 368-369
tumor suppressor genes in, 371-373
tyrosine kinase receptors and, 369-371
natural history of, 243-244
nonresectable, 327-344; *see also* Nonresectable differentiated cancer

Differentiated cancer—cont'd
papillary; *see* Papillary cancer
thallium-201 imaging for, 175
thyroidectomy for, partial *vs.* total, 244-245
total thyroidectomy for, 229-230, 232
iodine-131 scanning after, 234
Diffuse sclerosis variant papillary carcinoma, 70
Dissection, radical neck, in child, 251
Disseminated papillary cancer, 211, 215
DNA analysis, 366
predictive value of, 400-402
Doppler ultrasonography, color, 220-222
Dosimetry for iodine-131 therapy
ablative, 178-179
of differentiated thyroid cancer, 180-182
Doxorubicin, 335

E

Edema
percutaneous ethanol injection causing, 330
radiation-induced, 186
Electrocardiograph-gated image, 196, 207
Encapsulated papillary carcinoma, 68
Endocrine neoplasia, multiple; *see* Multiple endocrine neoplasia
Endostatin, 387-388
Endothelial growth factor, vascular, 383-385
thyroid-stimulating hormone and, 425-427
Environmental pollution, cancer incidence and, 6
Eosinophilia, 89
Epidemiology of thyroid cancer
autopsy studies in, 4
classification in, 6-8
etiologic factors in, 5-6
Graves' disease and, 10-12
Hashimoto's thyroiditis and, 12-13
pediatric carcinomas and, 9-10
Epidermal growth factor, 383
Epidermal growth factor receptor, 369
Epithelial cell, follicular, 39-40
Eriochrome Black T, 388
Ethanol injection, percutaneous intranodular, 33
for nonresectable cancer, 328-333, 340-341, 343
Ethnicity and cancer incidence, 4
External-beam radiation therapy, 323
Extracapsular deposit in follicular carcinoma, 111
Extracapsular invasion of microcancer, 117, 118

F

Familial medullary cancer, 85-86
genetic basis of, 393-406; *see also* Medullary cancer, genetic basis of
non-MEN, 284
management of, 289
Femur, follicular cancer in, 143
^{18}F-FDG-PET scan, after thyroidectomy, 177
Fibroblast growth factor in angiogenesis, 381-382
Fibrosarcoma, 91, 92
Fibrosis, pulmonary, 187
Fine-needle aspiration cytology, 39-93; *see also* Cytology, fine-needle aspiration
Flow cytometric analysis for Hürthle cell follicular carcinoma, 74-75
Follicle, anatomy of, 39-40
Follicular adenoma
characteristics of, 24
fine-needle aspiration cytology of, 54-57
histology of, 133
illustration of, 132
surgery for, 28-29
Follicular cancer
adenylase cyclase system in, 358
autonomously functioning nodules and, 32
classification of, 5-6
cytogenetic screening and, 366
diagnosis of, 21-22, 24-26
Follicular cancer—cont'd
fine-needle aspiration cytology of, 57-61, 142
histology of, 141
Hürthle cell, 72-75
illustration of, 140
microcarcinoma, 111-114
minimally invasive, 236
pelvic metastasis of, 143
percentage of malignancy in, 26
poorly differentiated, 76-77
postoperative MRI and, 203
radioiodine scan of, 144
recurrence of, 314
size of, at presentation, 14-15
solitary, 24-29
surgery for, 28
treatment of, 24-26
ultrasonography of, 218
color Doppler, 221-222
Follicular C-cell lesion, 87
Follicular epithelial cell, 39-40
Follicular hyperplasia, 51-61
adenoma and, 54-57
carcinoma and, 57-61
nodular goiter and, 51-54
Follicular nodule, 113
Follicular variant papillary carcinoma, 68, 69, 71
FR-118487, 387-388

G

Gadolinium imaging, postoperative, 203
Gadolinium-enhanced, fat-suppressed T1-weighted image, 199
Gallium-67, 177
Ganglioneuroma, mucosal, 155
Gastrointestinal complications of iodine-131 therapy, 186
Gating, magnetic resonance imaging and, 196
Gender
papillary cancer and, 67
as risk factor for recurrence, 321
Gene
mutations in; *see* Mutation
ras, 368-369
tumor suppressor
in differentiated cancer, 371-373

Gene—cont'd
tumor suppressor—cont'd
in medullary cancer, 287-288
thyroid-stimulating hormone and, 423
Genetic factors in thyroid cancer, 5; *see also* Molecular biology; Mutation
medullary, 8, 393-406
Genotype-phenotype correlation in medullary cancer, 400
Giant cell, 83
Giant cell variant anaplastic carcinoma, 78, 79
Glial-derived growth factor, 286
Glial-derived neurotrophic factor receptor-alpha, 286
Glycolysis, 177
Goiter
adenomatous, 115
anaplastic carcinoma and, 81
angiogenesis and, 382
multinodular, 29-32
massive, 130
ultrasonography of, 215-216
nodular, 131
thyroid follicular hyperplasia and neoplasia and, 51-54
Gonadal function, 186
Graves' disease
cancer incidence with, 10-12
microcancer and, 118
Growth, tumor, angiogenesis as prerequisite for, 380
Growth factor
angiogenesis and, 381-382
epidermal, angiogenesis and, 383
glial-derived, 286
transforming, 359
angiogenesis and, 383
vascular endothelial, 383-385
thyroid-stimulating hormone and, 425-427
Growth factor receptor
epidermal, 369
hepatocyte, 369
gsp oncogene, 358

H

Hashimoto's thyroiditis
cancer incidence with, 12-13
lymphoma *vs.*, 91
Hemangiopericytoma, 91
Hemorrhage
percutaneous ethanol injection causing, 330
radiation-induced, 186
Hepatocyte growth factor receptor, 369
Hereditary cancer
medullary, 8, 85-86, 281
multiple endocrine neoplasia and; *see* Multiple endocrine neoplasia
Heterozygosity, loss of, 366
Hexachlorobenzene, 6
Hirschsprung's disease, 405
Homologous desensitization, 419
Hormone, thyroid-stimulating; *see* Thyroid-stimulating hormone *entries*
Hormone receptor, thyroid-stimulating, 356, 358-359
mutations in physiologic pathways and, 367-368
Horner's syndrome
modified radical neck dissection and, 263
percutaneous ethanol injection causing, 329-330
Hot nodule, definition of, 164
Hürthle cell lesion, 72-76
adenoma, 74
carcinoma
diagnosis and treatment of, 24-25
fine-needle aspiration cytology of, 21, 72-76, 146
histology of, 145
surgery for, 28
technetium-99m sestamibi imaging of, 176
hyperplastic, 73-74
Hyperplasia
adenomatous, 197
C-cell, 86, 114
fine-needle aspiration cytology of
Hürthle cell, 73-74
papillary, 62-63
medullary carcinoma and, 86-87
Hyperthyroidism
autonomously functioning nodules and, 32
nodule with, 165-167
Hyperthyroidism—cont'd
thyroid-stimulating hormone suppression and, 428-429
Hypoparathyroidism after thyroidectomy, 250, 251

I

Imaging
after thyroidectomy, 168-177; *see also* Thyroidectomy, imaging after
magnetic resonance, 195-208; *see also* Magnetic resonance imaging
of nodules, 164-167
radionuclide, 161-188; *see also* Iodine *entries;* Radionuclide imaging
safety of, 187-188
Immunohistochemistry
anaplastic carcinoma and, 79
medullary carcinoma and, 84
Immunostaining for cytokeratins, 69-70
Infarct, Hürthle cell tumor, 73
Infiltration
by anaplastic carcinoma, 79
in papillary cancer, 68
Inflammatory infiltrate in papillary cancer, 68
Inflammatory lesion
cytology of, 46-51
thyroid metastasis *vs.*, 173-174
Informed consent for iodine-131 ablative therapy, 180
Infusion chemotherapy for nonresectable differentiated cancer, 335-338
Inhibitors of angiogenesis, 385-388
Injection, percutaneous ethanol
for autonomously functioning nodules, 33
for nonresectable cancer, 328-333, 343
Instrumentation
imaging, 162-164
for nuclear medicine, 162-164
Insular carcinoma, 76-77
Intraglandular disseminated papillary cancer, 211, 215

Intranodular ethanol injection, 33
Intranuclear oncogene, 373
Intraoperative radiation therapy
  nonresectable cancer and, 334-335, 343
  for nonresectable differentiated cancer, 334-335, 343
Invasion
  of primary tumor, 260
  as risk factor for recurrent, 320-321
  thyroid-stimulating hormone and, 424
Invasive cancer, minimally, 235
Iodine
  for autonomously functioning nodules, 32
  cancer incidence and, 6
  Hashimoto's thyroiditis and, 12
  high-risk cancer and, 244
  stunning effect and, 169-171
Iodine-123, stunning effect and, 170-171
Iodine-131
  stunning effect and, 171
  uses of, 163
Iodine-131 therapy, 178-187
  after thyroidectomy, 178-187
    ablative, of gland remnants, 178-180
    complications of, 184-187
    elevated thyroglobulin and, 182-184
    facilitation of, 233-234
    for metastatic differentiated cancer, 180-182
    partial, 249
  for recurrent cancer, 322-323
Iron oxide particle, ultrasmall supraparamagnetic, 200
Irsogladine, 388
Isthmectomy, total lobectomy with, 232-233

K

K ras mutation, 356-357
Ki-ras mutation, 369
Kocher, Theodore, experiments of, 350, 351

L

Lactate dehydrogenase, nodule and, 23
Landmarks in neck, 282
Laparoscopy in medullary cancer, 297, 299
Laxative, radionuclide imaging and, 169
Leukemia, 186-187
Levothyroxine therapy, postoperative, 249-250
Lithium, 182
Liver
  metastasis to, 299, 300
  radionuclide concentrated in, 173
Lobe, thyroid, lymphoma involvement in, 218
Lobectomy
  multinodular goiter and, 30-31
  thyroidectomy *vs.*, 244, 247
  total, 232-233
Locally recurrent thyroid carcinoma, 309-324; *see also* Recurrent cancer
Loss of heterozygosity, 366
Low-iodine diet, 169
L-T_4 therapy, 180
Lung metastasis, childhood cancer and, 10
Lymph node
  excision of, 260-263
  magnetic resonance imaging and, 198-200
  in medullary cancer, 292
  metastasis to; *see* Metastasis
  in neck and mediastinum, 282
  ultrasonography of, 219, 220
Lymphadenopathy
  magnetic resonance imaging and, 198
  thyroid nodules and, 22
Lymphoma
  anaplastic carcinoma *vs.*, 81
  clinical *vs.* microcancer, 108
  fine-needle aspiration cytology of, 90-91, 92, 150
  Hashimoto's thyroiditis and, 8
  illustration of, 149
  thyroiditis and, 115
  thyroid-related, 13
  ultrasonography of, 218

M

MACIS classification, 139, 243
Magnetic resonance imaging, 195-208
  of medullary cancer, 156
Magnetic resonance imaging—cont'd
  of nodules, 23-24, 197
  nonresectable cancer and, 340
  postoperative, 201-207
  in staging of carcinoma, 198-200, 201
  techniques of, 195-196
Malignancy, risk of, 134
Marker for papillary cancer, 67
Massive goiter, 130
Mediastinum, anatomic landmarks in, 282
Medullary cancer, 279-304
  anatomic landmarks in neck and, 282
  C-cell hyperplasia in, 114
  classification of, 8
  clinical management of, 289-291
  clinical *vs.* microcancer, 107
  familial non-MEN, 284
    management of, 289
  fine-needle aspiration cytology of, 82-86
  fine-needle cytology of, 153
  genetic basis of, 393-406
    C-cell stimulation test and, 394-395
    DNA testing and, 400-402
    genotype-phenotype correlation in, 400
    germline mutations and, 396-399
    RET mutations and, 399-400
    RET proto-oncogene and, 395-396
  histology of, 152
  illustration of, 151
  magnetic resonance imaging of, 156
  microvasculature and, 381
  molecular genetics in, 284-288
  in multiple endocrine neoplasia, 283-284
  persistent or recurrent, 295-296
  in series 1, 296-299
  in series 2, 299-304
  sporadic, 402-403
  surgery for, 291-292
    preventive, in MEN2A gene carriers, 292-295
  total thyroidectomy for, 235

Medullary cancer—cont'd
tumor characteristics in, 279-282
ultrasonography of, 218
MEN; *see* Multiple endocrine neoplasia
Menarche, 63
Metastasis
chest x-ray for, 139
in child, 9-10
of differentiated cancer, 180-182
fine-needle aspiration cytology of, 90, 91
of insular carcinoma, 77
liver, in medullary cancer, 299, 300
magnetic resonance imaging and, 198-200
of medullary cancer, 280-281, 292
microcancer and, 116, 119
of papillary cancer, 67
partial thyroidectomy for, 248-249
radionuclide imaging for, 167-177
surgical options for, 263-269
technetium-99m sestamibi imaging for, 177
thyroidectomy for, partial, 246, 248-249
ultrasonography in evaluation of, 219, 220
2-Methoxyoestradiol, 388
Microcancer, 105-120
benign lesions with, 115
clinical cancer incidence and, 106-109
histologic criteria for, 109-114
C-cell hyperplasia and, 114
follicular carcinoma and, 111-114
papillary carcinoma and, 109-110
incidence of, 105-106
papillary, 68, 69
prognosis for, 115-119
total thyroidectomy for, 235
ultrasonography of, 211, 215
Micrometastasis, 233
Micropapillary cancer, occult, 245
Microsarcoma, 108-109
Microvasculature, thyroid, 380-381
Minimally invasive cancer, total thyroidectomy for, 235
Mitosis, in anaplastic carcinoma, 79
Mixed follicular C-cell lesion, 87
Molecular biology, 349-433
angiogenesis and, 379-389; *see also* Angiogenesis
basic science research and, 349-360
historical background of, 349-352
impact of
on clinical management, 354-359
on surgical training, 352-354
of medullary cancer, 284-288
dominant oncogenes in, 287
RET proto-oncogene in, 284-286
tumor suppressor genes in, 287-288
oncogenes and; *see* Oncogene; RET proto-oncogene
tumor suppressor genes and
in differentiated cancer, 371-373
in medullary cancer, 287-288
Monitor, personnel radiation, 187
Mortality, 244
Mucoepidermoid carcinoma, 89
Mucosal ganglioneuroma, 155
Multicentricity, 245
Multifocal papillary carcinoma, cytology of, 67
Multinodular goiter, 29-32
massive, 130
ultrasonography of, 215-216
Multiple endocrine neoplasia
genetic basis of, 393-406; *see also* Medullary cancer, genetic basis of
medullary cancer in, 8, 85-86, 151
type 2A
basic science research and, 354-355
clinical management of, 289-290
medullary cancer in, 283
Multiple endocrine neoplasia—cont'd
type 2A—cont'd
preventive surgery in, 292-294
RET gene mutations in, 284-285
screening for, 353
type 2B
basic science research and, 354-355
clinical management of, 289-290
ganglioneuroma in, 155
medullary cancer in, 283-284
phenotype of, 154
preventive surgery in, 294-295
RET gene mutations in, 285-286
screening for, 353
Mutation, 355-356
in differentiated cancer
in physiologic pathways, 367-368
in ras genes, 368-369
tumor suppressor genes in, 371-373
tyrosine kinase receptors and, 369-371
K ras, 356-357
Ki-ras, 369
in medullary cancer, 396-399
RET, 399-400
somatic RET, 402-405
in multiple endocrine neoplasia, 396-399
type 2A, 284-285
type 2B, 285-286
p53, in anaplastic carcinoma, 80
ras gene, 368-369
in RET proto-oncogene
amino acids and, 399
biologic aspects of, 399-400
protein domains and, 355
somatic, 402-404
thyroid-stimulating hormone receptor and, 367-368

N

Nasal secretion, 175
Nausea, iodine-131 therapy causing, 184, 186

Neck
anatomic landmarks in, 282
modified radical dissection of, 260-263
radical dissection of, in child, 251
Necrosis in anaplastic carcinoma, 79
Neoplasia, multiple endocrine; *see* Multiple endocrine neoplasia
Nerve injury
partial thyroidectomy and, 250-251
percutaneous ethanol injection causing, 329-330
Nest, solid cell, 40
Neuroendocrine tumor, 405
Node, medullary cancer in, 156
Nodular goiter, 51-54, 131
Nodule, thyroid, 21-33
autonomously functioning, 32-33
benign
colloid, 129
ultrasonography of, 210-211
cytology of, 40-44
diagnosis and evaluation of, 22-24
follicular, 113
Hürthle cell, 73
imaging of, 164-167
magnetic resonance imaging of, 197
management of, 128
in medullary cancer, 289
multinodular goiter and, 29-32
papillary hyperplastic, 63
radioiodine scan of, 135
risk of malignancy of, 134
solitary follicular tumor and, 24-29
thyroidectomy *vs.* lobectomy for, 247
types of, 164
ultrasonography of
color Doppler, 221
fine-needle aspiration cytology with, 222
papillary cancer *vs.*, 210-211
Noncurative surgery, categories of, 328
Nonepithelial neoplasm, 90-92
Nonmedullary lesion
C-cell hyperplasia in, 114
chromosomal abnormality in, 355
Nonresectable differentiated cancer, 327-343
arterial infusion chemotherapy for, 335-338
intraoperative radiotherapy for, 334-335
multidisciplinary treatment for, 339-341
complications of, 341-343
efficacy of, 338
patient characteristics and, 328
percutaneous ethanol injection for, 328-334
Nonthyroid neoplasm *vs.* thyroid metastasis, 173-174
Nuclear medicine
agents and instrumentation for, 162-164
iodine-131 therapy
ablative, of gland remnants, 178-180
complications of, 184-187
elevated thyroglobulin and, 182-184
of metastatic differentiated cancer, 180-182
nodule evaluation with, 164-167
thyroidectomy and, 167-177; *see also* Thymectomy, imaging after
Nucleolus
in anaplastic carcinoma, 80
in papillary cancer, 66
Nucleus in papillary cancer, 65-66

O

Occult microcancer, 105-120; *see also* Microcancer
papillary, 245
Oncogene; *see also* RET proto-oncogene
intranuclear, 373
in medullary cancer, dominant, 287
Oncogene—cont'd
in parathyroid tumor, 157
thyroid-stimulating hormone and, 423
Options, surgical, 257-272; *see also* Surgical options
Osteosarcoma, 91
Overexpression of p53 in papillary microcarcinoma, 109
Oxyphilic cell; *see* Hürthle cell lesion

P

p16 tumor suppressor gene, 372
p53 tumor suppressor gene, 372
anaplastic carcinoma and, 80
in papillary microcarcinoma, 109
Pain from percutaneous ethanol injection, 329
Palliative surgery in medullary cancer, 301
Papillary cancer
adenylate cyclase system in, 358
anaplastic carcinoma and, 81
autonomously functioning nodules and, 32
chest x-ray for, 139
in child, 9-10
chromosomal abnormality in, 354-355
classification of, 7-8
clinical *vs.* microcancer, 107
cytogenetic screening and, 366
fine-needle aspiration cytology of, 63-68, 138
histology of, 137
Hürthle cell, 75-76
illustration of, 136
initial treatment of, 310-311
microcarcinoma, 109-110
multicentricity in, 245
patient characteristics with, 258-260
postoperative MRI and, 203
predicting death from, 243
recurrence of, 314
size of, 27-28
at presentation, 14
thyroidectomy for
partial, 246, 248

Papillary cancer—cont'd
thyroidectomy for—cont'd
total, 231-232
ultrasonography of
benign nodules *vs.*, 210-214
color Doppler, 221
intraglandular
disseminated, 211, 215
in multinodular goiter, 215-216
rare variant, 216-217
variants of, 68-72
Papillary hyperplastic lesion, 62-63
Paralysis
nerve
partial thyroidectomy and, 250-251
percutaneous ethanol injection causing, 329-330
vocal cord, 22
Parathyroid gland, in medullary cancer, 296-297
Parathyroid tumor, oncogenes and chromosomes in, 157
Parathyroidectomy in medullary cancer, 291
Parenchyma, 39-40
Partial thyroidectomy, 241-254; *see also* Thyroidectomy, partial
Percutaneous ethanol injection
for autonomously functioning nodules, 33
for nonresectable cancer, 328-333, 340-341, 343
Personnel monitor, radiation, 187
Pheochromocytoma, 287
Placental-derived growth factor, 382-383
Pollution and cancer incidence, 6
Polymerase chain reaction, 367
Poorly differentiated carcinoma, 76-77
Positron emission tomography
after thyroidectomy, 177
^{18}F-FDG-PET scan, 177
Postoperative magnetic resonance imaging, 201-207
Preventive surgery for MEN2 gene carriers, 292-294
Protein, ras, 368-369
Protein kinase C, 422-423
Proto-oncogene, RET; *see* RET proto-oncogene
Pseudofollicular appearance of medullary carcinoma, 82
Pseudopapillary appearance of medullary carcinoma, 82
Pulmonary fibrosis, radionuclide therapy causing, 187

R

Radiation therapy
external-beam, 323
intraoperative, for nonresectable cancer, 334-335, 342
for recurrent medullary cancer, 295, 323
relationship to cancer incidence, 5-6
safety of, 187-188
thyroiditis after, 184
Radical neck dissection
in child, 251
modified, 260-263
Radiographic evaluation of pelvis, 143
Radionuclide imaging, 161-188
after thyroidectomy
^{18}F-fluorodeoxyglucose for, 177
iodine-131 for, 178-187
patient preparation for, 168-169
radioiodine therapy and, 171-175
stunning effect and, 169-171
technetium-99m sestamibi for, 176-177
thallium-201 for, 175-176
agents and instrumentation for, 162-164
characteristics of, 162
of cold nodule, 135
of follicular cancer, 144
iodine-123, 162
of nodules, 23
whole-body, 164
Radionuclide therapy; *see also* Iodine *entries*
after thyroidectomy, 171-175
for autonomously functioning nodules, 32
iodine-131
ablative, of gland remnants, 178-180
complications of, 184-187
Radionuclide therapy—cont'd
iodine-131—cont'd
elevated thyroglobulin and, 182-184
of metastatic differentiated cancer, 180-182
for recurrent medullary cancer, 295
ras mutation, 356-357, 368-369
Receptor
epidermal growth factor, 369
hepatocyte growth factor, 369
retinoic acid, 373
thyroid hormone, 373
thyroid-stimulating hormone, 356, 358-359
mutations in physiologic pathways and, 367-368
vascular endothelial growth factor, 383
Recombinant human thyroid-stimulating hormone, 168-169
Recurrence
of medullary cancer, 295-296, 305-306
of microcancer, 116-118
in thyroid remnant, 231, 263
total thyroidectomy and, 233
iodine-131 scanning for, 233-234
Recurrent cancer, 309-324
diagnosis of, 312-313
initial treatment of cancer and, 310-311
results of, 311-312
nonresectable, 327-343; *see also* Nonresectable differential cancer
papillary, 314-321
follicular *vs.*, 314
risk factors for, 313
treatment of, 322-323
Recurrent laryngeal nerve
modified radical neck dissection and, 262
partial thyroidectomy and, 250-251
Remnant, thyroid gland
ablative therapy for, 178-180
recurrence and, 231, 246, 263
Reoperation for medullary cancer, 296, 303
Research, basic science, 349-360
historical background of, 349-352

Research, basic science—cont'd
impact of
on clinical management, 354-359
on surgical training, 352-354
RET proto-oncogene
biologic aspects of mutations of, 399-400
follicular variant papillary carcinoma and, 70
in medullary cancer, 86, 284-286, 395-396
preventive surgery and, 293
in multiple endocrine neoplasia type 4, 284-286
in papillary cancer, 357
papillary variant carcinoma and, 70
protein domains and mutations and, 355
somatic mutations of, 402-404
Retinoic acid receptor, 373
RET/PTC rearrangements, 357, 370-371
RhTSH, after thyroidectomy, 168-169
Risk factors for recurrence, 313

S

Safety, radiation, 187-188
Saliva, radionuclide scan and, 175
Salt, iodized, 6
Sarcoma
fine-needle aspiration cytology of, 91-92
microsarcoma, 108-109
Scalloping of tongue, 155
Scan; *see* Radionuclide imaging
Science research, basic, 349-360
historical background of, 349-352
impact of
on clinical management, 354-359
on surgical training, 352-354
Scintillation camera, 163
variables affecting scan sensitivity, 167-168
Sclerosing mucoepidermoid carcinoma, 89
Sclerosis variant papillary carcinoma, diffuse, 70
Score
AGES, 231, 243
MACIS, 139
Seafood, cancer incidence and, 6
Secretion, radionuclide scan and, 175
Serum thyroglobulin, 23
SETTLE lesion, 88
Sex differences in recurrence, 321
Sialadenitis, 184
Single-photon emission computed tomography
of nodule, 168
uses of, 164
Skin, cancer invading through, 148
Small cell *vs.* anaplastic carcinoma, 81
Sodium/iodide symporter, 372-373
Solid cell nest, 40
Solitary nodule
hyperplastic papillary, 63
thyroidectomy vs. lobectomy for, 247
Somatic RET mutation, 402-404
Spindle cell variant anaplastic carcinoma, 78-79
Spindle epithelial tumor with thymus-like differentiation, 88
Sporadic medullary cancer, 402-403
Squamoid variant anaplastic carcinoma, 78, 79
Squamous cell carcinoma, 88
ST 25989, 388
Staging of thyroid cancer, 242, 270
magnetic resonance imaging for, 198-200, 201
Stunning effect, 169-171
Suppression, bone marrow, 186
Suppression therapy
for recurrent cancer, 322
thyroid-stimulating hormone, 415-429; *see also* Thyroid-stimulating hormone suppression therapy
Supraparamagnetic iron oxide particle, ultrasmall, 200
Surgery
for autonomously functioning nodules, 32
for follicular carcinoma, 22
for follicular tumor, 25-26
Surgery—cont'd
for Hashimoto's thyroiditis, 11-12
multinodular goiter and, 30-31
Surgical options, 257-272
evaluating outcome of, 270-272
lymph node excision as, 260-263
for lymph node metastasis, 263-269
patient characteristics and, 258-269
recurrence from remnant thyroid and, 263
thyroidectomy as, 260

T

T-cell lymphoma, Hashimoto's thyroiditis and, 8
Tall cell cancer, recurrence of, 248
Tall cell variant papillary carcinoma, diffuse, 70-71
Technetium-99m, characteristics of, 162, 163
Technetium-99m diphosphonate, 177
bone scanning with, 177
Technetium-99m sestamibi, 176-177
Hürthle cell carcinoma and, 176
Technetium-99m tetrofosmin, 177
Telomerase, in follicular tumor, 25
Tetrachlorodibenzo-p-dioxin, 8
Thallium-201 imaging
after thyroidectomy, 175-176
for metastasis, 175-176
Therapeutic-dose radiation, relationship to cancer, 5-6
Thorax, 196
Thrombospondin-1, 388
Thymoma, 88-89
Thyrogen, 168
Thyroglobulin
negative iodine-131 scan and, 182-183
nodule and, 23
recurrent cancer and, 312-313
total thyroidectomy and, 234

Thyroid cancer; *see also* Follicular cancer; Microcancer; Papillary cancer
- angiogenesis and, 379-389; *see also* Angiogenesis
- autopsy studies in, 4
- in children, 9-10
- classification of, 6-8
- etiologic factors in, 5-6
- Graves' disease with, 10-12
- Hashimoto's thyroiditis with, 12-13
- incidence of, 135
- management of, 128
- natural history of, 242-246
- types of, 157

Thyroid gland anatomy, 39-40
Thyroid hormone receptor, 373
Thyroid hormone therapy, 180
Thyroid nodule, 21-33; *see also* Nodule, thyroid
Thyroidectomy
- argument for, 232-234
- conservative viewpoint on, 230-232
- imaging after
  - ^{18}F-fluorodeoxyglucose for, 177
  - iodine-131 for, 178-187
  - patient preparation for, 168-169
  - radioiodine therapy and, 171-175
  - stunning effect and, 169-171
  - technetium-99m sestamibi for, 176-177
  - thallium 201 for, 175-176
- magnetic resonance imaging after, 201-207
- in medullary cancer, 235
- in minimally invasive cancer, 235-236
- multinodular goiter and, 30, 31
- partial, 241-254
  - argument for, 246-248
  - complications of, 250-251
  - for metastatic cervical nodal disease, 248-249
  - natural history of thyroid cancer and, 242-246
  - postoperative management and, 249-250

Thyroidectomy—cont'd
- partial—cont'd
  - results of, 250-251
- as surgical option, 260
- total, 229-237
  - DNA analysis and, 401
  - lobectomy *vs.*, 244
  - for medullary cancer, 291
  - partial *vs.*, 311
  - recurrence after, 342

Thyroiditis
- Hashimoto's, 12-13, 91
- lymphoma and, 91, 108, 115
- radiation, iodine-131 therapy causing, 184
- suspicion of cancer and, 258

Thyroid-stimulating hormone
- ablative therapy and, 180
- angiogenesis and, 385
- follicular cancer and, 140
- mutations in physiologic pathways and, 367-368
- nodules and, 23, 165
- radionuclide imaging after thyroidectomy and, 168
- recurrent cancer and, 322

Thyroid-stimulating hormone receptor, 356
- mutations in physiologic pathways and, 367-368

Thyroid-stimulating hormone suppression therapy, 415-429
- adenylate cyclase and, 418-421
- angiogenesis and, 425-427
- apoptosis and, 427-428
- clinical background of, 416-418
- invasion and, 424
- oncogenes and tumor suppressor genes and, 423
- potential complications of, 428-429
- protein kinase C activation and, 422-423
- transgenic mice and, 428

Thyrotoxicosis, 10-12
Thyroxin, nodules and, 23
Thyroxine, suppression therapy with, 428-429
TNP-470, 386-387
Tomography; *see* Computed tomography
Tongue, scalloping of, 155
Total thyroidectomy, 229-237; *see also* Thyroidectomy, total
Toxic nodular goiter, 32
T3-R, 373
Trabecular cell variant papillary carcinoma, 70
Tracheostomy, 250
Transforming growth factor, angiogenesis and, 383
Transforming growth factor-beta, 359
Transgenic mice, thyroid-stimulating hormone and, 428
Transplantation of parathyroid glands, 291-292
Triiodothyronine, 234
Tumor growth, angiogenesis as prerequisite for, 380
Tumor size in papillary cancer, 67
Tumor suppressor gene
- in differentiated cancer, 371-373
- in medullary cancer, 287-288
- thyroid-stimulating hormone and, 423

Tumorlike lesion, cytology of
- congenital, 44-46
- inflammatory, 46-51

T1-weighted spin-echo image, 196
- cancer staging and, 198-199
- postoperative, 205

T2-weighted spin-echo image
- cancer staging and, 198-199
- postoperative, 206
- in postoperative evaluation, 203

Tyrosine kinase inhibitor, 387
Tyrosine kinase receptor, 369-371

U

Ultrasmall supraparamagnetic iron oxide particle, 200
Ultrasonography, 209-223
- aspiration cytology with, 222
- color Doppler, 220-222
- of follicular cancer, 218
- in initial evaluation, 310
- of lymph node metastasis, 219, 220
- of medullary cancer, 218

Ultrasonography—cont'd
of microcarcinoma, 211, 215
of papillary cancer
benign nodules *vs.*, 210-214
intraglandular disseminated, 211, 215
in multinodular goiter, 215-216
rare variant of, 216-217
of thyroid nodule, 22
Undifferentiated cancer, 78-82
clinical *vs.* microcancer, 108-109
Uptake, iodine, stunning effect and, 169-171

V

Variant of papillary cancer, 68-72
Variant of papillary cancer
ultrasonography of, 216, 217
Vascular endothelial growth factor, 383-385
angiogenesis and, 381
thyroid-stimulating hormone and, 425-427
Vasculogenesis *vs.* angiogenesis, 380
Vocal cord paralysis, 22
Vomiting after iodine-131 therapy, 186

W

Warm nodule, 164
Whole-body scan, 164